Maxillofacial Imaging

T. A. Larheim · P.-L. Westesson

T. A. Larheim
P.-L. Westesson

Maxillofacial Imaging

With 425 Figures (approx. 1450 Illustrations)

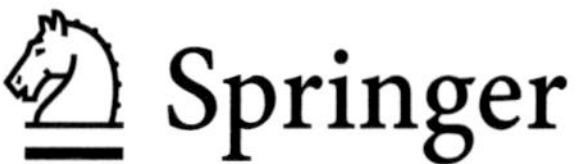

ISBN 10 3-540-25423-4
ISBN 13 978-3-540-25423-2
Springer Berlin Heidelberg New York

Library of Congress Control Number: 2005923311

Springer is a part of Springer Science+Business Media

springeronline.com

Editor: Dr. Ute Heilmann, Heidelberg
Desk editor: Dörthe Mennecke-Bühler, Heidelberg
Production editor: LE-TeX Jelonek, Schmidt & Vöckler GbR, Leipzig
Cover design: F. Steinen, eStudio Calamar, Spain
Reproduction and Typesetting: AM-productions GmbH, Wiesloch
Printing and bookbinding: Stürtz AG, Würzburg

21/3150 – 5 4 3 2 1 0
Printed on acid-free paper

To our wives
Sigrid and Ann-Margret
And our children
Tor Eirik and Arnstein
and
Karin, Oscar and Nils
Besides the fascinating field of radiology,
you mean everything to us.

Preface

There are substantial textbooks on head and neck imaging as well as on dental imaging, but since the early 1990s there has been no book focusing on the gap between imaging in dentistry and in medicine, namely maxillofacial imaging. Emanating from dentistry, maxillofacial radiology uses principles and techniques from medical radiology. There has been significant advance in imaging technology during the last 15 years, and this maxillofacial imaging book demonstrates how advanced medical imaging technology can be successfully applied to dental and maxillofacial conditions.

Dental radiology is mainly based on intraoral and panoramic examinations with an ongoing replacement of plain films with their digital counterparts. Medical radiology, on the other hand, is moving away from projectional radiography and is using more and more cross-sectional imaging modalities such as computed tomography (CT), magnetic resonance (MR) imaging, ultrasound, and positron emission tomography (PET). These contemporary and advanced techniques have not been widely applied to maxillofacial imaging and the purpose of this extensively illustrated book is to show how advanced imaging modalities, primarily CT and MRI, can be applied to maxillofacial imaging.

We have built this book around the images rather than an extensive text since we think others are like us – we like to see the images and read the text only if necessary. Thus, the book is atlas-like with a condensed and bulleted text. With all images of the patient on one or two pages, the reader will very quickly obtain an image overview of the specific condition. Demonstrating the use of advanced imaging techniques in dentistry is particularly important since maxillofacial radiology has been accepted as a specialty of dentistry in several countries and the international trend is a closer cooperation between professionals in dentistry and medicine to provide the best patient care. During the writing of this book it has evolved into a rather comprehensive description of maxillofacial imaging and could easily be used as the foundation for building a formal curriculum in maxillofacial radiology.

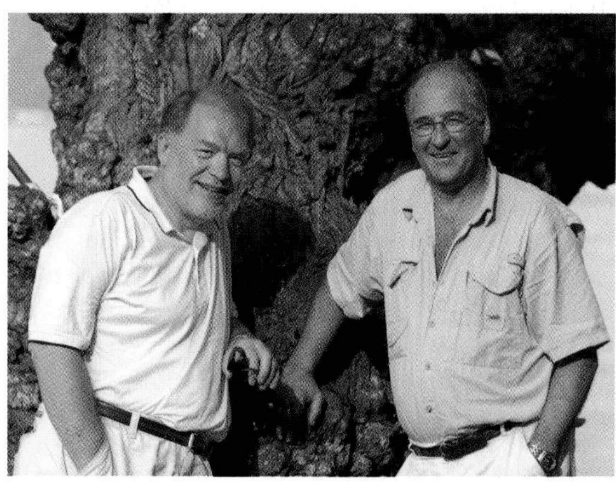

Dr. Westesson (left) and Dr. Larheim (right) relaxing after finishing the book

The book is divided into 14 chapters starting with a quite comprehensive chapter on normal imaging anatomy of the maxillofacial structures followed by four chapters on advanced imaging of conditions of dental or non-dental etiology, affecting the mandible and maxilla. When dentists get more and more involved in imaging of maxillofacial soft tissues, knowledge of both hard and soft tissues becomes mandatory. Although the majority of patients with jaw problems are diagnosed with intraoral and panoramic (film or digital) examinations, advanced imaging has become necessary for a reliable diagnostic assessment of a number of conditions. The sixth chapter is on the temporomandibular joint. This is valuable for professionals in both medicine and dentistry since many patients with facial pain seek any doctor who gives hope of being able to help them irrespective of training background and subspecialty. The four following chapters focus on dental implants, maxillofacial trauma and fractures, face and skull deformities, and paranasal sinuses. These regions are closely related to the jaw and many conditions involve both the dental structures proper and the adjacent regions.

The following two chapters cover soft-tissue imaging of the oral cavity and salivary glands. These are important topics, since traditional dental and maxillofacial imaging has been limited to evaluation of the hard tissue. In chapter 13 we have focused on imaging abnormalities of structures adjacent to the maxillofacial region, namely the cervical spine, neck, skull base, and orbit. It is not our intention to incorporate these areas into maxillofacial radiology, but we think it is important that the maxillofacial radiologist has a working understanding of what there is in the areas neighboring the maxillofacial region. At the end we have included a chapter on interventional maxillofacial radiology. Interventional radiology is the fastest growing area of general medical radiology, but has not been extensively applied to maxillofacial imaging. Our intention in this chapter is to show how minimally invasive interventional radiologic techniques can be successfully used for maxillofacial conditions.

This book is an attribute to the early work of Dr. Karl-Åke Omnell, who was the pioneer of maxillofacial radiology. Already in the late 1960's Dr. Omnell had the vision of centralized advanced maxillofacial imaging as a specialty of dentistry working closely with medical radiology. Dr. Omnell initiated the first hospital-based clinic for maxillofacial radiology in Sweden and he promoted the recognition of oral and maxillofacial radiology as a specialty of dentistry. His pioneer work has later been followed by many. We are proud to present this contemporary book on maxillofacial imaging as an attribute to his pioneer work.

This book has evolved from a friendship of more than 25 years and professional cooperation between Drs. Larheim and Westesson. It started around 1980 when Dr. Larheim from the dental school in Oslo, Norway, crossed the border to the neighboring country, Sweden, and visited Dr. Westesson at the dental school in Malmö to observe the performance of double-contrast arthrotomography of the temporomandibular joint. Both have been working as maxillofacial radiologists ever since. Dr. Larheim is currently the head of the first maxillofacial radiology department outside Japan that installed its own CT scanner, recently replaced with a multislice scanner. Dr. Westesson took another step and went through medical training, radiology residency and a neuroradiology fellowship, and eventually became chief of diagnostic and interventional neuroradiology at the University of Rochester. Their combined experience is reflected in this current book on maxillofacial imaging.

Dr. Larheim completed this work during a sabbatical stay at the University of Rochester Medical Center, Division of Diagnostic and Interventional Neuroradiology, and is highly grateful for the support he got from the Faculty of Dentistry, University of Oslo, Norway and the Research Council of Norway. Without this support the book would never have been accomplished.

We would like to express our sincere gratitude to our collaborators (in alphabetical order) Drs. Susan I. Blaser, Naoya Kakimoto, Alf Kolbenstvedt, Masaki Oka, Ravinder Sidhu, Hans-Jørgen Smith, Hanna Strømme-Koppang and Geir Støre, for the fruitful discussion of the text and contribution of good quality images. A special thanks goes to Dr. Kakimoto for his hard work in obtaining the best possible image quality throughout the book.

We thank Dr. Sven Ekholm at the University of Rochester Medical Center and Drs. Linda Arvidsson, Bjørn Mork Knutsen and medical radiographer Magne Borge at the Institute of Clinical Dentistry, University of Oslo, for supplying us with images when we were in need, as well as all others from whom we borrowed their images; they are acknowledged in the legends.

The secretarial work of Bjørg Jacobsen, Institute of Clinical Dentistry, University of Oslo, Norway, and Regina Cullen and Belinda De Libero, University of Rochester Medical Center, Rochester, NY is highly appreciated with special thanks to Bjørg reviewing the reference lists.

We are grateful to graphic designer Margaret Kowaluk, University of Rochester Medical Center, Rochester, NY and photographer Håkon Størmer, Faculty of Dentistry, University of Oslo, for professional work with the scanning of many images and obtaining some of the photos.

Editor Ute Heilman, desk editor Dörthe Mennecke-Bühler at the Springer, as well as production editor Michael Reinfarth and copy editor John Nicholson with their professional skill made this work to our satisfaction.

We are proud to present this maxillofacial imaging book and we hope that our work will serve you well.

Rochester, August 2005

Tore A. Larheim
Per-Lennart Westesson

Authors

Tore A. Larheim, DDS, PhD
(e-mail: larheim@odont.uio.no)
Professor of Maxillofacial Radiology
Department of Maxillofacial Radiology
Institute of Clinical Dentistry
Faculty School of Dentistry
University of Oslo, Oslo, Norway
Visiting Professor (2004–2005)
Division of Diagnostic
and Interventional Radiology
Department of Radiology
University of Rochester School of Medicine
and Dentistry, Rochester, New York, USA

Per-Lennart Westesson, MD, PhD, DDS
(e-mail: perlennart_westesson@urmc.rochester.edu)
Professor of Radiology, Director
Division of Diagnostic
and Interventional Radiology
Department of Radiology
University of Rochester School of Medicine
and Dentistry, Rochester, New York, USA
Professor of Oral Diagnostic Sciences
State University of New York at Buffalo
Buffalo, New York, USA
Associate Professor of Oral Radiology
University of Lund, Lund, Sweden

Collaborators

Susan I. Blaser, MD
(e-mail: susan.blaser@sickkids.ca)
Associate Professor of Neuroradiology
The Hospital for Sick Children
Division of Neuroradiology
Department of Medical Imaging
The University of Toronto
Toronto, Ontario, Canada

Naoya Kakimoto, DDS, PhD
(e-mail: kakimoto@dent.osaka-u.ac.jp)
Research Assistant
Department of Oral and Maxillofacial Radiology
Osaka University Graduate School of Dentistry
Osaka, Japan
Visiting Researcher (2004–2005)
Division of Diagnostic
and Interventional Radiology
Department of Radiology
University of Rochester School of Medicine
and Dentistry, Rochester, New York, USA

Alf Kolbenstvedt, MD, PhD
(e-mail: alf.kolbenstvedt@medisin.uio.no)
Professor of Radiology, Department of Radiology
Rikshospitalet University Hospital, Oslo, Norway

Masaki Oka, MD, PhD
(e-mail: okamasaki_1213@yahoo.com)
Staff Radiologist, Department of Radiology
Kikuna Memorial Hospital, Yokohama, Japan
Visiting Researcher (2004–2005)
Division of Diagnostic
and Interventional Neuroradiology
Department of Radiology
University of Rochester School of Medicine
and Dentistry, Rochester, New York, USA

Ravinder Sidhu, MD
(e-mail: ravinder_sidhu@urmc.rochester.edu)
Fellow, Division of Diagnostic
and Interventional Radiology
Department of Radiology
University of Rochester School of Medicine
and Dentistry, Rochester, New York, USA

Hans-Jørgen Smith, MD, PhD
(e-mail: h.j.smith@medisin.uio.no)
Professor of Radiology, Head, MRI Section
Department of Radiology
Rikshospitalet University Hospital, Oslo, Norway

Hanna Strømme-Koppang, DDS, PhD
(e-mail: hanna@odont.uio.no)
Professor of Pathology, Head
Department of Pathology and Forensic Odontology
Institute of Clinical Dentistry, Faculty of Dentistry
University of Oslo, Oslo, Norway

Geir Støre, MD, DDS, PhD
(e-mail: geir.store@rikshospitalet.no)
Head, Section for MaxilloFacial Surgery
ENT Department
Rikshospitalet University Hospital, Oslo, Norway

Contents

6 Temporomandibular Joint

7 Dentoalveolar Structures and Implants

8 Facial Traumas and Fractures

9 Facial Growth Disturbances

10 Paranasal Sinuses

11 Maxillofacial Soft Tissues

12 Salivary Glands

13 Adjacent Structures; Cervical Spine, Neck, Skull Base and Orbit

14 Interventional Maxillofacial Radiology

Maxillofacial Imaging Anatomy

In collaboration with N. Kakimoto · H.-J. Smith

Introduction

This chapter presents a series of high-quality images on maxillofacial imaging anatomy. The first intention is to familiarize those working in dental imaging with advanced maxillofacial imaging anatomy. Therefore we have included extensive soft tissue details on both CT and MR images. General radiologists will benefit from the detailed description of the anatomic structures of the jaws and oral cavity. The description of anatomic details of the jaws and teeth is primarily directed towards the medical profession since these areas are well known to dentists. The temporomandibular joint section with imaging features of asymptomatic volunteers should be valuable for both professions.

The anatomic structures in Figure 1.1:

1 Anterior fontanelle
2 Anterior nasal spine
3 Anterolateral fontanelle
4 Choanae
5 Coronal suture
6 Coronoid process
7 External auditory canal
8 Foramen magnum
9 Frontal bone
10 Frontozygomatic suture
11 Glenoid fossa
12 Hard palate
13 Incisive foramen
14 Infraorbital foramen
15 Lambdoid suture
16 Lateral pterygoid plate
17 Mandible
18 Mandibular condyle
19 Maxilla
20 Medial pterygoid plate
21 Mental foramen
22 Metopic suture
23 Nasal bone
24 Nasofrontal suture
25 Nasomaxillary suture
26 Occipital bone
27 Parietal bone
28 Posterolateral fontanelle
29 Sagittal suture
30 Squamosal suture
31 Temporal squama
32 Zygoma
33 Zygomatic arch

3D CT

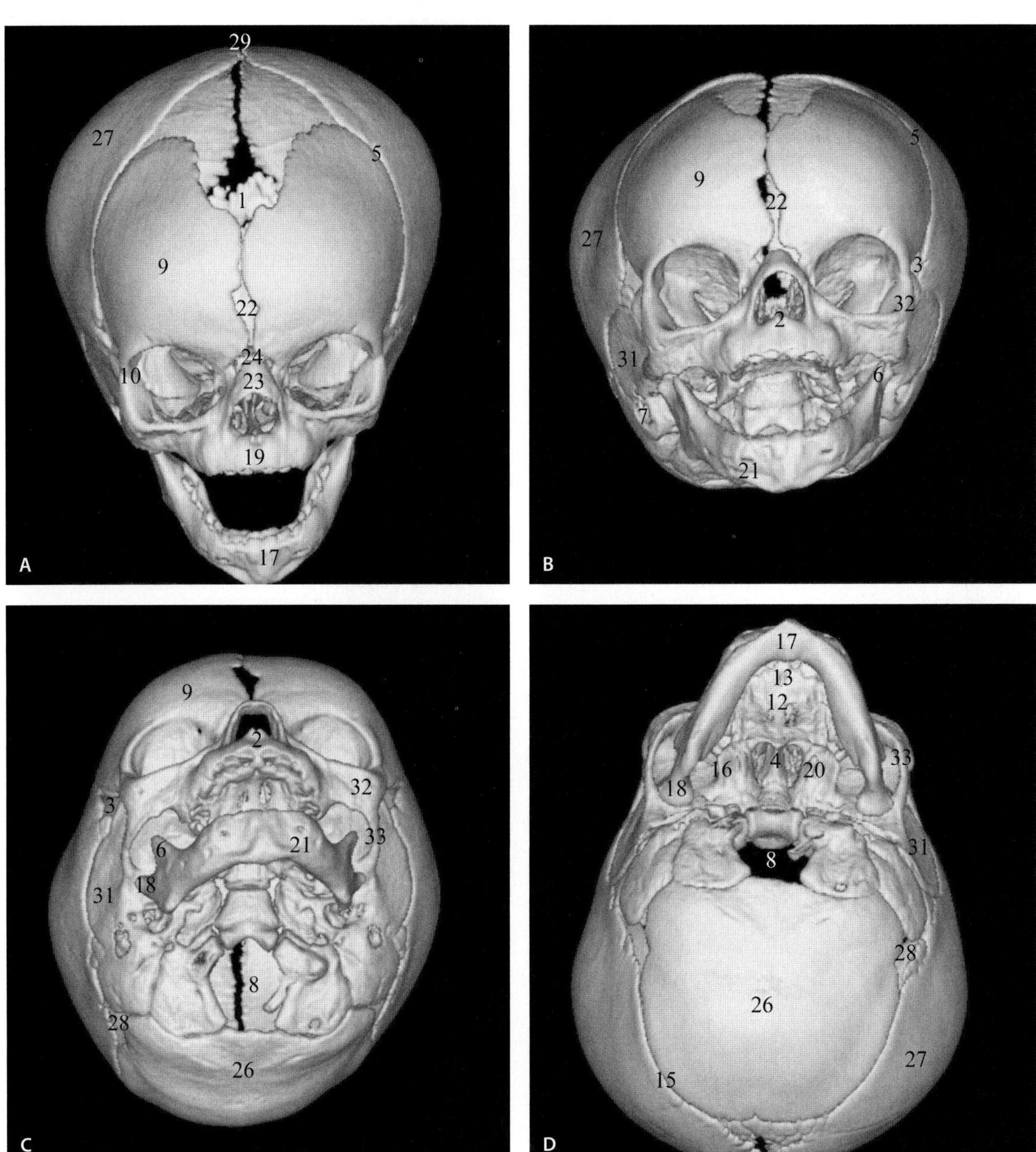

Figure 1.1

Normal 3D CT bone anatomy of the face and skull; **A–E** 7-month-old, **F–H** 8-year-old

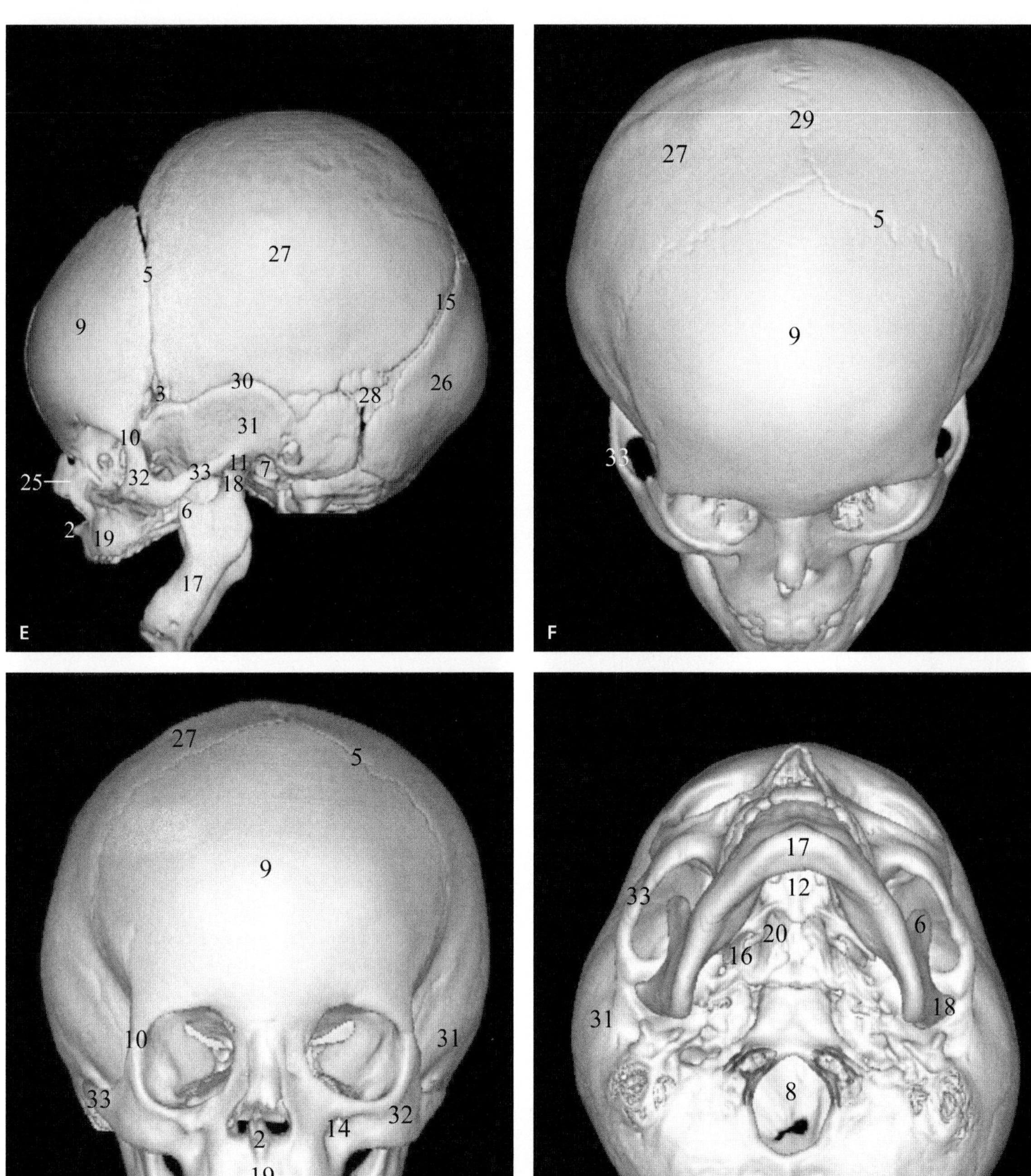
E
9
5
27
15
30
26
3
28
31
10
25
32
33
11
7
18
6
2
19
17
F
29
27
5
9
33
G
27
5
9
10
31
33
32
14
2
19
21
17
H
17
12
33
6
20
16
31
18
8
26

The anatomic structures in Figures 1.2–1.10:

1 Adenoidal tissue (nasopharyngeal tonsil)
2 Alveolar recess of maxillary sinus
3 Anterior belly of digastric muscle
4 Anterior nasal spine
5 Base of tongue
6 Buccal space fat
7 Buccinator muscle
8 Carotid canal
9 Clivus
10 Concha bullosa
11 Coronoid process
12 Crista galli
13 Dens axis
14 Epiglottis
15 Ethmoid sinus
15B Eustachian tube
16 External auditory canal
17 External carotid artery
18 External jugular vein
19 Facial vein
20 Foramen ovale
21 Foramen rotundum
22 Fossa of Rosenmüller (lateral pharyngeal fold)
23 Frontal bone
24 Frontal process of maxilla
25 Frontal sinus
26 Genial process of mandible
27 Genioglossus muscle
28 Geniohyoid muscle
29 Glenoid fossa
30 Greater palatine canal
31 Greater palatine foramen
32 Greater wing of sphenoid bone
33 Hamulus of medial pterygoid plate
34 Hard palate
35 Hyoglossus muscle
36 Hyoid bone
37 Incisive artery canal
38 Incisive canal
39 Incisive foramen
40 Inferior meatus
41 Inferior orbital fissure
42 Inferior turbinate
43 Infraorbital canal
44 Infratemporal fossa
45 Internal carotid artery
46 Internal jugular vein
47 Lacrimal bone
48 Lacrimal sac fossa
49 Lamina papyracea of ethmoid
50 Lateral pterygoid muscle
51 Lateral pterygoid plate
52 Lateral recess of sphenoid sinus
53 Lesser palatine canal
54 Levator labii superioris muscle
55 Lingual septum
56 Longus colli muscle
57 Major zygomatic muscle
58 Mandible
59 Mandibular alveolar bone
60 Mandibular canal
61 Mandibular condyle
62 Mandibular foramen
63 Mandibular notch
64 Mandibular ramus
65 Mandibular tooth
66 Mandibular tooth 1, central incisor
67 Mandibular tooth 2, lateral incisor
68 Mandibular tooth 3, canine
69 Mandibular tooth 4, first premolar
70 Mandibular tooth 5, second premolar
71 Mandibular tooth 6, first molar
72 Mandibular tooth 7, second molar
73 Mandibular tooth 8, third molar
74 Mandibular tooth crown pulp
75 Mandibular tooth root
76 Mandibular tooth root canal
77 Masseter muscle
78 Mastoid process
79 Maxilla
80 Maxillary alveolar bone
81 Maxillary sinus
82 Maxillary tooth
83 Maxillary tooth 1, central incisor
84 Maxillary tooth 2, lateral incisor
85 Maxillary tooth 3, canine
86 Maxillary tooth 4, first premolar
87 Maxillary tooth 5, second premolar
88 Maxillary tooth 6, first molar
89 Maxillary tooth 7, second molar
90 Maxillary tooth 8, third molar
91 Maxillary tooth crown pulp
92 Maxillary tooth root
93 Maxillary tooth root canal
94 Maxillary tuberosity
95 Medial pterygoid muscle
96 Medial pterygoid plate
97 Medial wall of maxillary sinus
98 Mental foramen
99 Middle meatus
100 Middle turbinate
101 Middle suture of hard palate
102 Mylohyoid line (ridge)
103 Mylohyoid muscle
104 Nasal ala
104B Nasal bone
105 Nasal cavity airway

106 Nasal septum
107 Nasal vestibule
108 Nasofrontal suture
109 Nasolacrimal canal
110 Nasopharynx
111 Olfactory recess
112 Orbicularis oris muscle
113 Orbit
114 Oropharynx
115 Palatal recess of maxillary sinus
116 Palatine tonsil
117 Parapharyngeal space
118 Parotid gland
119 Parotid gland, accessory
120 Parotid gland, deep lobe
121 Parotid gland, superficial lobe
122 Perpendicular plate of ethmoid bone
123 Platysma muscle
124 Posterior belly of digastric muscle
125 Pterygoid fossa
126 Pterygoid process of sphenoid
127 Pterygomandibular space
128 Pterygopalatine fossa
129 Retromandibular vein
130 Retromolar trigone
131 Soft palate
132 Sphenoid bone
133 Sphenoid sinus
134 Sphenoid sinus septum
135 Sphenozygomatic suture
136 Stensen's duct
137 Sternocleidomastoid muscle
138 Styloid process
139 Sublingual gland
140 Sublingual space
141 Submandibular gland
142 Submandibular space
143 Submental space
144 Superior turbinate
145 Temporalis muscle
146 Tongue, oral
147 Torus tubarius
148 Uvula
149 Vomer
150 Zygoma
151 Zygomatic arch

Cone Beam 3D CT

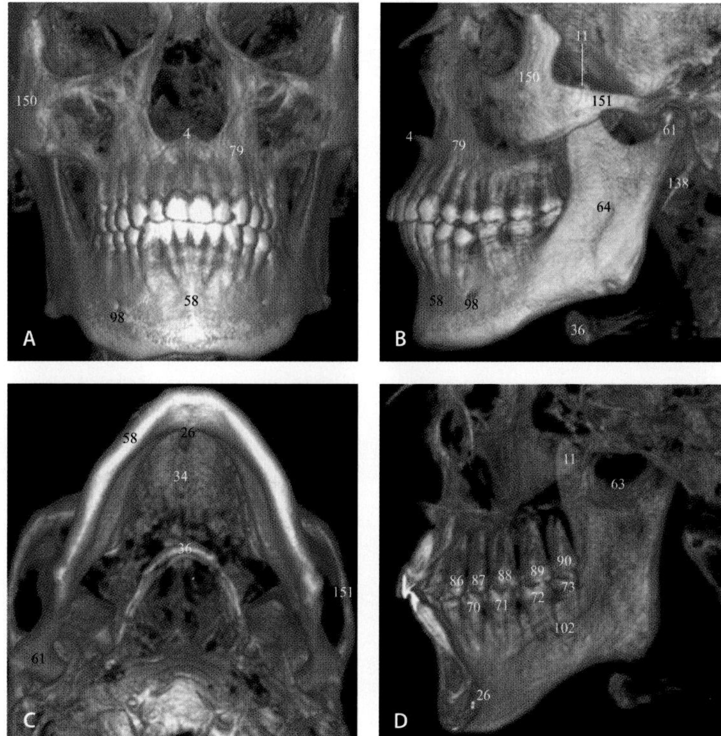

Figure 1.2

Normal 3D cone beam CT anatomy of the facial skeleton (courtesy of Drs. A. G. Farman and W. C. Scharfe, University of Louisville School of Dentistry)

CT Sections, Bone Structures

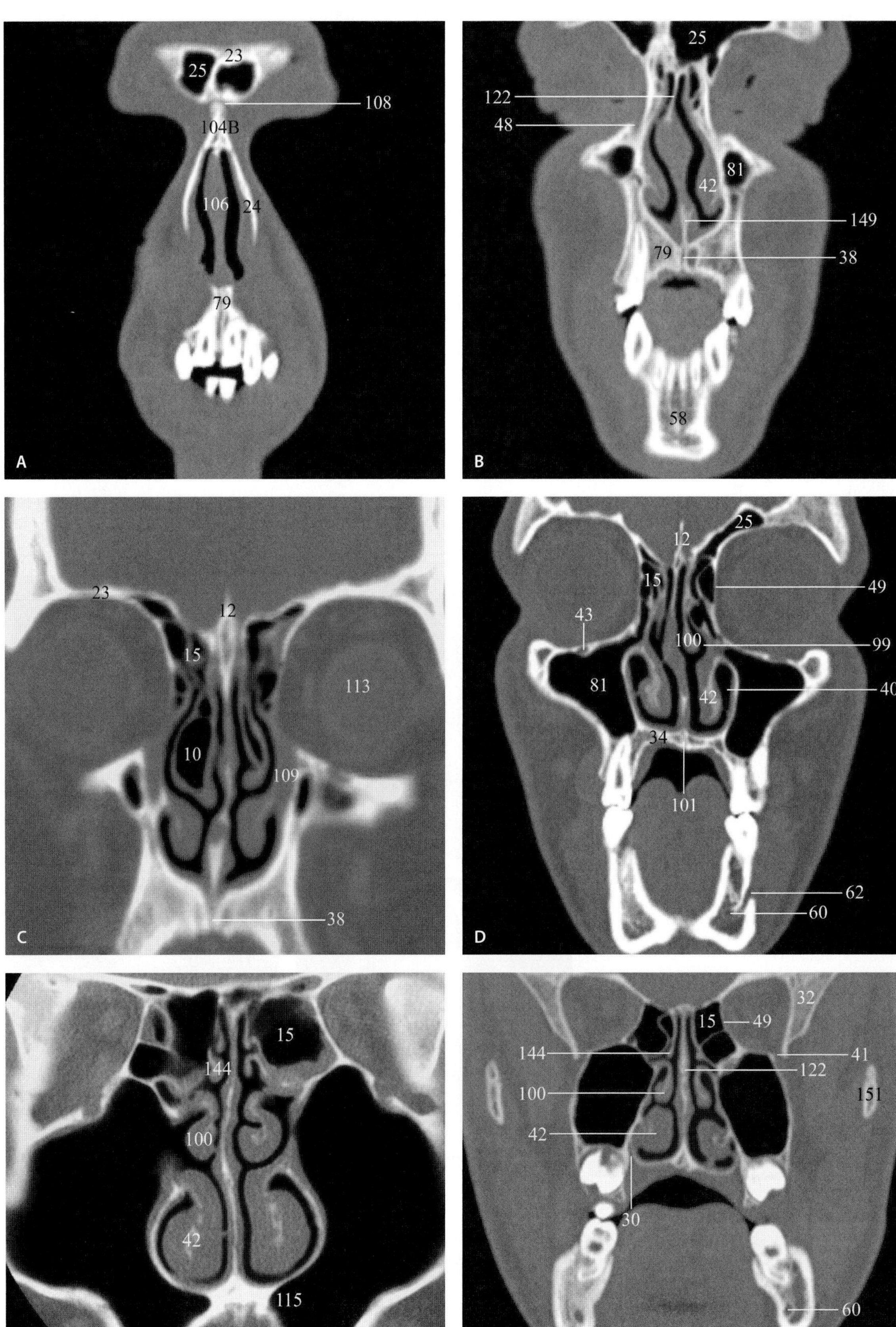

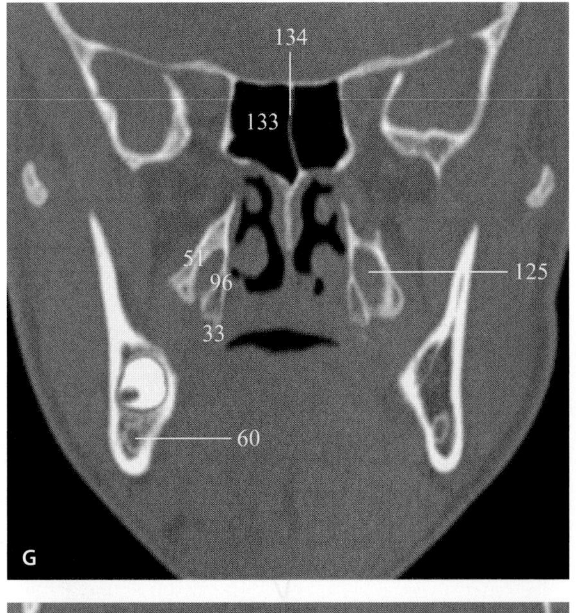

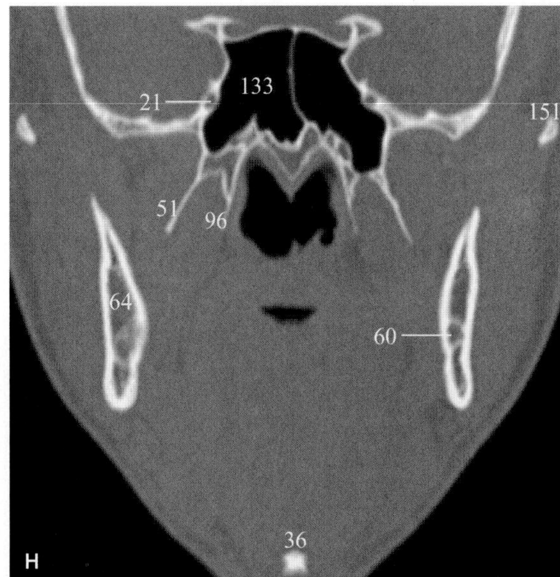

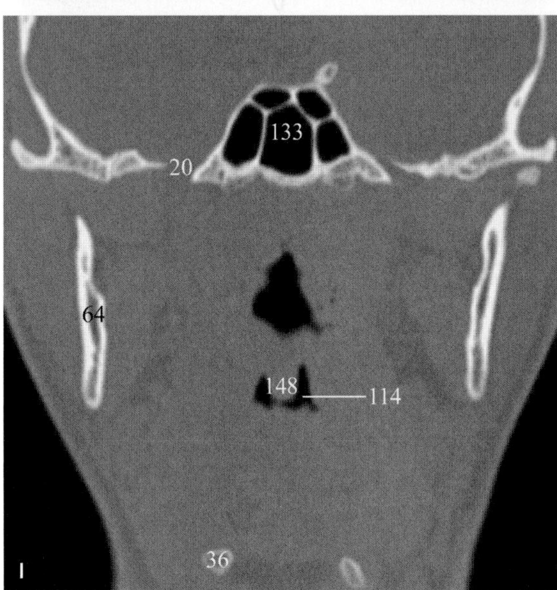

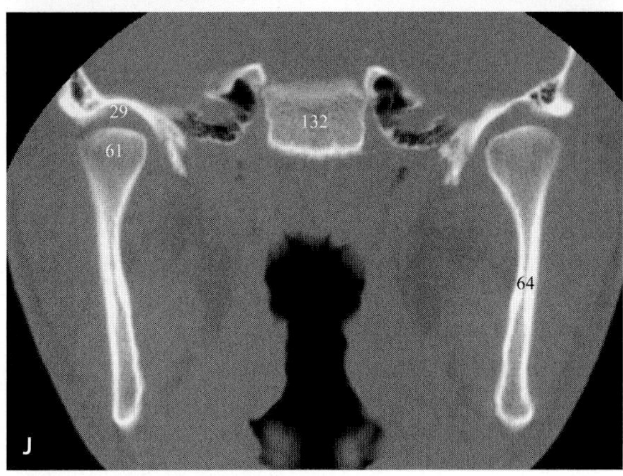

Figure 1.3

Normal coronal CT bone anatomy of the face from anterior to posterior

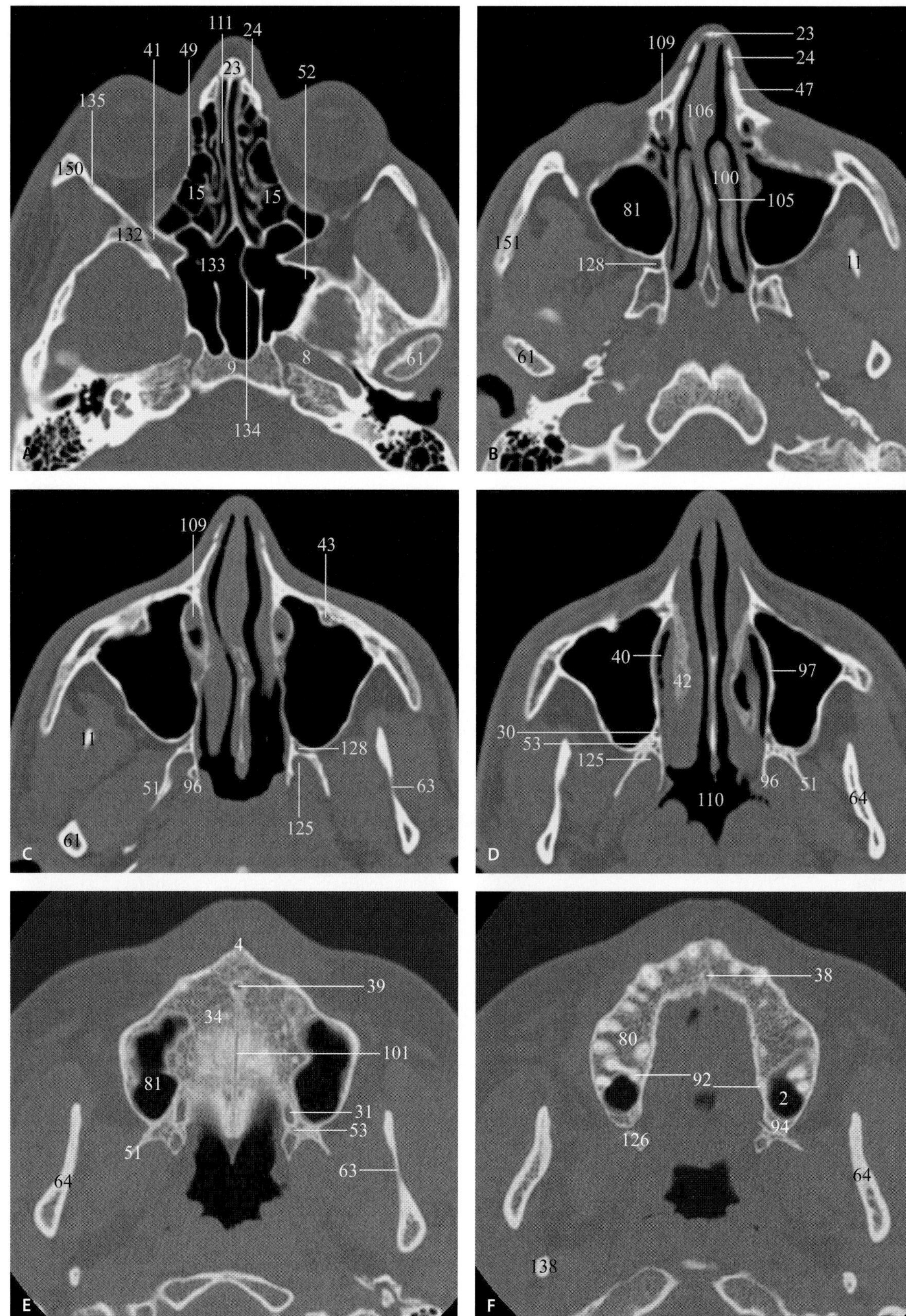

A
111
24
41
49
23
52
135
150
15
15
132
133
61
8
9
134
B
109
23
24
47
106
100
81
105
151
128
11
61
C
109
43
11
128
51
96
63
125
61
D
40
97
42
30
53
125
96
51
110
64
E
4
39
34
101
81
31
53
51
63
64
F
38
80
92
2
94
126
64
138

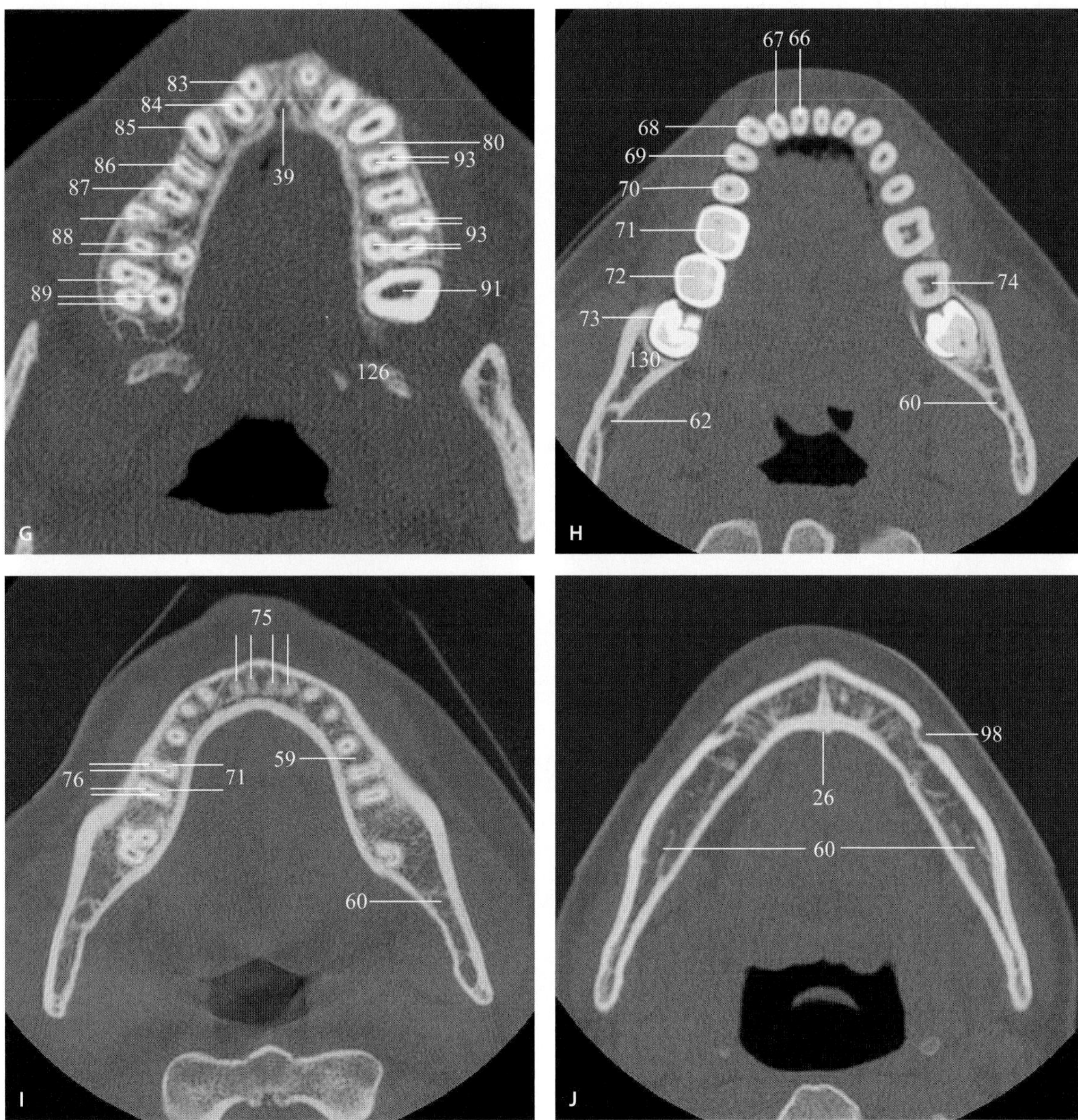

Figure 1.4

Normal axial CT bone anatomy of the lower face from superior to inferior

Cone Beam CT Sections

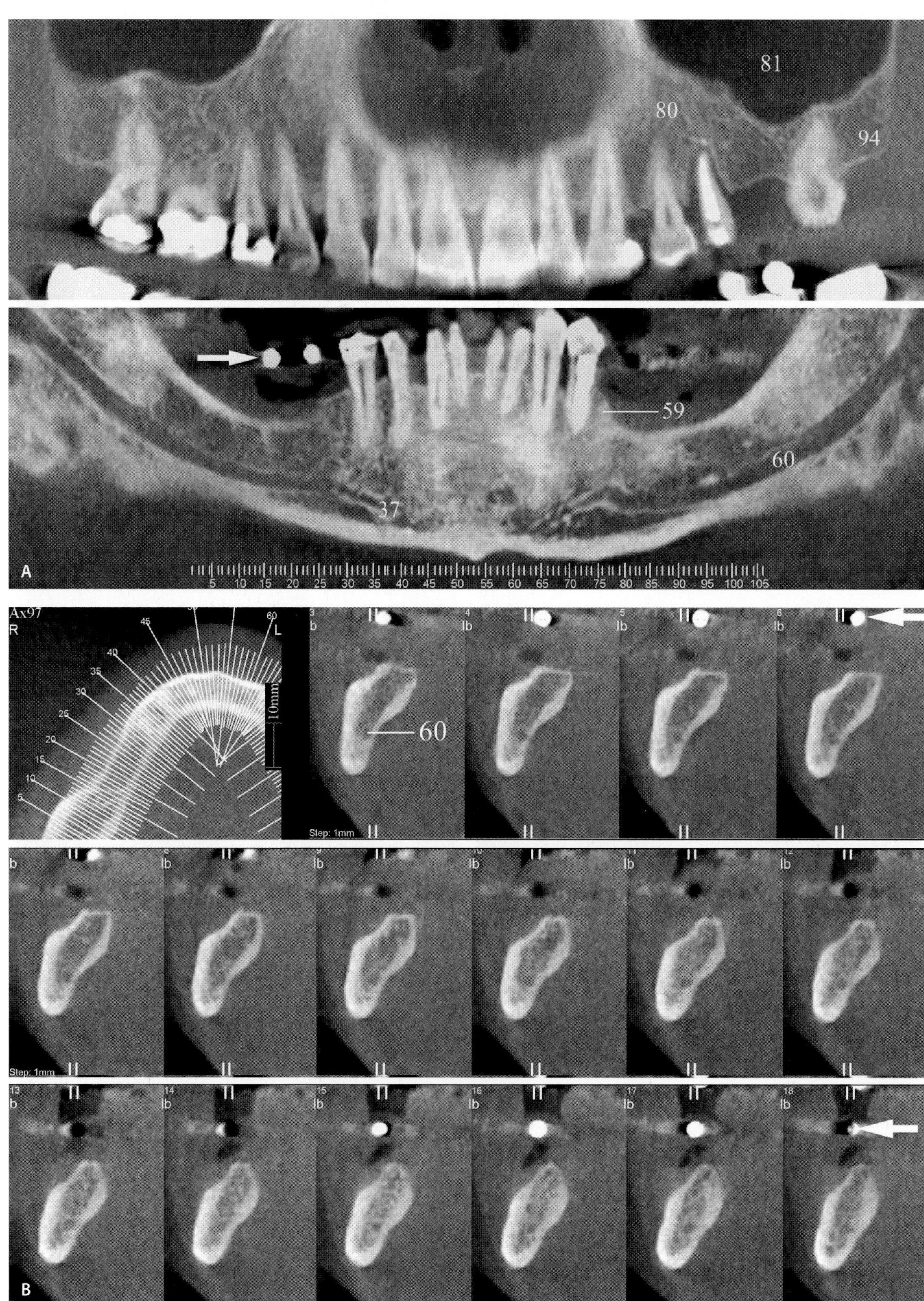

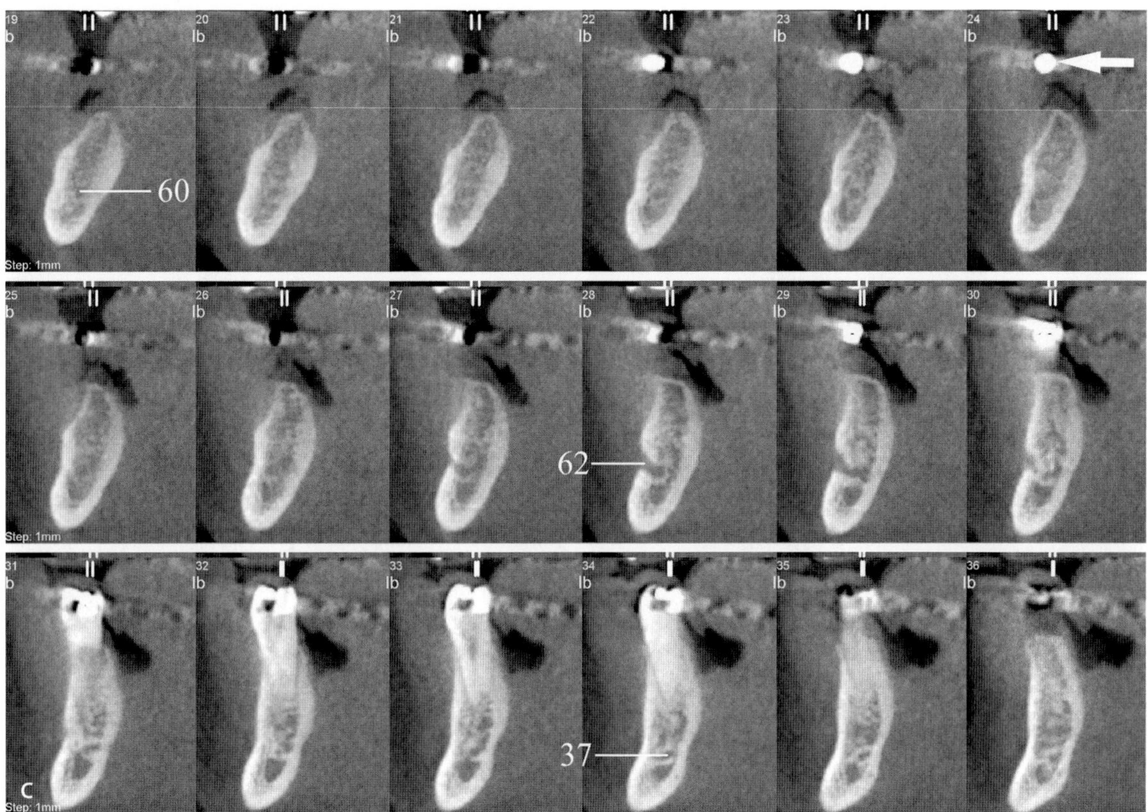

Figure 1.5

Normal cone beam CT bone anatomy of the maxilla and mandible. **A** Panoramic view of the maxilla (*upper*) and mandible (*lower*); *arrow* metallic reference ball. **B** Scout view with cross-sectional images of the posterior part of the right mandible. **C** Cross-sectional images of the anterior part of the right mandible (courtesy of Drs. S. C. White and S. Tetradis, UCLA School of Dentistry)

Schematic Drawing, Floor of Mouth

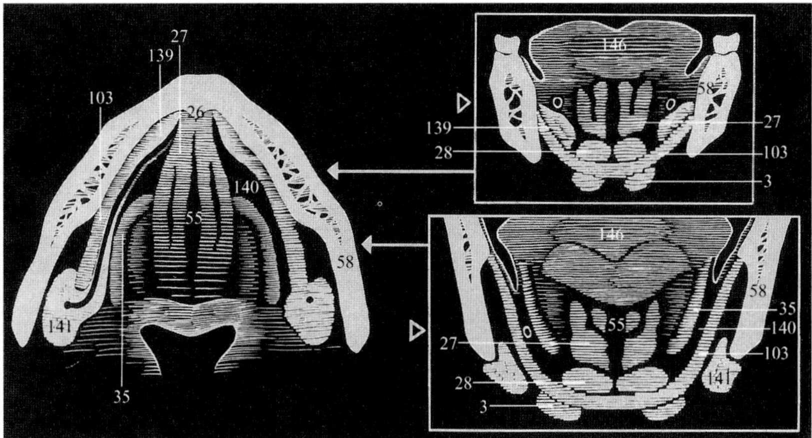

Figure 1.6

Schematic drawing of the floor of the mouth (reproduced with permission from Aasen and Kolbenstvedt 1992)

CT Sections, Soft Tissue Structures

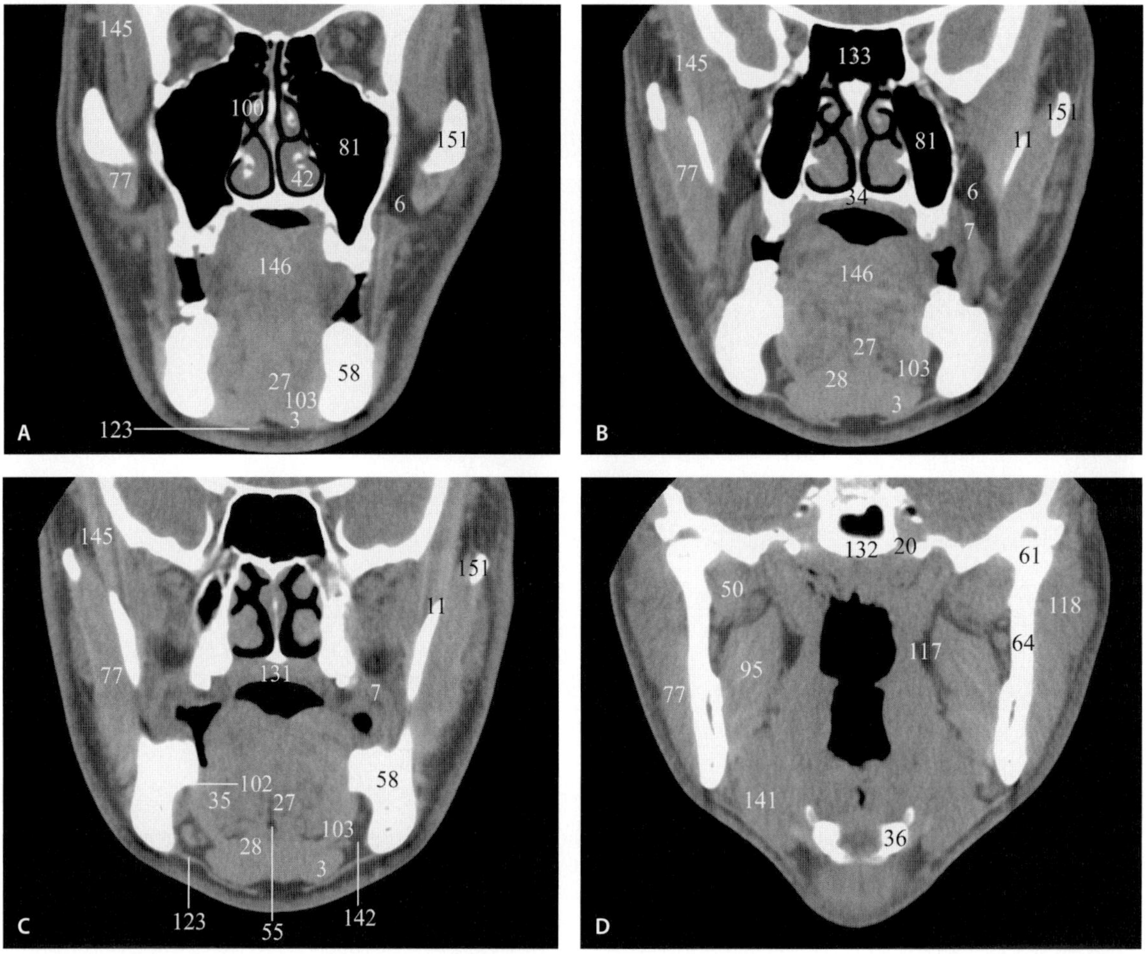

Figure 1.7

Normal coronal CT soft-tissue anatomy of the face from anterior to posterior

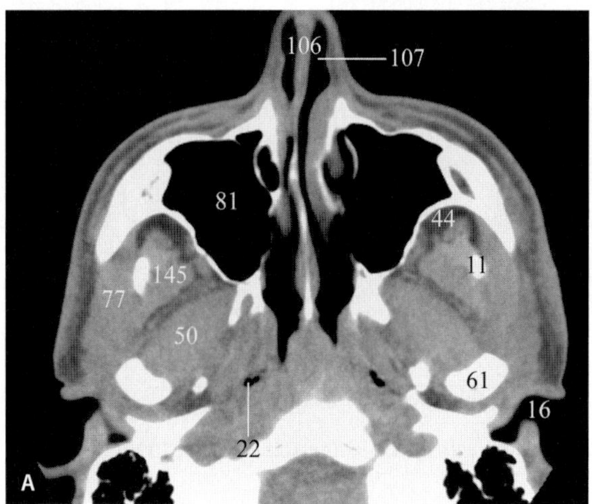

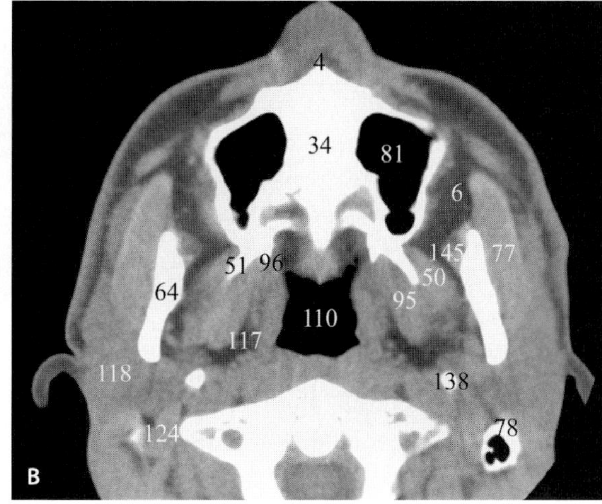

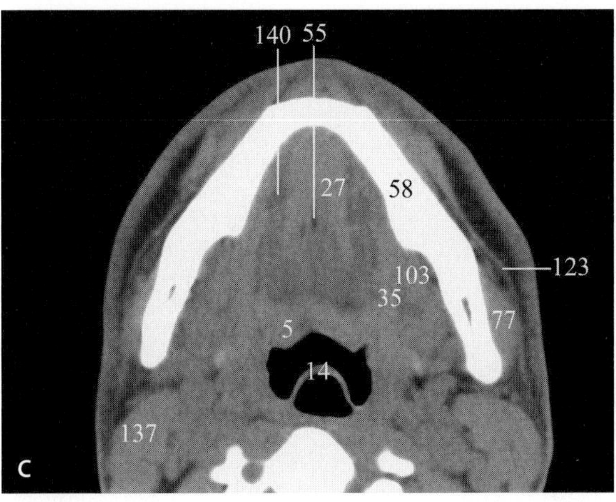

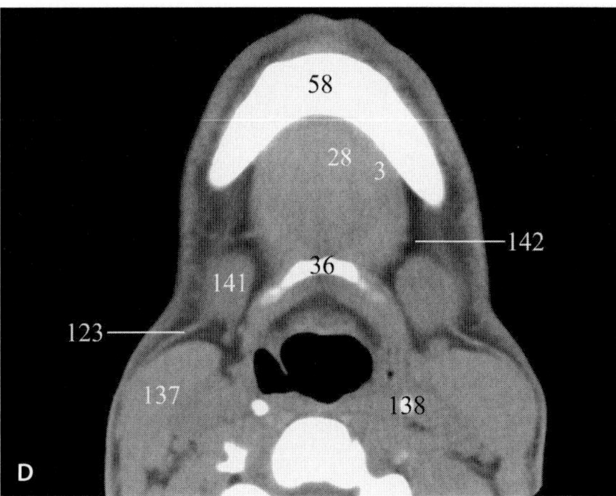

Figure 1.8

Normal axial CT soft-tissue anatomy of the lower face from superior to inferior

MR Sections

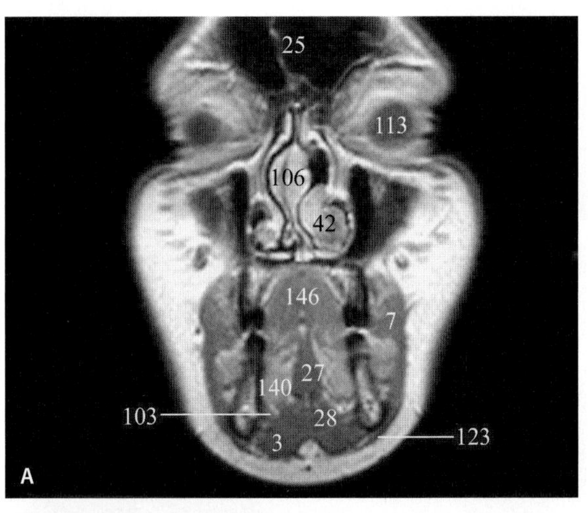

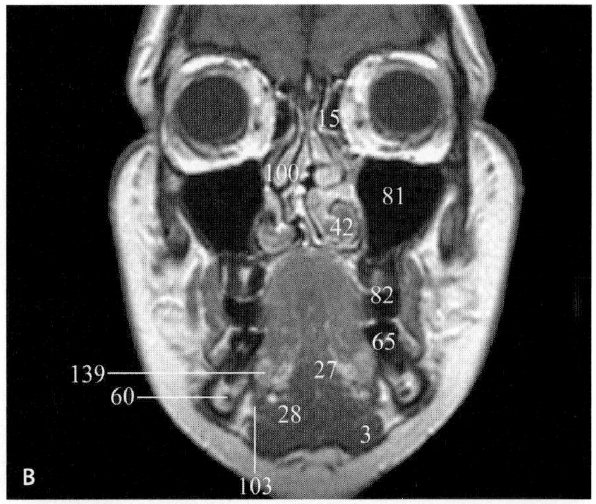

Figure 1.9

Normal coronal T1-weighted post-Gd MRI anatomy of the face from anterior to posterior

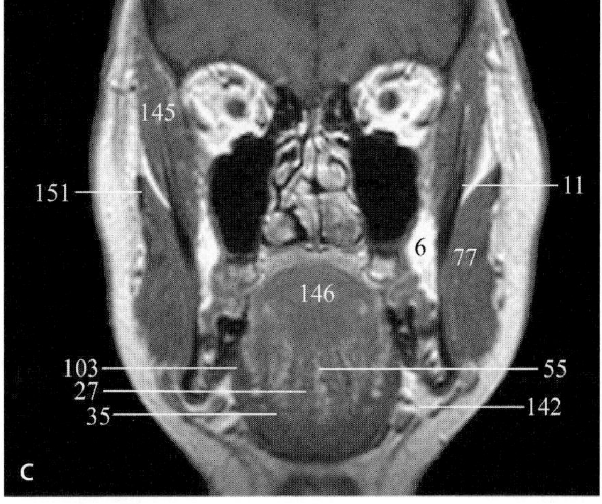

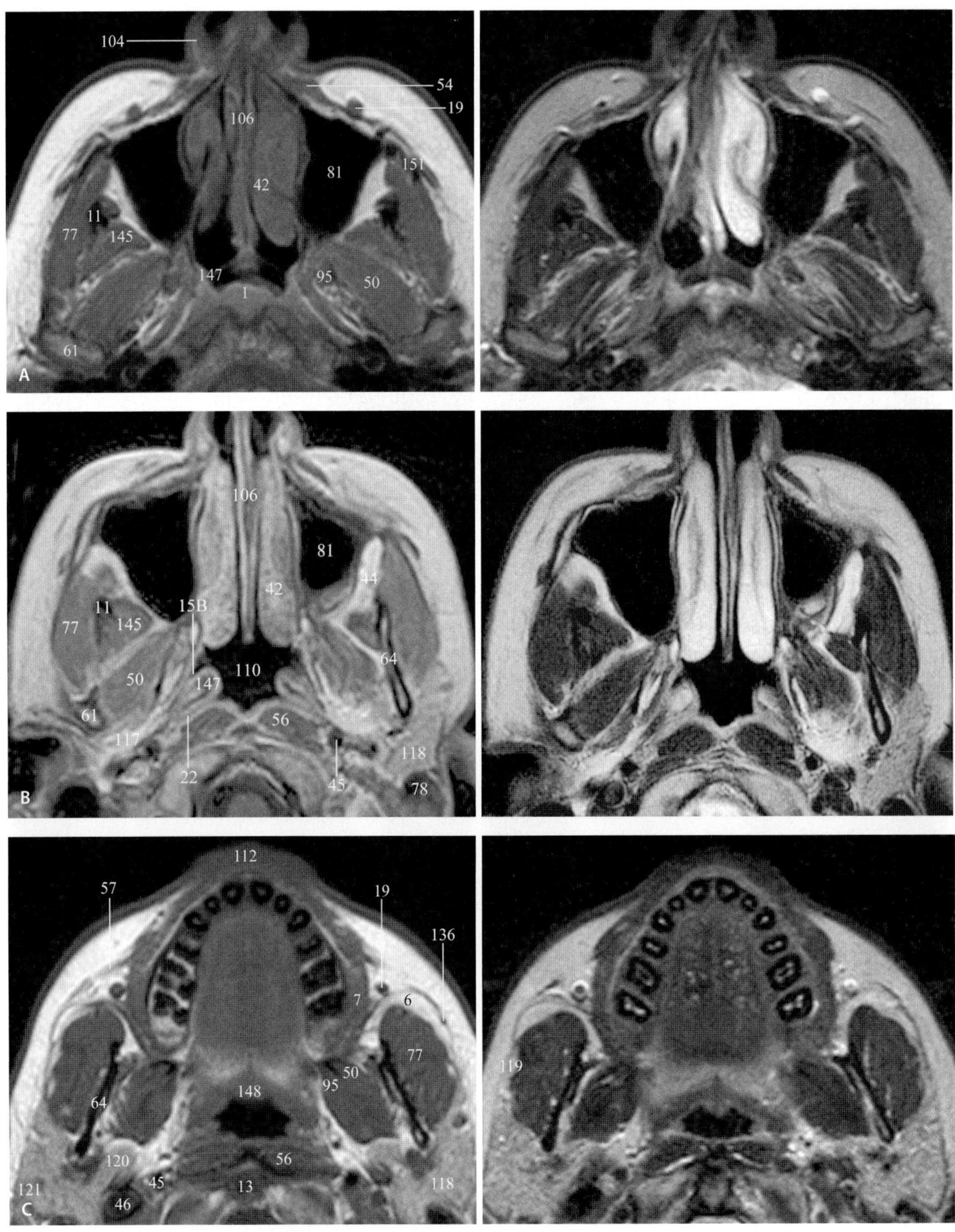

Figure 1.10

Normal axial T1- and T2-weighted MRI anatomy of the lower face from superior to inferior

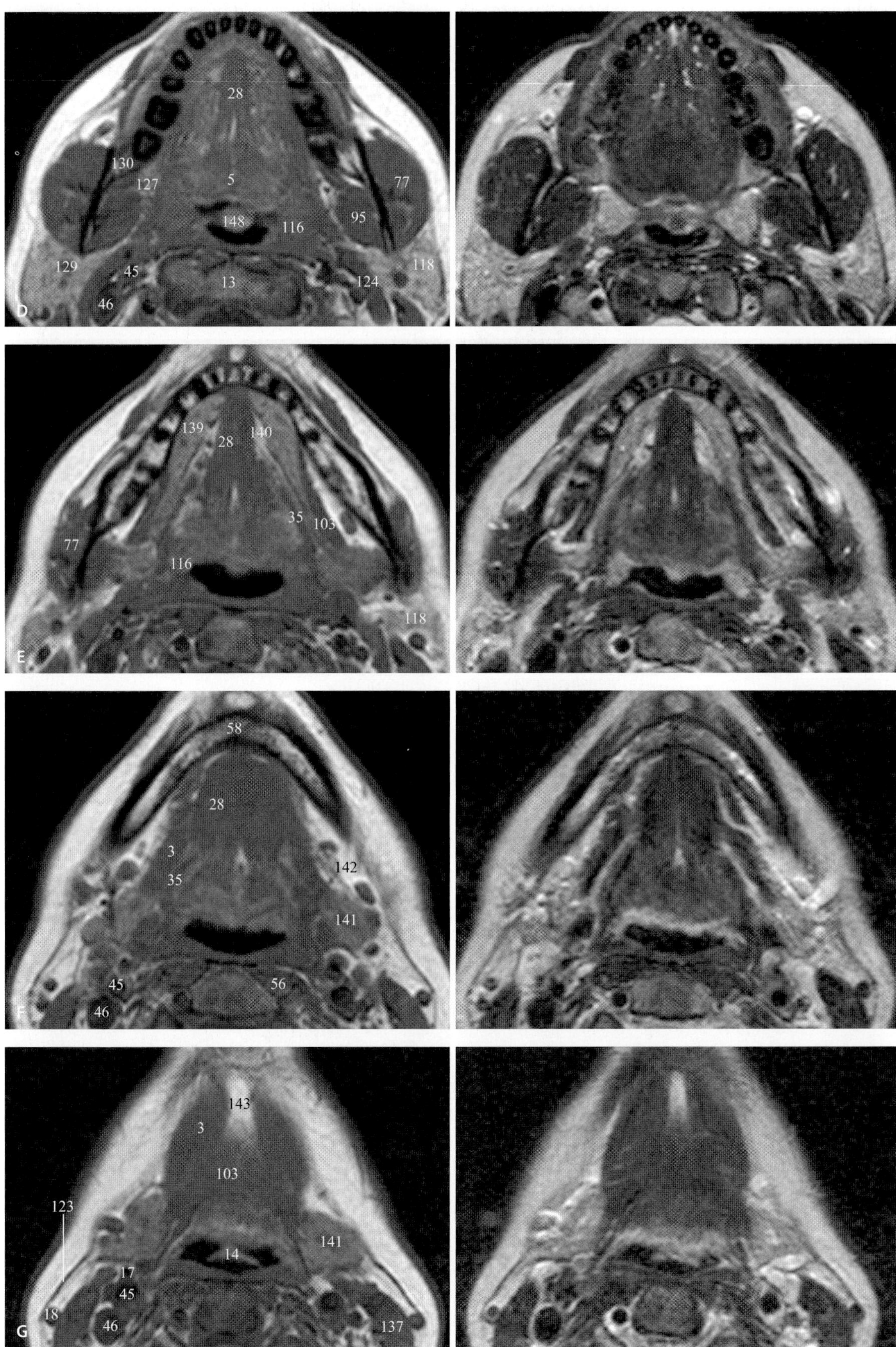
28
130
127
5
77
148
116
95
129
45
13
124
118
46
D
139
28
140
35
103
77
116
118
E
58
28
3
35
142
141
45
56
46
F
143
3
103
123
141
14
17
45
18
46
137
G

The anatomic structures in Figures 1.11–1.18:

1 Anterior band of articular disc
2 Articular disc
3 Articular tubercle (eminence)
4 Glenoid fossa
5 Inferior joint space
6 Intermediate (central) thin zone
7 Lateral pterygoid muscle raphe
8 Lower head of lateral pterygoid muscle
9 Mandibular condyle (head)
10 Mandibular condyle articulating surface
11 Mandibular condyle marrow
12 Posterior band of articular disc
13 Posterior disc attachment
14 Superior joint space
15 Upper head of lateral pterygoid muscle.

Temporomandibular Joint

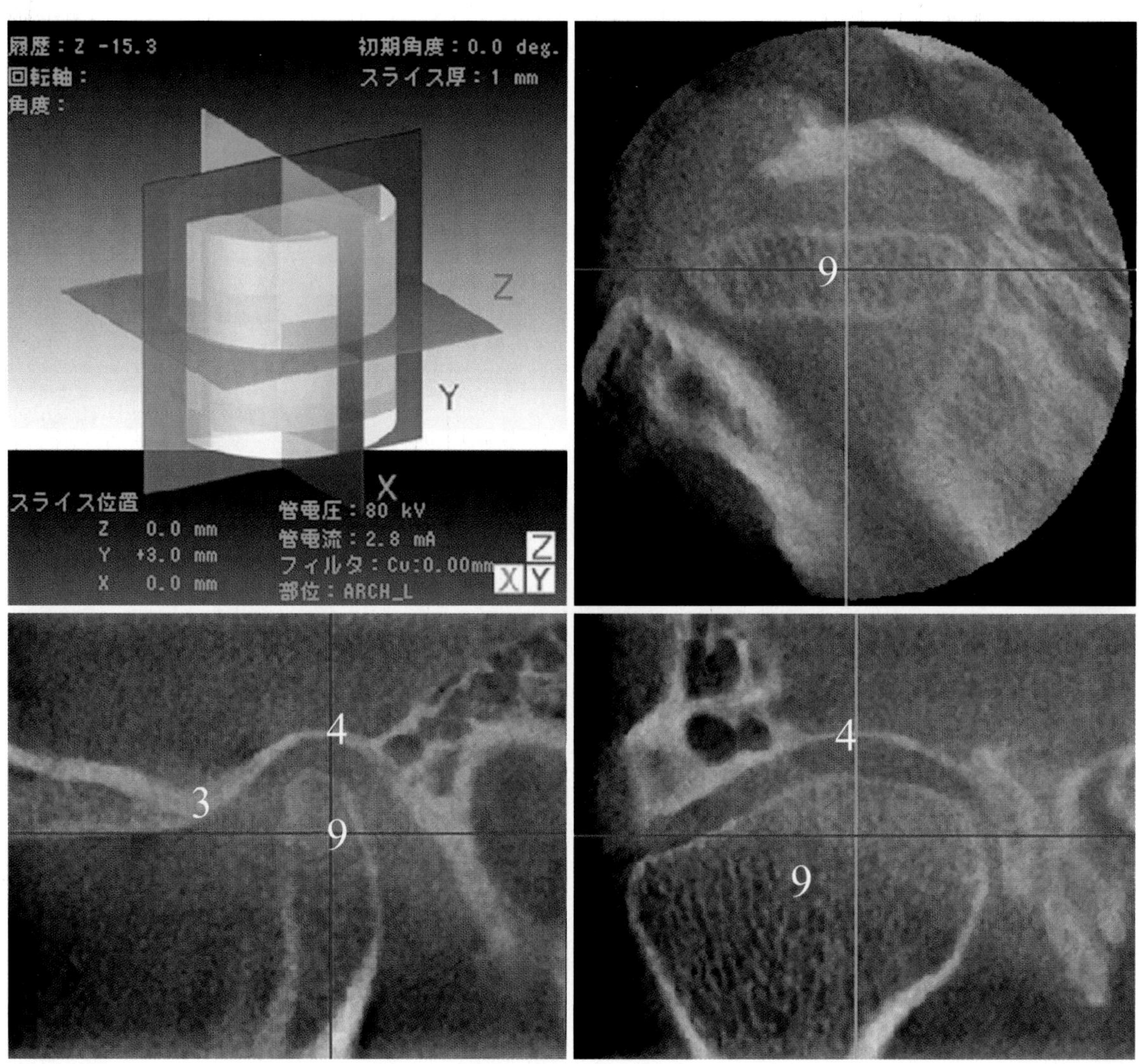

Figure 1.11

Cone beam CT bone anatomy of normal temporomandibular joint (*upper left* three image planes indicated by different colors, *upper right* axial, *lower left* oblique sagittal, *lower right* oblique coronal) (courtesy of Dr. K. Honda, Nihon University School of Dentistry, Tokyo, Japan)

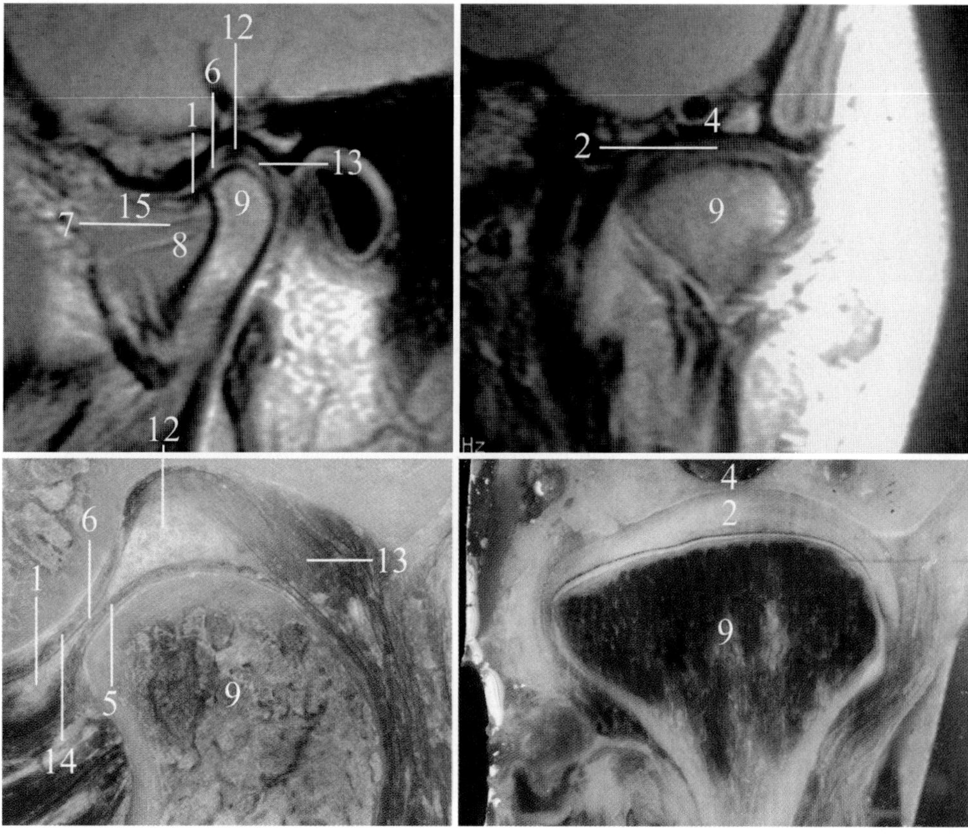

Figure 1.12

MRI and autopsy midcondyle anatomy of normal temporomandibular joint: *upper left* oblique sagittal MRI, *upper right* oblique coronal MRI, *lower left* oblique sagittal section, *lower right* oblique coronal section

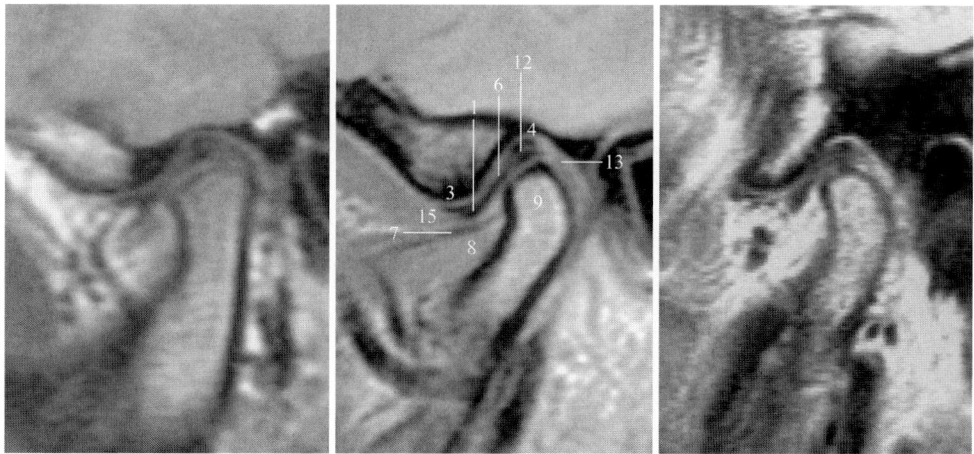

Figure 1.13

Oblique sagittal MRI, asymptomatic volunteers: *left* 9-year-old, *middle* 40-year-old, *right* 56-year-old (*right image* reproduced with permission from Larheim et al. 2001)

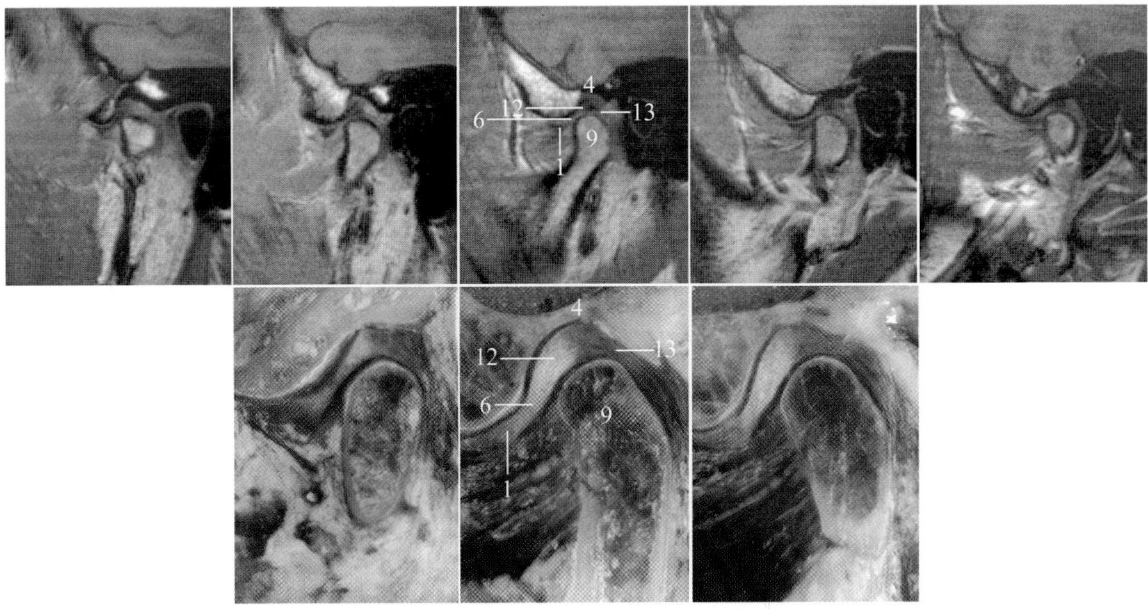

Figure 1.14

MRI and autopsy sections: *upper row* oblique sagittal MRI, asymptomatic volunteer, from lateral (*left*) to medial (*right*); *lower row* oblique sagittal, autopsy specimen, from lateral (*left*) to medial (*right*)

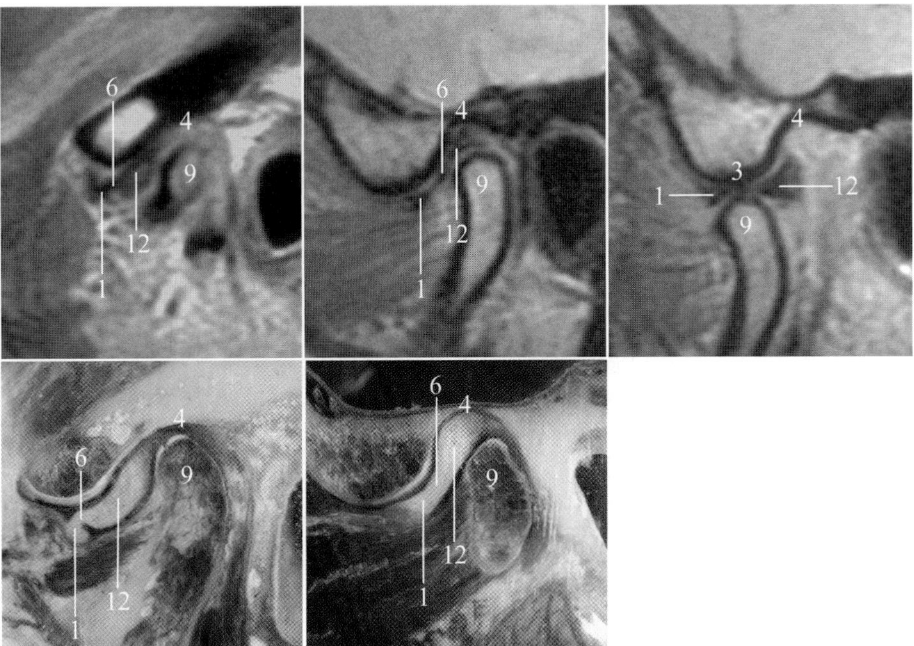

Figure 1.15

MRI and autopsy sections: *upper row* oblique sagittal MRI, asymptomatic volunteer: *left* lateral, *middle* medial, *right* opened mouth; *lower row* oblique sagittal, autopsy specimen, *left* lateral, *right* medial (*upper row images* reproduced with permission from Larheim et al. 2001)

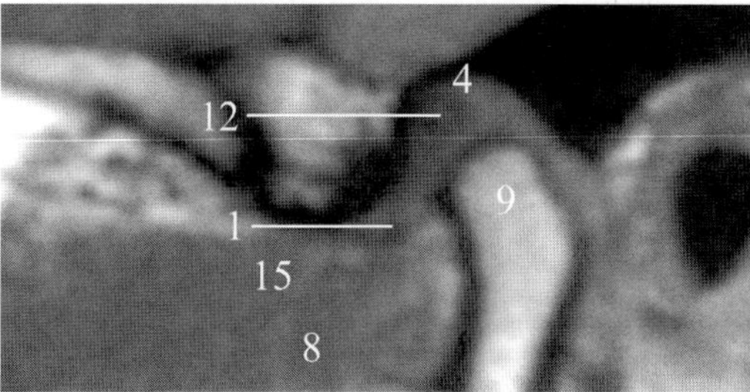

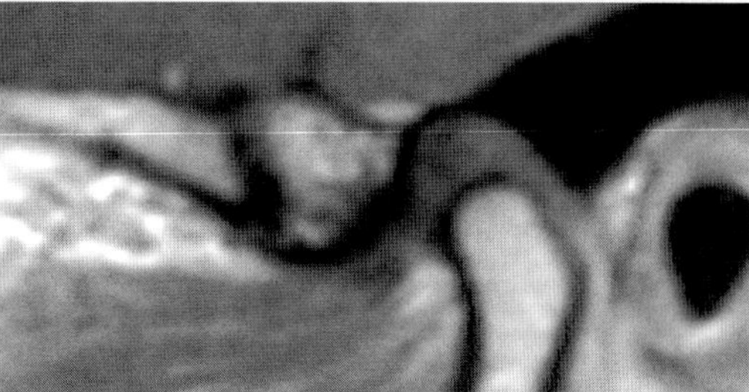

Figure 1.16

Oblique sagittal T1-weighted MRI, asymptomatic volunteer: *left* pre-Gd, *right* post-Gd

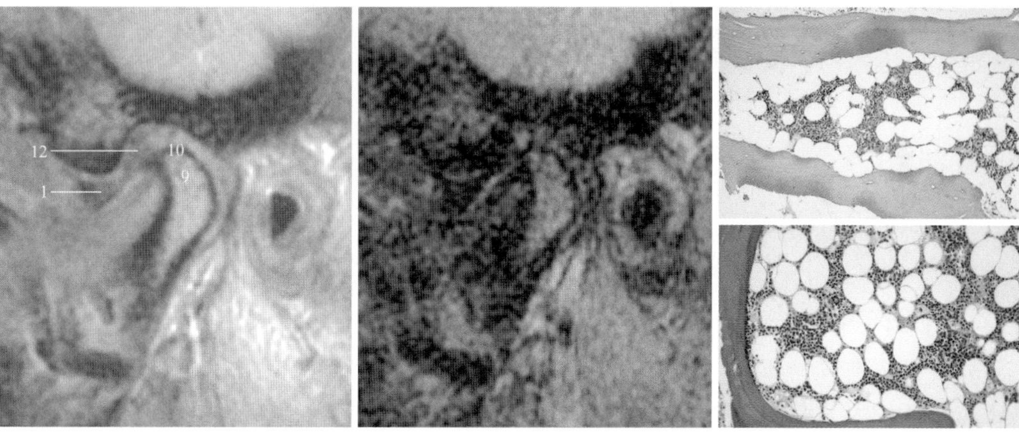

Figure 1.17

MRI and bone marrow biopsies: *left* oblique sagittal T1-weighted MRI, *middle* oblique sagittal T2-weighted MRI, *right upper* normal bone marrow from mandibular condyle of same patient, *right lower* normal bone marrow from hip for comparison (all images except right lower reproduced with permission from Larheim et al. 1999)

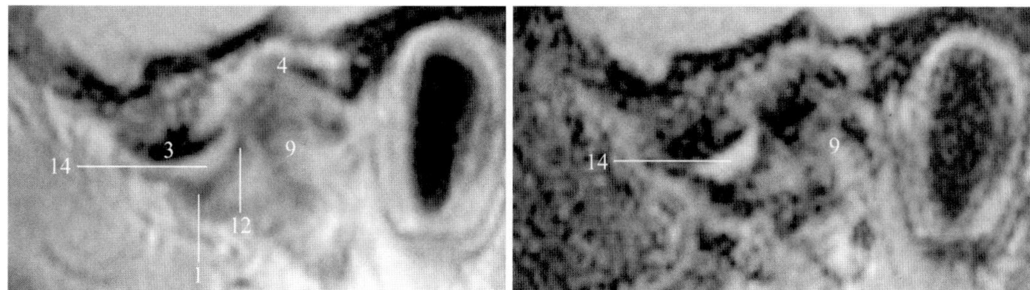

Figure 1.18

Oblique sagittal MRI, asymptomatic volunteer with joint fluid in upper joint space: *left* T1-weighted MRI, *right* T2-weighted MRI (reproduced with permission from Larheim et al. 2001)

Suggested Reading

Aasen S, Kolbenstvedt A (1992) CT appearances of normal and obstructed submandibular duct. Acta Radiol 33:414–419

Abrahams JJ, Rock R, Hayt MW (2003) Embryology and anatomy of the jaw and dentition. In: Som PM, Curtin HD (eds) Head and neck imaging, 4th edn, Mosby, St. Louis, pp 889–906

Brooks SL, Westesson P-L, Eriksson L, Hansson LG, Barsotti JB (1992) Prevalence of osseous changes in the temporomandibular joint of asymptomatic persons without internal derangement. Oral Surg Oral Med Oral Pathol 73:118–122

Katzberg RW, Westesson P-L, Tallents RH, Drake CM (1996) Anatomic disorders of the tempromandibular joint disc in asymptomic subjects J Oral Maxillofac Surg 54:147–153

Larheim TA, Katzberg RW, Westesson P-L, Tallents RH, Moss ME (2001) MR evidence of temporomandibular joint fluid and condyle marrow alterations: occurrence in asymptomatic volunteers and symptomatic patients. Int J Oral Maxillofac Surg 30:113–117

Larheim TA, Westesson P-L, Hicks DG, Eriksson L, Brown DA (1999) Osteonecrosis of the temporomandibular joint: correlation of magnetic resonance imaging and histology. J Oral Maxillofac Surg 57:888–898

Larheim TA, Westesson P-L, Sano T (2001) Temporomandibular joint disk displacement: comparison in asymptomatic volunteers and patients. Radiology 218:428–432

Smoker WRK (2003) The oral cavity. In: Som PM, Curtin HD (eds) Head and neck imaging, 4th edn. Mosby, St. Louis, pp 1377–1464

Som PM, Shugar JMA, Brandwein MS (2003) Sinonasal cavities: anatomy and physiology. In: Som PM, Curtin HD (eds) Head and neck imaging, 4th edn. Mosby, St. Louis, pp 87–147

Som PM, Smoker WRK, Balboni A, Reidenberg JS, Hudgins PA, Weissman JL, Laitman J (2003) Embryology and anatomy of the neck. In: Som PM, Curtin HD (eds) Head and neck imaging, 4th edn. Mosby, St. Louis, pp 1757–1827

Jaw Cysts

In collaboration with H.-J. Smith · H. Strømme Koppang

Introduction

Cysts in the jaws are common and mostly diagnosed and managed by general dental practitioners and dental specialists using intraoral or panoramic (film or digital) radiography. However, advanced imaging modalities are increasingly used to assess more precisely those which are larger and cannot be adequately diagnosed with conventional radiography. We present a number of cases richly illustrated with CT and MR images to give specialists both in the dental and in the medical fields an opportunity to become familiar with both their appearances and the spectrum they represent.

Definition

Epithelium-lined cavity containing fluid or semifluid material, surrounded by fibrous tissue.

Most jaw cysts originate from odontogenic epithelial residues after tooth development.

Clinical Features

- Usually an incidental radiographic finding
- Occasional swelling and jaw asymmetry
- No pain if not secondarily infected

Imaging Features

- Radiolucency in bone (density in maxillary sinus)
- Unilocular round, oval or scalloped, or influenced by surrounding structures
- Border well-defined thin, uniform, intact and sclerotic
- May expand bone
- May displace or resorb teeth
- May displace walls of maxillary sinus, nasal cavity, and mandibular canal
- When secondarily infected, border may become destroyed or more sclerotic
- Rarely, border may show defect also without infection
- Rarely, calcified tissue may be produced
- T1-weighted MRI: homogeneous intermediate signal (fluid content) or occasionally, homogeneous high signal (cholesterol content)
- T2-weighted and STIR MRI: homogeneous high or occasionally homogeneous low signal or occasionally heterogeneous signal (high to intermediate to low), consistent with fluid or semifluid (large molecules, granulation tissue) content
- T1-weighted post-Gd MRI: no enhancement, or enhancement of peripheral thin rim (partial or complete), consistent with cyst capsule
- T1-weighted and T2-weighted MRI: homogeneous high signal reported to be specific for nasopalatine duct cyst

Periapical Cyst

Synonyms: Radicular cyst, apical periodontal cyst

Definition

Cyst arising from epithelial residues (rests of Malassez) in periodontal ligament as a consequence of inflammation, usually following death of dental pulp (WHO).

Clinical Features

- Odontogenic
- Inflammatory
- At or around a tooth root or lateral to root
- Nonvital tooth
- Most common type of jaw cyst
- Maxilla and mandible
- Anterior region of maxilla in particular
- Males more frequent than females
- All ages, particularly third and fourth decades, but seldom in deciduous dentition

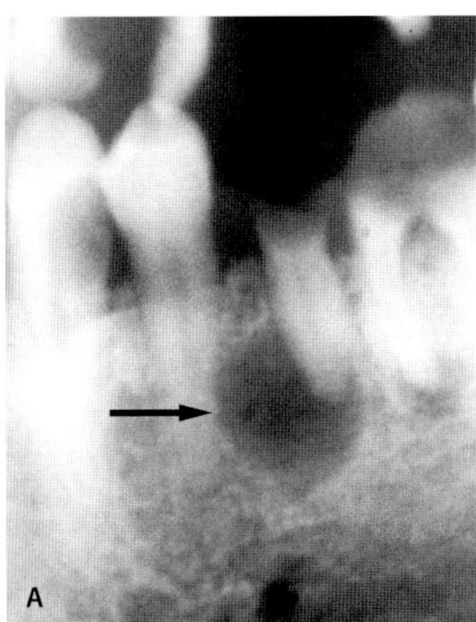

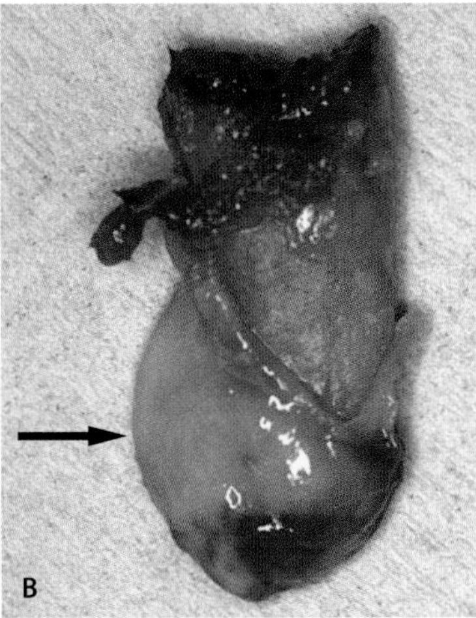

Figure 2.1

Periapical cyst, mandible; asymptomatic, nonvital tooth root. **A** Panoramic view shows round radiolucency with sclerotic border (*arrow*). **B** Surgically removed tooth with cyst (*arrow*)

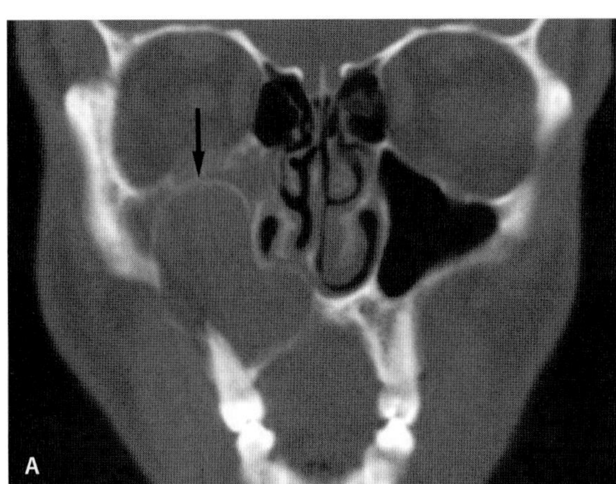

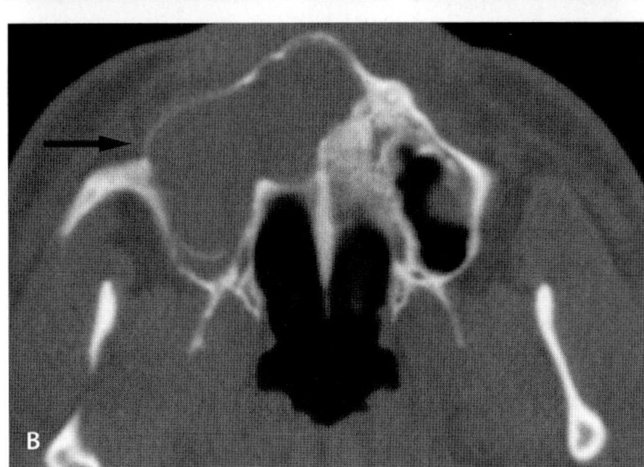

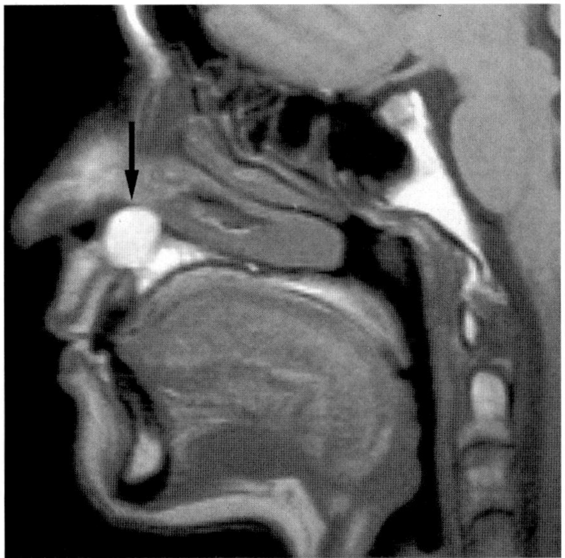

Figure 2.2

Periapical cyst, maxilla; 38-year-old male with some discomfort and swelling of mucobuccal fold; nonvital right lateral incisor. **A** Coronal CT image shows expansive process displacing part of nasal cavity, with intact and sclerotic border, occupying most of right maxillary sinus (*arrow*). **B** Axial CT image shows scalloped process destroying alveolar bone and hard palate (*arrow*)

Figure 2.3

Periapical cyst, maxilla; 58-year-old female with incidental finding at routine dental radiography, nonvital central incisor. Sagittal T1-weighted MRI shows oval expansive process with homogeneous high signal (*arrow*)

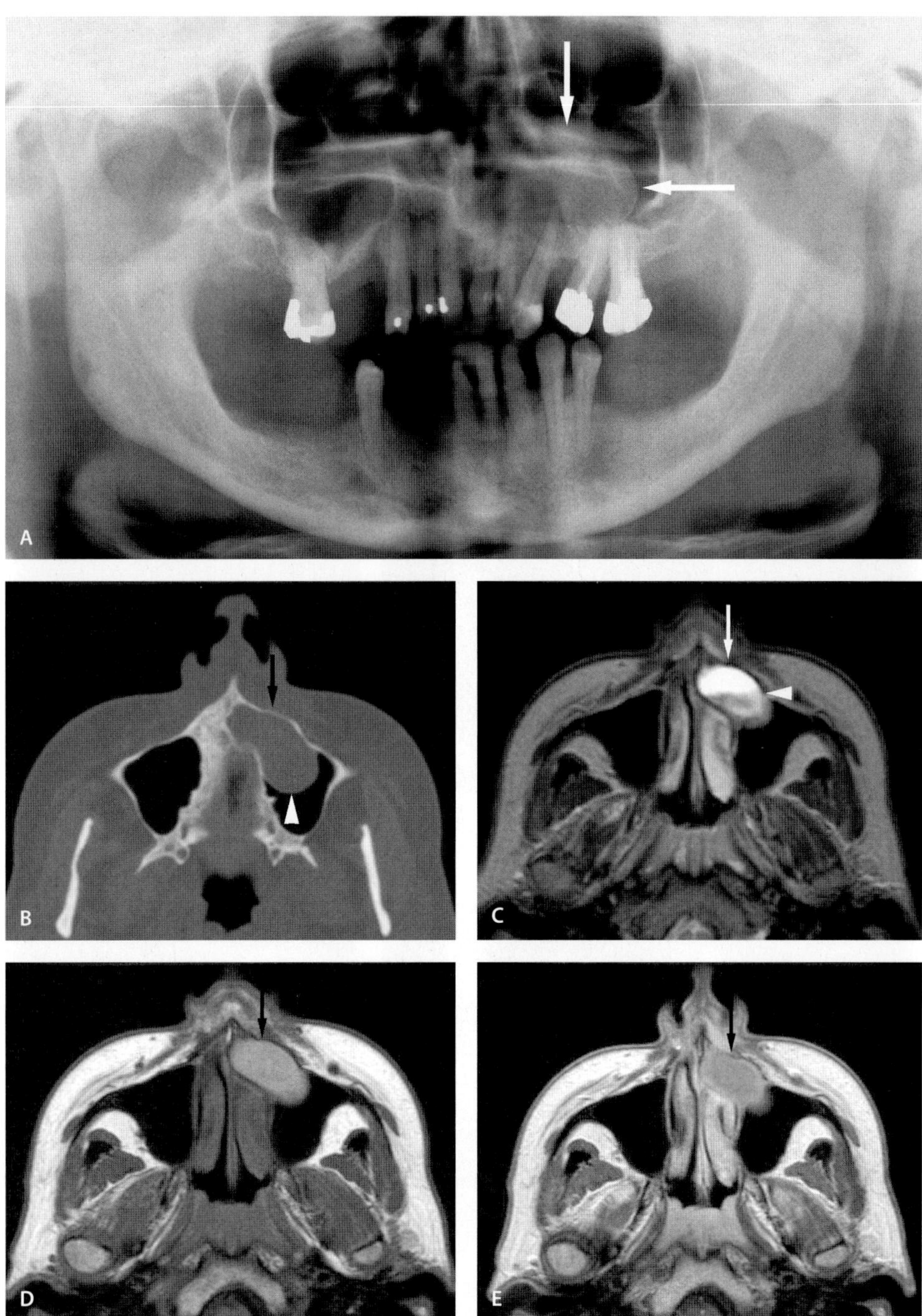

Figure 2.4

Periapical cyst, maxilla; 45-year-old female with incidental finding at routine dental radiography, nonvital lateral left incisor. A Panoramic view shows round process (more dense than air) with sclerotic border (*arrows*). B Axial CT image shows expansive process (*arrow*) with intact sclerotic border in maxillary sinus (*arrowhead*). C Axial T2-weighted MRI shows high signal content (*arrow*) above intermediate signal content in dependent part; *arrowhead* fluid level. D Axial T1-weighted pre-Gd MRI shows homogeneous intermediate signal (*arrow*). E Axial T1-weighted post-Gd MRI shows no enhancement except a thin peripheral rim (*arrow*)

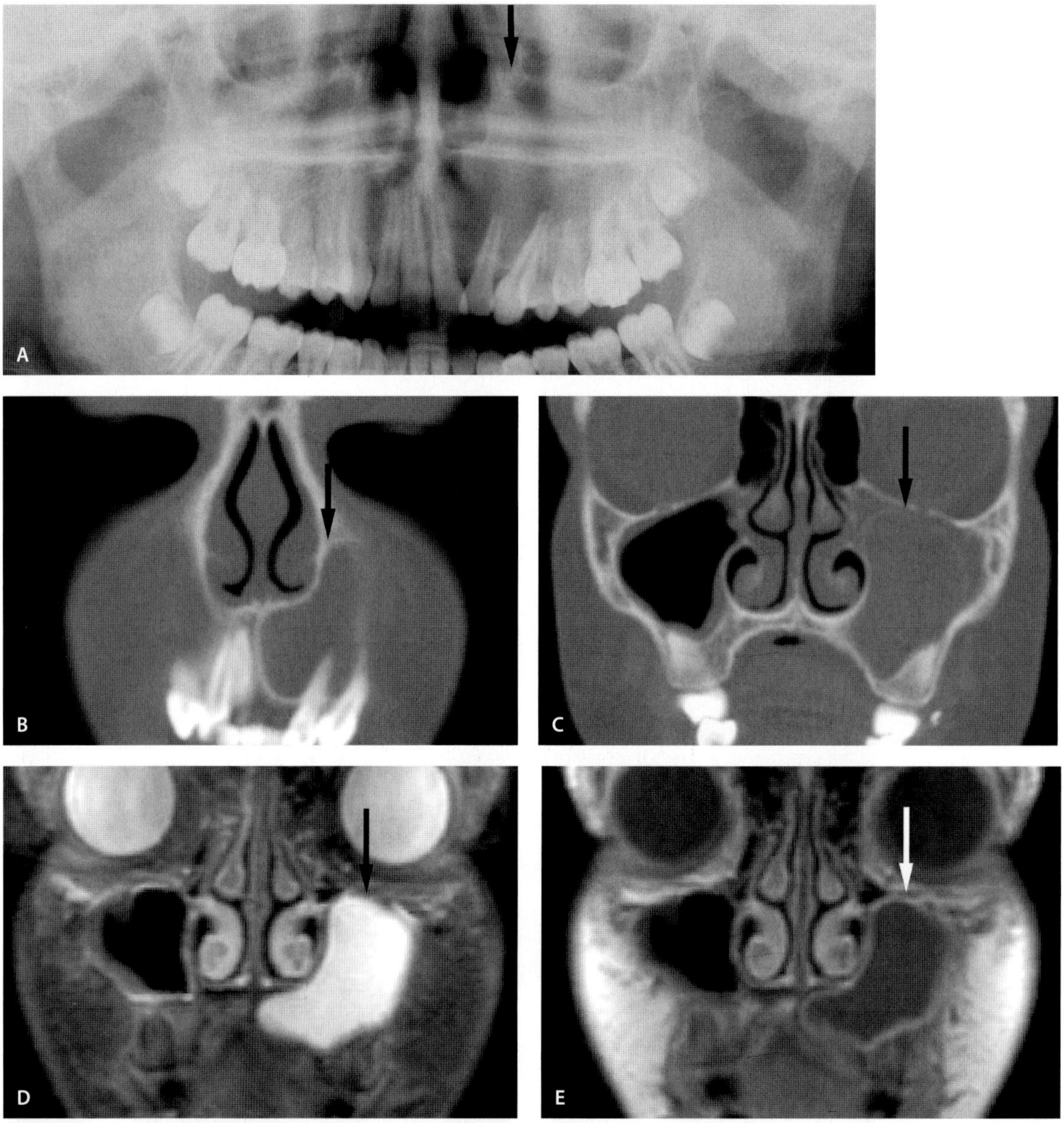

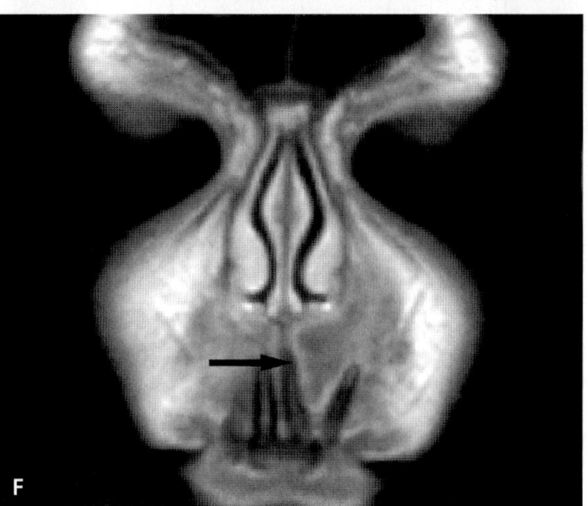

Figure 2.5

Periapical cyst, maxilla; 13-year-old female with painless swelling of mucobuccal fold and nonvital left lateral incisor, with previous pain from incisor. **A** Panoramic view shows radiolucency with partially sclerotic border in alveolar process around left lateral incisor and lack of sinus demarcation (*arrow*), and deviation of central incisor and canine. **B** Coronal CT image shows expansive process with sclerotic border around incisor (*arrow*). **C** Coronal CT image shows process occupying most of maxillary sinus with a very thin sclerotic border (*arrow*). **D** Coronal STIR MRI shows homogeneous high signal content (*arrow*). **E** Coronal T1-weighted post-Gd MRI shows no enhancement except peripheral rim (arrow). **F** Coronal T1-weighted post-Gd MRI shows rim of enhancement and displacement of teeth (*arrow*)

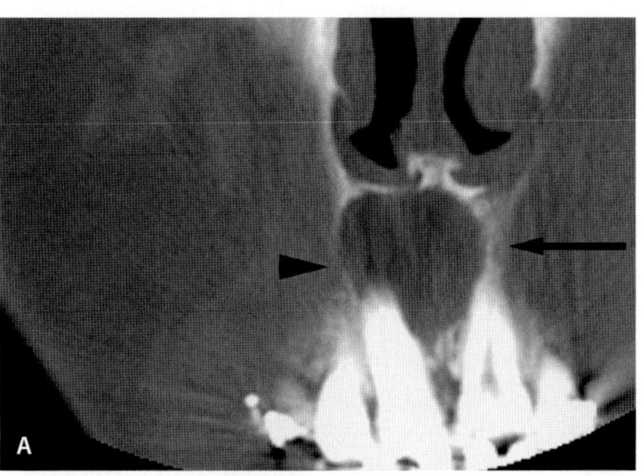

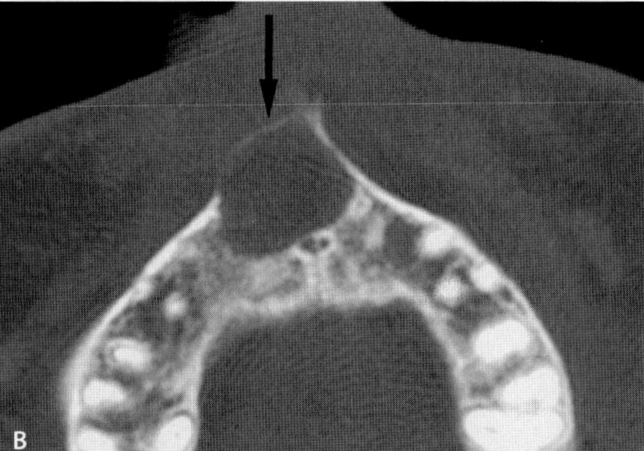

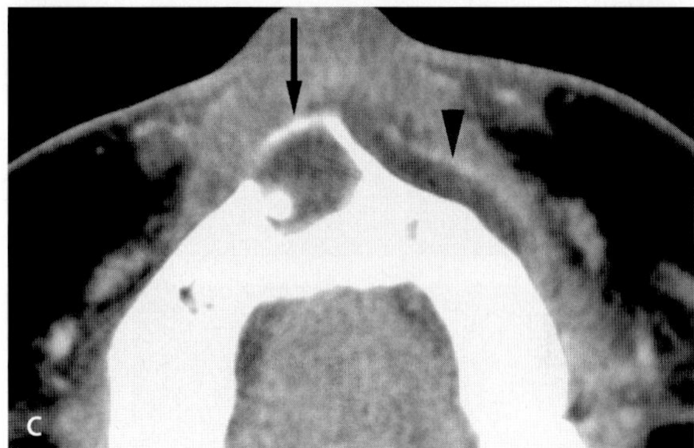

Figure 2.6

Periapical cyst, maxilla, with abscess development; 14-year-old male with swelling of mucobuccal fold, pain, foul odor, and nonvital right central incisor. A Coronal CT image shows expansive process with well-defined border (*arrow*), thin and perforated on right side (*arrowhead*). B Axial CT image shows process (*arrow*) with no sclerotic border in alveolar bone on right side. C Axial CT image, soft-tissue window shows cyst in alveolar process (*arrow*) with inflammatory exudate (*hypodense area*) along buccal surface and elevation of periosteum (*arrowhead*)

Residual Cyst

Definition

Periapical cyst which is retained in jaw after removal of associated tooth (WHO).

Clinical Features

- Odontogenic
- see Periapical cyst

Figure 2.7

Residual cyst, mandible; asymptomatic, teeth were extracted many years previously. Intraoral view shows round radiolucency with sclerotic border (*arrow*)

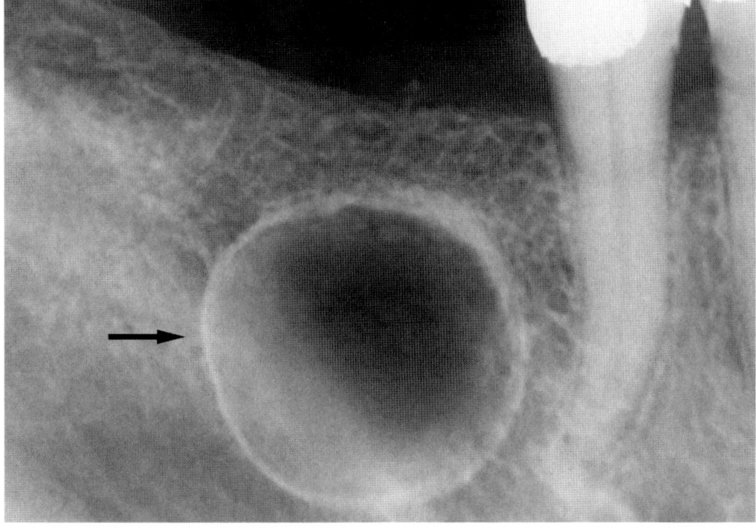

Paradental (Mandibular Infected Buccal) Cyst

Definition

Cyst occurring near to cervical margin of lateral aspect of root as a consequence of inflammatory process in periodontal pocket (WHO).

Clinical Features

- Odontogenic
- Inflammatory
- Mandible, usually first molars
- Unilateral or bilateral
- Vital teeth
- 6–8 years of age
- Distinctive form may occur at mandibular molars, most commonly third molars associated with a history of pericoronitis

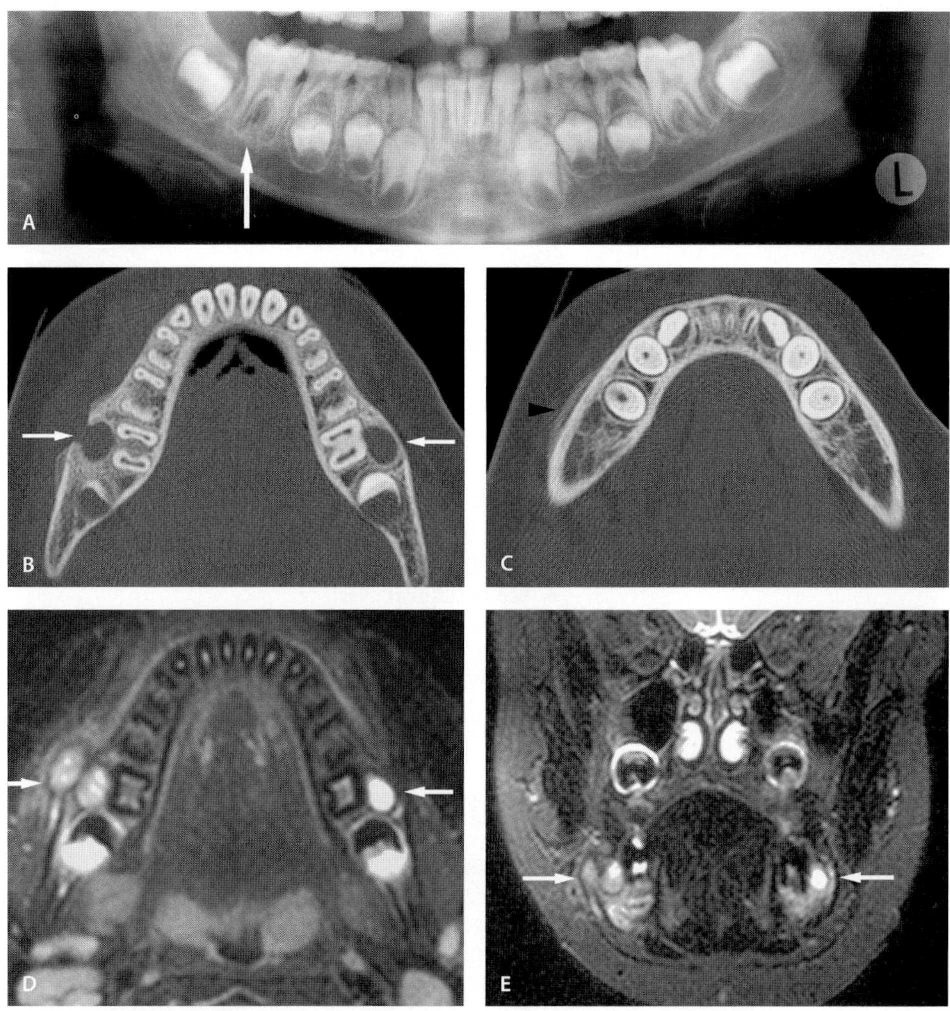

Figure 2.8

Paradental cyst, mandible; 8-year-old male with right perimandibular swelling and pain. A Panoramic view suggests small radiolucency in root area of first molar (*arrow*). B Axial CT image shows buccal oval bone cavities bilaterally at first molars (*arrows*), with sclerotic outline on left side and with cortical defect on more severely inflamed right side. C Axial CT image shows periosteal bone reaction (*arrowhead*). D Axial STIR MRI shows bilateral high signal at first molars (*arrows*); homogeneous signal on left side and double contour with heterogeneous signal on right side. E Coronal STIR MRI shows bilateral cysts with different shapes and signals (*arrows*)

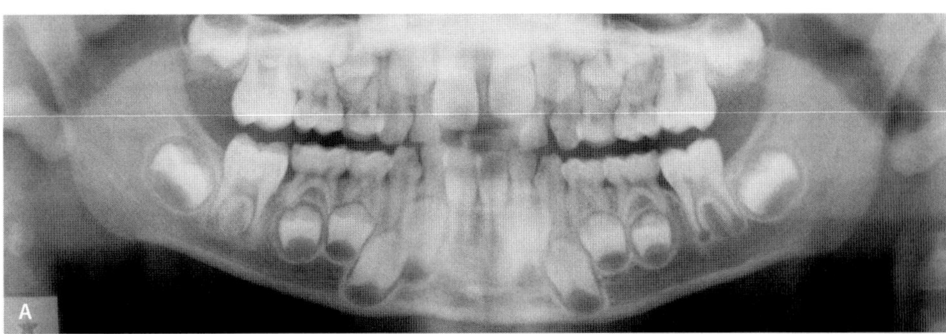

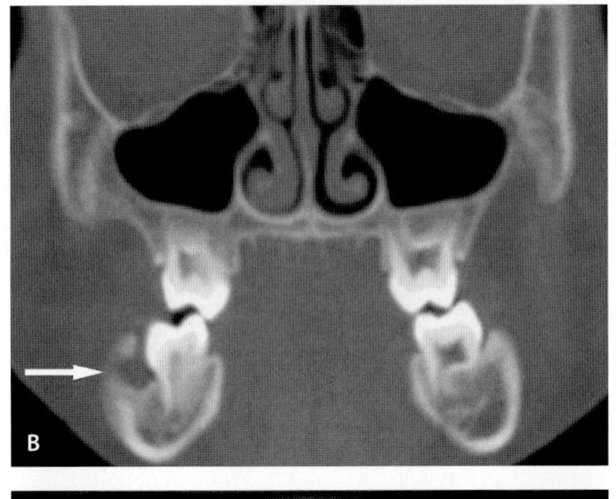

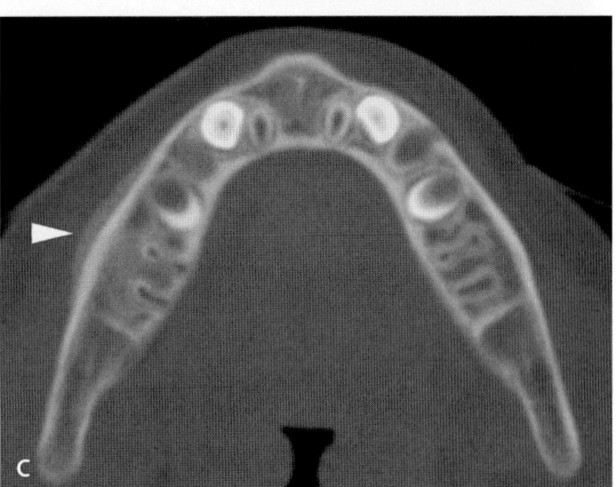

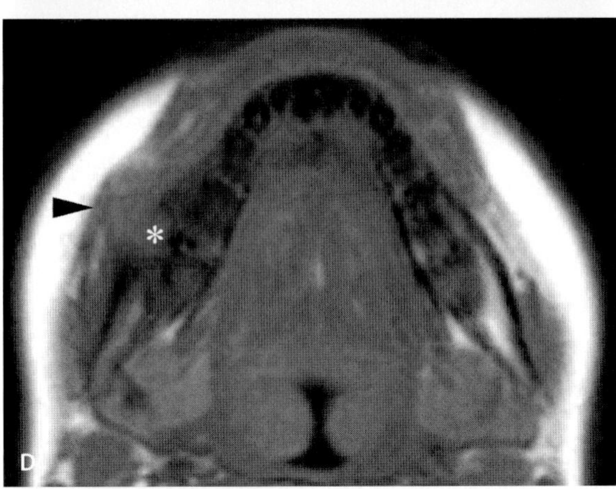

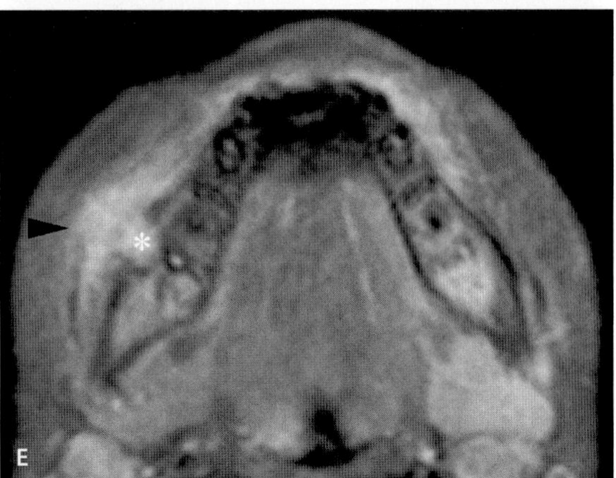

Figure 2.9

Paradental cyst, mandible; 7-year-old male with right perimandibular swelling and pain. A Panoramic view shows no abnormalities. B Coronal CT image shows buccal cystic radiolucency in molar area (*arrow*). C Axial CT image shows periosteal reaction (*arrowhead*). D Axial T1-weighted pre-Gd MRI shows intermediate (to low) signal (*arrowhead*); *asterisk* area of bone destruction. E Axial T1-weighted fat suppressed post-Gd MRI shows contrast enhancement in bone destruction (*asterisk*) and in buccal soft tissue (*arrowhead*). F Axial STIR MRI shows diffuse but intense signal in buccal soft tissue, indicating inflammatory response (*arrowhead*); *asterisk* area of bone destruction

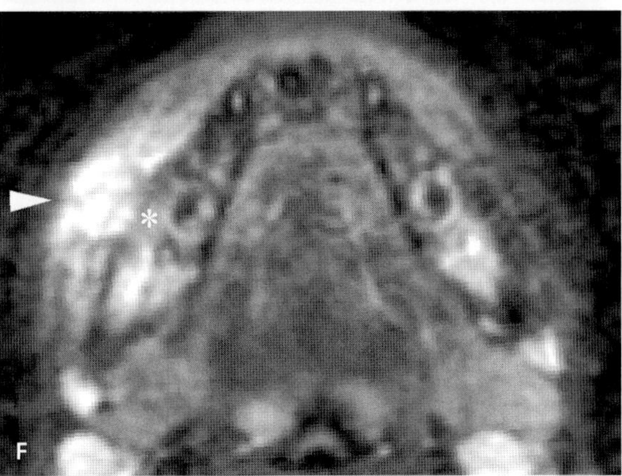

Lateral Periodontal Cyst

Definition

Cyst occurring on lateral aspect or between roots of vital teeth and arising from odontogenic epithelial remnants, but not as a result of inflammatory stimuli (WHO).

Clinical Features

- Odontogenic cyst
- Developmental
- Vital teeth with normal periodontal ligament
- Mandibular premolar and maxillary anterior regions in particular
- Wide age distribution

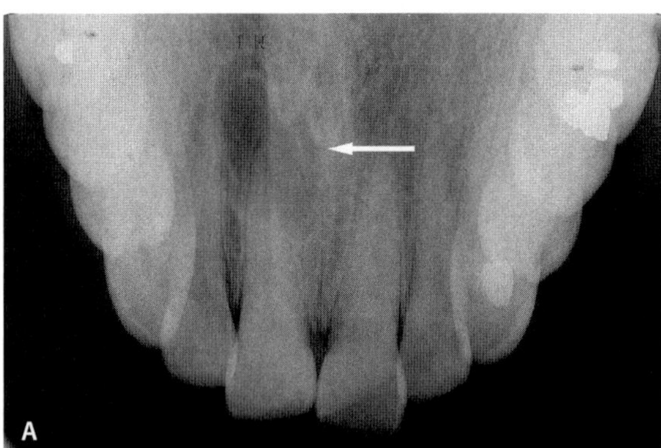

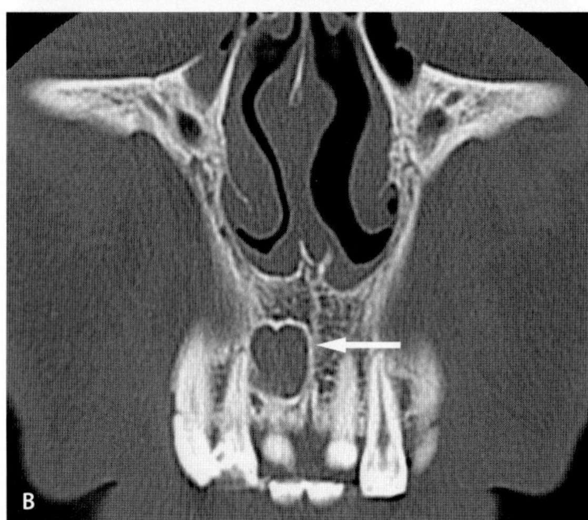

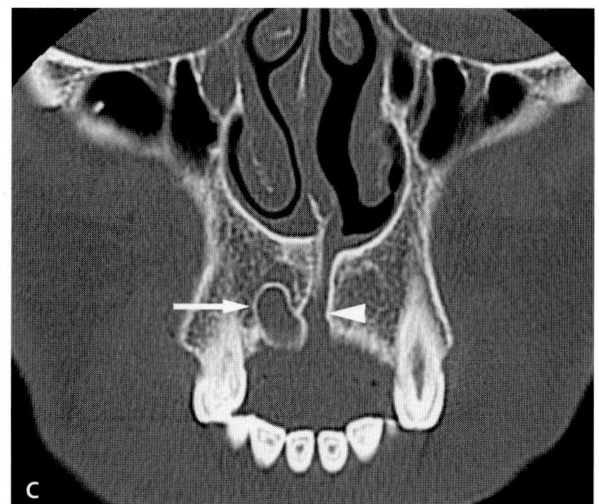

Figure 2.10

Lateral periodontal cyst, maxilla; 35-year-old male with incidental finding at routine dental radiography; vital teeth. **A** Intraoral view shows oval periapical radiolucency with sclerotic border (*arrow*) and normal apical periodontal ligament of teeth. **B** Coronal CT image shows oval radiolucency with sclerotic border in alveolar process medial to incisor (*arrow*). **C** Coronal CT image shows radiolucency (*arrow*) separate from incisive canal (*arrowhead*)

Incisive Canal Cyst

Synonym: Nasopalatine duct cyst

Definition

Cyst arising from epithelial residues in nasopalatine (incisive) canal (WHO).

Clinical Features

- Non-odontogenic
- Developmental
- Located in nasopalatine canal
- Vital teeth
- Males more frequent than females
- Fourth decade and older

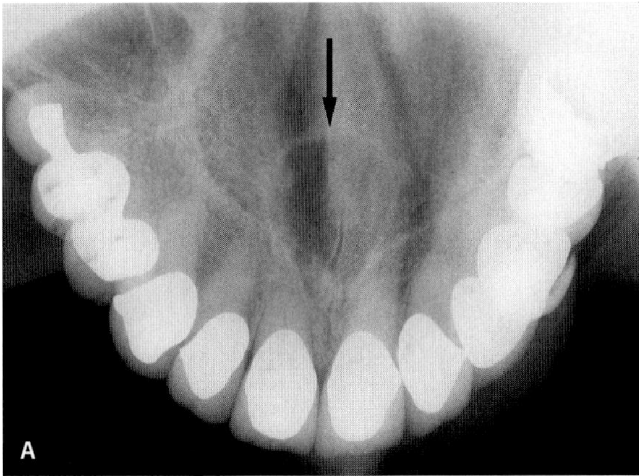

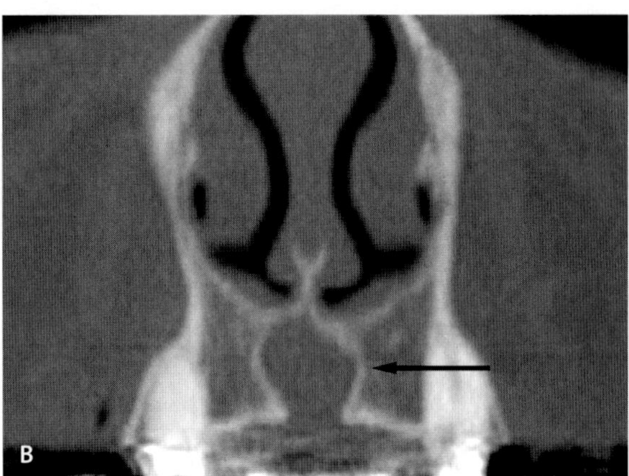

Figure 2.11

Incisive canal cyst, maxilla; 60-year-old male with incidental finding at routine dental radiography. A Intraoral occlusal view shows round radiolucency in midline with sclerotic border (*arrow*) and normal apical periodontal ligament. B Coronal CT image shows radiolucency with sclerotic border (*arrow*)

Figure 2.12

Incisive canal cyst, maxilla; 27-year-old male with incidental finding at routine dental radiography. Axial CT image shows radiolucency in midline with sclerotic border (*arrow*) and communication to bone destruction at incisor. Also bone destruction at other incisor (*arrowhead*)

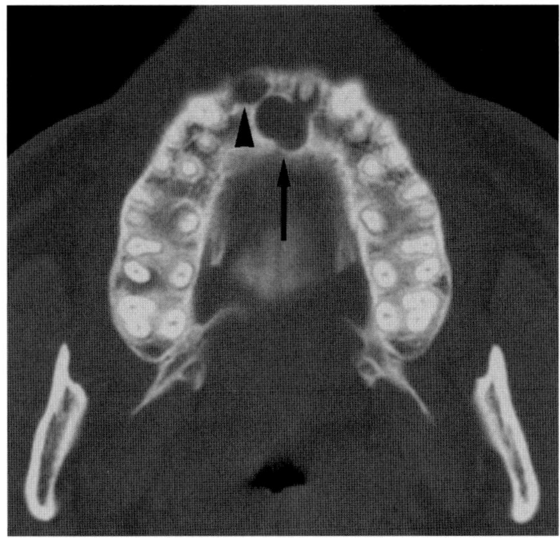

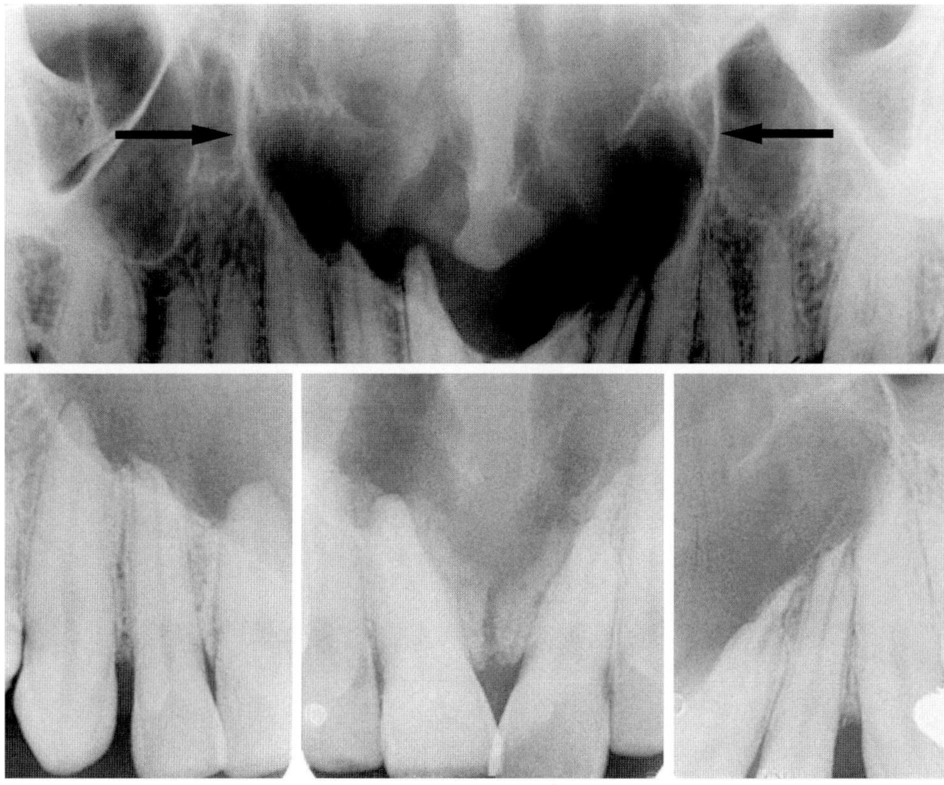

Figure 2.13

Incisive canal cyst; painless swelling of palate, vital teeth. Panoramic and intraoral views show large cyst (*arrows*) resorbing tooth roots

Follicular Cyst

Synonym: Dentigerous cyst

Definition

Cyst which encloses crown and is attached to neck of unerupted tooth. It develops by accumulation of fluid between reduced enamel epithelium and crown, or between layers of reduced enamel epithelium (WHO).

Clinical Features

- Odontogenic
- Developmental
- Around tooth crown
- Mandibular third molar, maxillary canine and third molar, mandibular second premolar
- Males more frequent than females
- All ages, particularly second to fourth decades
- **Eruption cyst** surrounds crown of an erupting tooth

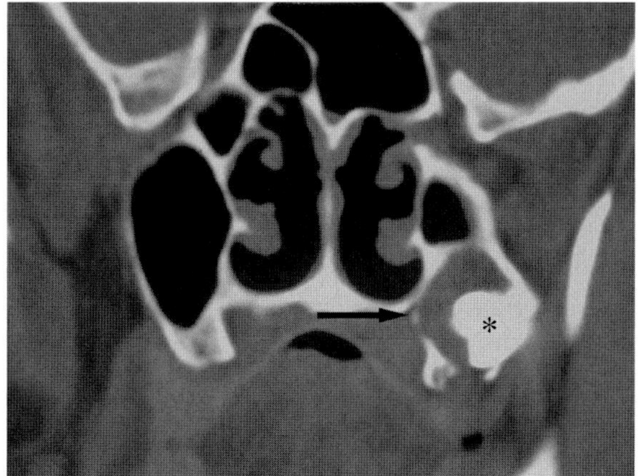

Figure 2.14

Follicular cyst, maxilla; 54-year-old male with incidental finding at paranasal sinus examination. Coronal CT image shows expansive process (*arrow*) around crown of impacted third molar (*asterisk*)

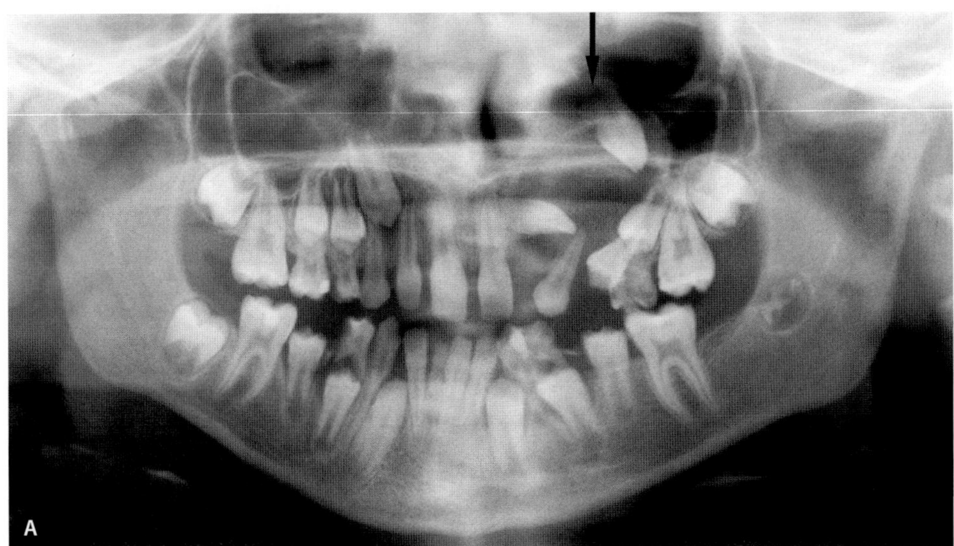

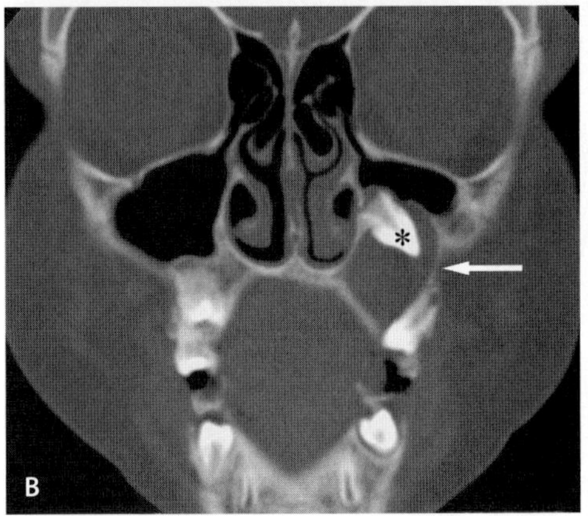

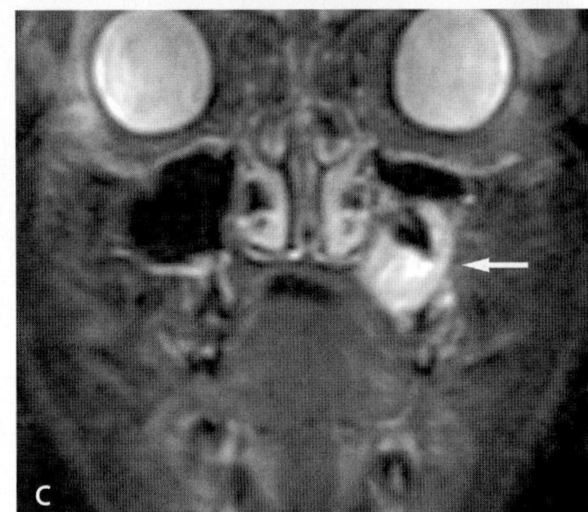

Figure 2.15

Follicular cyst, maxilla; 8-year-old male with incidental finding when examined for an unerupted lateral incisor. A Panoramic view shows radiolucency and two unerupted teeth (*arrow*). B Coronal CT image shows process with sclerotic border (*arrow*) around crown of canine (*asterisk*). C Coronal STIR MRI shows homogeneous high signal content (*arrow*). D Coronal CT image shows cyst (*arrow*) around crown of lateral incisor (*asterisk*)

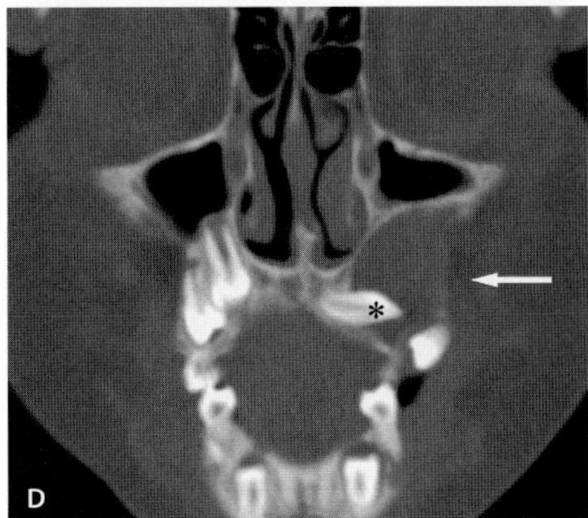

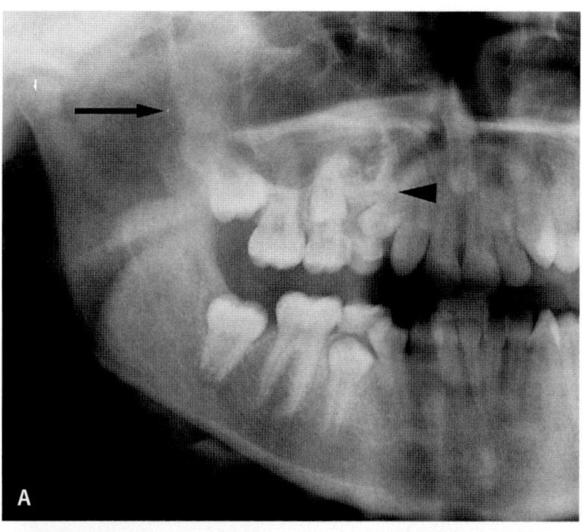

Figure 2.16

Follicular cyst, maxilla; 13-year-old female examined for unerupted maxillary right first premolar. A Panoramic view shows expansive process, partially with sclerotic outline (*arrow*) in right maxillary sinus, and an odontoma (*arrowhead*). B Axial CT image shows expansive radiolucency and root resorption (*arrow*), and complex odontoma (*arrowhead*) in alveolar process. C Axial CT image shows process occupying entire maxillary sinus with expanded walls (*arrow*). D Axial T2-weighted MRI shows homogeneous high signal (*arrow*). E Coronal STIR MRI shows homogeneous high signal (*arrow*). F Axial T1-weighted pre-Gd MRI shows homogeneous intermediate signal (*arrow*). G Axial T1-weighted post-Gd MRI shows no enhancement except peripheral rim (*arrow*). H Coronal T1-weighted post-Gd MRI shows no enhancement except peripheral rim (*arrow*)

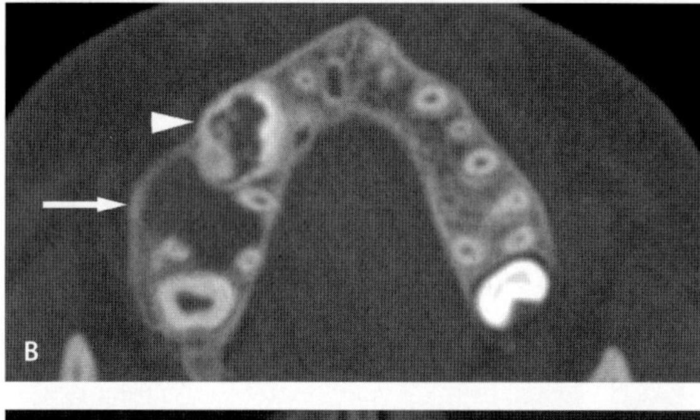

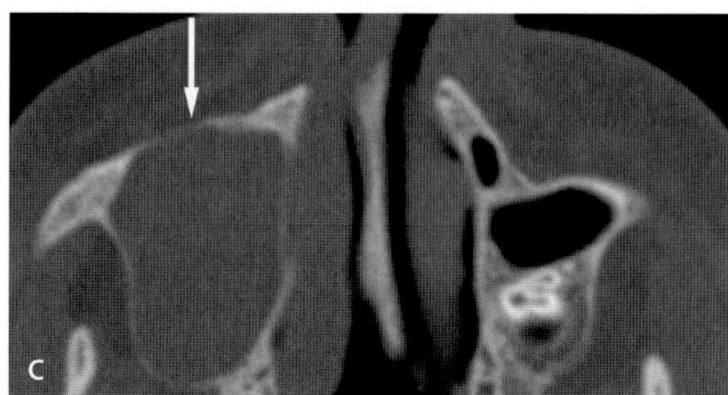

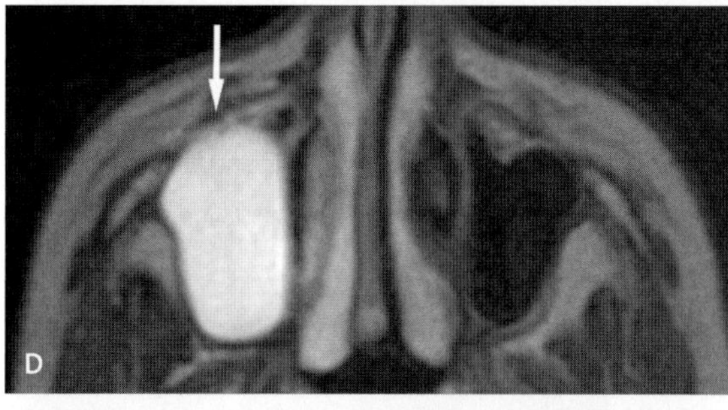

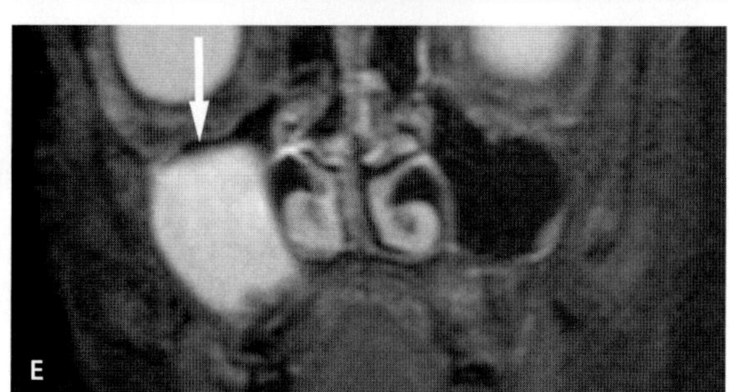

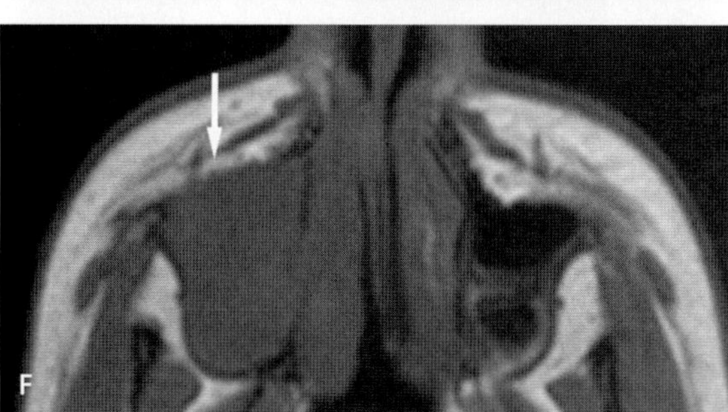

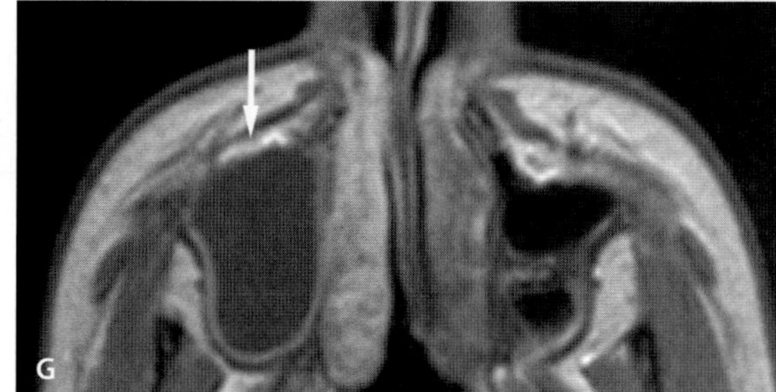

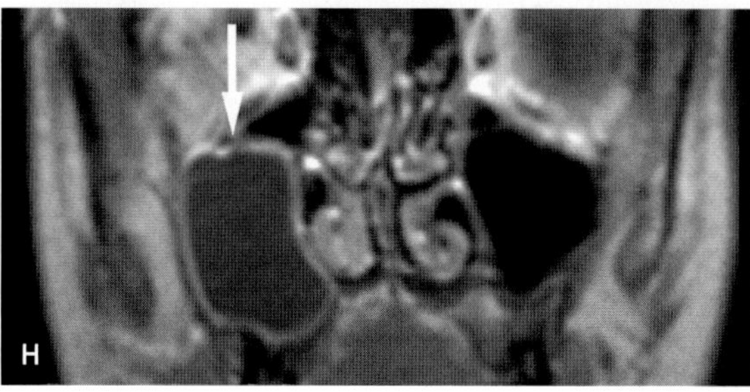

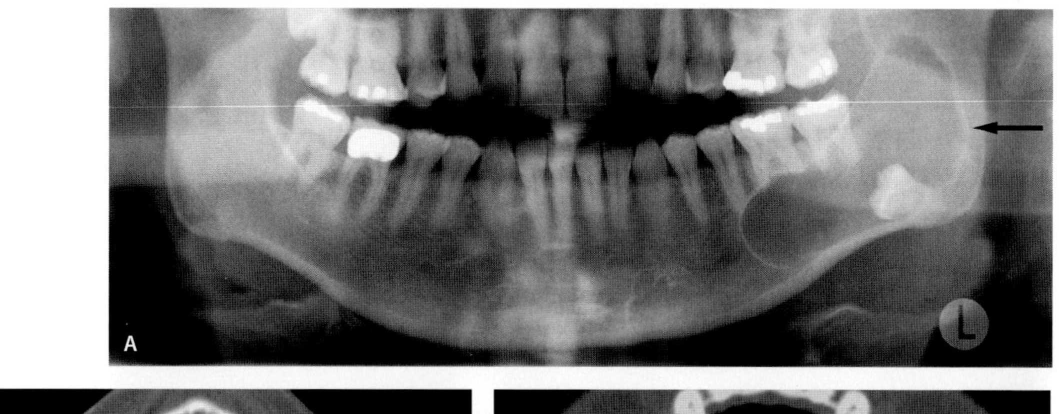

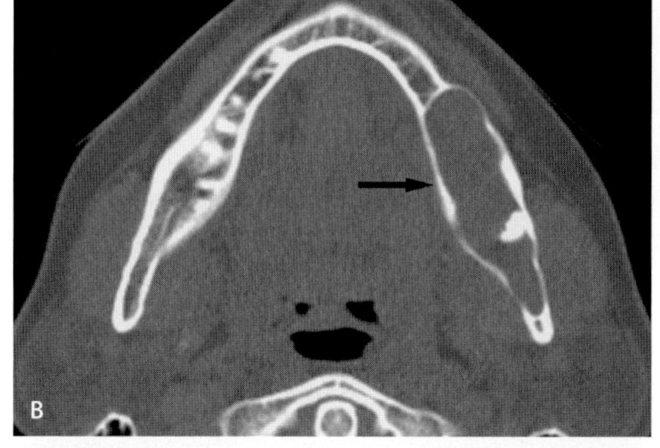

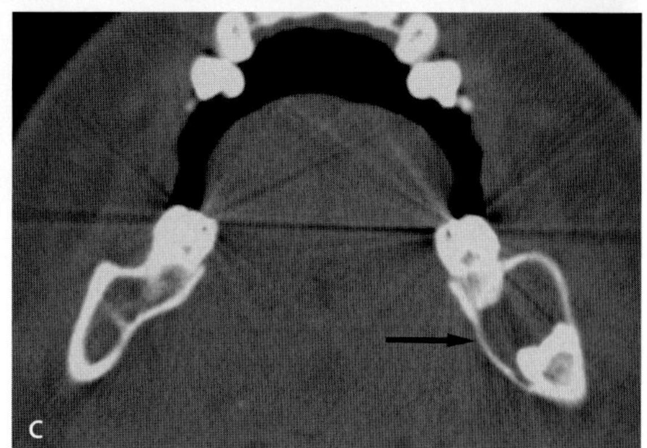

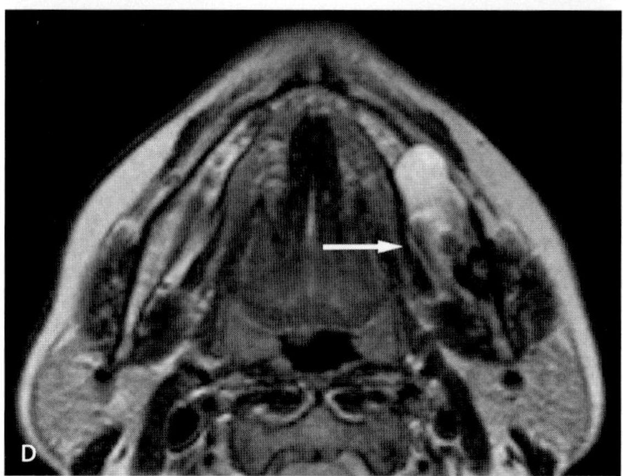

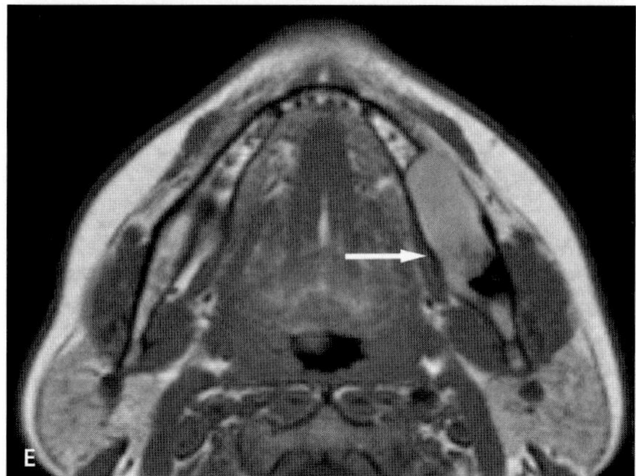

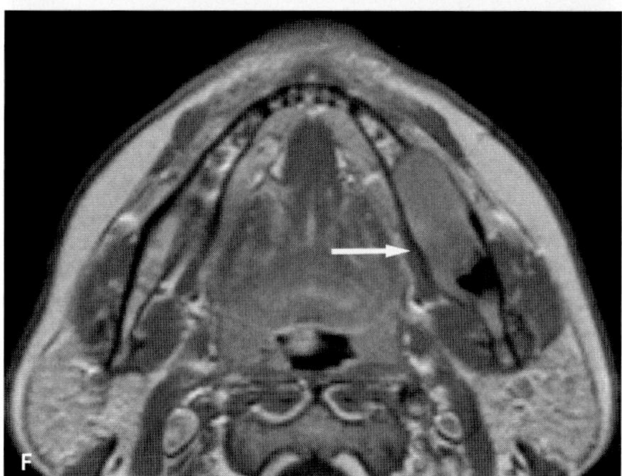

Figure 2.17

Follicular cyst, mandible; 38-year-old female with incidental finding at routine dental radiography. A Panoramic view shows radiolucency with sclerotic border around crown of impacted third molar, and root resorption of molars (*arrow*). B Axial CT image shows process with intact cortical bone (*arrow*) and part of impacted third molar. C Oblique coronal CT image shows process around crown of third molar with intact cortical bone expanding lingually (*arrow*) and buccally. D Axial T2-weighted MRI shows heterogeneous signal content; homogeneous high signal in one part and heterogeneous low to intermediate signal close to impacted tooth (*arrow*). E Axial T1-weighted pre-Gd MRI shows homogeneous intermediate signal content (except small area close to impacted tooth) (*arrow*). F Axial T1-weighted post-Gd MRI shows no contrast enhancement (*arrow*)

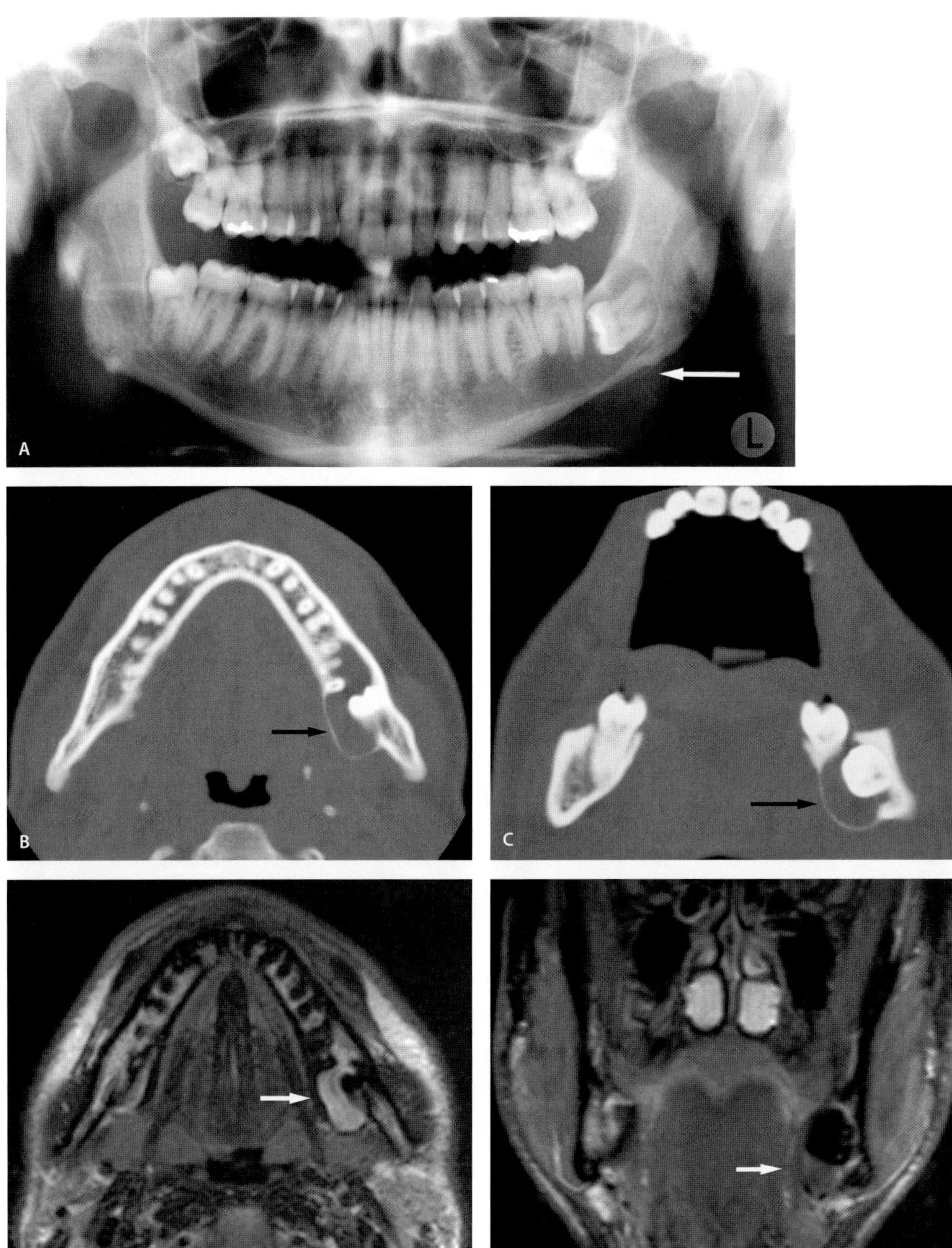
A
L
B
C
D
E

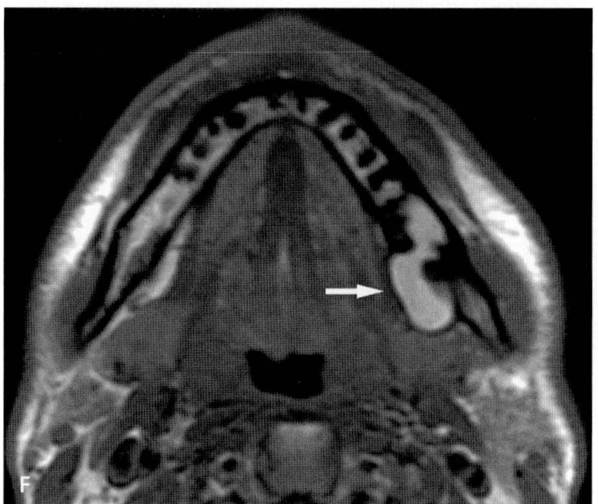

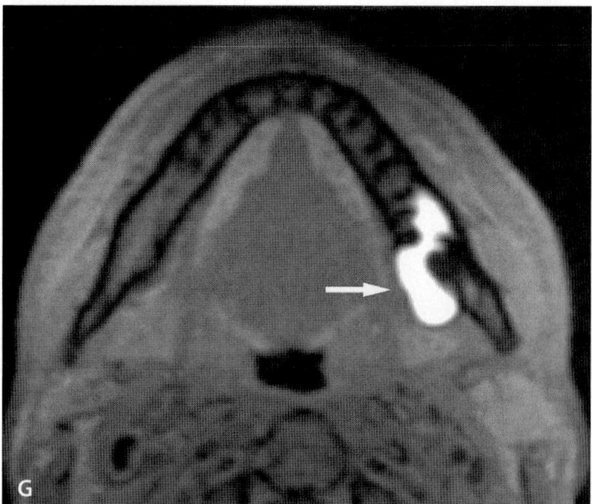

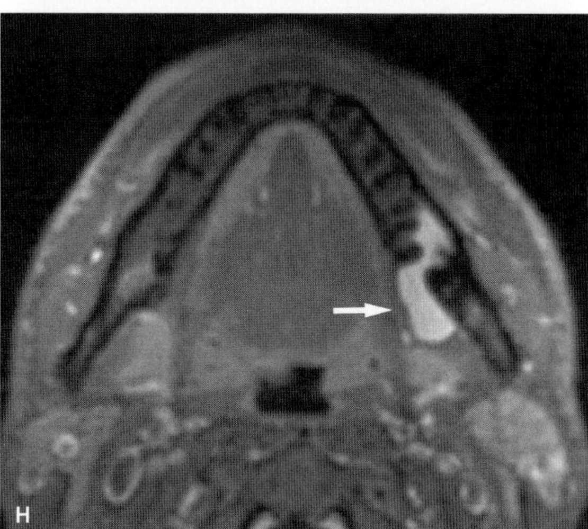

Figure 2.18

Follicular cyst, mandible; 40-year-old male with incidental finding at routine dental radiography. A Panoramic view shows radiolucency with sclerotic border (*arrow*), and impacted third molar. B Axial CT image shows expansive process with thinned, intact cortical bone, partially around crown of impacted third molar (*arrow*). C Oblique coronal CT image shows process with intact cortical outline expanding lingually (*arrow*). D Axial T2-weighted MRI shows homogeneous intermediate to high signal content (*arrow*). E Coronal STIR MRI shows homogeneous low signal content (*arrow*). F Axial T1-weighted pre-Gd MRI shows homogeneous intermediate to high signal (*arrow*). G Axial T1-weighted fat-suppressed pre-Gd MRI shows homogeneous high signal (*arrow*). H Axial T1-weighted fat-suppressed post-Gd MRI shows no contrast enhancement when compared to G (*arrow*)

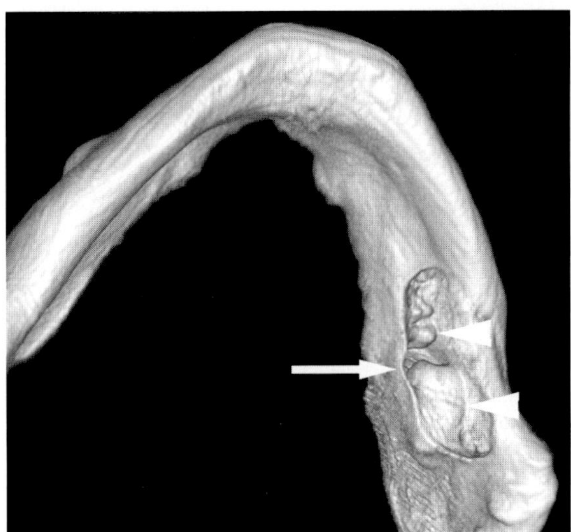

Figure 2.19

Follicular cyst, mandible; 56-year-old male with incidental finding at routine dental radiography. 3D CT image shows large cortical defect on lingual side (*arrow*) and within cavity an impacted third molar (*lower arrowhead*) and roots of second molar (*arrowhead*)

Glandular Odontogenic Cyst

Synonym: Sialo-odontogenic cyst

Definition

Cyst arising in tooth-bearing areas and characterized by epithelial lining with cuboidal or columnar cells both at surface and lining crypts or cyst-like spaces within thickness of epithelium (WHO).

Clinical Features

- Odontogenic
- Developmental
- Mandible more often than maxilla, anterior region in particular
- Vital teeth
- Unilocular or multilocular (also bilocular reported)
- Border may be destroyed and penetrated, indicating some aggressivity
- High recurrence reported (about 20% in one study)

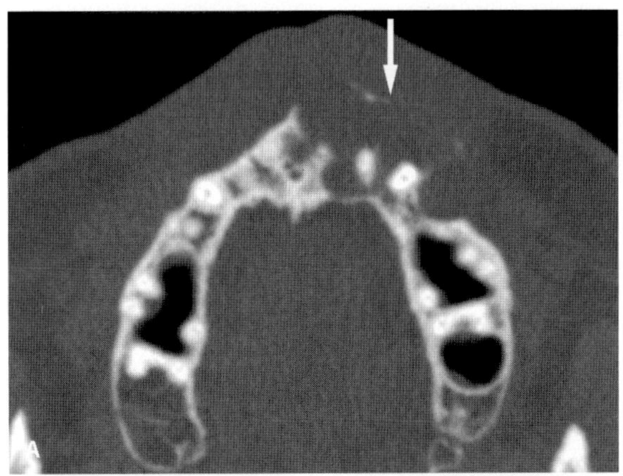

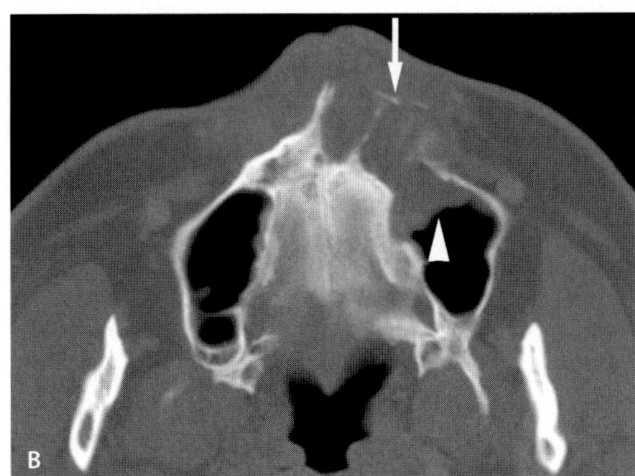

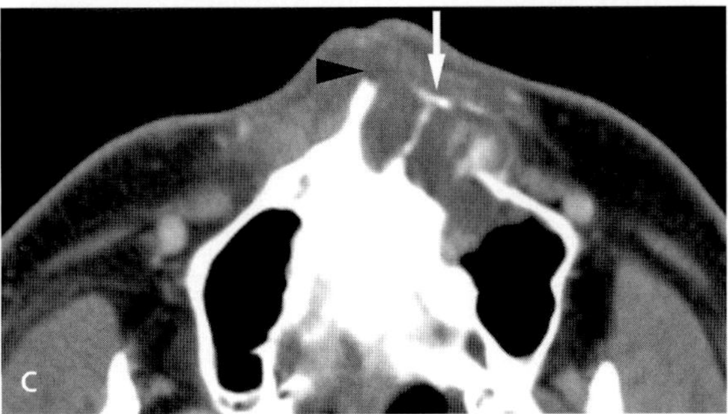

Figure 2.20

Glandular odontogenic cyst, maxilla; 47-year-old male with painless swelling of mucobuccal fold. **A** Axial CT image shows radiolucency between teeth with expanded, destroyed cortical outline (*arrow*). **B** Axial CT image shows process (*arrow*) with no cortical outline in maxillary sinus (*arrowhead*). **C** Axial post-contrast CT image with soft-tissue window shows process (*arrow*) with no demarcation from surrounding soft tissue (*arrowhead*) and no contrast enhancement

Suggested Reading

Farman AG, Nortje CJ, Wood RE (eds) (1993) Cysts of the jaws. In: Oral and maxillofacial diagnostic imaging. Mosby, St. Louis, pp 210–238

Hisatomi M, Asaumi J-I, Konouchi H, Shigehara H, Yanagi Y, Kishi K (2003) MR imaging of epithelial cysts of the oral and maxillofacial region. Eur J Radiol 48:178–182

Koppang HS, Johannessen S, Haugen LK, Haanaes HR, Solheim T, Donath K (1998) Glandular odontogenic cyst (sialo-odontogenic cyst): report of two cases and literature review of 45 previously reported cases. J Oral Pathol Med 27:455–462

Kramer IRH, Pindborg JJ, Shear M (1992) World Health Organisation International Histological Classification of Tumours. Histological typing of odontogenic tumours, 2nd edn. Springer, Berlin, pp 34–42

Lovas JGL (1991) Cysts. In: Miles DA, Van Dis M, Kaugars GE, Lovas JGL (eds) Oral and maxillofacial radiology. Radiologic/pathologic correlations. Saunders, Philadelphia, pp 21–50

Minami M, Kaneda T, Ozawa K, Yamamoto H, Itai Y, Ozawa M, Yoshikawa K, Sasaki Y (1996) Cystic lesions of the maxillomandibular region: MR imaging distinction of odontogenic keratocysts and ameloblastomas from other cysts. AJR Am J Roentgenol 166:943–949

Spinelli HM, Isenberg JS, O'Brien M (1994) Nasopalatine duct cysts and the role of magnetic resonance imaging. J Craniofac Surg 5:57–60

Weber AL, Kaneda T, Scrivani, Aziz S (2003) Jaw: cysts, tumors, and nontumorous lesions. In: Som PM, Curtin HD (eds) Head and neck imaging, 4th edn. Mosby, St. Louis, pp 930–994

White SW, Pharoah MJ (eds) (2004) Cysts of the jaws. In: Oral radiology. Principles and interpretation, 5th edn. Mosby, St. Louis, pp 384–409

Benign Jaw Tumors and Tumor-like Conditions

In collaboration with H.-J. Smith · H. Strømme Koppang

Introduction

Benign processes in the jaws represent a wide spectrum of conditions, many of which are small and therefore adequately diagnosed with intraoral and panoramic (film or digital) radiography. However, larger processes may expand jaw bone extensively and grow into neighboring structures. Since some types of benign processes may be locally aggressive and may even be difficult to distinguish from malignant neoplasms, advanced imaging should be applied to precisely assess their structure, extent and demarcation to surrounding tissues. We present a number of different conditions so that specialists both in the dental and the medical fields can become familiar with their wide range of imaging appearances.

Bone-destructive Tumors

Keratocystic Odontogenic Tumor

Synonyms: Odontogenic keratocyst, primordial cyst

Definition

Benign uni- or multicystic, intraosseous tumor of odontogenic origin, with a characteristic lining of parakeratinized stratified squamous epithelium and potential aggressive, infiltrative behavior. It may be solitary or multiple. The latter is usually one of the stigmata of the inherited nevoid basal cell carcinoma syndrome (WHO).

Usually contains thick yellow, cheesy material (keratin).

Clinical Features

- Frequently asymptomatic
- May be very large before detected since swelling not prominent
- Frequently with an impacted tooth
- Two-thirds to more than 80% occur in mandible
- About one-half at angle of mandible, extending anteriorly and superiorly
- Second and third decades
- Males more frequent than females
- Recurrence rate up to 60% reported
- Gorlin-Goltz syndrome; multiple tumors

Imaging Features

- Radiolucency
- Unilocular round, oval, scalloped (with or without bone septa) or occasionally, multilocular
- Border usually sclerotic, may be thinned, intact or perforated, even diffuse in parts
- Bone expansion or not; frequently not prominent
- Soft-tissue extension through cortical perforation
- May displace teeth, mandibular canal
- Tooth resorption rare
- Frequently located with, but unrelated to, impacted third molar
- T1-weighted MRI: homogeneous or heterogeneous intermediate signal
- T2-weighted and STIR MRI: heterogeneous high signal
- T1-weighted post-Gd MRI: no enhancement or enhancement of thin peripheral rim; more evident if secondarily inflamed

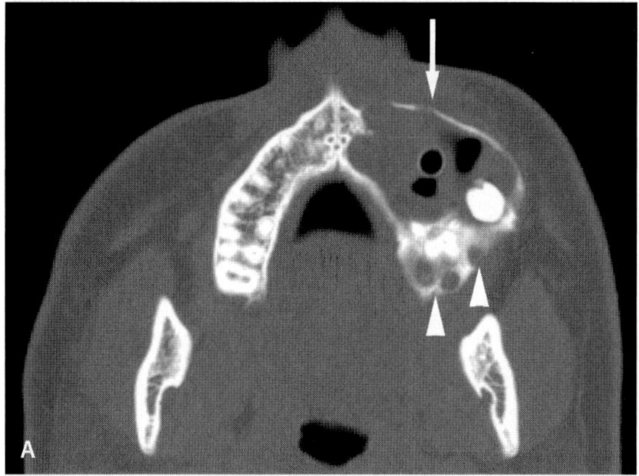

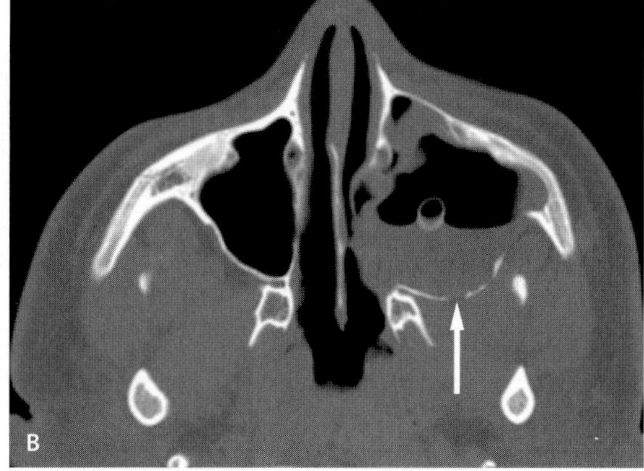

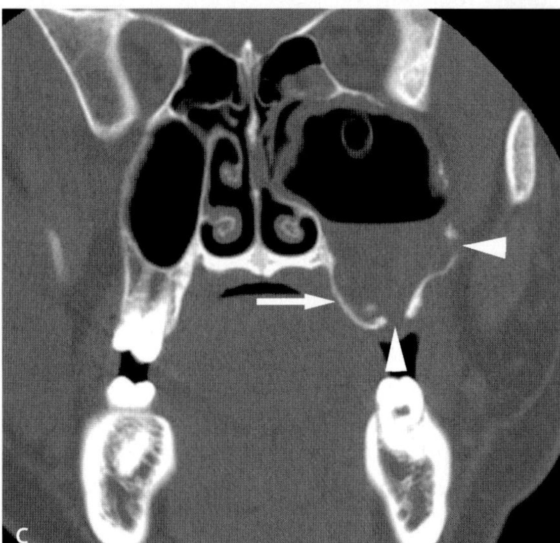

Figure 3.1

Keratocystic odontogenic tumor, maxilla; 16-year-old male with painless expansion of maxilla, complicated by sinusitis. **A** Axial CT image (after biopsy with a drain in place) shows expansive process in left maxillary sinus (*arrow*), multilocular in posterior part (*arrowheads*). **B** Axial CT image shows expansion of posterior thinned sinus wall with cortical defects (*arrow*), and fluid. **C** Coronal CT image shows expansion of palatal sinus wall (*arrow*), and cortical defects both in lateral and alveolar sinus walls (*arrowheads*), and fluid

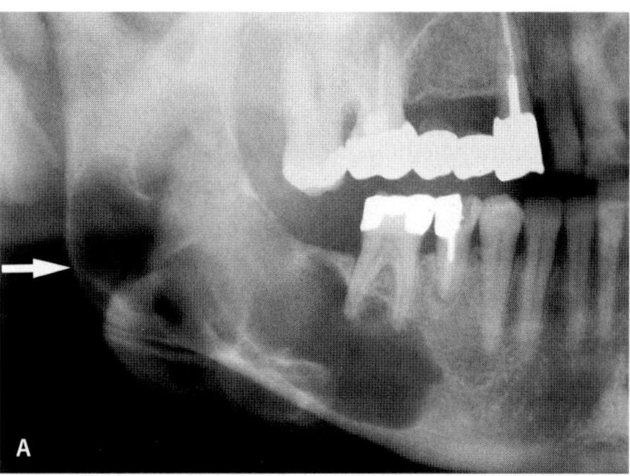

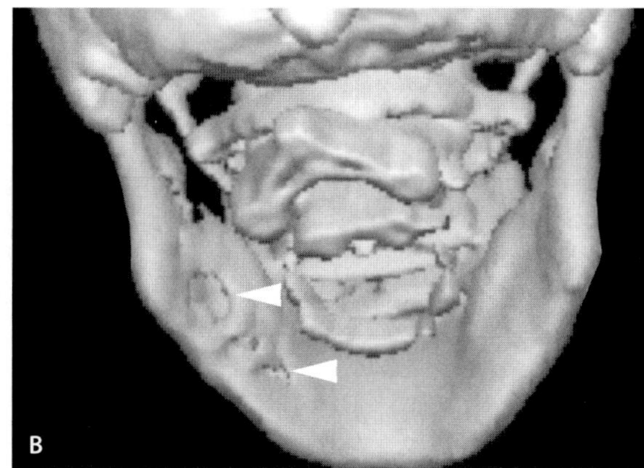

Figure 3.2

Keratocystic odontogenic tumor, mandible; 52-year-old female with incidental finding at routine dental radiography. **A** Panoramic view shows scalloped radiolucency with bone septa and sclerotic border (*arrow*). **B** 3D CT image shows cortical defects on lingual side of mandible (*arrowheads*)

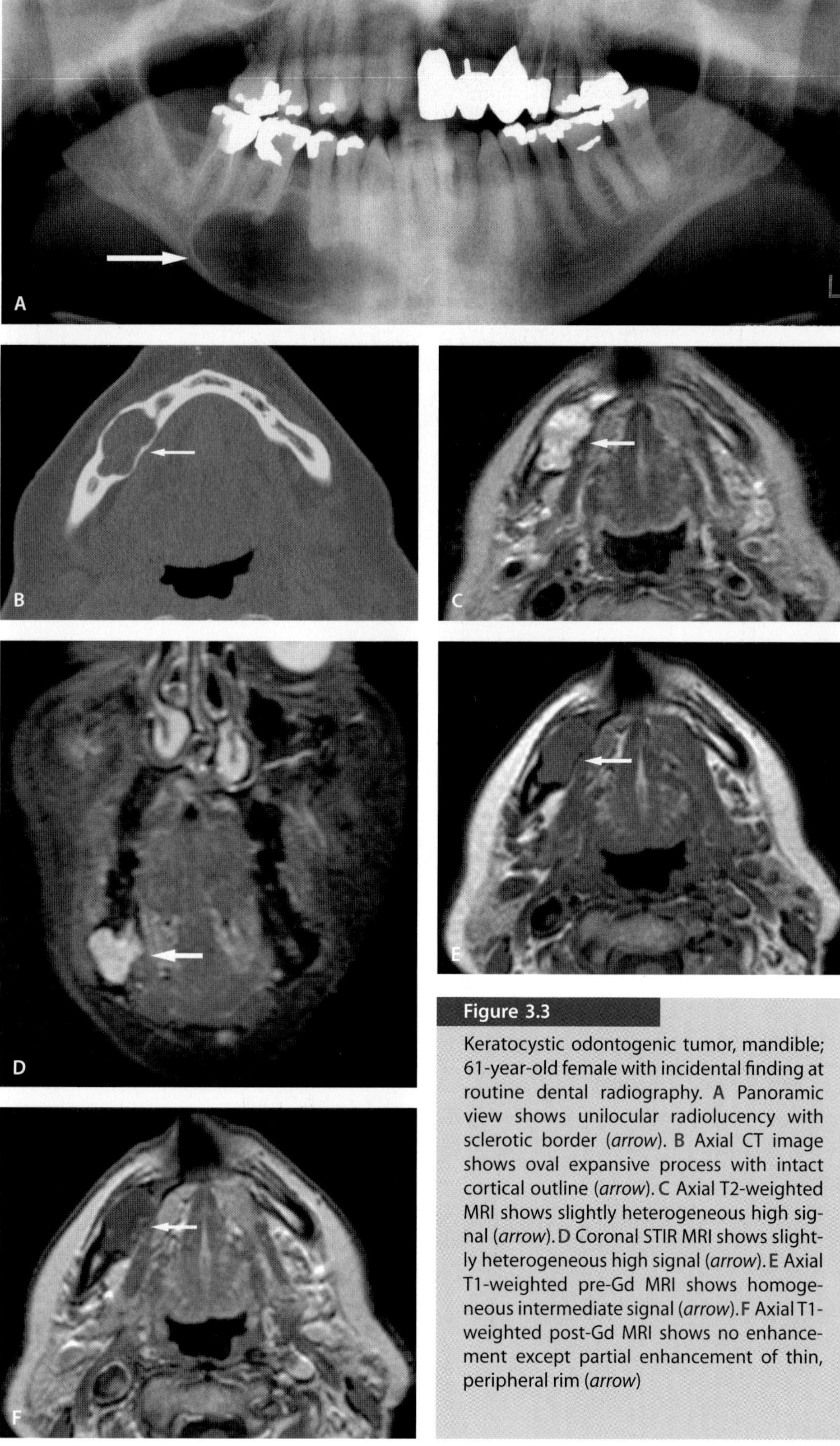

Figure 3.3

Keratocystic odontogenic tumor, mandible; 61-year-old female with incidental finding at routine dental radiography. A Panoramic view shows unilocular radiolucency with sclerotic border (*arrow*). B Axial CT image shows oval expansive process with intact cortical outline (*arrow*). C Axial T2-weighted MRI shows slightly heterogeneous high signal (*arrow*). D Coronal STIR MRI shows slightly heterogeneous high signal (*arrow*). E Axial T1-weighted pre-Gd MRI shows homogeneous intermediate signal (*arrow*). F Axial T1-weighted post-Gd MRI shows no enhancement except partial enhancement of thin, peripheral rim (*arrow*)

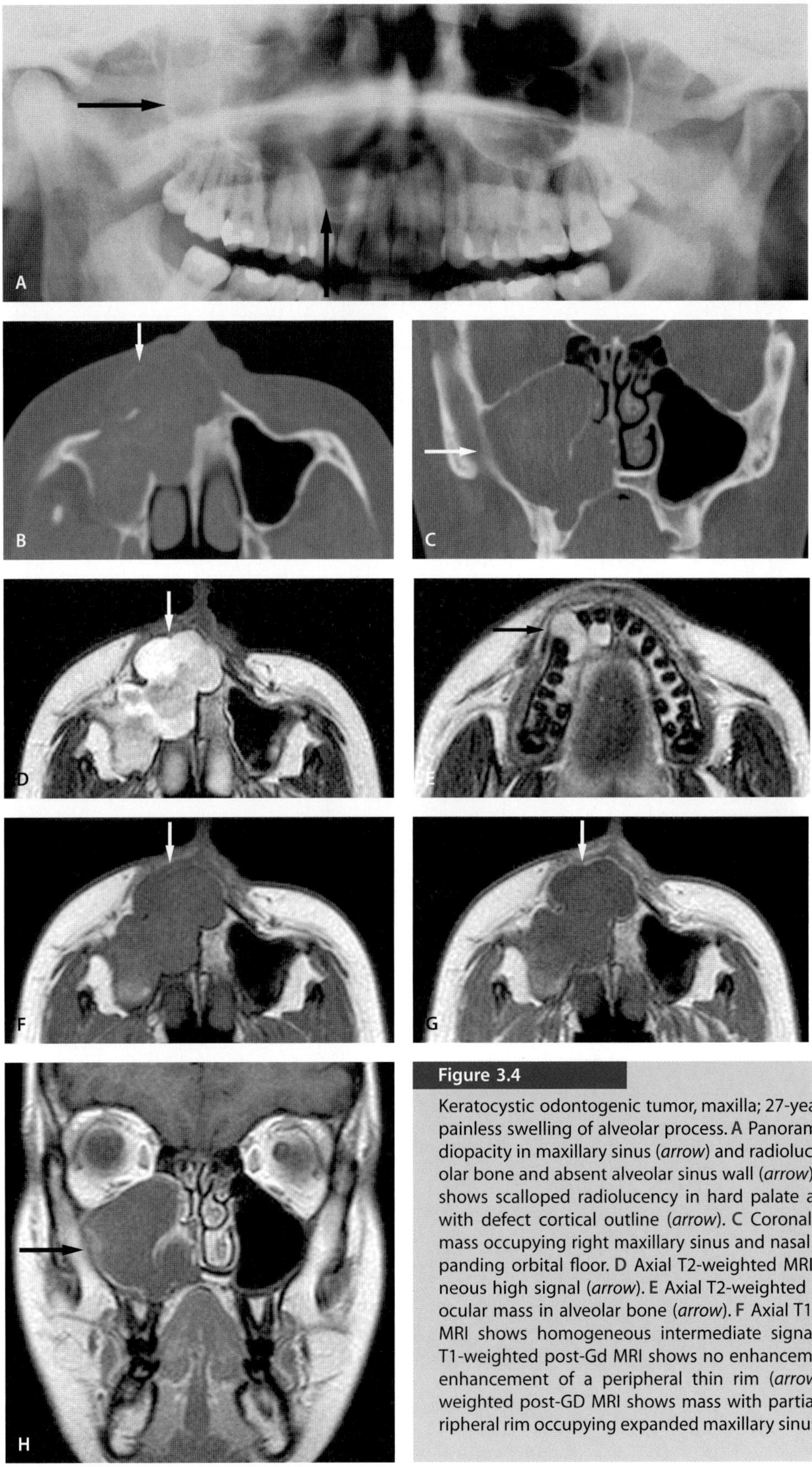

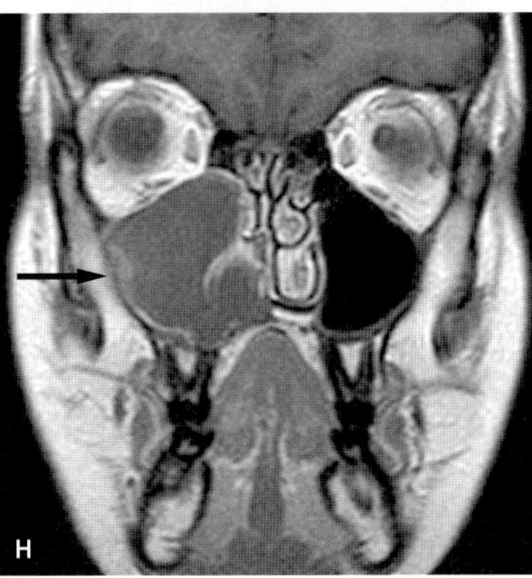

Figure 3.4

Keratocystic odontogenic tumor, maxilla; 27-year-old female with painless swelling of alveolar process. **A** Panoramic view shows radiopacity in maxillary sinus (*arrow*) and radiolucency in right alveolar bone and absent alveolar sinus wall (*arrow*). **B** Axial CT image shows scalloped radiolucency in hard palate and alveolar bone with defect cortical outline (*arrow*). **C** Coronal CT image shows mass occupying right maxillary sinus and nasal cavity (*arrow*), expanding orbital floor. **D** Axial T2-weighted MRI shows heterogeneous high signal (*arrow*). **E** Axial T2-weighted MRI shows multilocular mass in alveolar bone (*arrow*). **F** Axial T1-weighted pre-Gd MRI shows homogeneous intermediate signal (*arrow*). **G** Axial T1-weighted post-Gd MRI shows no enhancement except partial enhancement of a peripheral thin rim (*arrow*). **H** Coronal T1-weighted post-GD MRI shows mass with partially enhancing peripheral rim occupying expanded maxillary sinus (*arrow*)

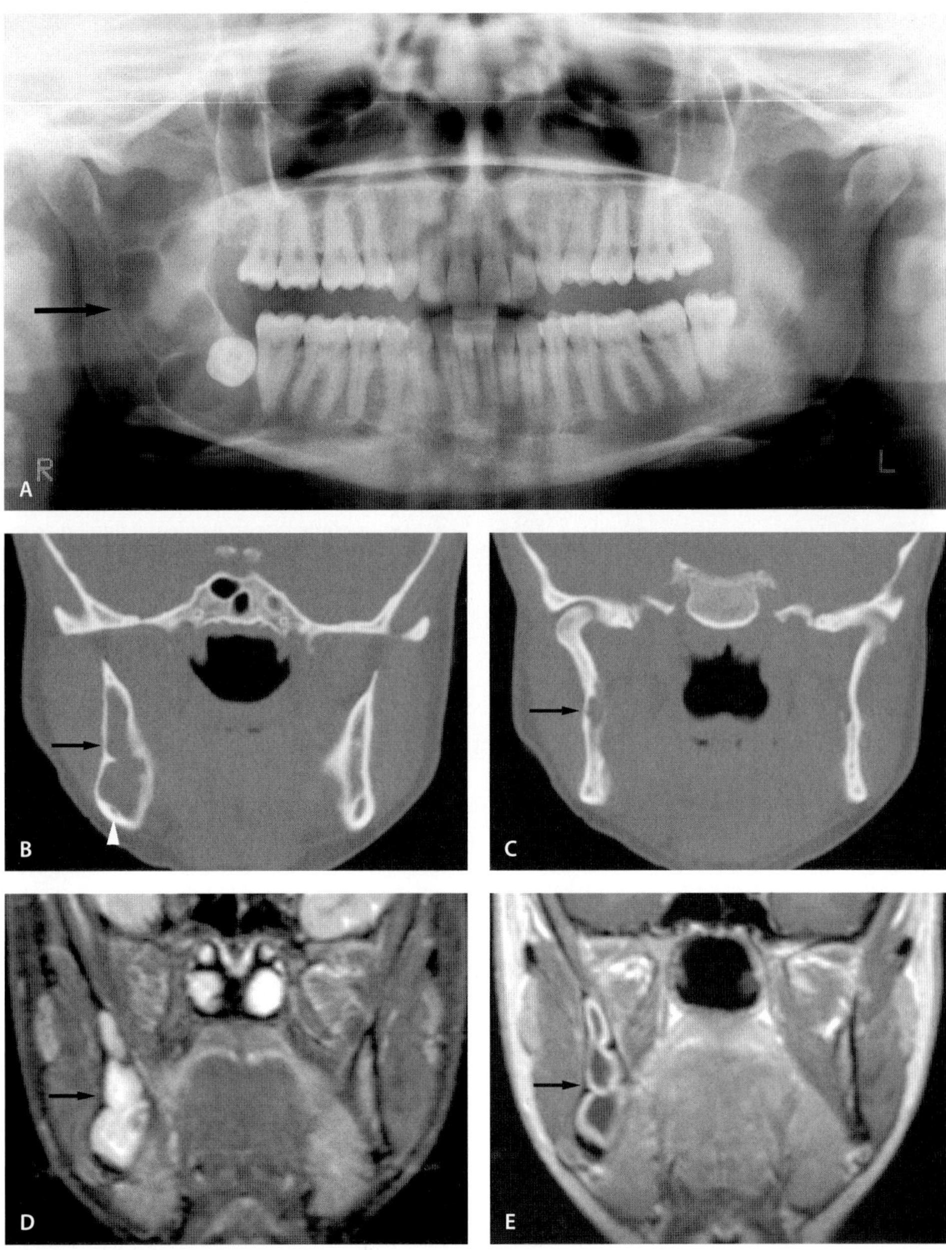

Figure 3.5

Keratocystic odontogenic tumor, mandible; 42-year-old female with incidental finding at routine dental radiography. **A** Panoramic view shows scalloped radiolucency with bone septa and impacted third molar (*arrow*). **B** Coronal CT image shows expansive radiolucency with intact cortical bone (*arrow*), and mandibular canal displaced peripherally (*arrowhead*). **C** Coronal CT image shows scalloped border in ramus (*arrow*). **D** Coronal STIR MRI shows high signal (*arrow*) and possibly two compartments. **E** Coronal T1-weighted post-Gd MRI shows no enhancement except peripheral rim (*arrow*) and possibly three compartments. MRI was performed a few days after a biopsy was taken, probably with subsequent inflammatory reaction

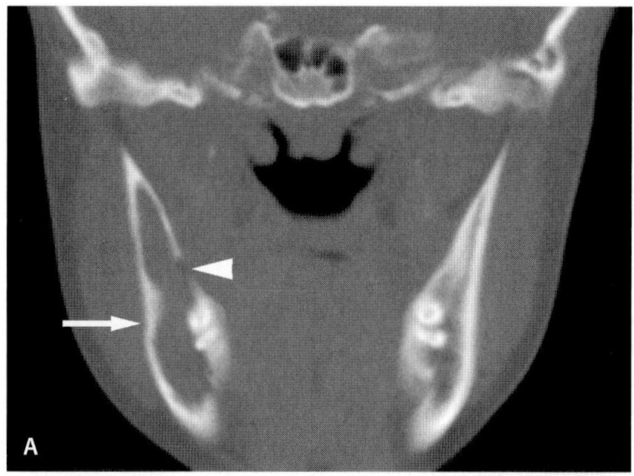
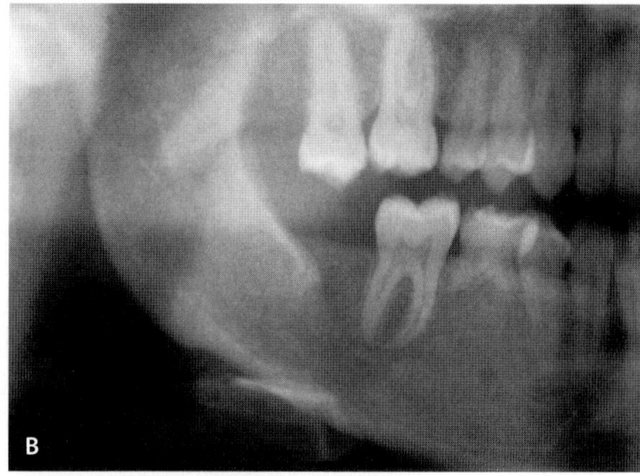
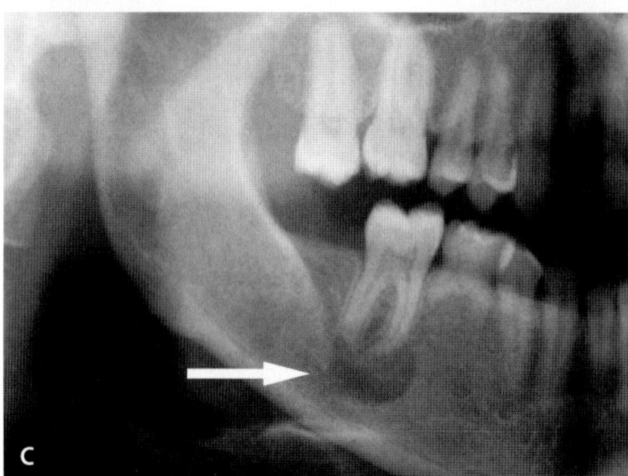

Figure 3.6

Keratocystic odontogenic tumor, mandible; 19-year-old female with incidental finding at routine dental radiography, followed for 6 years, never symptomatic. **A** Coronal CT image shows radiolucency (*arrow*) with cortical defect (*arrowhead*). **B** Panoramic view, 4 years postoperatively shows bone regeneration. **C** Panoramic view, 6 years postoperatively shows recurrence of tumor (*arrow*)

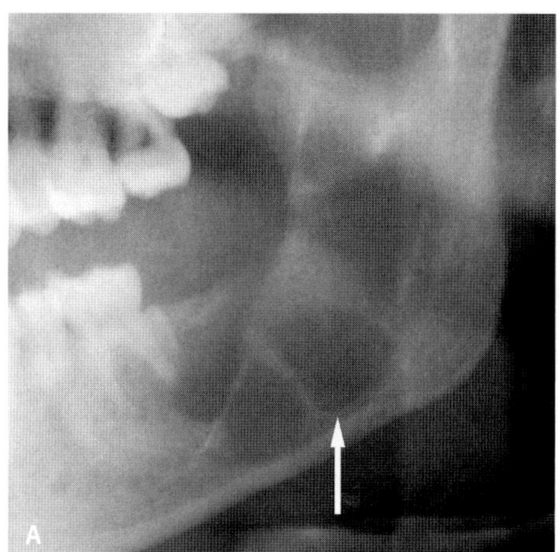
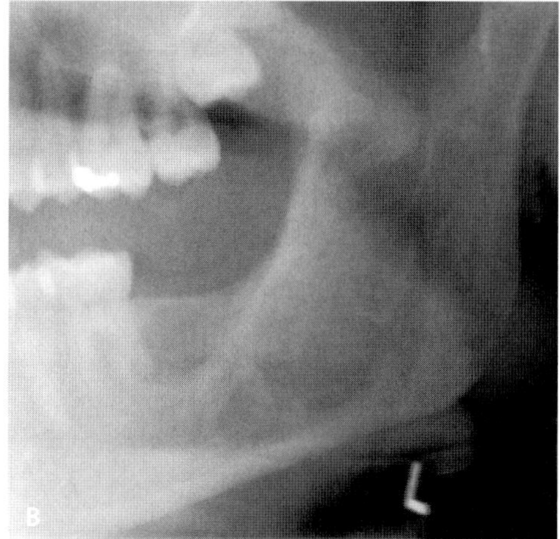

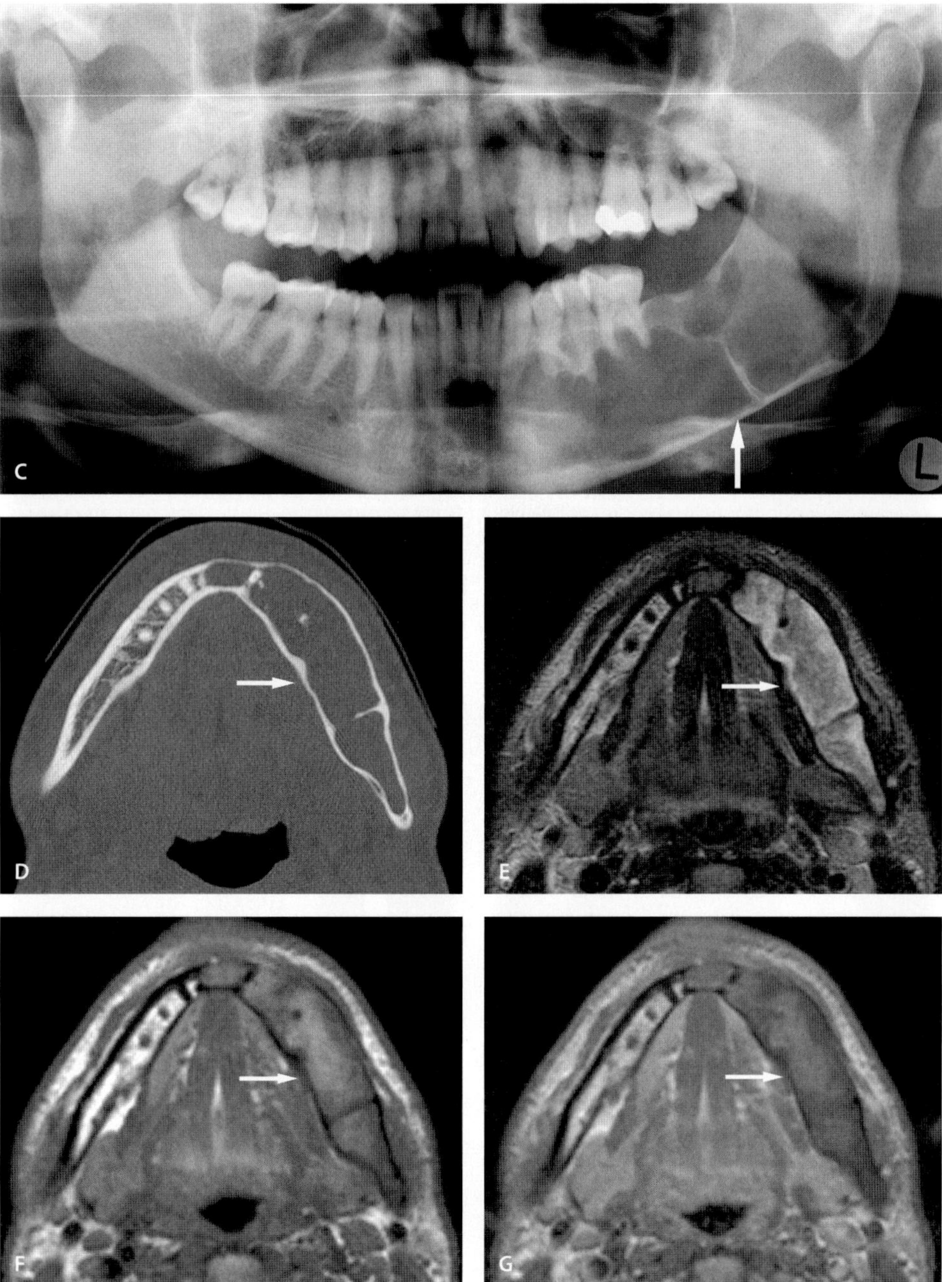

Figure 3.7

Keratocystic odontogenic tumor, mandible; 33-year-old male, painless perimandibular swelling 12 years after first surgery. **A** Panoramic view shows multilocular radiolucency (*arrow*). **B** Panoramic view 9 months postoperatively shows nearly complete regeneration. **C** Panoramic view 12 years after surgery shows recurrence of tumor, now crossing midline, being more extensive than initially (*arrow*). **D** Axial CT image shows expansive radiolucency with intact cortical bone (*arrow*). **E** Axial T2-weighted MRI shows heterogeneous high to intermediate signal (*arrow*). **F** Axial T1-weighted pre-Gd MRI shows heterogeneous intermediate to low signal (*arrow*). **G** Axial T-weighted post-Gd MRI shows no contrast enhancement (*arrow*)

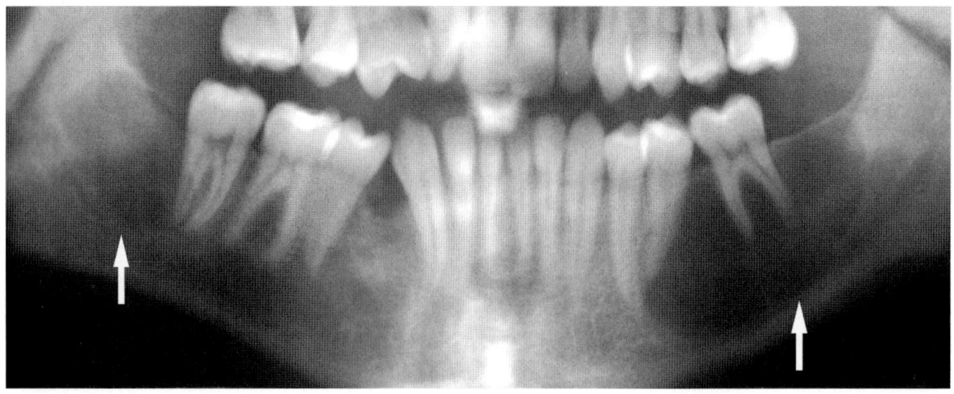

Figure 3.8

Keratocystic odontogenic tumor, mandible; Gorlin-Goltz syndrome, previously treated for maxillary cystic tumors. Panoramic view shows cystic tumors bilaterally (*arrows*)

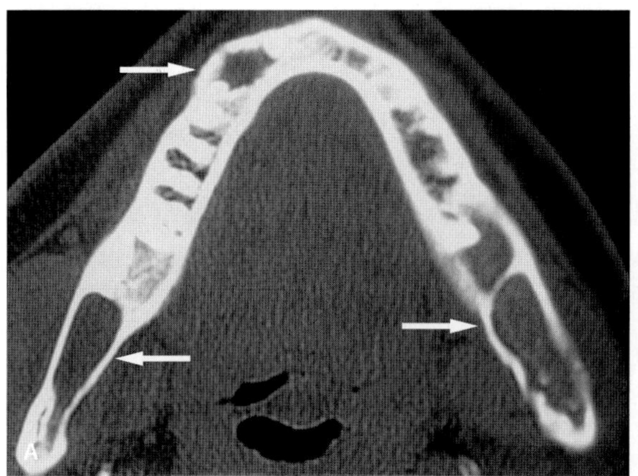

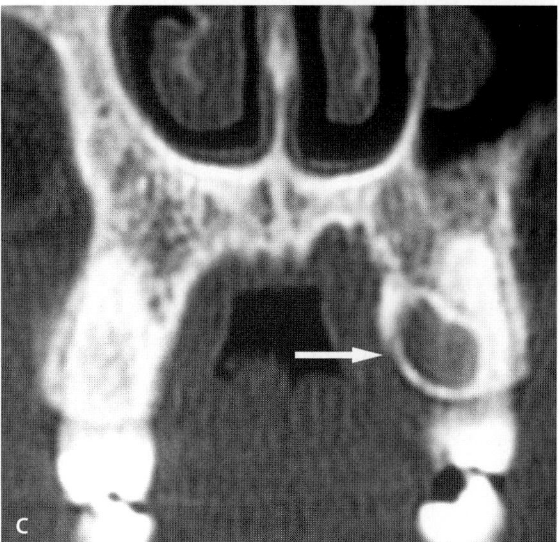

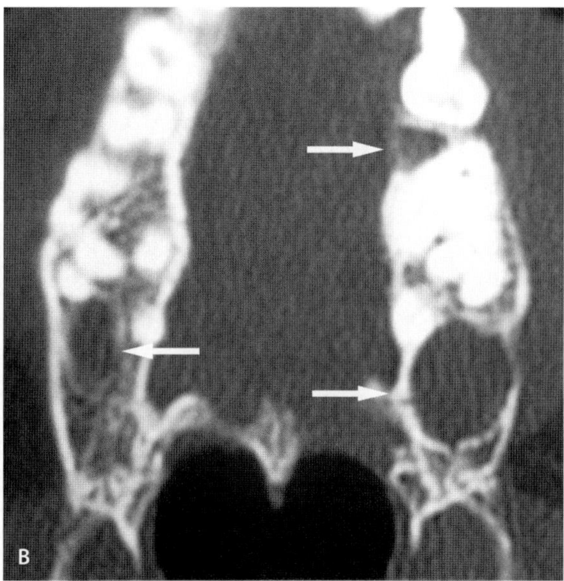

Figure 3.9

Keratocystic odontogenic tumor, maxilla and mandible; Gorlin-Goltz syndrome. **A** Axial CT image shows three cystic tumors in mandible (*arrows*). **B** Axial CT image shows three cystic tumors in maxilla (*arrows*). **C** Coronal CT image shows better cystic tumor in anterior part of maxilla (*arrow*)

Ameloblastomas

Ameloblastoma, Solid/Multicystic Type

Synonyms: Conventional or classic intraosseous ameloblastoma

Definition

Slowly growing, locally invasive epithelial odontogenic tumor of the jaws with a high rate of recurrence, but with virtually no tendency to metastasize (WHO).

Clinical Features

- Usually painless swelling (80%)
- Pain if secondarily inflamed
- Small; incidental radiographic finding
- No sex predilection
- Fourth to sixth decades, but wide range of age
- Malignancy very rare

Imaging Features

- Radiolucency
- Unilocular round, oval, scalloped, or multilocular
- Border sclerotic or not, thinned, expanded
- Defect border, soft tissue extension
- Tooth root resorption common
- Mandible clearly more frequent than maxilla, at least 80%, mostly in molar region and ramus
- T1-weighted MRI: intermediate signal
- T2-weighted and STIR MRI: intermediate to high signal
- T1-weighted post-Gd MRI: contrast enhancement of solid components

Ameloblastoma, Unicystic Type

Definition

Variant of ameloblastoma, presenting as a cyst (WHO).

Imaging Features

- Represents 5–15% of all ameloblastomas; mean age significantly lower than solid/multicystic type
- More than 90% in mandible, mostly posterior region
- Frequently, unilocular corticated radiolucency
- Up to 80% associated with an unerupted mandibular third molar
- May have similar appearance to a follicular cyst

Ameloblastoma, Desmoplastic Type

Definition

Variant of ameloblastoma, characterized by specific clinical, radiologic and histologic features (WHO).

Imaging Features

- Mandible and maxilla ratio 1:1
- Less than 10% in mandibular molar region as opposed to nearly 40% of solid/multicystic type
- About 50% with mixture of radiolucency/radioopacity due to bone formation
- May show diffuse border

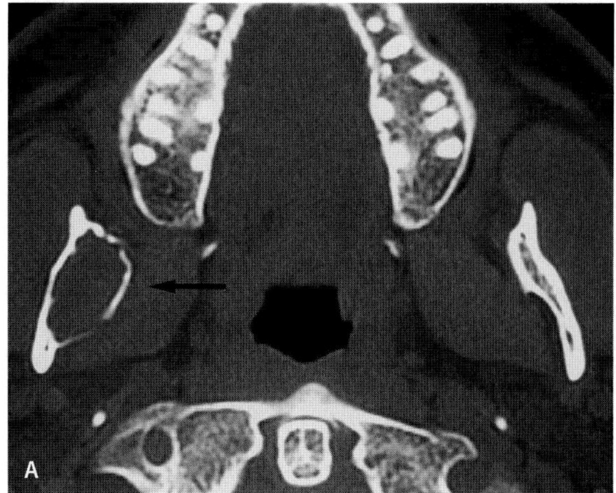

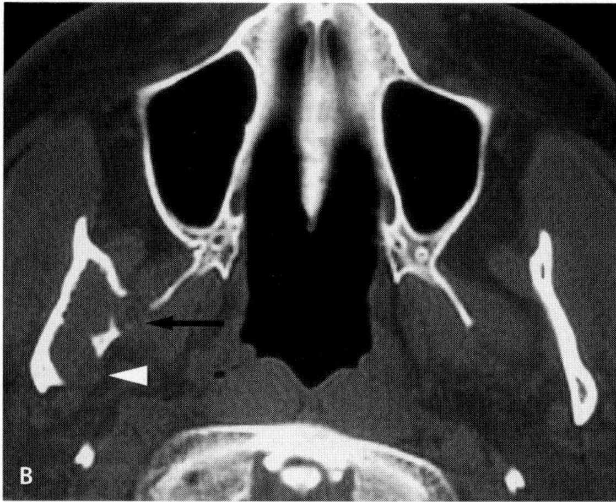

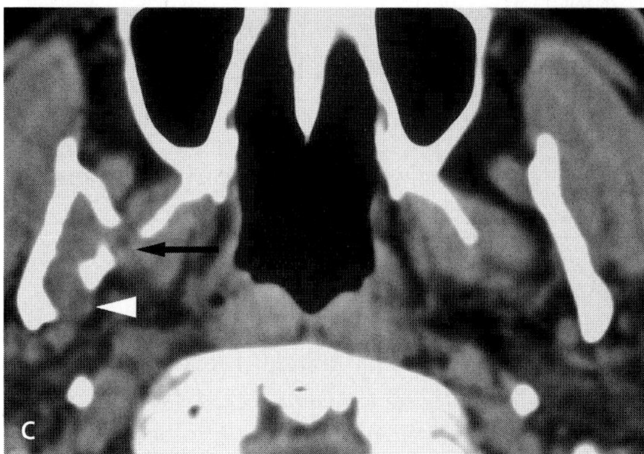

Figure 3.10

Ameloblastoma, solid/multicystic, mandible; 45-year-old male with incidental finding at routine dental radiography. **A** Axial CT image shows unilocular expansive process with nearly intact cortical bone (*arrow*). **B** Axial CT image, another section, shows cortical defects (*arrow* and *arrowhead*). **C** Axial CT image, soft-tissue window, shows soft-tissue mass at cortical defects well demarcated from surrounding soft tissue (*arrow* and *arrowhead*)

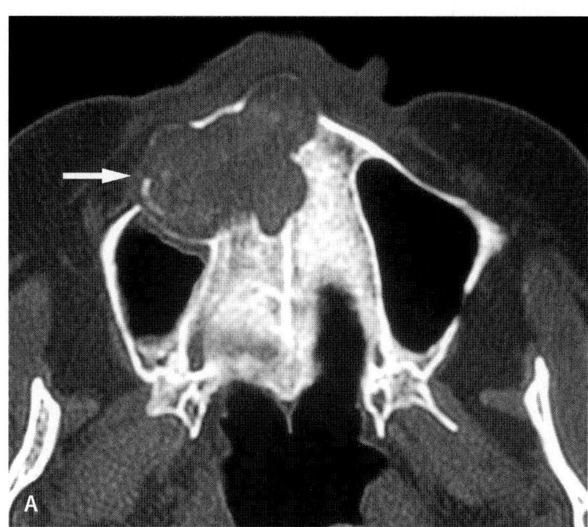

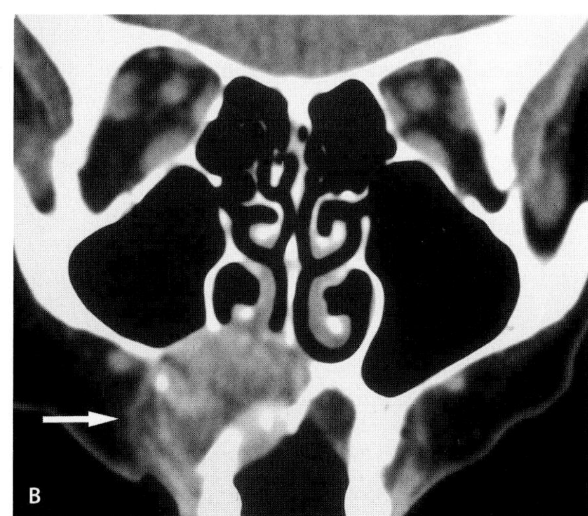

Figure 3.11

Ameloblastoma, solid/multicystic, maxilla; 80-year-old female with painless swelling in vestibulum and palate. **A** Axial CT image shows scalloped expansive process with destruction of palate and cortical bone defects (*arrow*). **B** Coronal CT image, soft-tissue window, shows well-defined soft-tissue mass without cortical outline palatally or buccally (*arrow*)

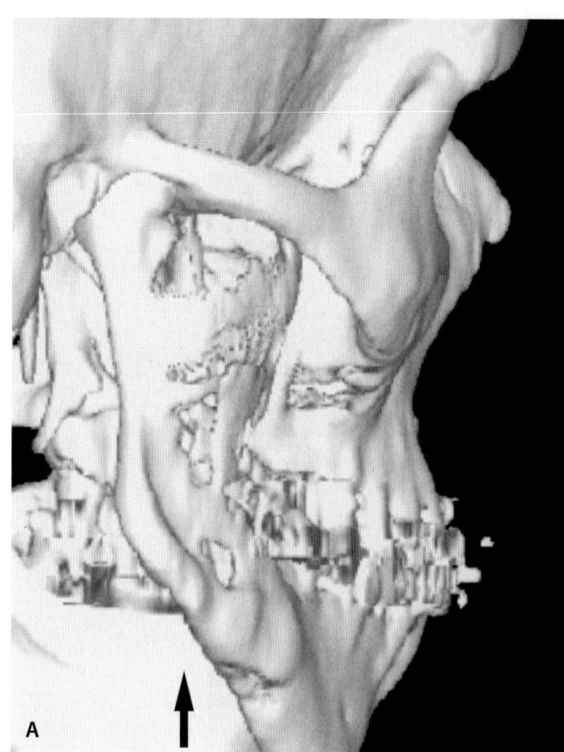

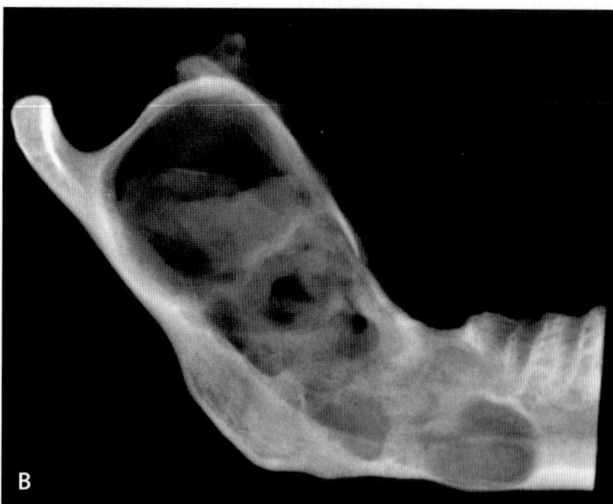

Figure 3.12

Ameloblastoma, solid/multicystic, mandible; 57-year-old male, painless swelling of mandibular ramus. A 3D CT image shows expansive tumor in entire mandibular ramus and part of body (*arrow*) with cortical defects. B Conventional radiograph of surgical specimen after hemimandible resection, with multilocular appearance

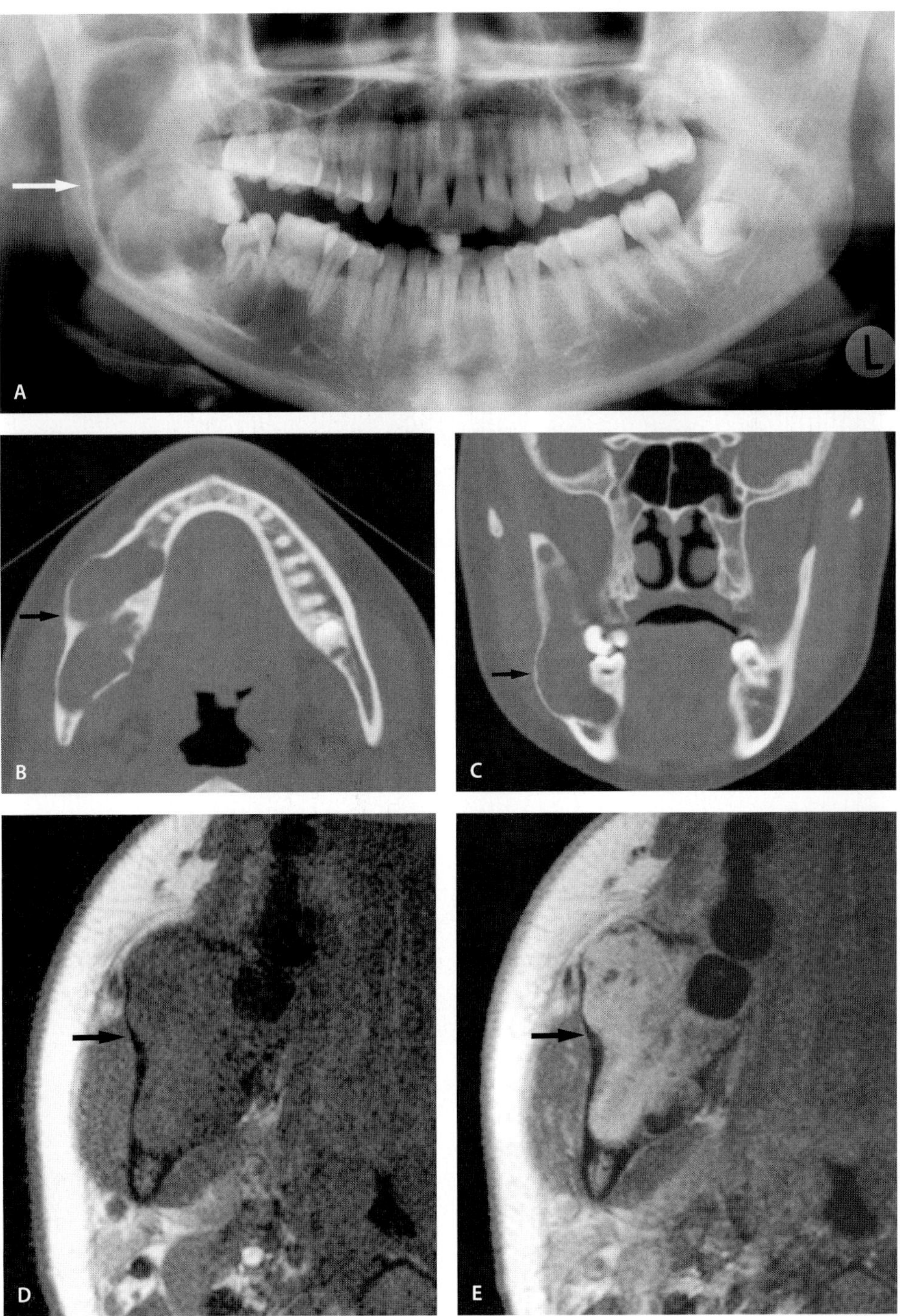

Figure 3.13

Ameloblastoma, solid/multicystic, mandible; 21-year-old female with painless swelling of right ramus. **A** Panoramic view shows expansive radiolucency and impacted third molar (*arrow*). **B** Axial CT image shows expanded cortical bone and partially scalloped border (*arrow*). **C** Coronal CT image shows expanded and thinned, intact cortical bone and root resorption (*arrow*). **D** Axial T1-weighted pre-Gd MRI shows homogeneous intermediate signal (*arrow*). **E** Axial T1-weighted post-Gd MRI shows homogeneous contrast enhancement (*arrow*)

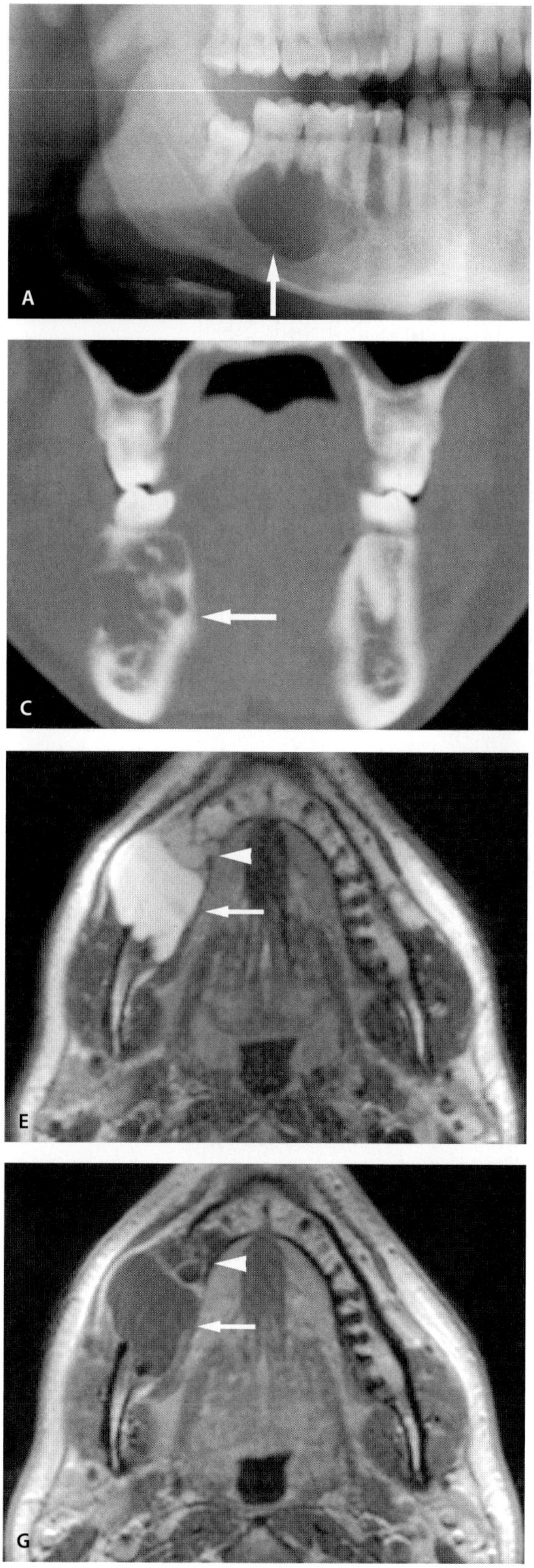

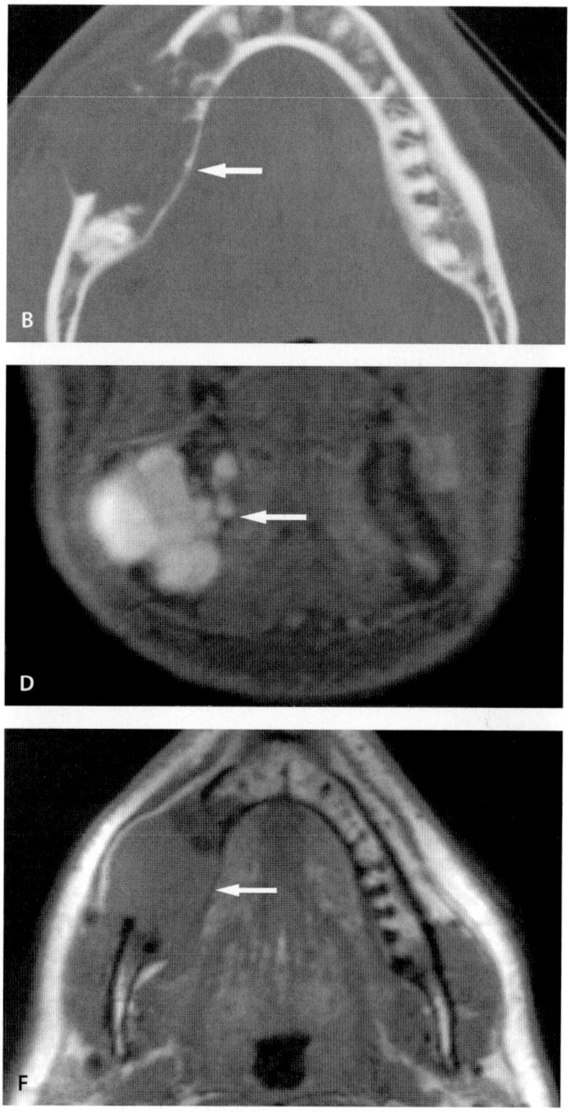

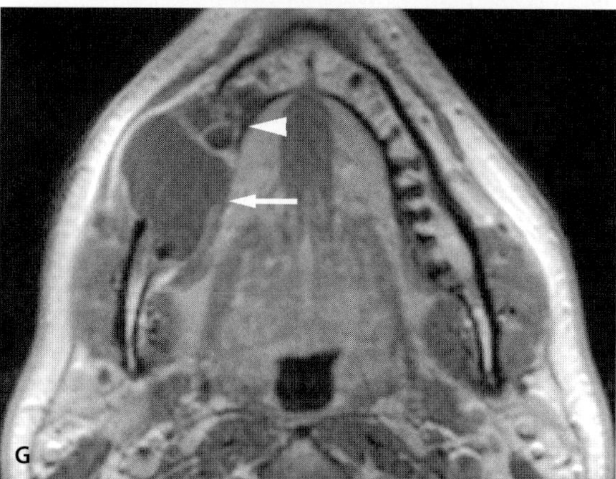

Figure 3.14

Ameloblastoma, unicystic, mandible; 22-year-old male with painless perimandibular swelling. A Panoramic view shows radiolucency and root resorption (*arrow*). B Axial CT image shows destroyed bone with expansion of buccal cortical bone, which is very thin and partially absent (*arrow*). C Coronal CT image shows multilocular appearance in anterior part without cortical outline buccally (*arrow*). D Coronal STIR MRI shows multilocular appearance and heterogeneous intermediate to high signal (*arrow*). E Axial T2-weighted MRI shows high signal in posterior part (*arrow*) and intermediate signal in anterior part (*arrowhead*). F Axial T1-weighted pre-Gd MRI shows intermediate signal in posterior part (*arrow*) and intermediate to low signal in anterior part. G Axial T1-weighted post-Gd MRI shows no contrast enhancement in posterior part (*arrow*) except partially in periphery, and septal enhancement in anterior part (*arrowhead*)

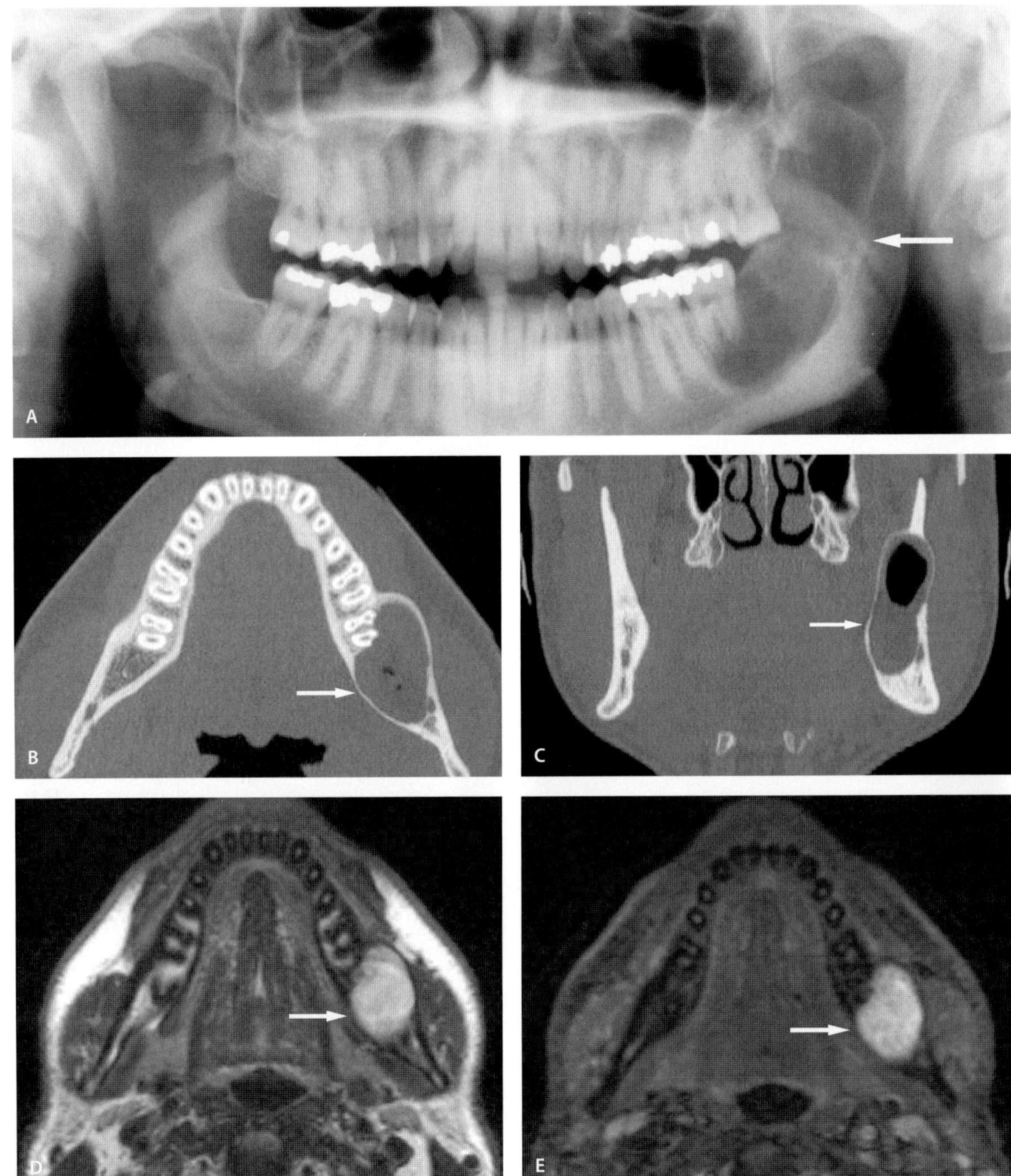
A
B
C
D
E

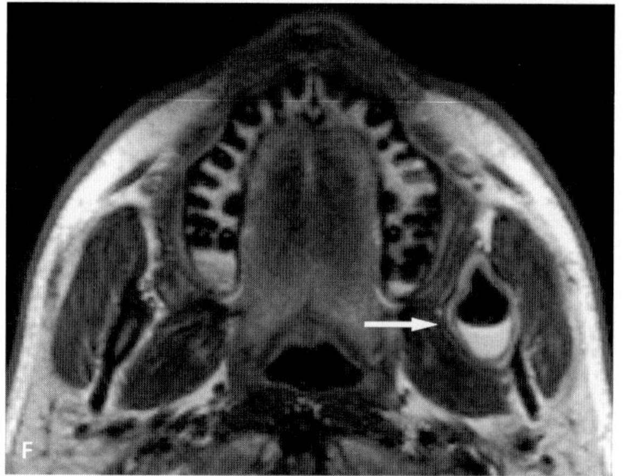

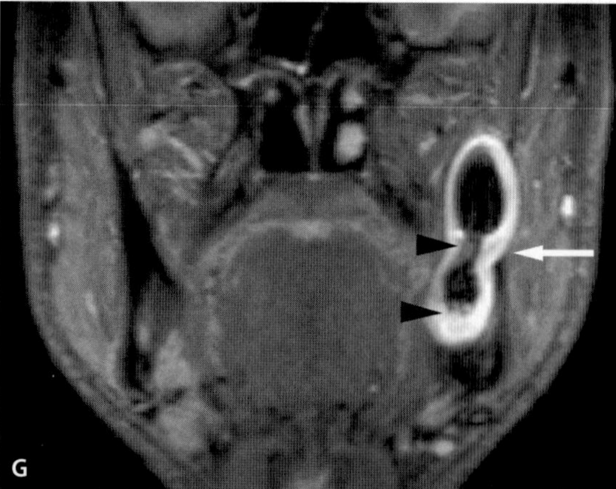

Figure 3.15

Ameloblastoma, unicystic, mandible; 33-year-old male with drainage into oral cavity as only symptom several months after third molar surgery. **A** Panoramic view shows unilocular radiolucency with sclerotic border (*arrow*). **B** Axial CT image shows expansive process with intact, sclerotic cortical outline, and with mandibular canal in periphery (*arrow*). Note root resorption. **C** Coronal CT image shows expansion of thin intact, cortical outline (*arrow*), and some air. **D** Axial T2-weighted MRI shows homogeneous intermediate to high signal (*arrow*). **E** Axial STIR MRI shows homogeneous high signal (*arrow*). **F** Axial T2-weighted MRI shows soft-tissue capsule and fluid level (*arrow*). **G** Coronal STIR MRI shows high signal soft-tissue capsule (*arrow*) with intraluminal tumor noduli (*arrowheads*). **H** Panoramic view 3 months postoperatively shows that only one molar was extracted and that tumor was enucleated with intact mandibular canal (no paresthesia)

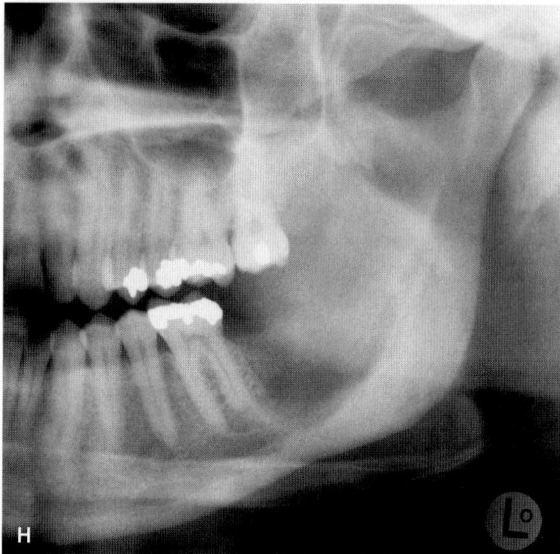

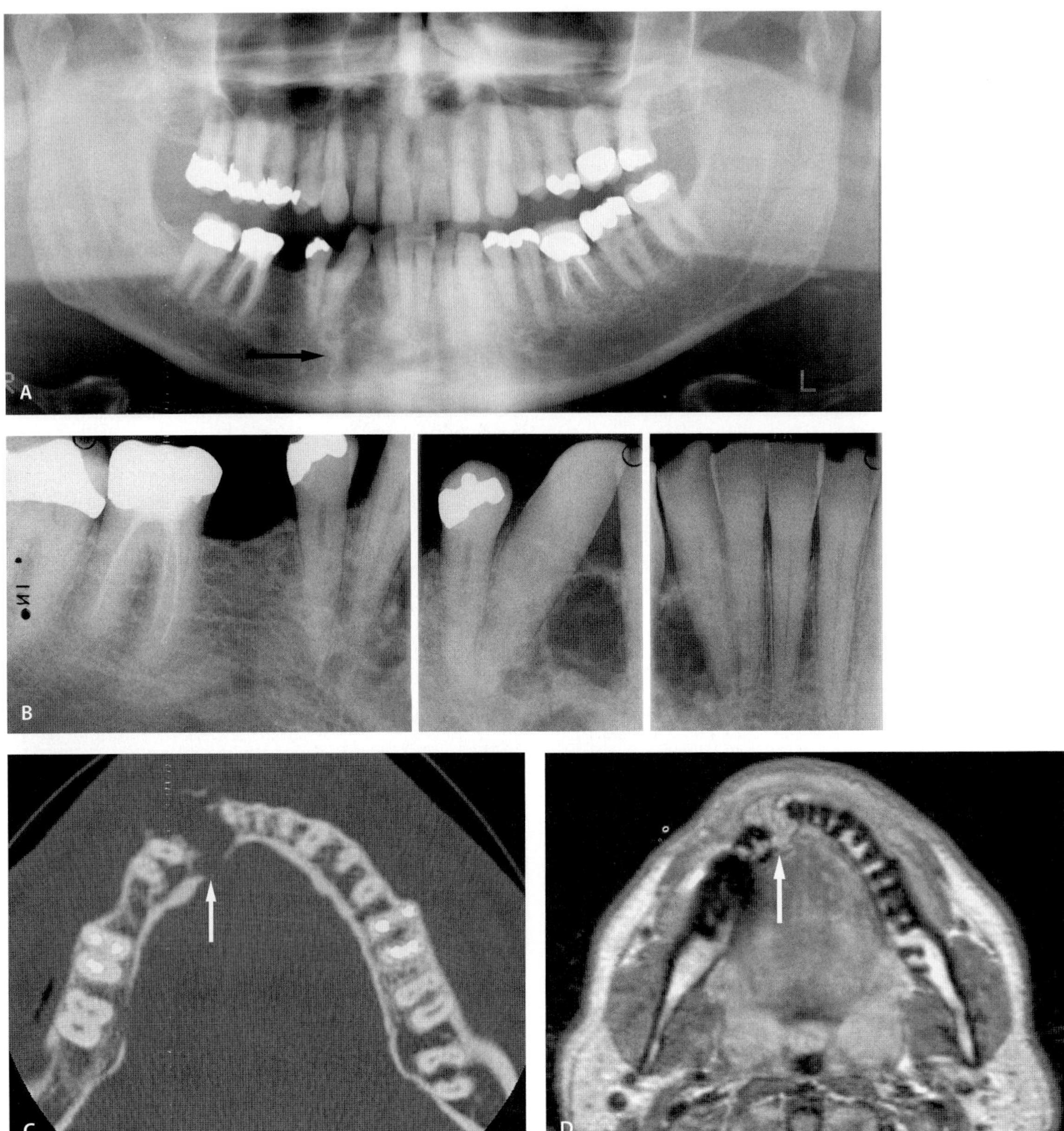
A
B
C
D
R
L

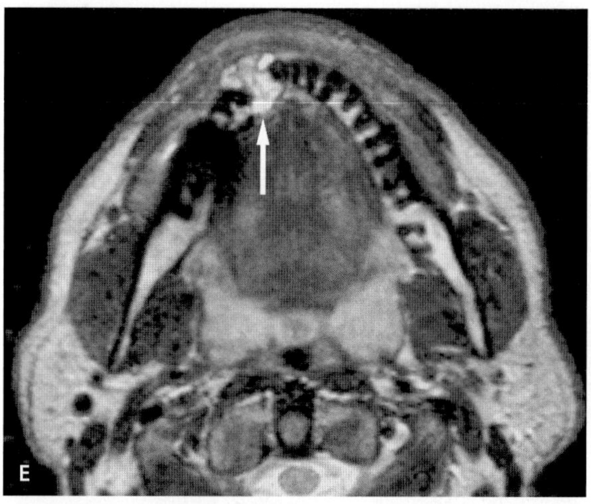

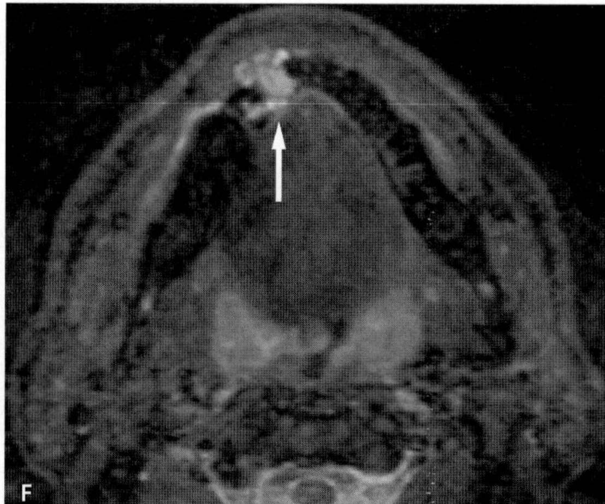

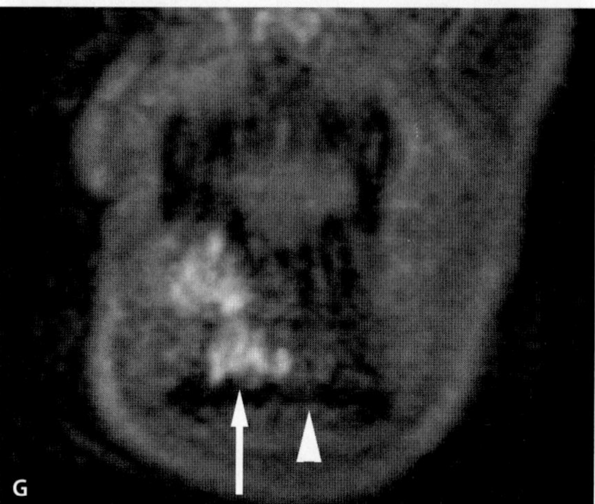

Figure 3.16

Ameloblastoma, desmoplastic, mandible; 52-year-old male with painless swelling in anterior part. A Panoramic view shows radiolucency (*arrow*) and displacement of canine and incisor. B Intraoral views show apparently multilocular radiolucency and displaced teeth. C Axial CT image shows cortical expansion and destruction buccally and lingually (*arrow*). D Axial PD MRI shows intermediate signal and septal appearance (*arrow*). E Axial T2-weighted MRI shows high signal content and septal appearance (*arrow*). F Axial STIR MRI shows intermediate to high signal and septal appearance (*arrow*). G Coronal STIR MRI of anterior region shows intermediate to high signal of bilocular septate tumor (*arrow*); most caudal part reaches mandibular border (*arrowhead*), surgically confirmed at tumor resection

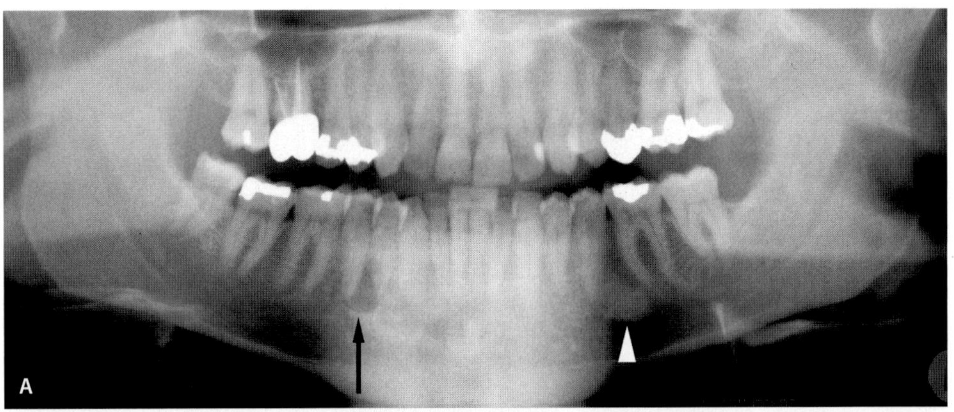

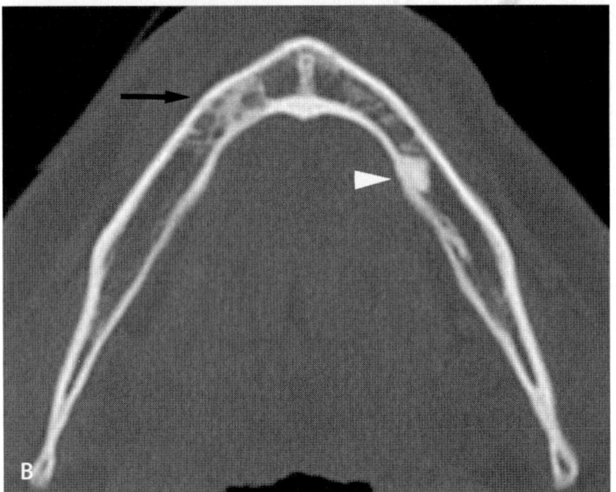

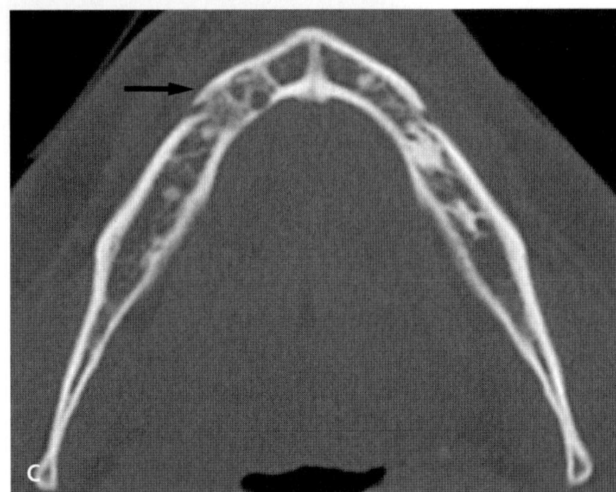

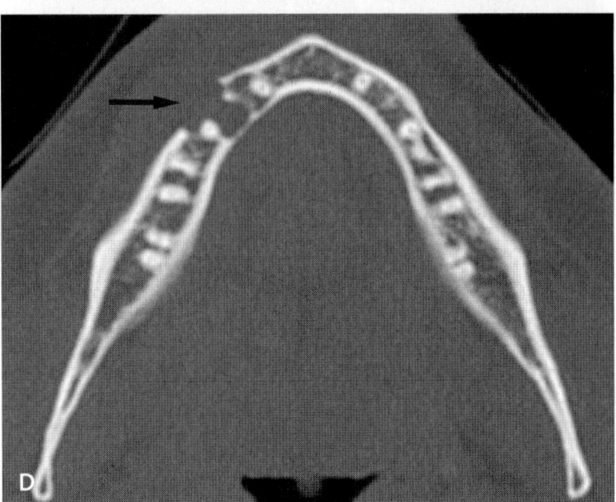

Figure 3.17

Ameloblastoma, desmoplastic, mandible; 40-year-old male with recurrence of ameloblastoma 2 years after surgery. **A** Panoramic view shows small unilocular radiolucency (*arrow*), and small radiopacity as an incidental finding (*arrowhead*). **B** Axial CT image shows multilocular radiolucency caudal to mental foramina with diffuse osteosclerosis (*arrow*), and well defined osteosclerosis, probably idiopathic (*arrowhead*). **C** Axial CT image shows two radiolucencies with some sclerosis at level of mental foramina (*arrow*). **D** Axial CT image shows destroyed cortical bone buccally in tooth-bearing area (*arrow*)

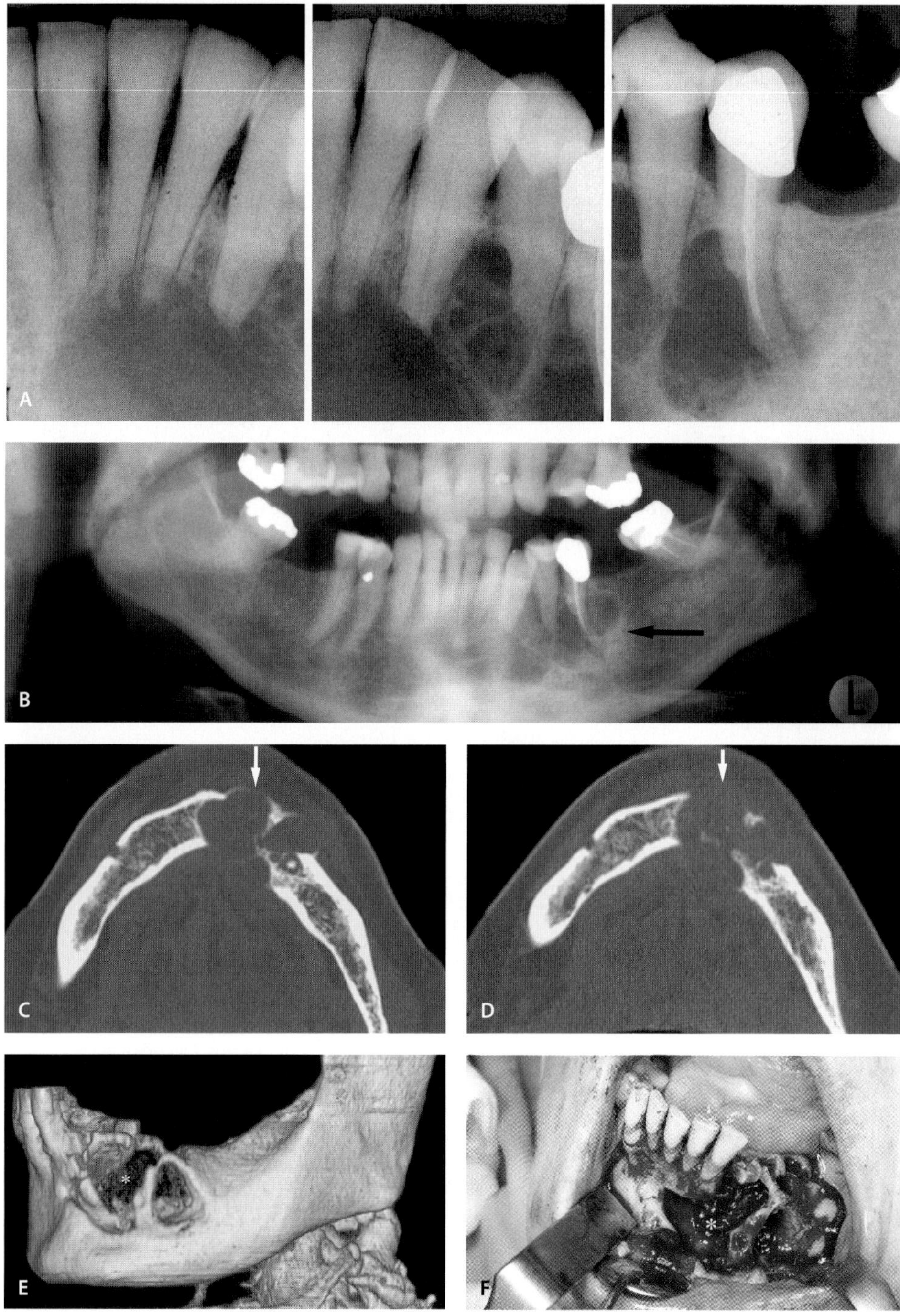

Figure 3.18

Ameloblastoma, mandible; 64-year-old female with painless swelling, then abscess development with swelling and pain. A Intraoral views show multilocular radiolucency and root resorptions. B Panoramic view indicates size of radiolucency (*arrow*). C Axial CT image shows expanded, intact cortical bone buccally (*arrow*) and destroyed bone lingually. D Axial CT image, 6 weeks later with abscess development, and destruction of buccal cortical bone (*arrow*). E 3D CT image shows severe buccolingual destruction (*asterisk*). F Photograph at surgery confirms severe buccolingual bone destruction (F: courtesy of Dr. B. B. Herlofson, University of Oslo, Norway)

Odontogenic Myxoma/Myxofibroma

Synonyms: Odontogenic fibromyxoma

Definition

Odontogenic myxoma is an intraosseous neoplasm characterized by stellate and spindle-shaped cells embedded in an abundant myxoid or mucoid extracellular matrix. When a relatively greater amount of collagen is evident, the term myxofibroma may be used (WHO).

Clinical Features

- Painless swelling or incidental finding (small)
- About two-thirds in mandible
- Second to fourth decades, but wide range of age
- Recurrence rate about 25% after curettage, but good prognosis
- Third most frequent odontogenic tumor (3–20%) after odontoma and ameloblastoma
- Slightly more common in females

Imaging Features

- Radiolucency
- Unilocular, scalloped or multilocular
- Border can be well-defined and corticated or not so well-defined and sclerotic
- May expand bone, but usually not prominent
- Tooth displacement or root resorption may occur
- T1-weighted MRI: homogeneous intermediate (to low) signal
- T2-weighted and STIR MRI: homogeneous high signal
- T1-weighted post-Gd MRI: homogeneous contrast enhancement

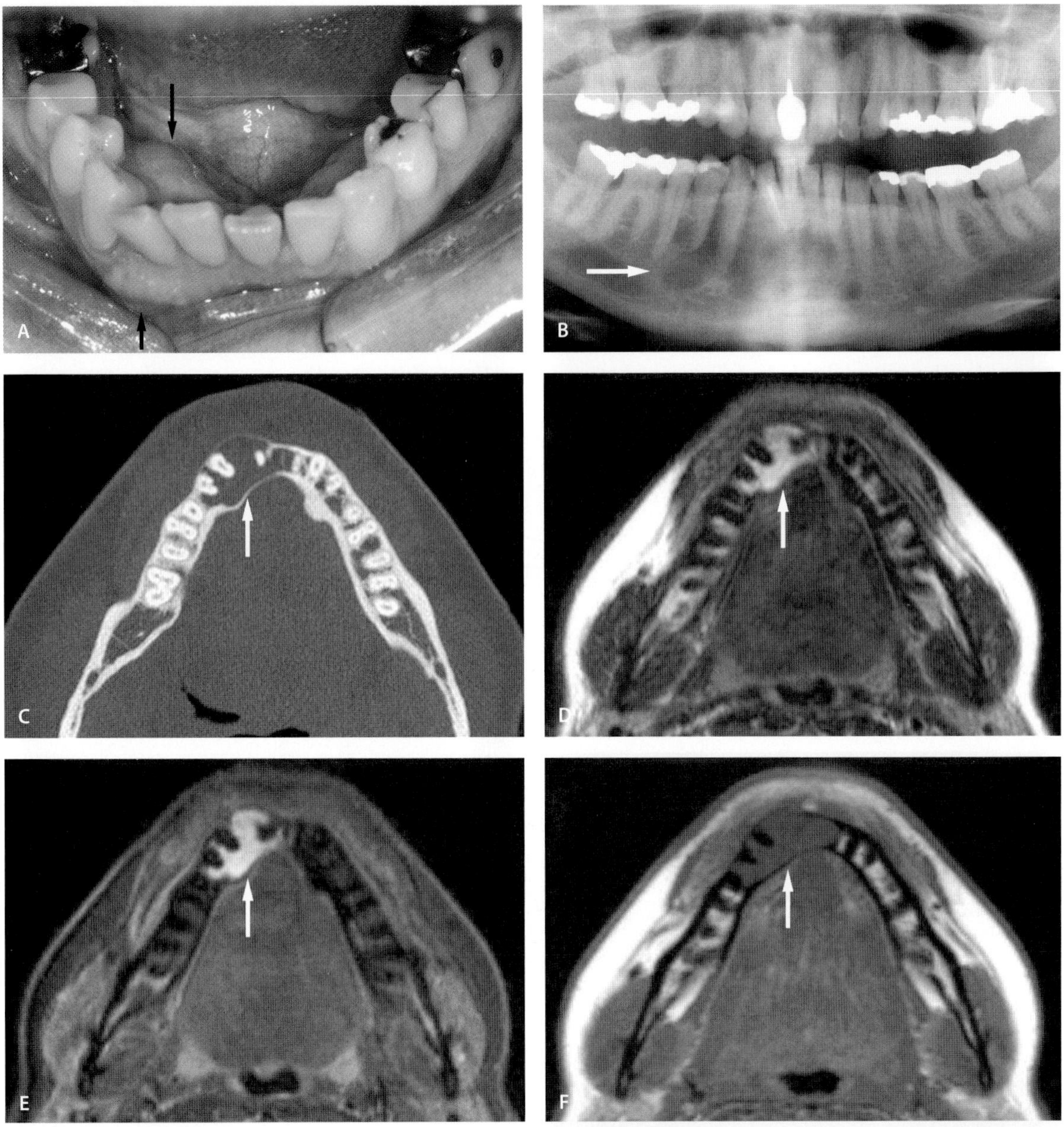

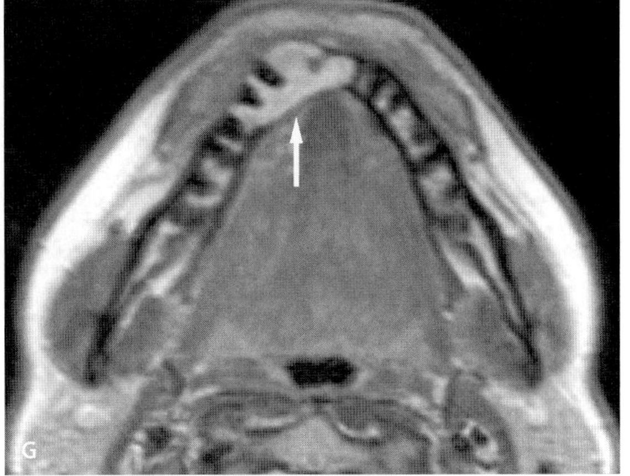

Figure 3.19

Odontogenic myxoma, mandible; 45-year-old female with painless swelling which the patient did not notice because tumor was "filling out" mandibular torus on right side. **A** Clinical photograph shows buccal and lingual jaw expansion (*arrows*). **B** Panoramic view shows scalloped radiolucency without sclerotic outline (*arrow*). **C** Axial CT image shows expanded but intact buccal and lingual cortical bone. Note tumor occupies mandibular torus on right side (*arrow*). **D** Axial T2-weighted MRI shows homogeneous high signal (*arrow*). **E** Axial STIR MRI shows homogeneous high signal (*arrow*). **F** Axial T1-weighted pre-Gd MRI shows intermediate (to low) signal (*arrow*). **G** Axial T1-weighted post-Gd MRI shows homogeneous contrast enhancement (*arrow*)

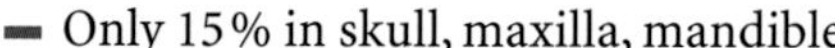

Bone-destructive and Bone-productive Tumors

Osteoblastoma

Definition

Mesenchymal tumor characterized by well-vascularized connective tissue stroma in which active production of osteoid or primitive woven bone occurs.

Osteoid osteoma is a similar tumor, but of much smaller size (a nidus usually less than 1 cm), and associated with nocturnal pain.

Clinical Features

- Swelling, usually painful, but also without pain
- Mandible more frequent than maxilla
- Males more frequent than females
- Peak incidence in second decade
- Most common site of occurrence is vertebrae, flat bones, femur, tibia, but generally considered a rare tumor
- Only 15% in skull, maxilla, mandible
- Nearly 15% recurrence rate has been reported for conventional mandibular osteoblastomas, without histologic atypia
- Juvenile aggressive osteoblastoma has high recurrence (close to 50%) after surgery and/or histologic atypia

Imaging Features

- Highly variable; osteolytic to osteoblastic (ground-glass appearance)
- Coarse trabecular pattern
- Expansive growth, may resemble aneurysmal bone cyst
- Distinction between aggressive osteoblastoma and low-grade osteosarcoma may be difficult, but osteoblastoma has more well-defined border
- If close to teeth it may cause displacement but not fuse with cementum (in contrast to benign cementoblastoma)

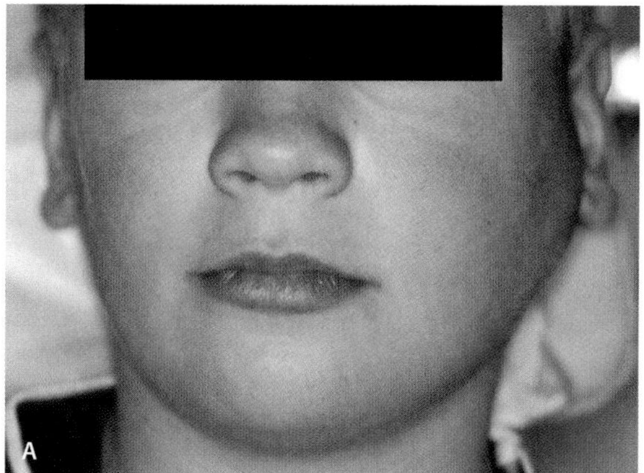

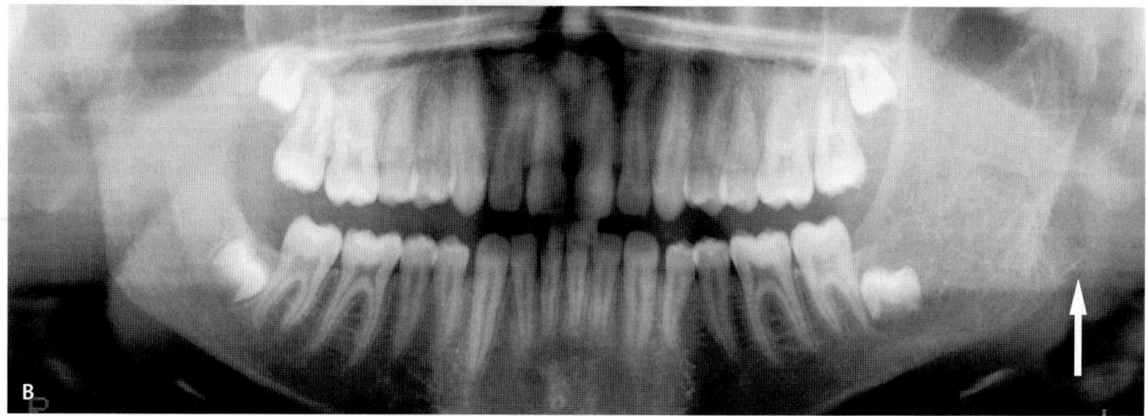

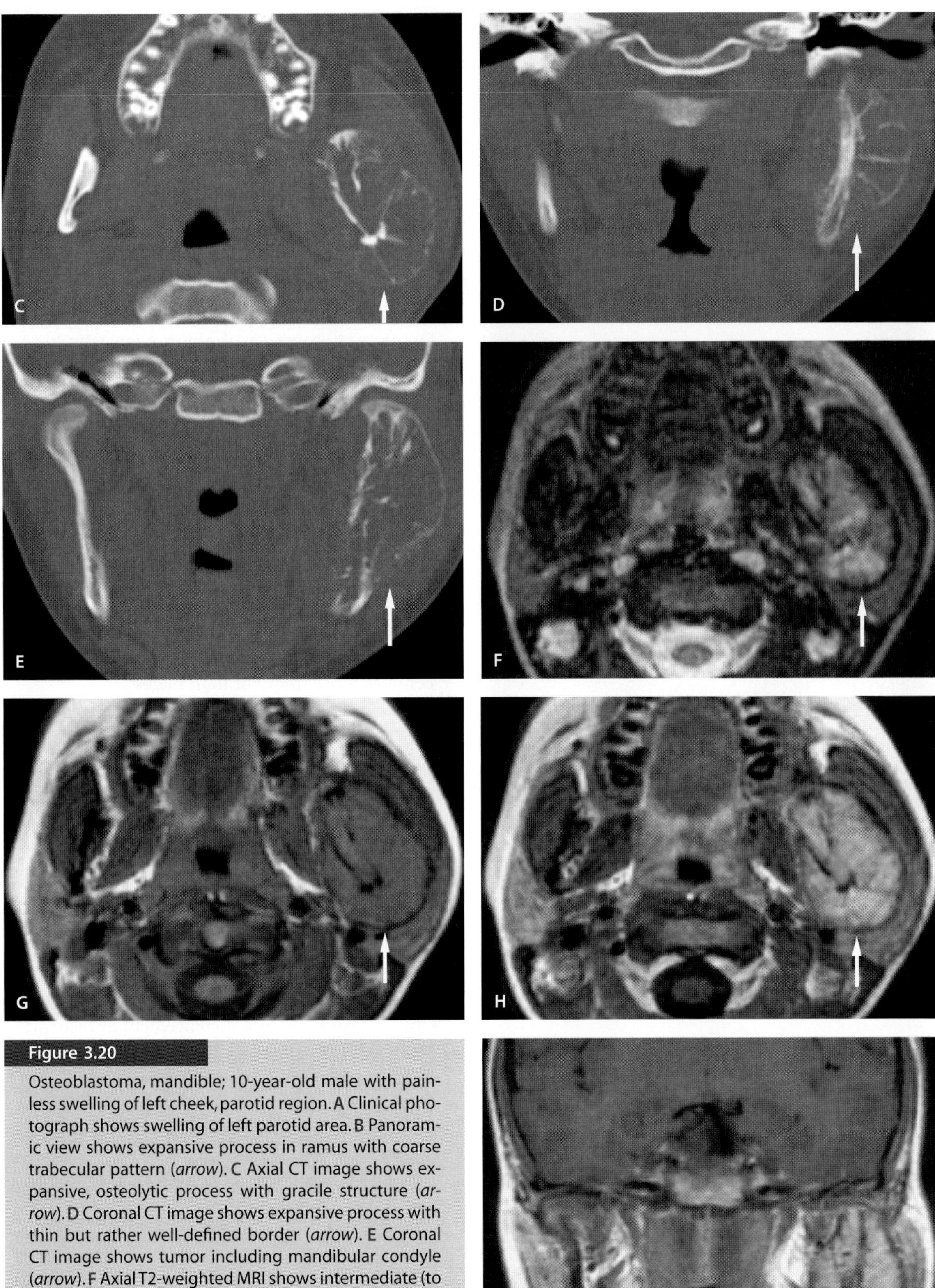

Figure 3.20

Osteoblastoma, mandible; 10-year-old male with painless swelling of left cheek, parotid region. A Clinical photograph shows swelling of left parotid area. B Panoramic view shows expansive process in ramus with coarse trabecular pattern (*arrow*). C Axial CT image shows expansive, osteolytic process with gracile structure (*arrow*). D Coronal CT image shows expansive process with thin but rather well-defined border (*arrow*). E Coronal CT image shows tumor including mandibular condyle (*arrow*). F Axial T2-weighted MRI shows intermediate (to high) signal (*arrow*). G Axial T1-weighted pre-Gd MRI shows intermediate signal (*arrow*). H Axial T1-weighted post-Gd MRI shows contrast enhancement (*arrow*). I Coronal T1-weighted post-Gd MRI shows contrast enhancement (*arrow*) (A: courtesy of Dr. T. Bjørnland, Rikshospitalet University Hospital, Oslo, Norway)

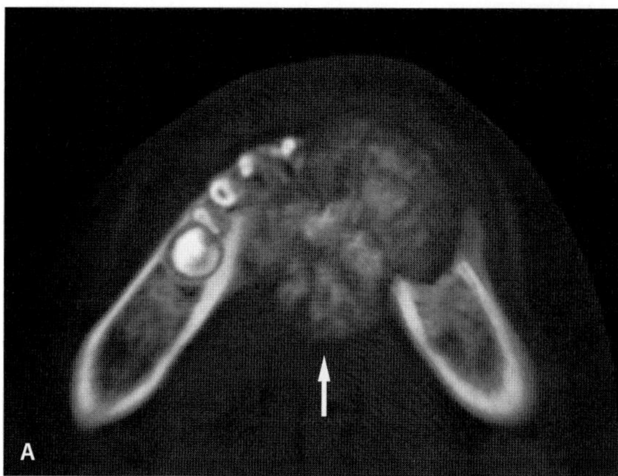

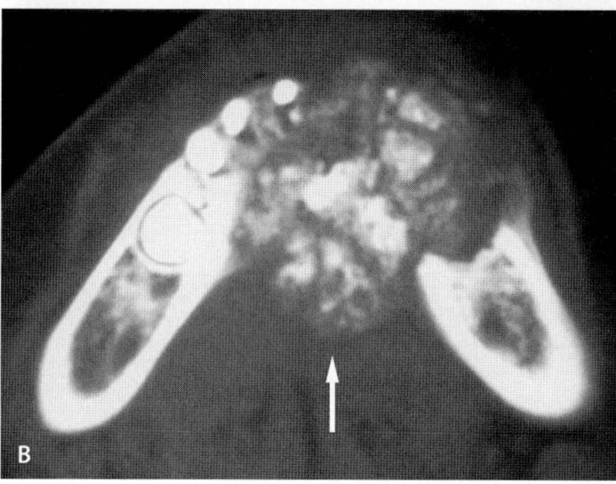

Figure 3.21

Osteoblastoma, mandible; 3-year-old male, painless swelling of anterior part of mandible. **A** Axial CT image shows extensive bone production (*arrow*). **B** Axial CT image, soft-tissue window, shows rather well-defined mass (*arrow*)

Ossifying Fibroma

Synonyms: Cemento-ossifying fibroma, cementifying fibroma, juvenile (active/aggressive) ossifying fibroma

Definition

Well-demarcated lesion composed of fibrocellular tissue and mineralized material of varying appearances. Juvenile trabecular ossifying fibroma and juvenile psammomatoid ossifying fibroma are two histologic variants of ossifying fibroma (WHO).

Ossifying fibroma (or the non-neoplastic fibrous dysplasia or giant cell granuloma) may occur as 'hybrid lesions' with the non-neoplastic aneurysmal bone cyst (see Figure 3.25)

Clinical Features

- Painless swelling
- Mostly in mandible, posterior region
- Juvenile variants mostly in maxilla
- Second to fourth decades; mean age about 35 years
- Mean age of juvenile variants about 10 and 20 years
- Females more frequent than males
- Tumor more active/aggressive in young patients

Imaging Features

- Radiolucency, radiopacity, or mixed appearance; about half of cases have been reported to be radiolucent
- Border usually well-defined, may be multilocular
- Bone expansion may be evident and in more than half of cases
- May displace maxillary sinus, nasal cavity, mandibular canal
- Majority shows no relationship to tooth apices
- Only occasionally root displacement or resorption
- May be impossible to distinguish from fibrous dysplasia (ground-glass appearance)
- Discrete zones of variable amounts of either osseous or fibrous tissue give variable signal pattern on MRI
- T1-weighted MRI: Low to intermediate to high signal
- T2-weighted and STIR MRI: low to intermediate to high signal
- T1-weighted post-Gd MRI: rather homogeneous contrast enhancement or contrast-enhanced areas interspersed with non-enhanced areas

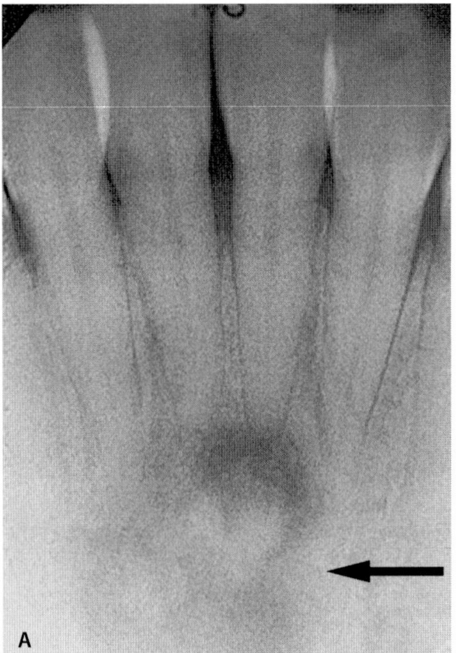

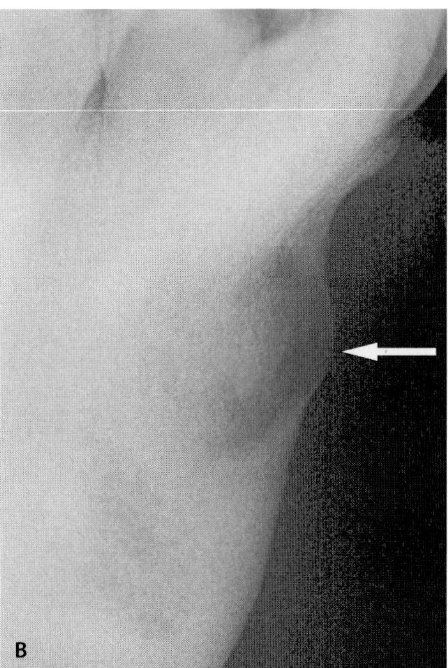

Figure 3.22

Ossifying fibroma, mandible; painless swelling in anterior part of mandible. A Intraoral view shows radiolucency with diffuse, somewhat sclerotic border and central mineralization (*arrow*). B Side view shows expanded and intact buccal cortical bone (*arrow*)

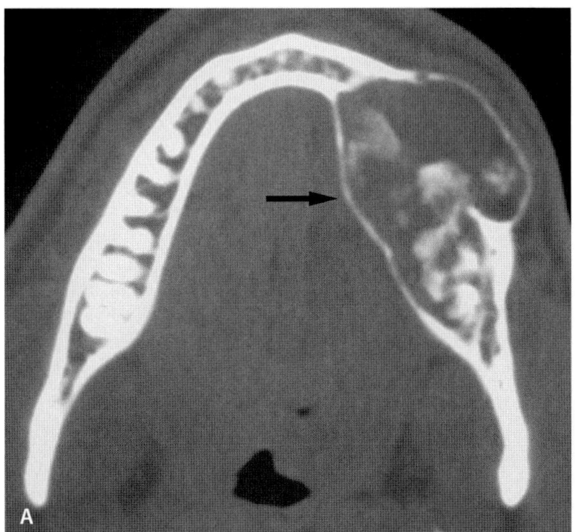

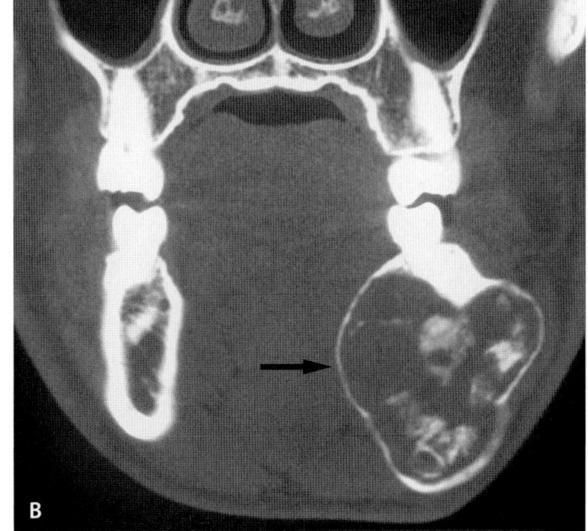

Figure 3.23

Ossifying fibroma, mandible; 22-year-old male with painless swelling of left mandible. A Axial CT image shows expansion with intact cortical border and central mineralization (*arrow*). B Coronal CT image shows expanded, intact cortical bone and central mineralization (*arrow*)

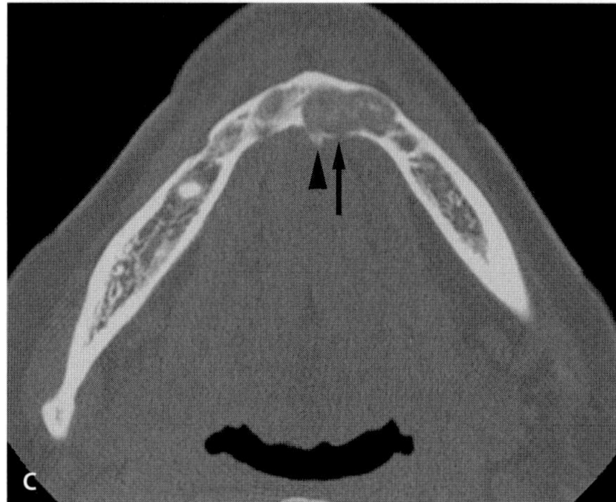
C

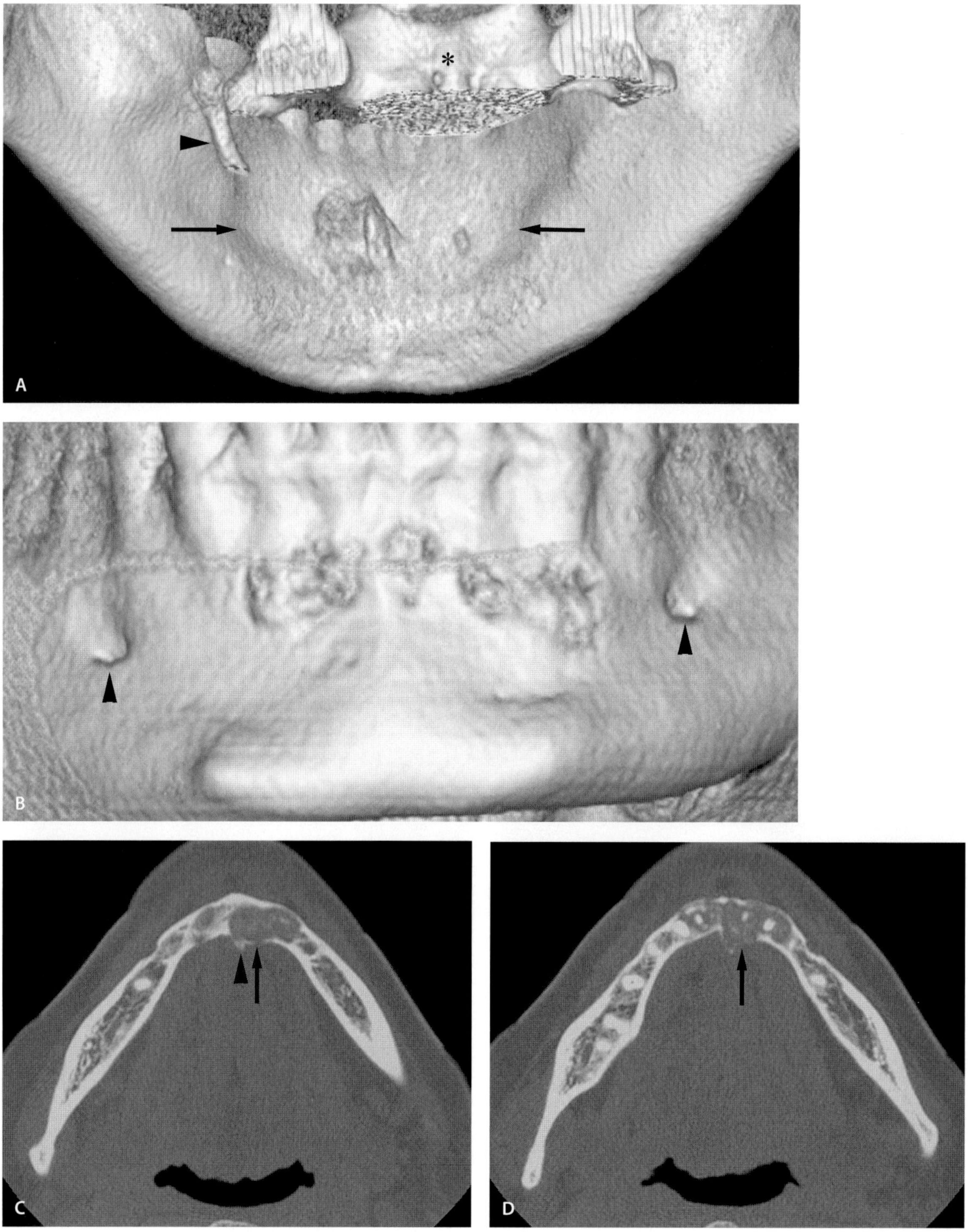

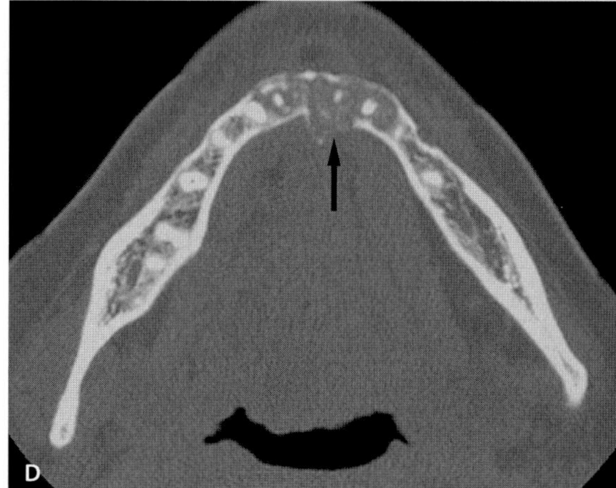
D

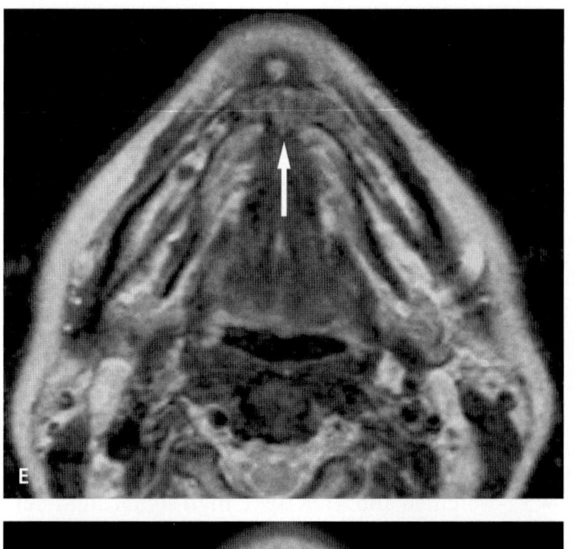

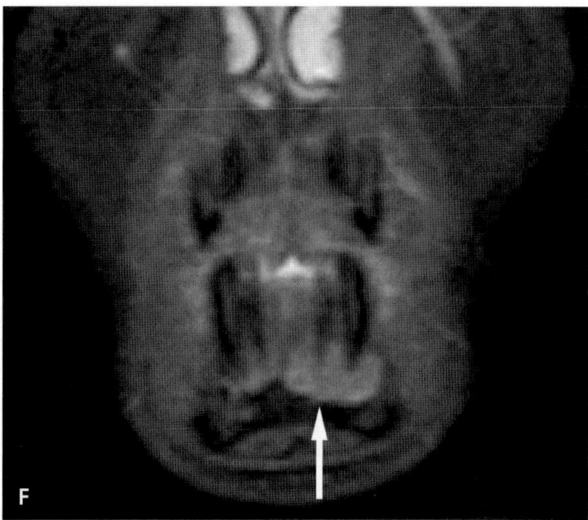

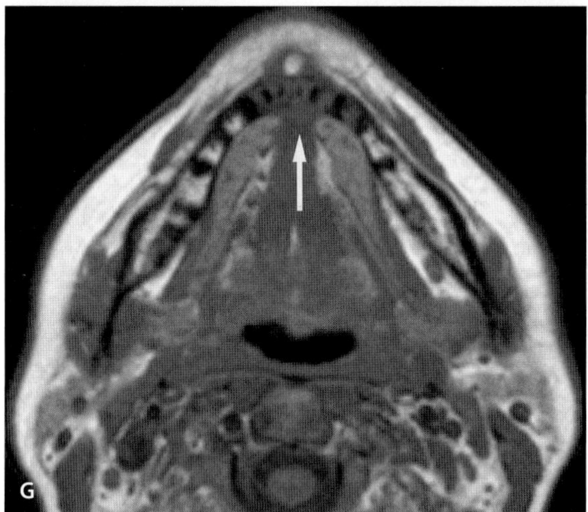

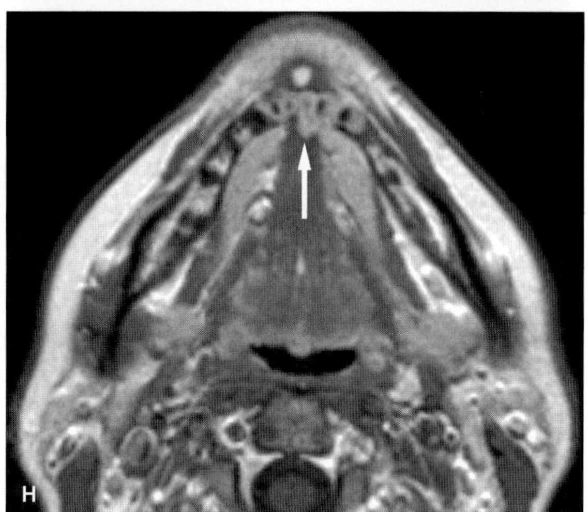

Figure 3.24

Ossifying fibroma, mandible; 41-year-old female with painless swelling of lingual aspect of anterior mandible. **A** 3D CT image shows swelling on lingual side with cortical defects (*arrows*). Note styloid process (*arrowhead*) and cervical spine (*asterisk*). **B** 3D CT image shows cortical defects on buccal side between mental foramina (*arrowheads*). **C** Axial CT image shows well-defined radiolucency with some expansion and intact cortical bone lingually (*arrow*). Note lingual crista (*arrowhead*) and small mineralizations. **D** Axial CT image shows tumor with small mineralizations and more expansion lingually (*arrow*). **E** Axial T2-weighted MRI shows intermediate, slightly heterogeneous signal (*arrow*). **F** Coronal STIR MRI shows intermediate signal (*arrow*). **G** Axial T1-weighted pre-Gd MRI shows intermediate signal (*arrow*). **H** Axial T1-weighted post-Gd MRI shows moderate contrast enhancement (*arrow*). **I** Coronal T1-weighted post-Gd MRI shows moderate contrast enhancement (*arrow*)

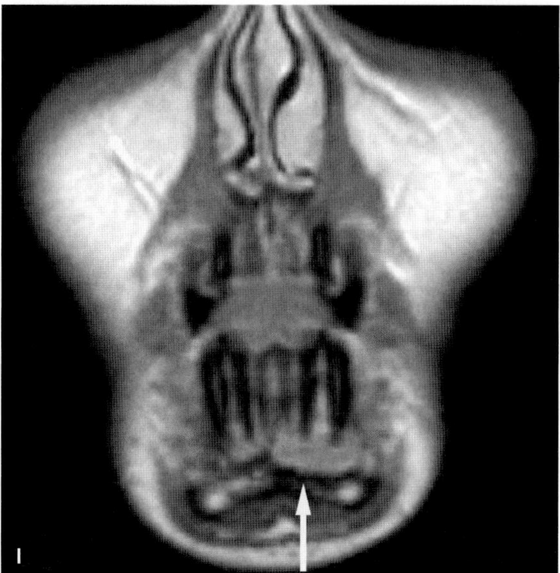

Ossifying Fibroma with Aneurysmal Bone Cyst

Aneurysmal Bone Cyst

Definition

Expansile osteolytic lesion often multilocular, containing blood-filled spaces separated by fibrous septa containing osteoclast-type giant cells and reactive bone (WHO).

Clinical Features

- Painless swelling, usually few symptoms
- Mandible more often than maxilla, mostly in posterior regions including ramus
- Usually below 30 years of age, but may present at any age in jaws
- No sex predominance, or slight female
- Can occur anywhere in skeleton; most frequently in long bones, followed by spine
- In a large series of children (1.5–17 years) more than 60% occurred in long bones

Imaging Features

- Highly variable radiologic appearance in jaws
- Mostly radiolucent (close to 90%), but also mixed or rarely radiopaque
- Unilocular (less than half) or multilocular
- Usually expansile, ballooning (about 50% in jaws)
- Border well-defined and corticated in about one-third, thus majority without sclerosis or even diffuse in jaws
- Cortical perforation may occur
- Tooth displacement and root resorption may occur
- T1-weighted MRI: intermediate-low signal surrounded by low-signal well-defined rim, and fluid–fluid level
- T2-weighted and STIR MRI: high signal, fluid–fluid level
- T1-weighted post-Gd MRI: enhancement of internal septations

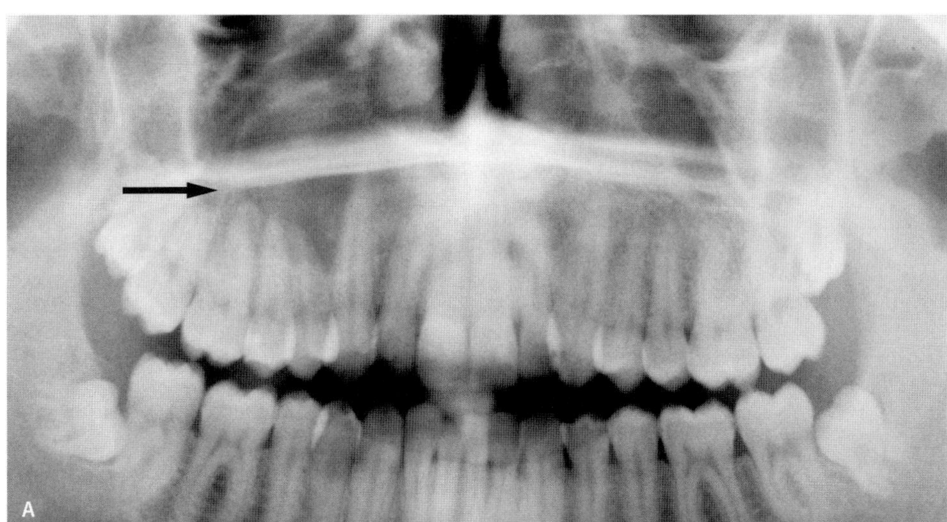

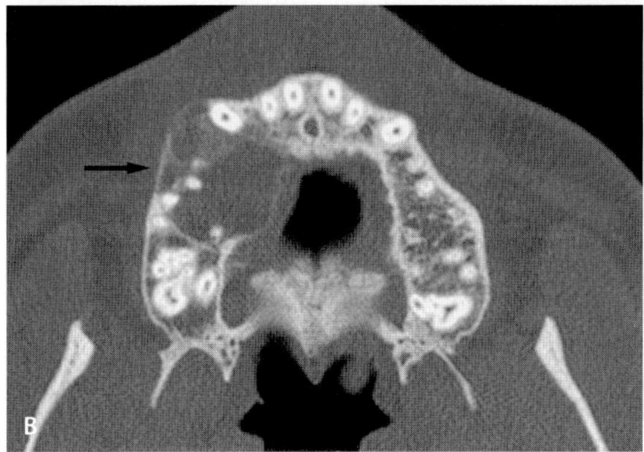

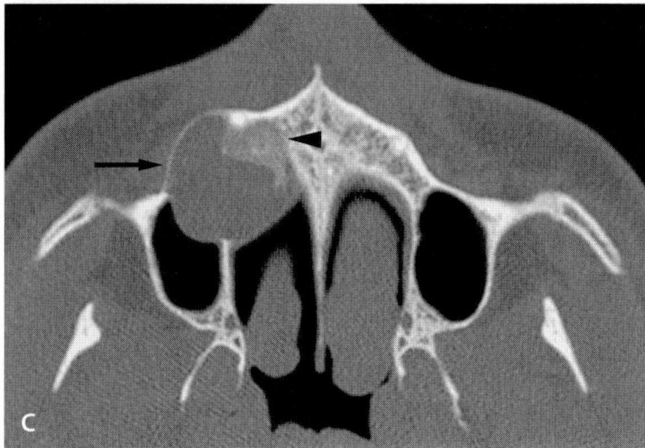

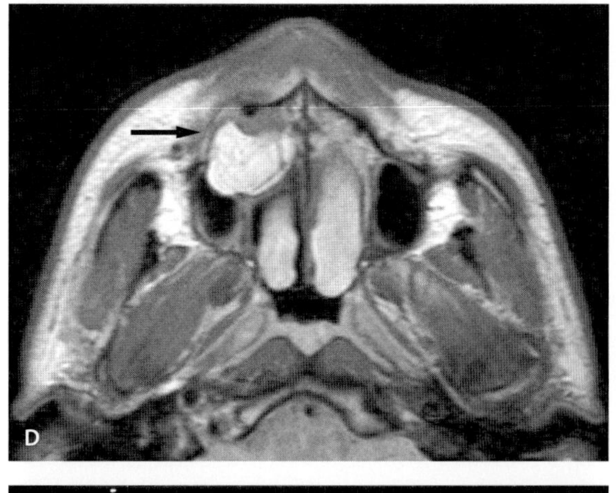

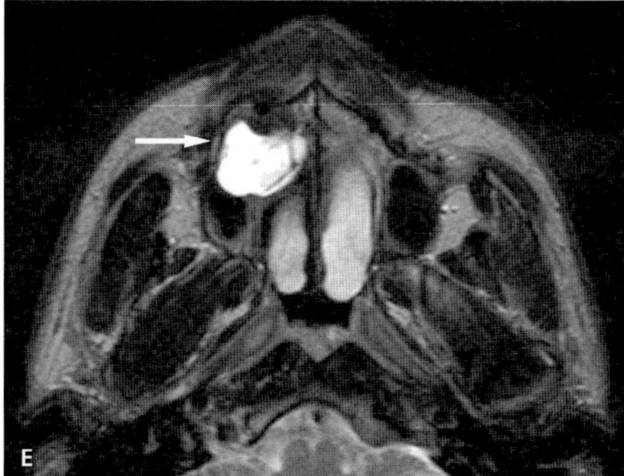

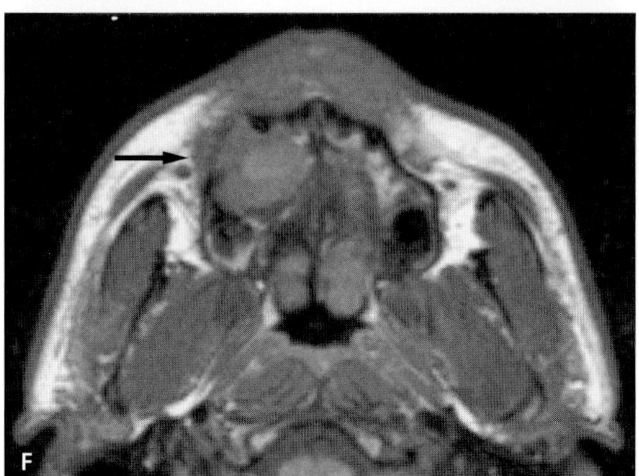

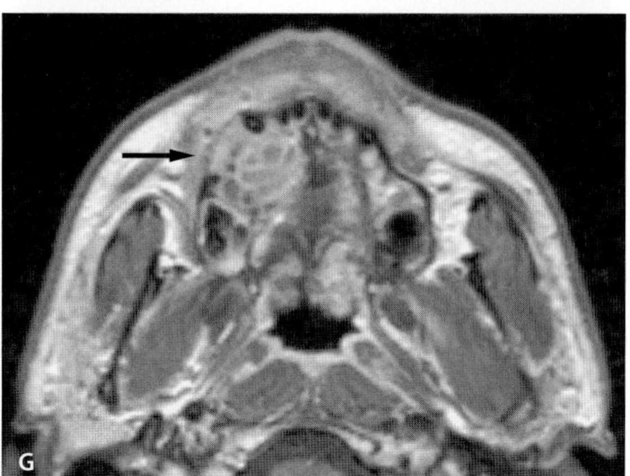

Figure 3.25

Ossifying fibroma with aneurysmal bone cyst, maxilla; 22-year-old male with painless swelling of mucobuccal fold. A Panoramic view shows radiolucency with sclerotic border in maxilla (*arrow*). B Axial CT image shows well-defined tumor with expanded, intact cortical delineation (*arrow*) with some mineralization in anterior part. C Axial CT image shows well-defined expanded tumor with intact cortical plate (*arrow*) and more mineralization than in B (*arrowhead*). D Axial PD MRI shows high signal in a large portion and intermediate signal in a small portion of tumor (*arrow*). E Axial T2-weighted MRI shows high signal in a large portion (*arrow*) and low signal in a small portion. F Axial T1-weighted pre-Gd MRI shows intermediate signal (*arrow*). G Axial T1-weighted post-Gd MRI shows septal contrast enhancement (*arrow*). H Coronal T1-weighted post-Gd MRI shows septal contrast enhancement (*arrow*)

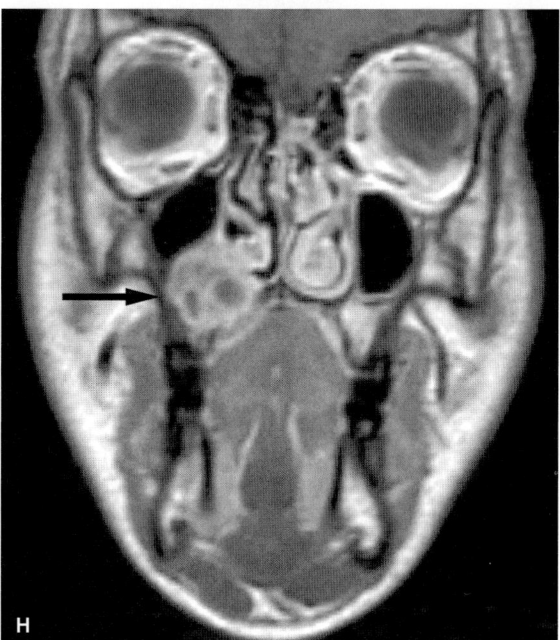

Hard Tissue-producing Tumors, Exostoses, and Malformations

Osteoma

Definition

Benign, slowly growing lesion consisting of well-differentiated mature bone, with a predominantly lamellar structure (WHO).

Clinical Features

- Incidental finding or painless hard swelling
- Mandible and maxilla
- All facial bones and paranasal sinuses
- Most frequent (more than one-third) in a large series of jaw lesions with hard-tissue formation

Imaging Features

- Variable amount of compact bone
- Variable amount of cancellous bone

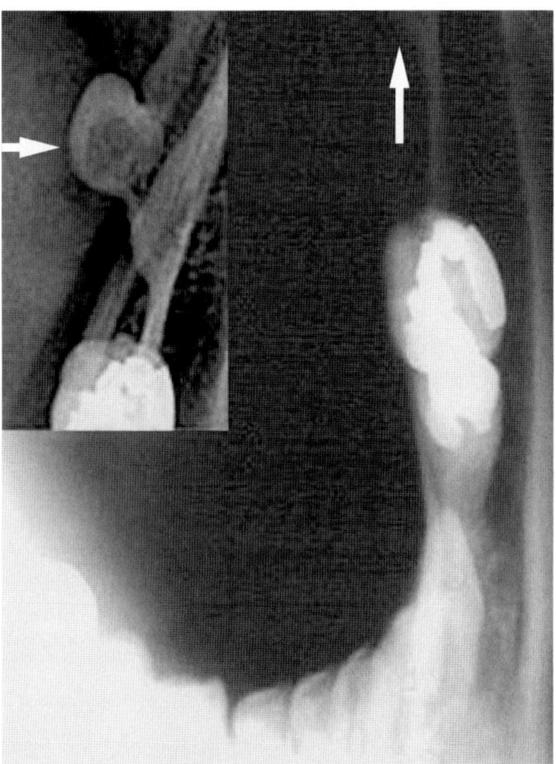

Figure 3.26

Osteoma, mandible; painless swelling lingually at mandibular angle. Intraoral views show exostotic tumor of cortical and cancellous bone (*arrows*)

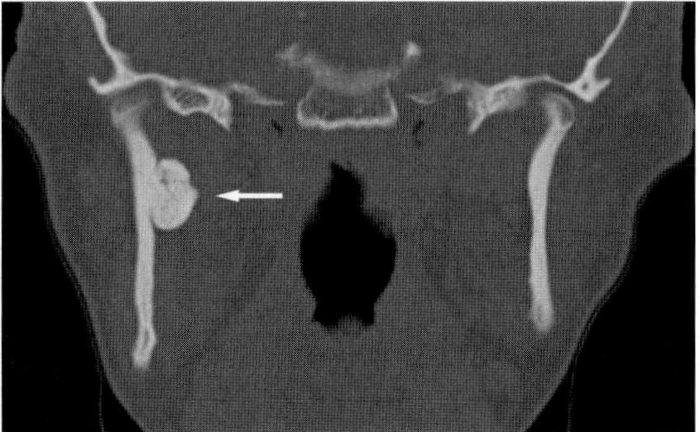

Figure 3.27

Osteoma, mandible; 23-year-old male with incidental finding at routine dental radiography. Coronal CT image shows exostotic tumor predominantly of cortical bone (*arrow*) at lingual aspect of mandibular ramus

Exostoses

Definition

Outgrowth of normal cancellous and compact bone in certain areas.

Clinical Features

- Mandible; torus mandibularis in premolar regions lingually and bilaterally
- Maxilla; torus palatinus in midline
- Maxilla; multiple exostoses in premolar region bilaterally; more common buccally than palatally

Imaging Features

- See **Osteoma**

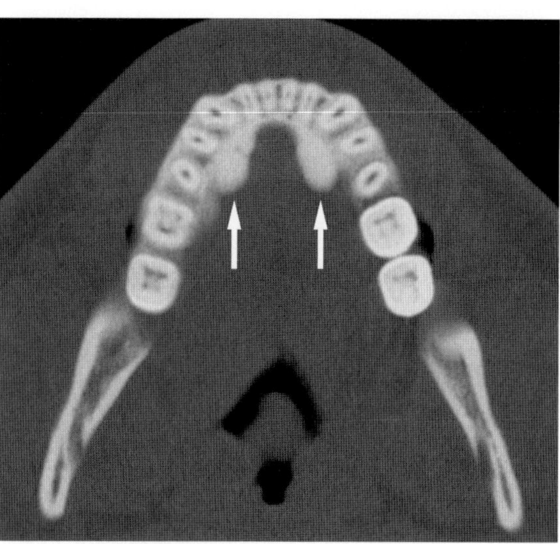

Figure 3.28

Torus mandibularis; painless hard lingual swellings. Axial CT image shows bilateral exostoses (*arrows*)

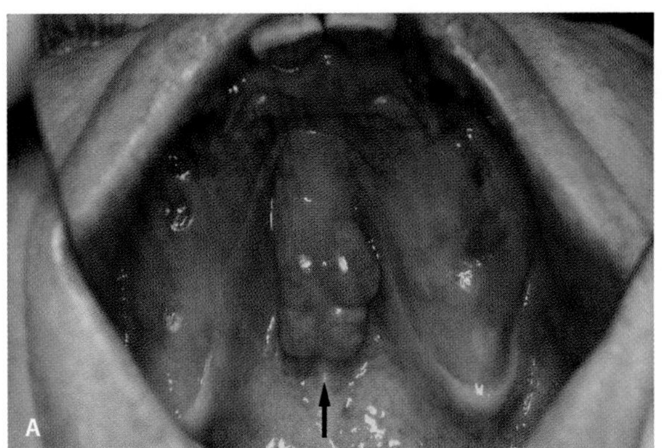

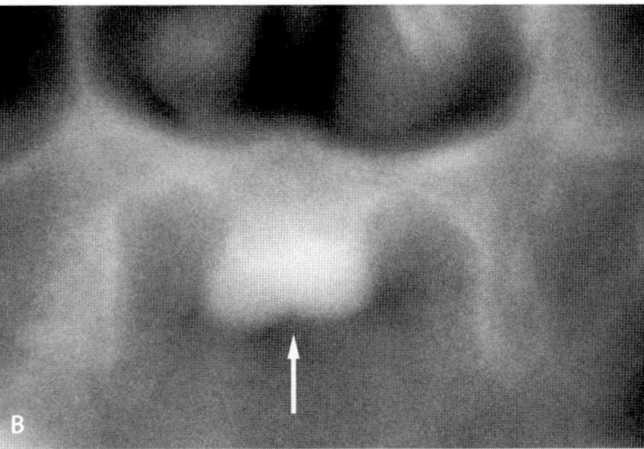

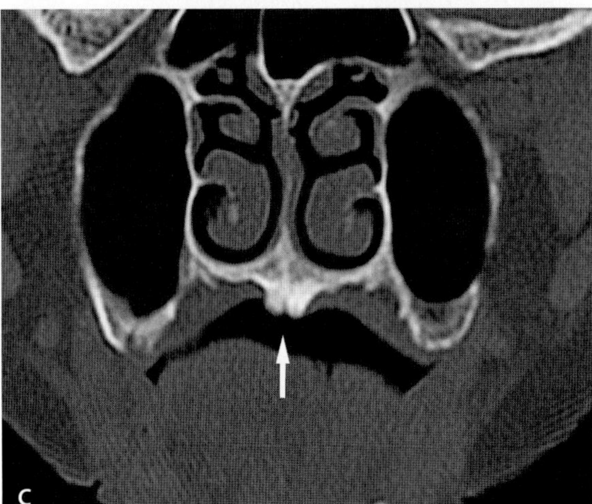

Figure 3.29

Torus palatinus; painless hard swelling. **A** Clinical photograph shows large torus with normal mucosa in midline of palate (*arrow*). **B** Coronal tomography of same patient shows exostosis with thick layer of compact bone (*arrow*). **C** Coronal CT of smaller torus in another patient (*arrow*)

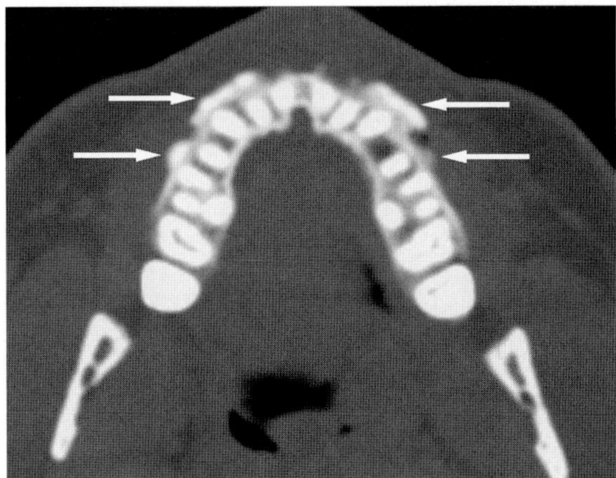

Figure 3.30

Multiple exostoses in maxilla; painless hard swellings buccally in premolar region. Axial CT image shows multiple buccal exostoses bilaterally (*arrows*)

Odontoma, Complex Type

Definition

Tumor-like malformation (hamartoma) in which enamel and dentin, and sometimes cementum is present (WHO).

Characteristically surrounded by a fibrous capsule.

Clinical Features

- Incidental finding
- Tooth-bearing regions of maxilla or mandible, mostly in posterior part of mandible
- Usually found during second decade
- No sex predilection

Imaging Features

- Predominantly an amorphous radiopacity, including enamel, but also soft tissue
- Surrounded by a radiolucent zone; fibrous capsule
- Compound type, more similar to teeth, consisting of several individual odontoids

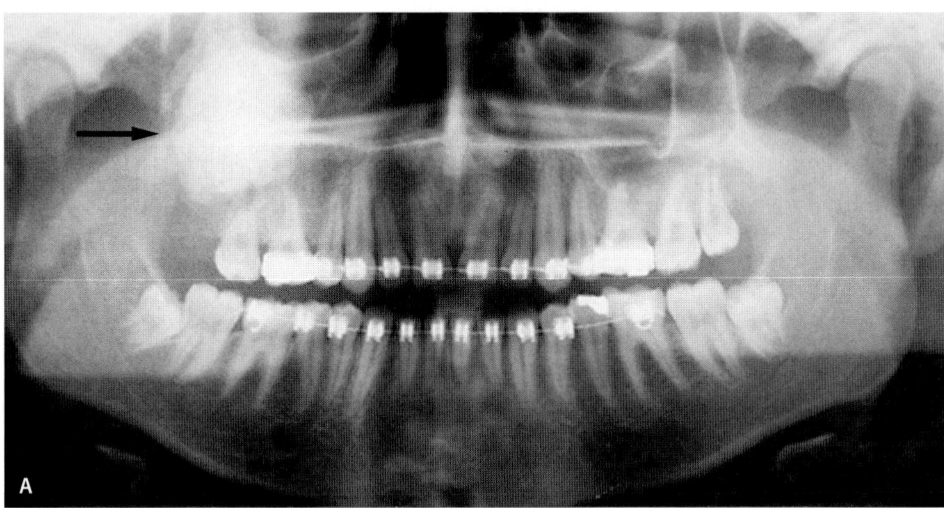

Figure 3.31

Odontoma, maxilla; 15-year-old female with incidental finding at orthodontic consultation. **A** Panoramic view shows large radiopaque mass in right maxillary sinus (*arrow*). **B** Coronal CT image shows large mass of cortex or enamel density in right maxillary sinus (*arrow*), surrounded by fibrous capsule, with destroyed lateral sinus wall and root resorption

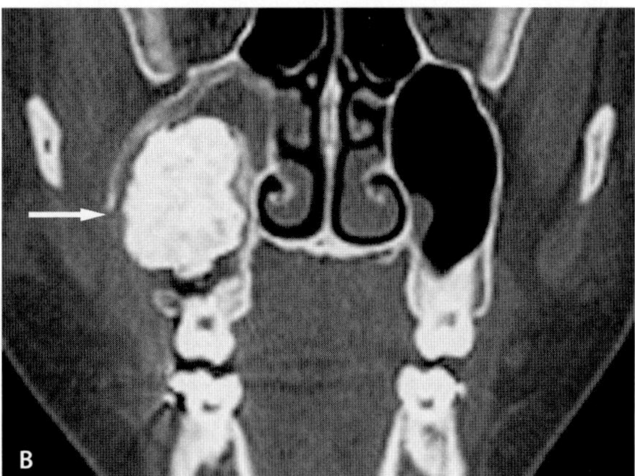

Bone-destructive and/or Bone-productive Tumor-like Conditions

This is a heterogeneous group of conditions not characterized as cysts, tumors or malformation.

Simple Bone Cyst

Synonyms: Solitary bone cyst, traumatic bone cyst, hemorrhagic bone cyst, hemorrhagic cyst, idiopathic bone cavity, unicameral bone cyst

Definition

Intraosseous pseudocyst devoid of an epithelial lining, either empty or filled with serous or sanguinous fluid (WHO).

Clinical Features

- Incidental radiographic finding
- Second decade
- Mandible, usually body or anterior (most frequent) areas
- Vital teeth
- No sex predilection in jaws (in contrast to long bones; males more frequent)

Imaging Features

- Radiolucency
- Unilocular, usually rounded in anterior region, often scalloped between teeth or roots in molar region
- Multilocular appearance may occur but rare
- Bilateral cases are reported
- Border usually well-defined and corticated, but may be less well-defined and non-corticated
- Usually no expansion of bone
- If expanding bone, only slightly with cortical thinning
- Usually no displacement or resorption of teeth
- Occasionally, may persist or even expand following surgical fenestration
- T1-weighted MRI: homogeneous intermediate signal
- T2-weighted and STIR MRI: homogeneous high signal
- T1-weighted post-Gd MRI: no contrast enhancement or in peripheral thin rim

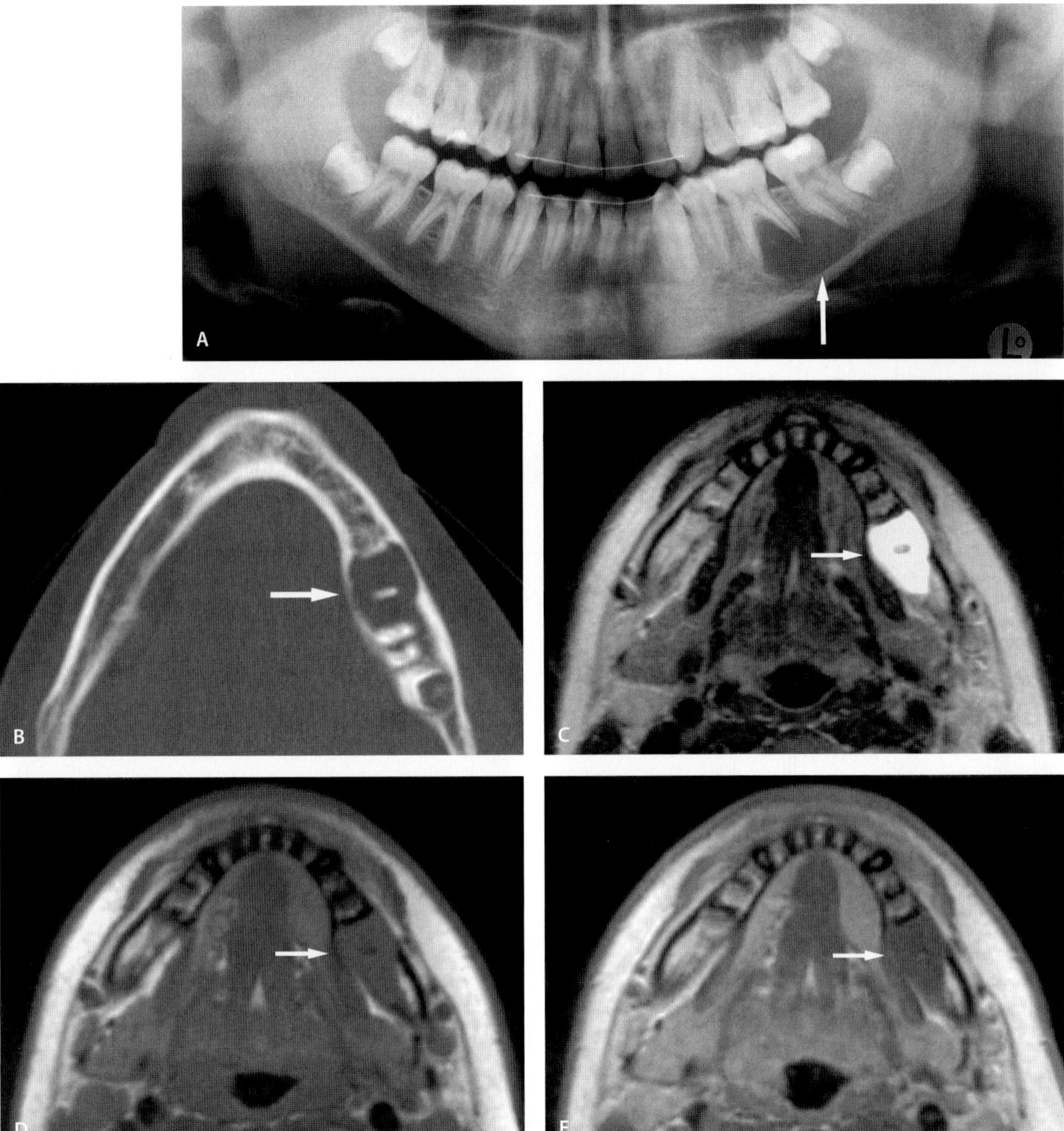

Figure 3.32

Simple bone cyst, mandible; 15-year-old male with incidental finding at routine dental radiography. **A** Panoramic view shows well-defined radiolucency with no sclerotic border (*arrow*). **B** Axial CT image shows expanded, thinned and intact cortical bone (*arrow*). **C** Axial T2-weighted MRI shows homogeneous high signal (*arrow*). **D** Axial T1-weighted pre-Gd MRI shows homogeneous intermediate signal (*arrow*). **E** Axial T1-weighted post-Gd MRI shows no contrast enhancement (*arrow*)

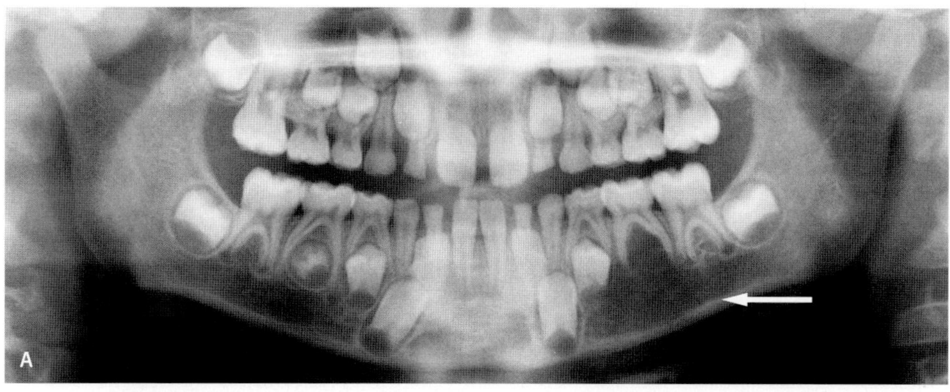
A

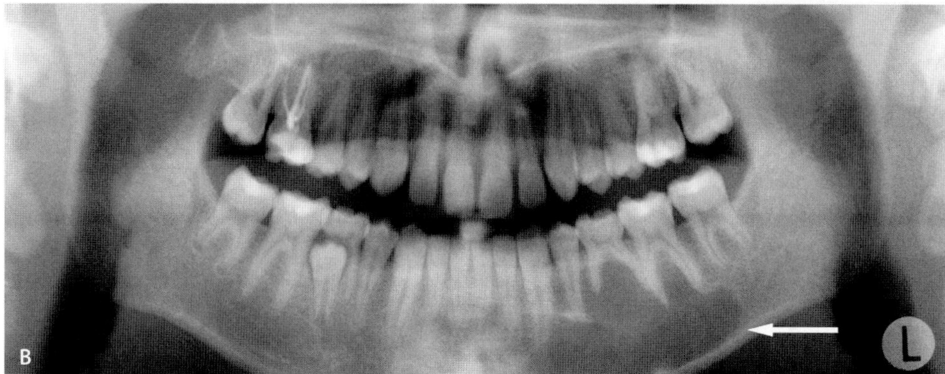
B
L

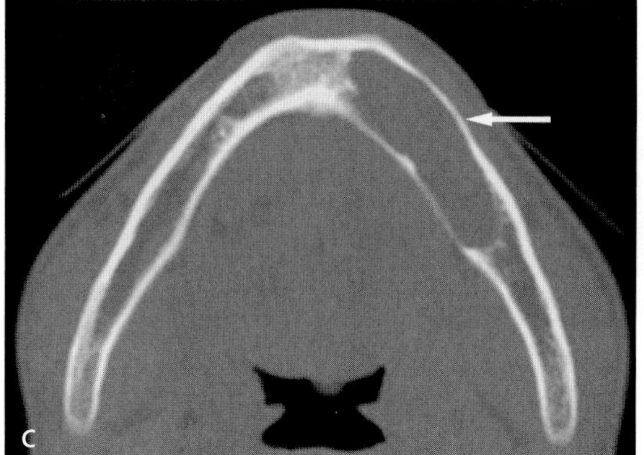
C

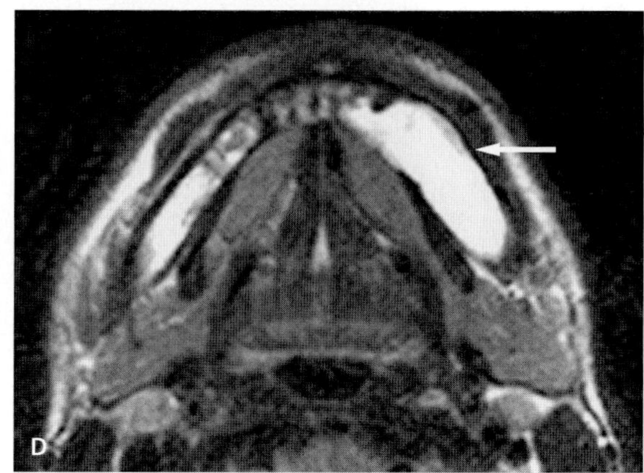
D

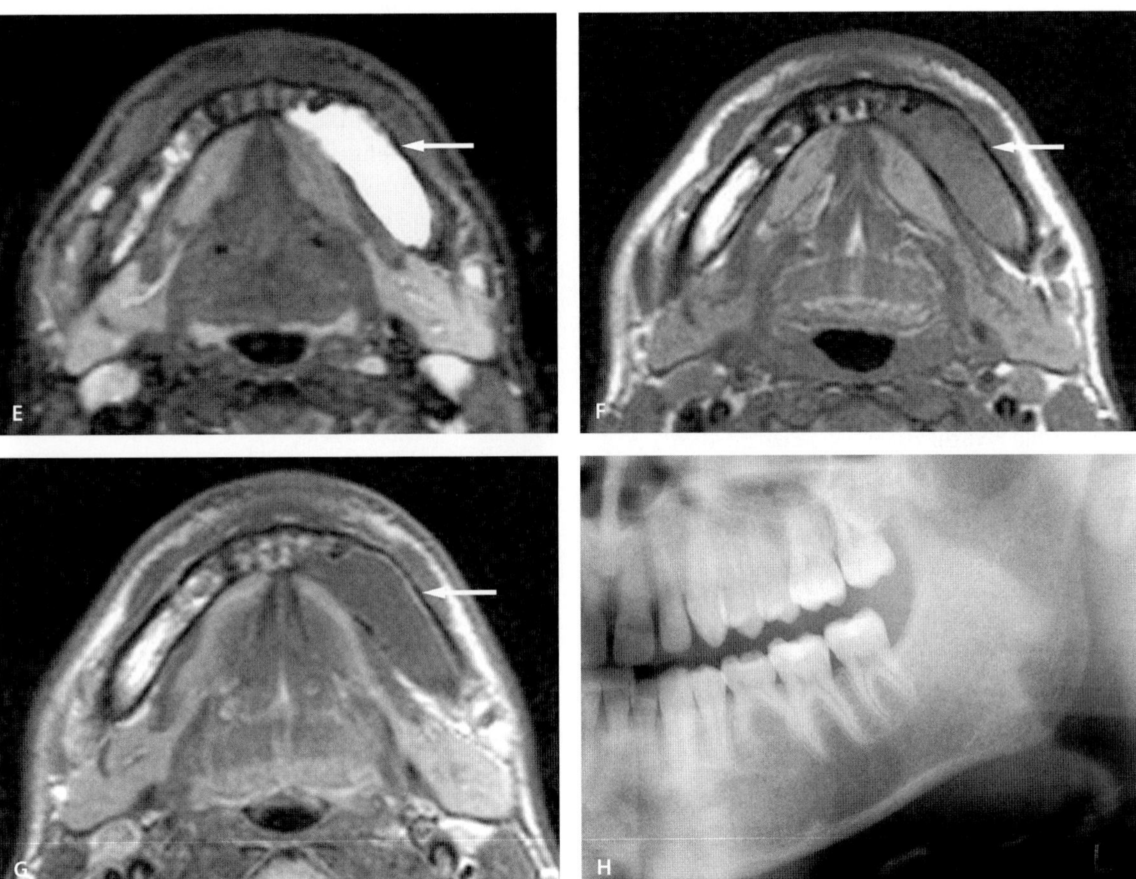

Figure 3.33

Simple bone cyst, mandible; 8-year-old male at baseline with incidental finding at routine dental radiography, and followed for 8 years. A Panoramic view shows poorly defined radiolucency with no sclerotic border (*arrow*). B Panoramic view shows enlarged radiolucency (*arrow*) at 6-year follow-up, after two surgical interventions. C Axial CT image shows expanded, thinned and intact cortical bone (*arrow*). D Axial T2-weighted MRI shows homogeneous high signal (*arrow*). E Axial STIR MRI shows homogeneous high signal (*arrow*). F Axial T1-weighted pre-Gd MRI shows homogeneous intermediate signal (*arrow*). G Axial T1-weighted post-Gd MRI shows no enhancement except thin peripheral rim buccally (*arrow*). H Panoramic view 8 years after presentation (2 years after third surgery) shows complete regeneration

Giant Cell Granuloma

Definition

Localized benign but sometimes aggressive osteolytic proliferation consisting of fibrous tissue with hemorrhage and hemosiderin deposits, presence of osteoclast-like giant cells and reactive bone formation (WHO).

Clinical Features

- Incidental finding or painless swelling
- First to third decades, but wide age range
- Females more frequent than males
- Mandible two-thirds, maxilla one-third
- Most often in posterior region, less frequently in anterior region (but also crossing midline)
- May behave aggressively in younger patients, with recurrence after surgical treatment
- Noonan syndrome; bilateral abnormalities

Imaging Features

- Radiolucency
- Unilocular or more often, multilocular; may be scalloped
- Border well defined or poorly defined, may be sclerotic but usually not
- May expand bone
- May displace or, less frequently, resorb teeth
- T1-weighted MRI: homogeneous or slightly heterogeneous intermediate signal
- T2-weighted and STIR MRI: homogeneous or slightly heterogeneous intermediate signal
- T1-weighted post-Gd MRI: contrast enhancement

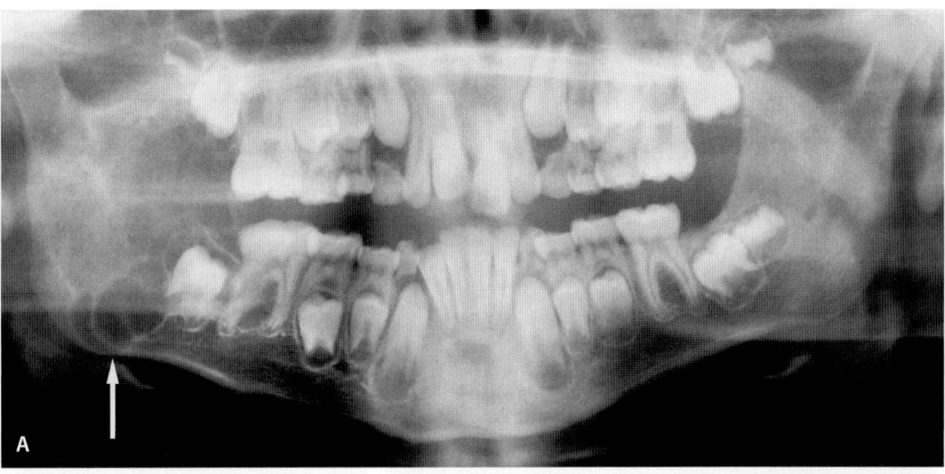

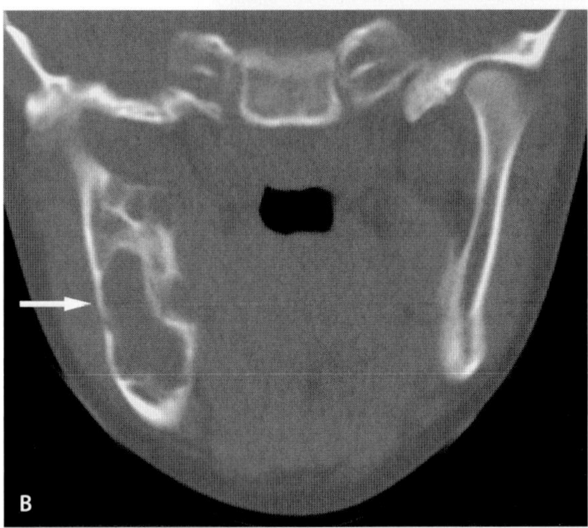

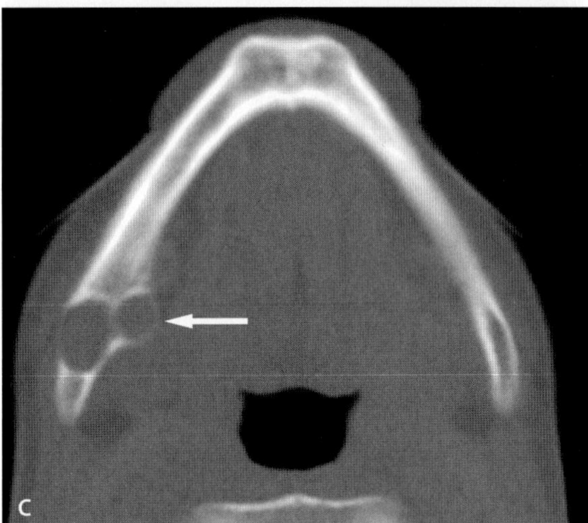

Figure 3.34

Giant cell granuloma, mandible; 10-year-old male at presentation with painless jaw swelling. **A** Panoramic view shows multilocular radiolucency with sclerotic border (*arrow*). **B** Coronal CT image shows expansive, multilocular process (*arrow*). **C** Axial CT image shows two "compartments" at lower mandibular border (*arrow*). **D** Panoramic view at 6-year follow-up shows complete regeneration after two surgical interventions

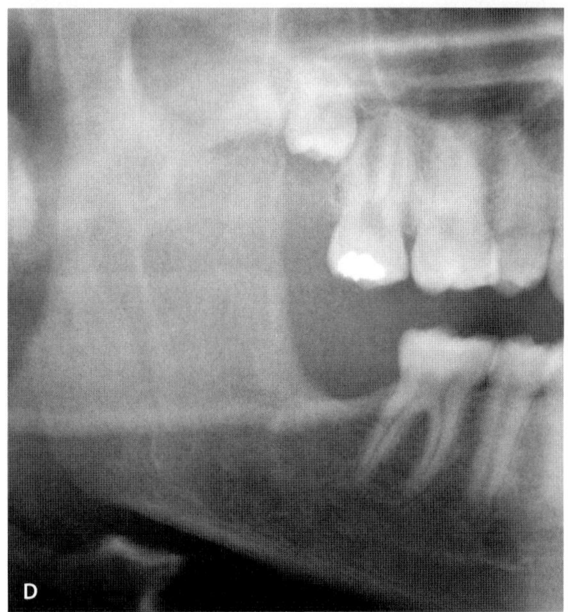

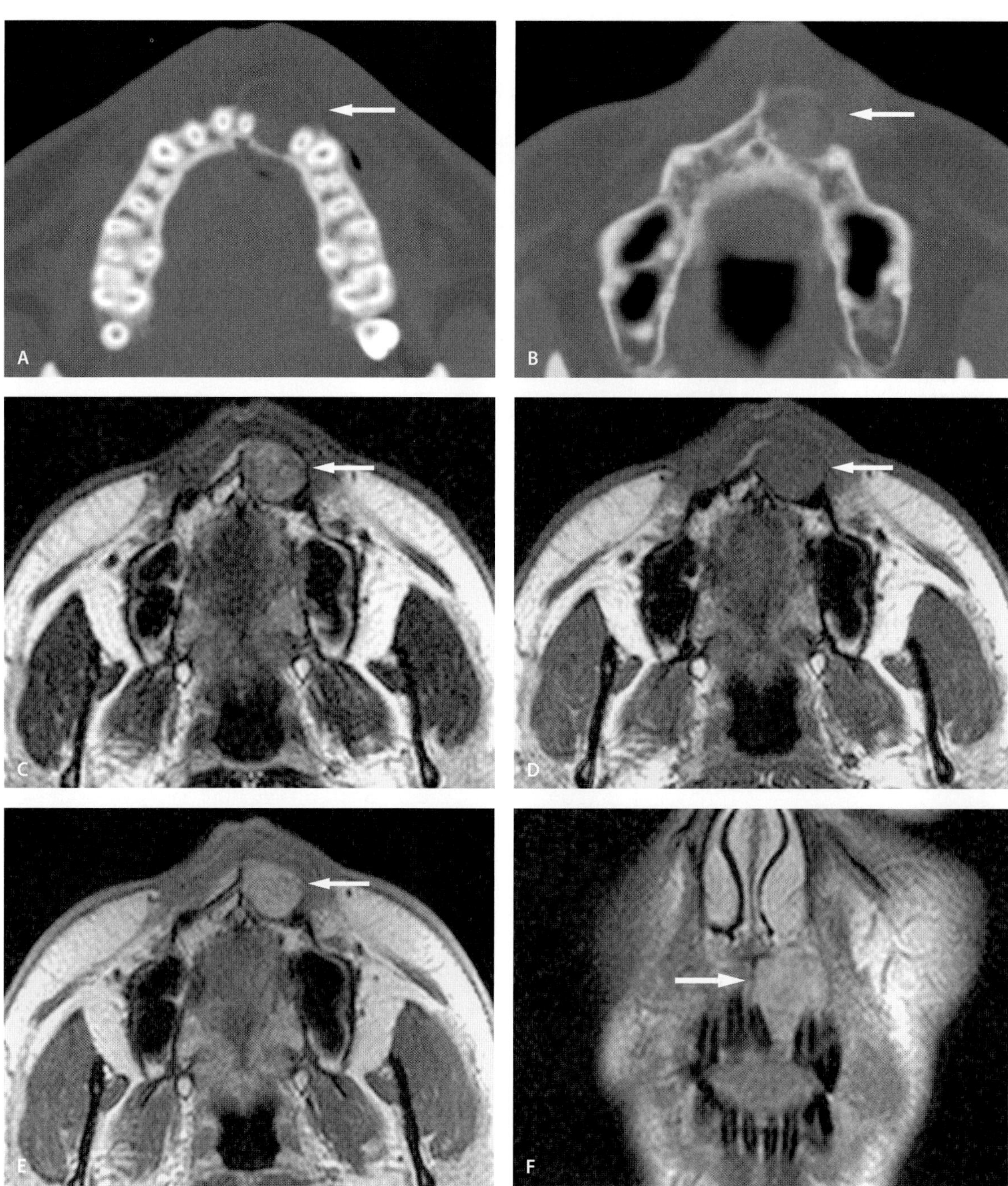

Figure 3.35

Giant cell granuloma, maxilla; 22-year-old male with recurrence (painless swelling) after previous surgery. **A** Axial CT image shows well-defined expansive process (*arrow*). **B** Axial CT image shows no sclerotic outline (*arrow*). **C** Axial T2-weighted MRI shows slightly heterogeneous intermediate signal (*arrow*). **D** Axial T1-weighted pre-Gd MRI shows homogeneous intermediate signal (*arrow*). **E** Axial T1-weighted post-Gd MRI shows homogeneous contrast enhancement (*arrow*). **F** Coronal T1-weighted post-Gd MRI shows contrast-enhanced and well-defined mass (*arrow*) displacing teeth

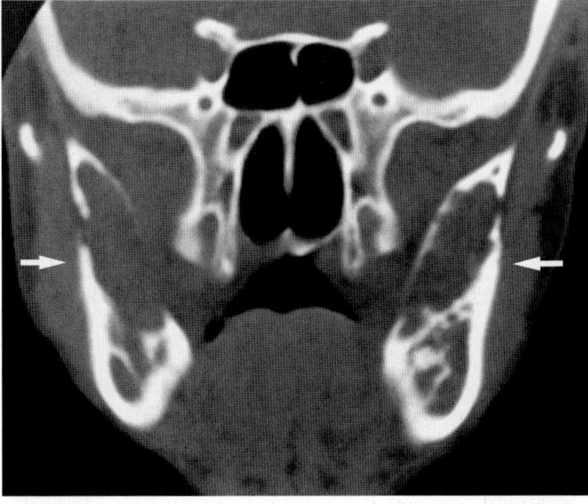

Figure 3.36

Giant cell granuloma, bilateral, mandible; patient with Noonan syndrome. Coronal CT image shows bilateral, expansive radiolucencies with cortical defects (*arrows*)

Langerhans Cell Histiocytosis

Synonyms: Langerhans cell granulomatosis, eosinophilic granuloma

Definition

Localized form of proliferation of Langerhans cells (histiocytes); a hemorrhagic lesion consisting of reticulum cells, multinucleated giant cells, eosinophils, lymphocytes, and plasma cells (inflammatory or reparative non-neoplastic nature).

Clinical Features

- Swelling, pain, tenderness
- Fever, general malaise
- Most common sites skull, mandible, spine, ribs, long bones
- Mandible more often than maxilla, posterior regions in particular
- Male predilection, 1–10 years of age
- Also generalized forms

Imaging Features

- Punched out bone destruction, sharply demarcated, not corticated
- No reactive sclerosis, but periosteal reaction
- Associated soft-tissue mass
- Usually no tooth resorption, may give a 'floating teeth' appearance

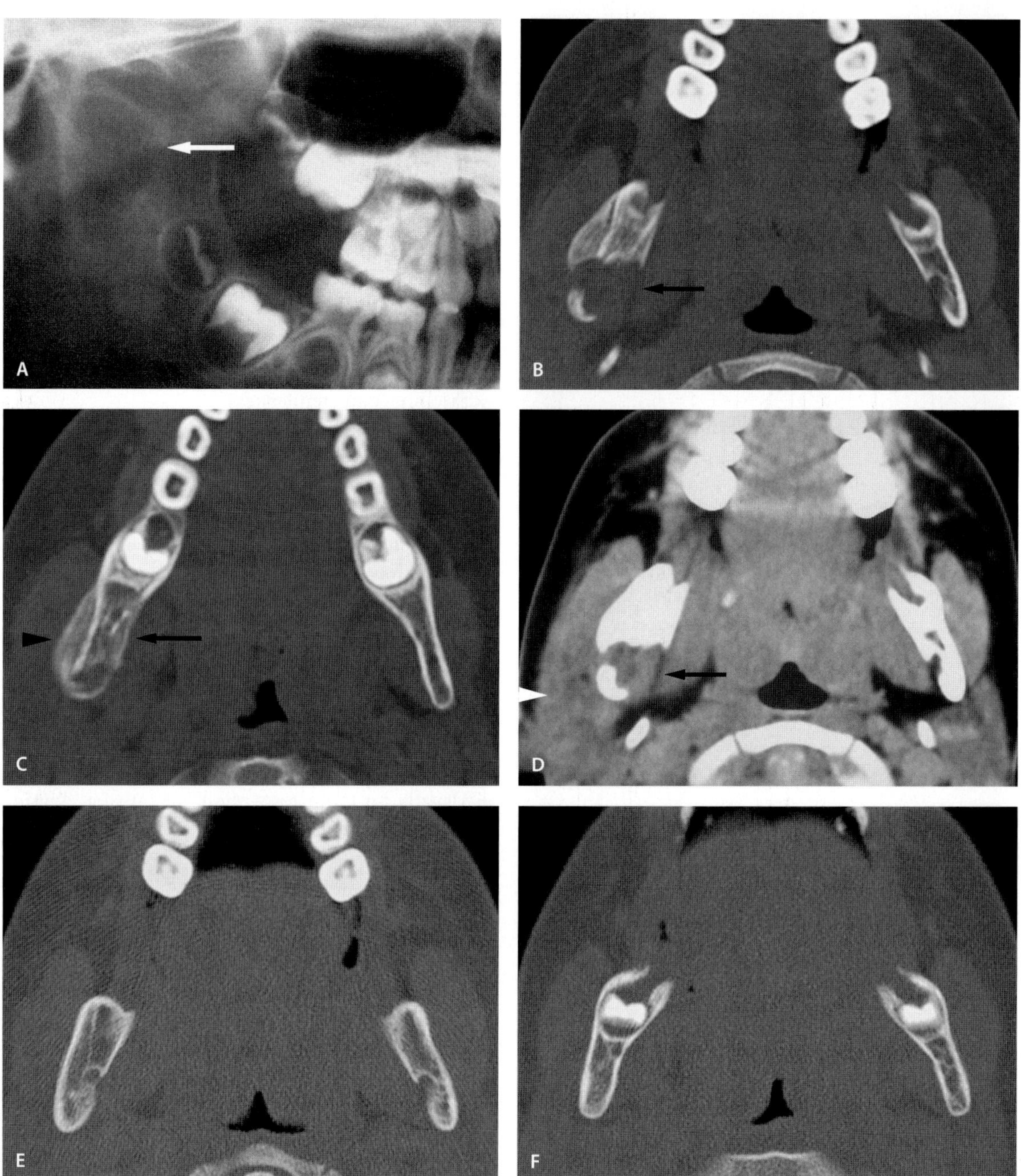

Figure 3.37

Eosinophilic granuloma, mandible; 4-year-old male with pain and swelling in the right cheek and jaw (ramus). **A** Panoramic view shows rather well-defined radiolucency (*arrow*). **B** Axial CT image shows punched-out bone destruction at level of mandibular foramina (*arrow*). **C** Axial CT image shows onion-skin periosteal reaction lingually (*arrow*) and buccally (*arrowhead*). **D** Axial CT image, soft-tissue window, shows well-defined soft-tissue mass lingually (*arrow*) and inflammatory infiltrate in connective tissue space laterally (*arrowhead*). **E** Axial CT image 1 year after treatment (surgery, cortisone medication) shows somewhat thickened right ramus and remnant of original buccal cortex at level of mandibular foramina, but otherwise normalized bone (*arrow*). **F** Axial CT image shows normalized bone also at another level (*arrow*)

Fibrous Dysplasia

Definition

Genetically based sporadic disease of bone that may affect single or multiple bones (monostotic or polyostotic). Fibrous dysplasia occurring in multiple adjacent craniofacial bones is regarded as monostotic (craniofacial fibrous dysplasia). May be part of the McCune-Albright syndrome (WHO).

Non-neoplastic, self-limiting but non-capsulated lesion occurring mainly in young subjects, showing replacement of normal bone by cellular tissue containing islands or trabeculae of metaplastic bone.

Clinical Features

- Monostotic most common (70–80%, femur, ribs)
- Craniofacial bones up to 25% of monostotic forms
- Maxilla, lateral region in particular, more frequent than mandible
- Painless swelling, jaw asymmetry
- Second and third decades
- No sex predilection
- McCune-Albright syndrome; polyostotic, café-au-lait spots

Imaging Features

- Radiolucency
- Mixture of radiolucency and radiopacity
- Radiopacity; ground-glass appearance
- Unilocular or multilocular
- Border poorly defined; blend into normal bone, but may be more well defined (and thus difficult to distinguish from ossifying fibroma; same histopathology)
- Usually expanded bone
- May displace teeth, walls of nasal cavity, paranasal sinuses, orbits
- Mandibular canal may be displaced cranially
- Tooth resorption rare
- T1-weighted MRI: intermediate signal
- T2-weighted MRI and STIR: heterogeneous low signal
- T1-weighted MRI: contrast enhancement

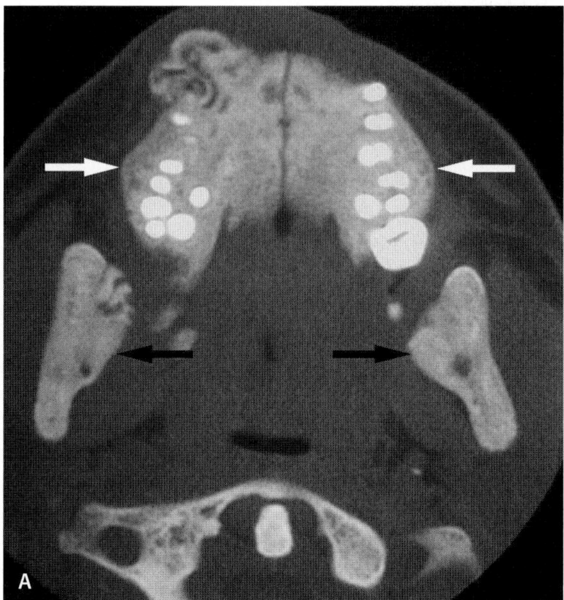

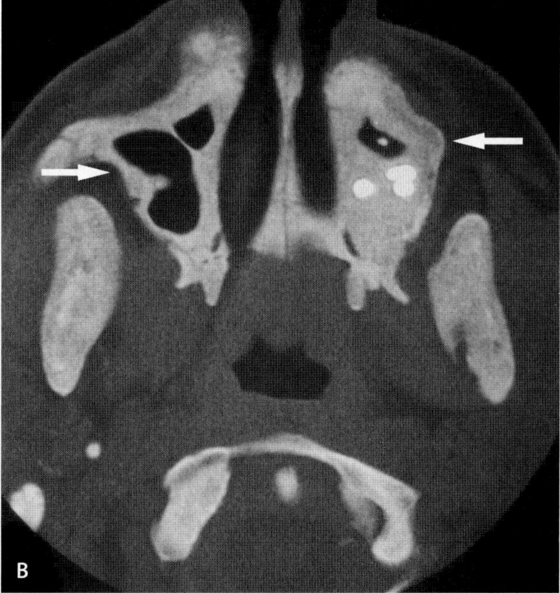

Figure 3.38

Fibrous dysplasia, maxilla and mandible; 21-year-old male with chronic renal failure, end-stage, and several months history of slowly enlarging maxillary mass. **A** Axial CT image shows maxilla and mandible with bilateral ground-glass appearance (*arrows*). **B** Axial CT image shows maxillary sinus involvement bilaterally (*arrows*)

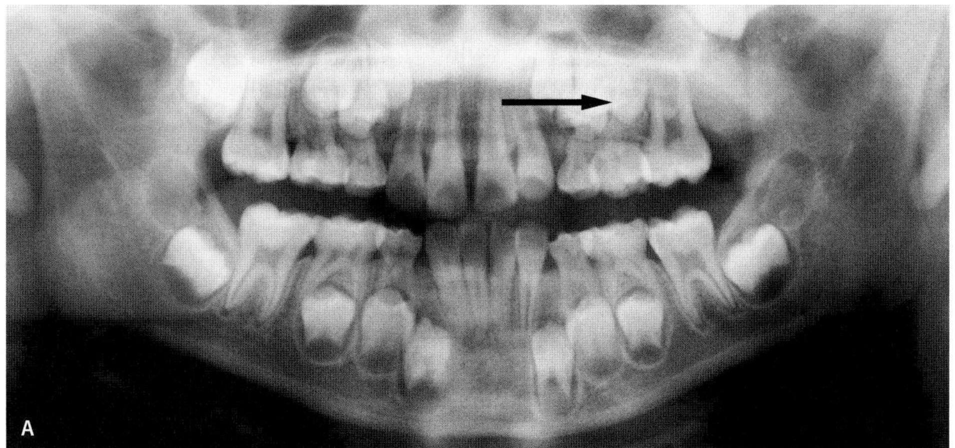

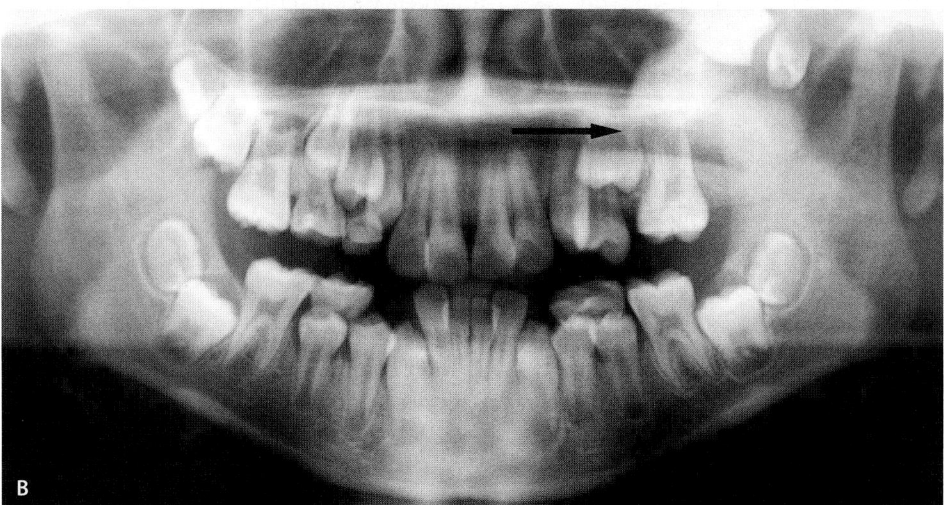

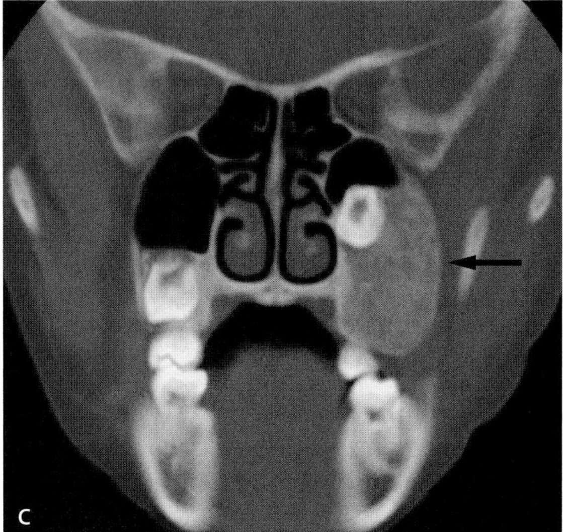

Figure 3.39

Fibrous dysplasia, maxilla; 10-year-old male with unilateral painless swelling of maxilla. **A** Panoramic view shows radiopaque expansive process (*arrow*) with displaced second molar. **B** Panoramic view at 2.5-year follow-up shows progression of process (*arrow*). **C** Coronal CT image shows well-defined process with typical ground-glass appearance (*arrow*); this could have been diagnosed as an ossifying fibroma

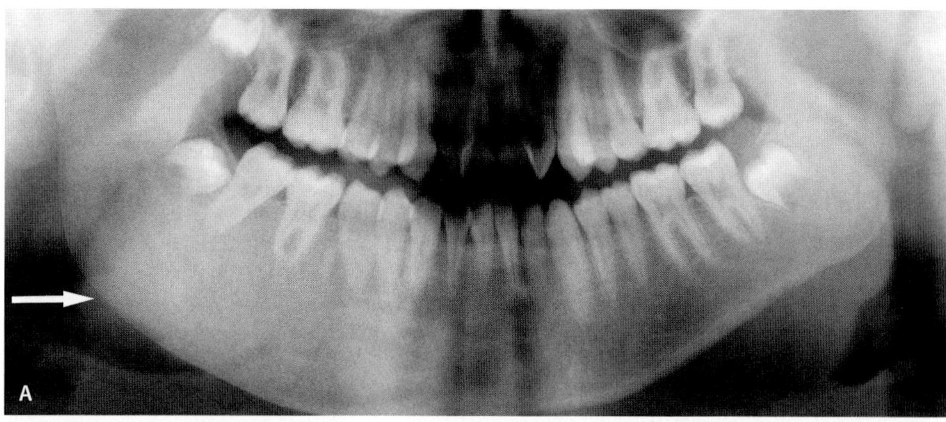

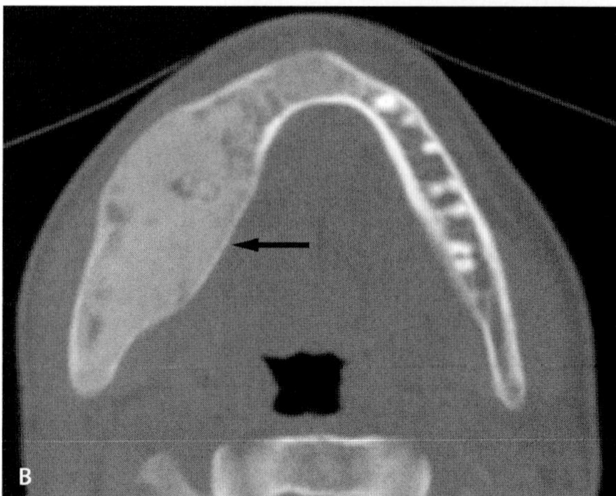

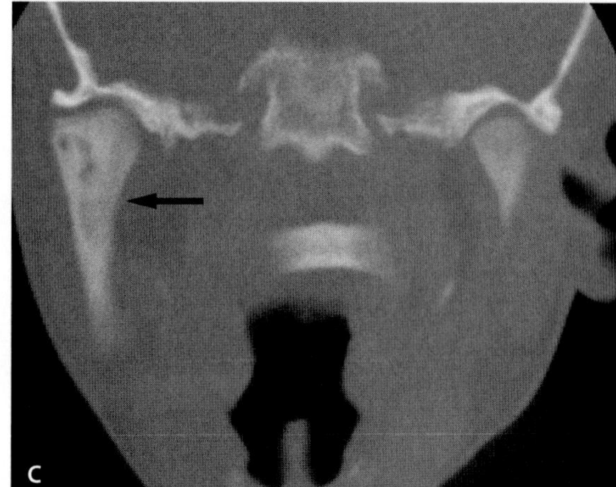

Figure 3.40

Fibrous dysplasia, mandible; 14-year-old male with painless facial asymmetry. A Panoramic view shows enlarged mandible with ground-glass appearance (*arrow*). B Axial CT image shows expanded mandible with ground-glass appearance (*arrow*). C Coronal CT image shows process involving mandibular collum and condyle (*arrow*). D Coronal CT image shows process involving coronoid process (*arrow*)

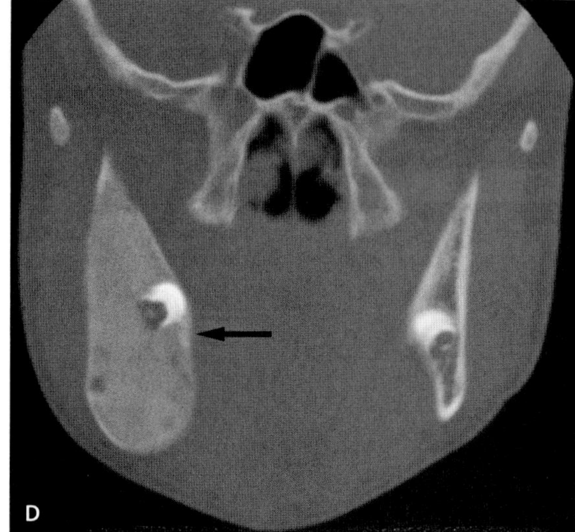

Cherubism

Definition

Autosomal dominant inherited disease characterized by a symmetrical distension of the jaw, often leading to a typical facial expression. The histology is indistinguishable from giant cell granuloma (WHO)

Clinical Features

- Familial disease affecting 100% of males and up to 70% of females
- Diagnosis often made in early childhood or preadolescence, depending on severity
- Lesions regress with age
- Usually mandible, posterior regions, but all four jaw quadrants may be affected
- Symmetric painless swellings
- Tooth displacement and loosening
- Delayed tooth eruption

Imaging Features

- Well-delineated, bilateral multilocular radiolucencies; soap-bubble appearance
- Thin corticated outline, may be perforated
- More sclerotic abnormalities with increasing age

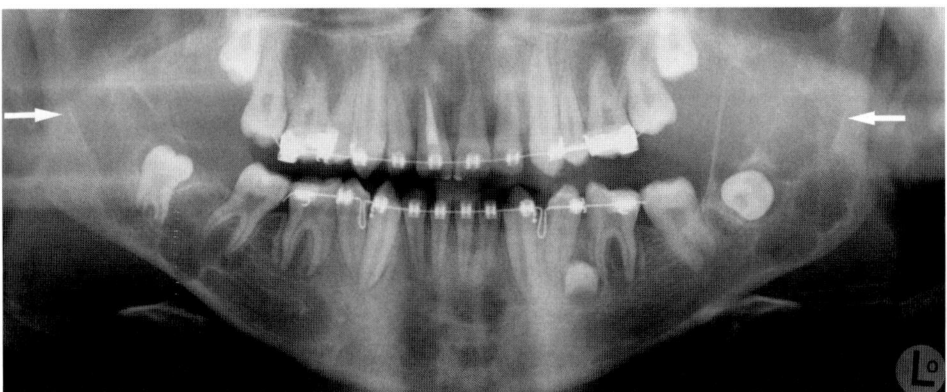

Figure 3.41

Cherubism (familiar fibrous jaw dysplasia); 13-year-old male with incidental finding at orthodontic consultation. Panoramic view shows bilateral multilocular radiolucencies with sclerotic border in mandible (*arrows*)

Suggested Reading

Asaumi J-I, Matsuzaki H, Hisatomi M, Konouchi H, Shigehara H, Kishi K (2002) Application of dynamic MRI to differentiating odontogenic myxomas from ameloblastomas. Eur J Radiol 43:37–41

Auclair PL, Cuenin P, Kratochvil FJ, Slater LJ, Ellis GL (1988) A clinical and histomorphologic comparison of the central giant cell granuloma and the giant cell tumor. Oral Surg Oral Med Oral Pathol 66:197–208

Barnes L, Eveson JW, Reichart P, Sidransky D (eds) (2005) World Health Organization Classification of Tumours. Pathology and genetics of head and neck tumours. IARC Press, Lyon

Beltran J, Simon DC, Levy M, Herman L, Weis L, Mueller CF (1986) Aneurysmal bone cysts: MR imaging at 1.5 T Radiology 158:689–690

Cottalorda J, Kohler R, Sales de Gauzy J, Chotel F, Mazda K, Lefort G, Louahem D, Bourelle S, Dimeglio A (2004) Epidemiology of aneurysmal bone cyst in children: a multicenter study and literature review. J Pediatr Orthop B 13:389–394

DelBalso AM, Werning JT (1986) The role of computed tomography in the evaluation of cemento-osseous lesions. Oral Surg Oral Med Oral Pathol 62:354–357

Eriksson L, Hansson LG, Akesson L, Stahlberg F (2001) Simple bone cyst: a discrepancy between magnetic resonance and surgical observations. Oral Surg Oral Med Oral Pathol Oral Radiol Endod 92:694–698

Eversole LR, Merrell PM, Strub D (1985) Radiographic characteristics of central ossifying fibroma. Oral Surg Oral Med Oral Pathol 59:522–527

Farman AG, Nortje C, Wood RE (1993) Benign tumors of the jaws. In: Oral and maxillofacial diagnostic imaging. Mosby, St. Louis, pp 239–279

Farman AG, Nortje C, Wood RE (1993) Fibro-osseous lesions. In: Oral and maxillofacial diagnostic imaging. Mosby, St. Louis, pp 316–330

Gardner DG, Heikinheimo K, Shear M, Philipsen HP, Coleman H (2005) Ameloblastomas. In: Barnes L, Eveson JW, Reichart P, Sidransky D (eds). World Health Organization Classification of Tumours. Pathology and genetics of head and neck tumours. 6. Odontogenic tumours. IARC Press, Lyon, p 296

Gordon SC, MacIntosh RB, Wesley RKA (2001) A review of osteoblastoma and case report of metachronous osteoblastoma and unicystic ameloblastoma. Oral Surg Oral Pathol Oral Med Oral Radiol Endod 91:570–575

Hisatomi M, Asaumi J-I, Konouchi H, Shigehara H, Yanagi Y, Kishi K (2003) MR imaging of epithelial cysts of the oral and maxillofacial region. Eur J Radiol 48:178–182

Jundt G (2005) Fibrous dysplasia. Central giant cell lesion/granuloma. Cherubism. Aneurysmal bone cyst. Simple bone cyst. In: Barnes L, Eveson JW, Reichart P, Sidransky D (eds). World Health Organization Classification of Tumours. Pathology and genetics of head and neck tumours. 6. Odontogenic tumours. IARC Press, Lyon, pp 321, 324, 325, 326, 327

Kaffe I, Naor H, Calderon S, Buchner A (1999) Radiological and clinical features of aneurysmal bone cysts of the jaws. Dentomaxillofac Radiol 28:167–172

Kaugars G (1991) Odontogenic tumors. In: Miles DA, Van Dis M, Kaugars GE, Lovas JGL (eds) Oral and maxillofacial radiology. Radiologic/pathologic correlations. Saunders, Philadelphia, pp 51–95

Kaugars G (1991) Benign fibro-osseous lesions. In: Miles DA, Van Dis M, Kaugars GE, Lovas JGL (eds) Oral and maxillofacial radiology. Radiologic/pathologic correlations. Saunders, Philadelphia, pp 125–154

Knutsen BM, Larheim TA, Johannessen S, Hillestad J, Solheim T, Koppang HS (2002) Recurrent conventional cemento-ossifying fibroma of the mandible. Dentomaxillofac Radiol 31:65–68

Kramer IRH, Pindborg JJ, Shear M (1992) World Health Organisation International Histological Classification of Tumours. Histological typing of odontogenic tumours, 2nd edn. Springer, Berlin, pp 11–33

MacDonald-Jankowski DS (2004) Fibro-osseous lesions of the face and jaws (review). Clin Radiol 59:11–25

Matsumura S, Murakami S, Kakimoto N, Furukawa S, Kishino M Ishida T, Fuchihata H (1998) Histopathologic and radiographic findings of the simple bone cyst. Oral Surg Oral Med Oral Pathol Oral Radiol Endod 85:619–625

Matsuura S, Tahara T, Ro T, Masumi T, Kasuya H, Yokota T (1999) Aneurysmal cyst of the coronoid process of the mandible. Dentomaxillofac Radiol 28:324–326

Matsuzaka K, Shimono M, Uchiyama T, Noma H, Inoue T (2002) Lesions related to the formation of bone, cartilage or cementum arising in the oral area: a statistical study and review of the literature. Bull Tokyo Dent Coll 43:173–180

McLeod RA, Dahlin DC, Beabout JW (1976) The spectrum of osteoblastoma. AJR Am J Roentgenol 126:321–325

Miles D (1991) Vascular and reactive lesions. In: Miles DA, Van Dis M, Kaugars GE, Lovas JGL (eds) Oral and maxillofacial radiology. Radiologic/pathologic correlations. Saunders, Philadelphia, pp 155–186

Minami M, Kaneda T, Ozawa K, Yamamoto H, Itai Y, Ozawa M, Yoshikawa K, Sasaki Y (1996) Cystic lesions of the maxillomandibular region: MR imaging distinction odontogenic keratocysts and ameloblastomas from other cysts. AJR Am J Roentgenol 166:943–949

Minami M, Kaneda T, Yamamoto H, Ozawa K, Itai Y, Ozawa M, Yoshikawa K, Sasaki Y (1992) Ameloblastoma in the maxillomandibular region: MR imaging. Radiology 184:389–393

Perdigao PF, Silva EC, Sakurai E, Soares de Araujo N, Gomez RS (2003) Idiopathic bone cavity: a clinical, radiographic, and histological study. Br J Oral Maxillofac Surg 41:407–409

Philipsen HP, Reichart PA, Sciubba JJ, van der Waal I, Buchner A, Odell EW (2005) Odontogenic fibroma/myxoma. In: Barnes L, Eveson JW, Reichart P, Sidransky D (eds). World Health Organization Classification of Tumours. Pathology and genetics of head and neck tumours. 6. Odontogenic tumours. IARC Press, Lyon, p 316

Praetorius F, Piattelli A (2005) Odontoma, compound type. In: Barnes L, Eveson JW, Reichart P, Sidransky D (eds). World Health Organization Classification of Tumours. Pathology and genetics of head and neck tumours. 6. Odontogenic tumours. IARC Press, Lyon, p 311

Resnick D (1996) Bone and joint imaging, 2nd edn. Saunders, Philadelphia, pp 615, 616, 998

Schajowicz F (1993) World Health Organisation. Histological typing of bone tumors, 2nd edn. Springer, Berlin, p 7

Shear M, Philipsen HP (2005) Keratocystic odontogenic tumour. In: Barnes L, Eveson JW, Reichart P, Sidransky D (eds). World Health Organization Classification of Tumours. Pathology and genetics of head and neck tumours. 6. Odontogenic tumours. IARC Press, Lyon, p 306

Slootweg PJ, El Mofty S (2005) Ossifying fibroma. In: Barnes L, Eveson JW, Reichart P, Sidransky D (eds). World Health Organization Classification of Tumours. Pathology and genetics of head and neck tumours. 6. Odontogenic tumours. IARC Press, Lyon, p 319

Slootweg PJ, Takeda Y, Tomich CE, Praetorius F, Piattelli A (2005) Odontoma, complex type. In: Barnes L, Eveson JW, Reichart P, Sidransky D (eds). World Health Organization Classification of Tumours. Pathology and genetics of head and neck tumours. 6. Odontogenic tumours. IARC Press, Lyon, p 310

Su L, Weathers DR, Waldron CA (1997) Distinguishing features of focal cemento-osseous dysplasia and cemento-ossifying fibroma. II: A clinical and radiologic spectrum of 316 cases. Oral Surg Oral Med Oral Pathol Oral Radiol Endod 84:540–549

Sullivan RJ, Meyer JS, Dormans JP, Davidson RS (1999) Diagnosing aneurysmal and unicameral bone cysts with magnetic resonance imaging. Clin Orthop 366:186–190

Weber AL, Kaneda T, Scrivani SJ, Aziz S (2003) Jaw: cysts, tumors, and non-tumorous lesions. In: Som PM, Curtin HD (eds) Head and neck imaging, 4th edn. Mosby, St. Louis, pp 930–994

White SW, Pharoah MJ (2004) Benign tumors of the jaws. In: Oral radiology. Principles and interpretation, 5th edn. Saunders, Philadelphia, pp 410–457

White SW, Pharoah MJ (2004) Diseases of bone manifested in the jaws. In: Oral radiology. Principles and interpretation, 5th edn. Saunders, Philadelphia, pp 485–515

Yoshiura K, Higuchi Y, Ariji Y, Shinohara M, Yuasa K, Nakayama E, Ban S, Kanda S (1994) Increased attenuation in odontogenic keratocysts with computed tomography: a new finding. Dentomaxillofac Radiol 23:138–142

Malignant Tumors in the Jaws

In collaboration with H.-J. Smith · G. Støre

Introduction

Malignant tumors of the jaws are relatively uncommon in most parts of the world. When they occur they should be examined with advanced imaging modalities to achieve the most precise diagnosis and hence the best possible treatment. This chapter is divided into tumors which are bone-destructive and in those which are bone-destructive and bone-productive to emphasize their principal difference in imaging appearance. The listing of malignant tumors is rather representative but far from complete.

Many cases in this chapter include a panoramic view and a few cases even intraoral views because specialists and practitioners in the dental field are familiar with conventional (film or digital) jaw radiography. In selected patients, follow-up images, clinical photos and surgical specimens are shown

Bone-destructive Tumors

Squamous Cell Carcinoma

Synonyms: Epidermoid carcinoma

Definition

Malignant epithelial neoplasm exhibiting squamous differentiation as characterized by formation of keratin and/or presence of intercellular bridges (WHO).

Clinical Features

- Most common malignancy of oral cavity
- 2–4% of all malignancies in the US and Europe
- Much higher prevalence in certain countries (due to habits such as inverse smoking)
- Males more frequent than females
- Older age groups (50 years and older), but also younger than 30 years
- Most frequent in tongue, floor of mouth, mandibular gingiva; retromolar trigone, and anterior tonsillar pillar, soft palate
- Erythroplakia developing in leukoplakia
- Ulceration surrounded by indurated or sharply defined border
- Predominantly white and warty growth
- Advanced stage: pain, paresthesia, pathologic fracture

Imaging Features

- Soft-tissue mass
- Bone radiolucency, secondary invasion of bone
- Border of bone destruction ill-defined
- Bone invasion frequent in gingival mandibular cancers, generally considered to be about 50%, but up to 85% reported in upper jaw; maxillary sinus frequently involved
- Floating teeth; tooth resorption uncommon
- Advanced stage: pathologic fracture
- T1-weighted MRI: intermediate-low signal
- T2-weighted and STIR MRI: high signal
- T1-weighted MRI: contrast enhancement

Most carcinomas found in jaws have invaded from lesions of the oral cavity. However, primary intraosseous carcinoma may arise within the jaw 'having no initial connection with oral mucosa, and presumably developing from residues of odontogenic epithelium' (WHO).

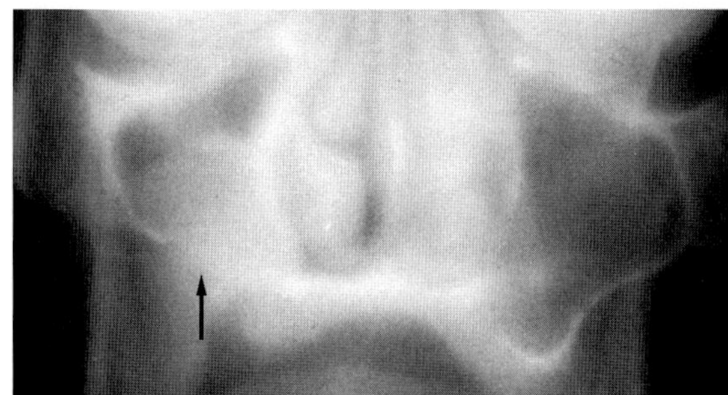

Figure 4.1

Squamous cell carcinoma, maxilla; 65-year-old female with ulcer beneath upper denture. Coronal tomogram shows destruction of alveolar bone with tumor growth into maxillary sinus (arrow)

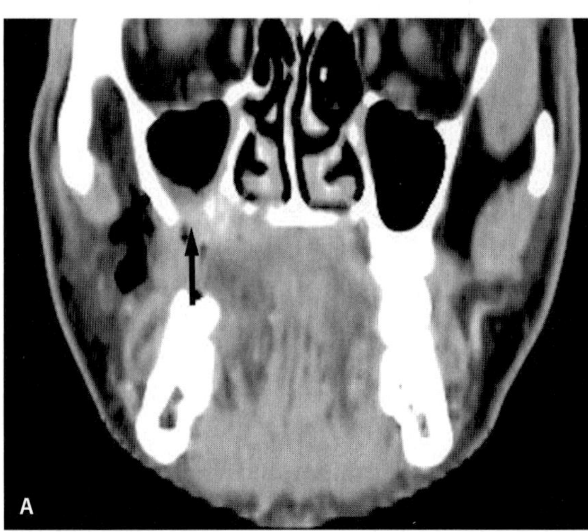

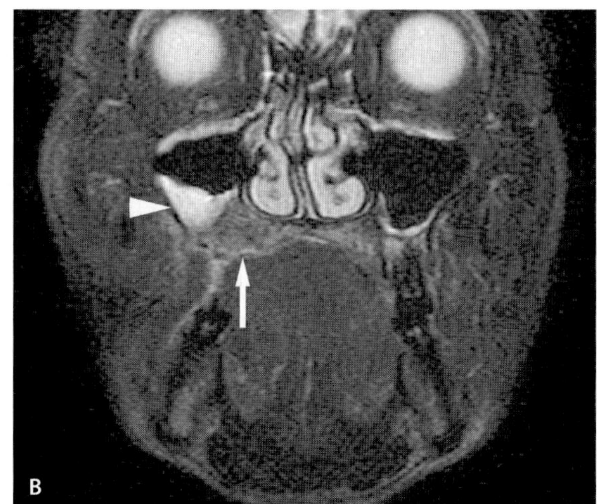

Figure 4.2

Squamous cell carcinoma, maxilla; 70-year-old female with some bleeding from tender soft tissue mass of right gingival mucosa. **A** Coronal CT image shows destruction of maxillary sinus delineation (arrow) and soft tissue mass. **B** Coronal T2-weighted fat suppressed MRI shows soft tissue tumor invading maxillary sinus (arrow) and high signal mucosal thickening (arrow head). (Courtesy of Dr N Kakimoto, Osaka University Graduate School of Dentistry)

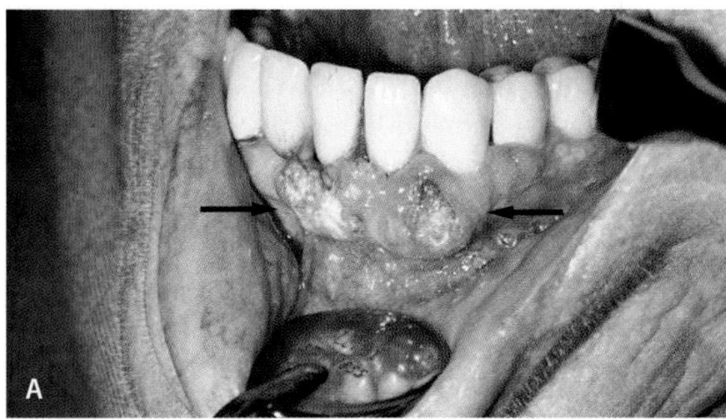

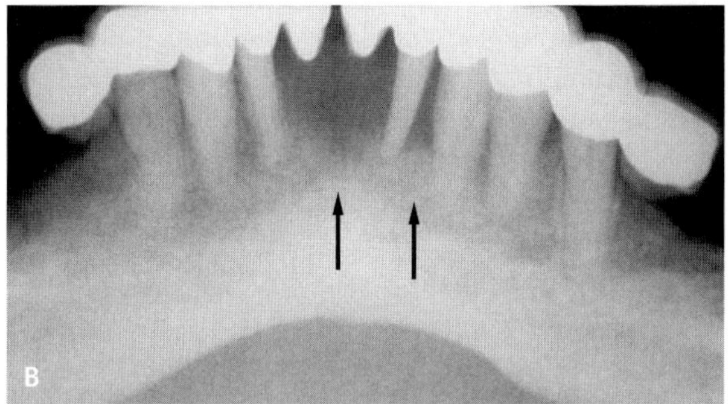

Figure 4.3

Squamous cell carcinoma, mandible; 70-year-old female with previous oral leukoplakia that developed erythroplakia and soreness. **A** Clinical photograph shows leukoplakia that transformed to gingival cancer (*arrows*). **B** Intraoral panoramic view shows diffuse bone destruction (*arrows*) due to tumor infiltration

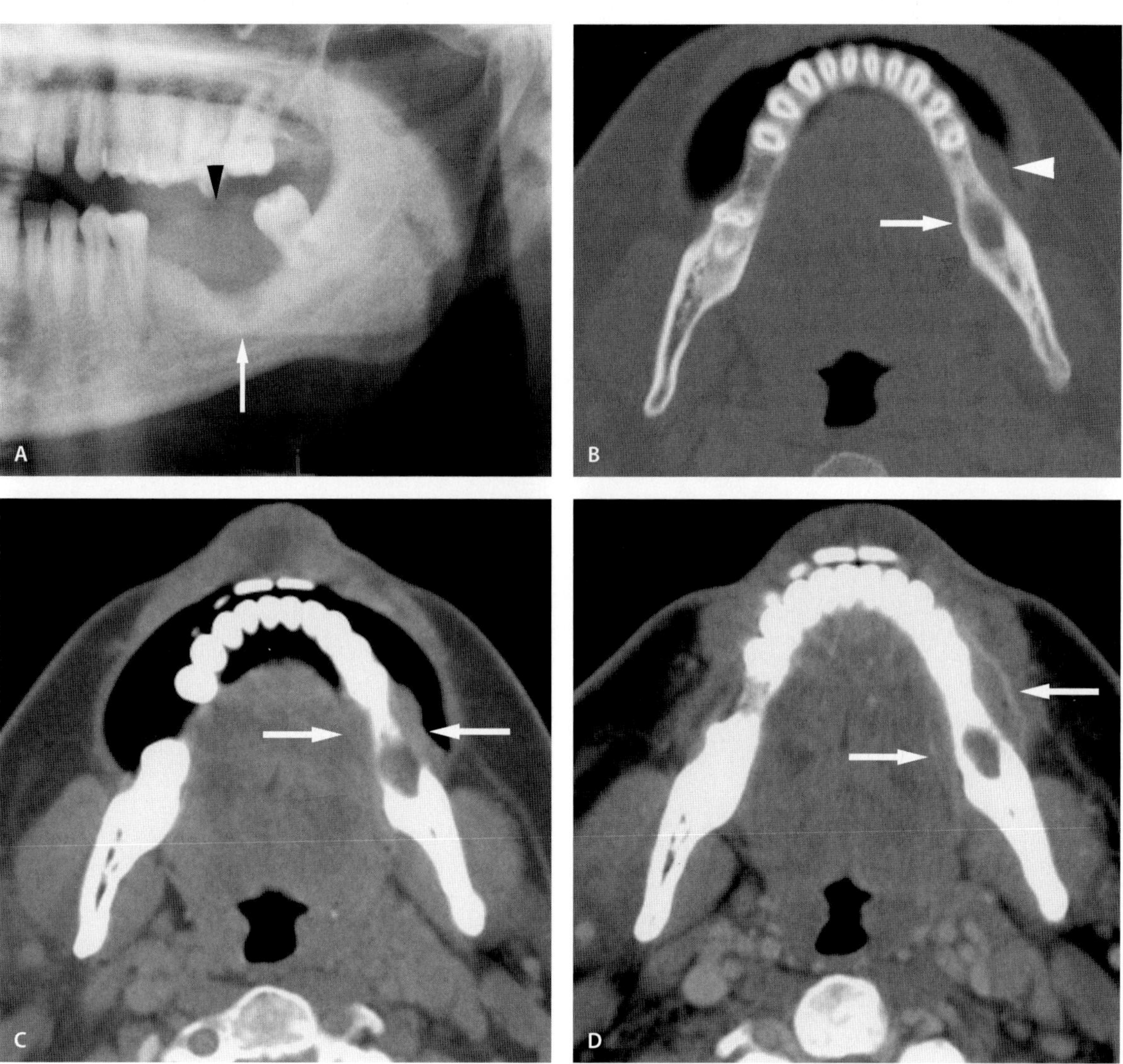

Figure 4.4

Squamous cell carcinoma, mandible; 37-year-old male with painless gingival soft-tissue swelling. **A** Panoramic view shows diffuse bone destruction (*arrow*) and soft-tissue mass (*arrowhead*). **B** Axial CT image with cheek blowing shows bone destruction (*arrow*) and soft-tissue mass (*arrowhead*) adherent to mandible. **C** Axial CT image, soft-tissue window, with cheek blowing shows soft-tissue mass (*arrows*) adherent to mandible. **D** Axial contrast-enhanced CT image, soft-tissue window, shows contrast-enhanced soft-tissue mass (*arrows*)

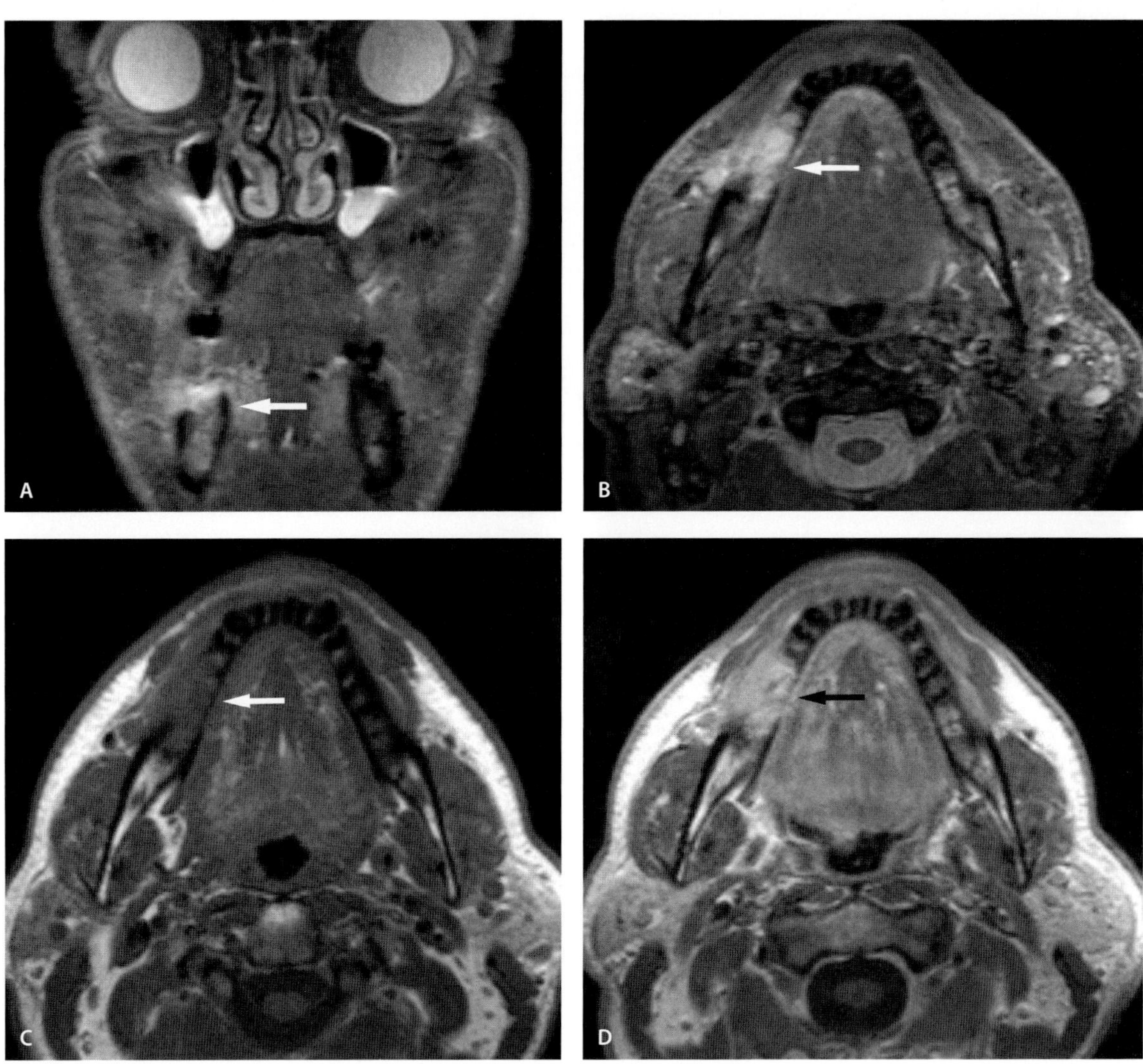

Figure 4.5

Squamous cell carcinoma, mandible; 55-year old male with oral leukoplakia several locations in oral cavity for many years, then developed pain and soreness, and cancer in tooth socket after molar extraction (panoramic view and CT were negative). A Coronal STIR MRI shows small area of high signal in cranial part of alveolar bone and gingival tissue (*arrow*). B Axial STIR MRI shows high signal in alveolar bone and buccally (*arrow*). C Axial T1-weighted pre-Gd MRI shows reduced signal in bone marrow (*arrow*). D Axial T1-weighted post-Gd MRI shows contrast enhancement in bone marrow and buccal mass (*arrow*)

Mucoepidermoid Carcinoma

Definition

Tumor characterized by presence of squamous cells, mucus-producing cells, and cells of intermediate type (WHO).

Malignant epithelial neoplasm arising in bone likely originating from odontogenic epithelium residues or from cyst lining.

Clinical Features

- Swelling with or without pain, or incidental finding at routine dental radiography
- Mandible, posterior regions, more frequent than maxilla
- Females more frequent than males (unlike most oral carcinomas)
- Fourth and fifth decades, but may occur in any age group
- Spread to regional lymph nodes in less than 10% and only occasionally, metastasis

Imaging Features

- Unilocular or multilocular radiolucency
- Border well defined and sclerotic
- Cortical plates as well as lower mandibular border may be intact
- May be expansive and resembles ameloblastoma or odontogenic cyst; thus predominantly benign appearance
- Frequently associated with cyst and/or impacted tooth (30–50%)
- T1-weighted MRI: intermediate–low signal
- T2-weighted and STIR MRI: high signal
- T1-weighted post-Gd MRI: predominantly none; only contrast enhancement in thin peripheral rim of cyst and areas of solid tumor

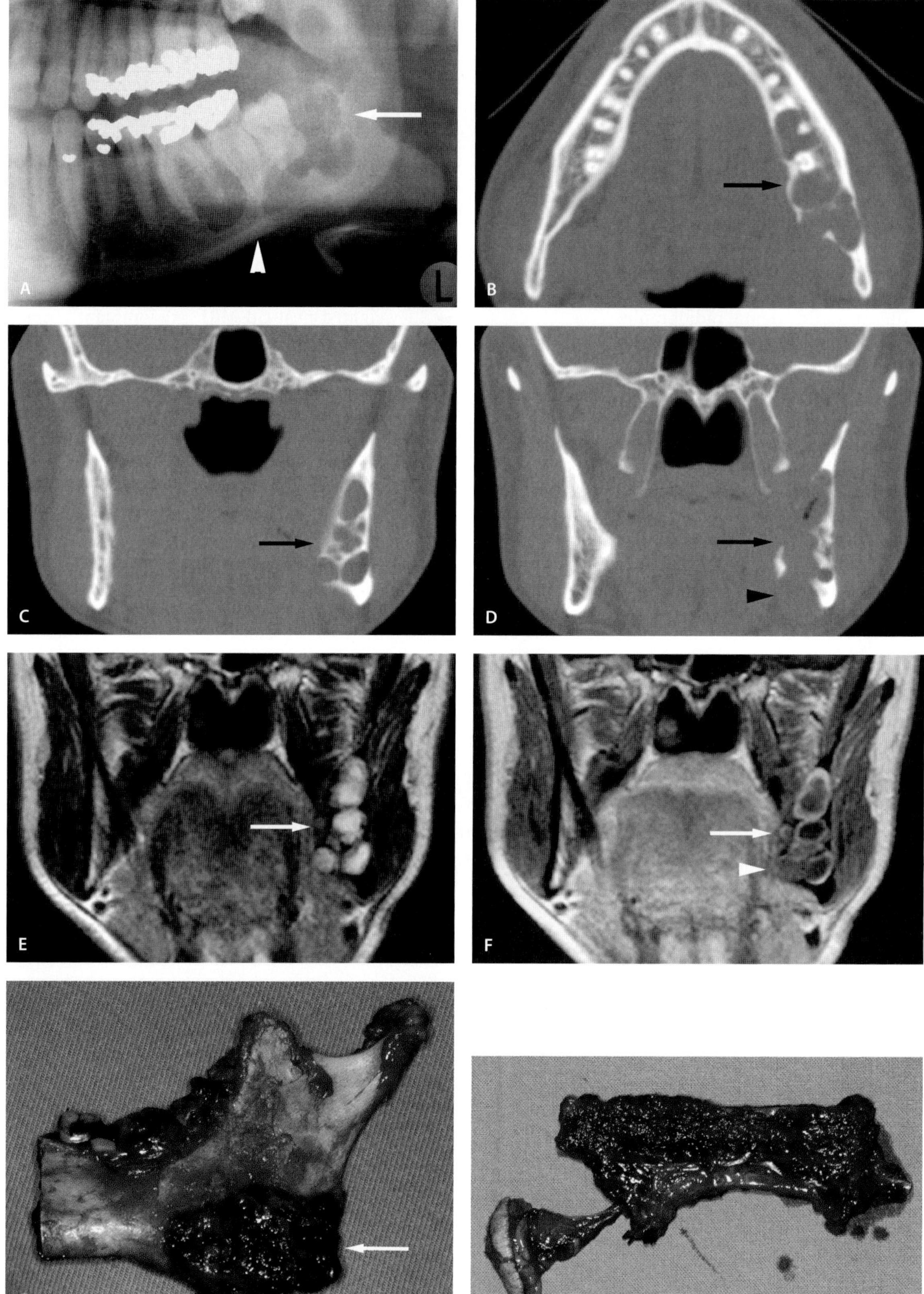
A
L
B
C
D
E
F
G
H

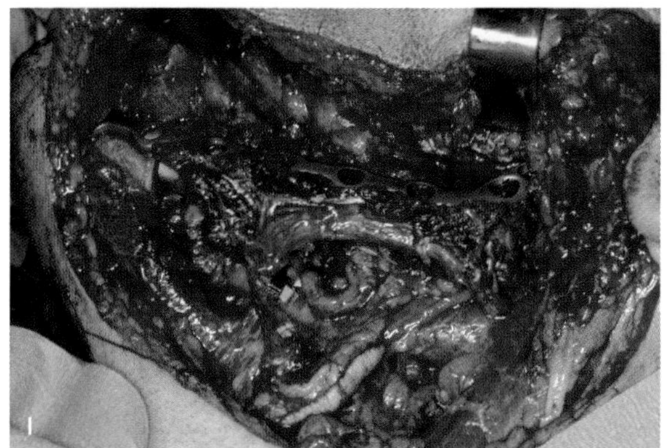

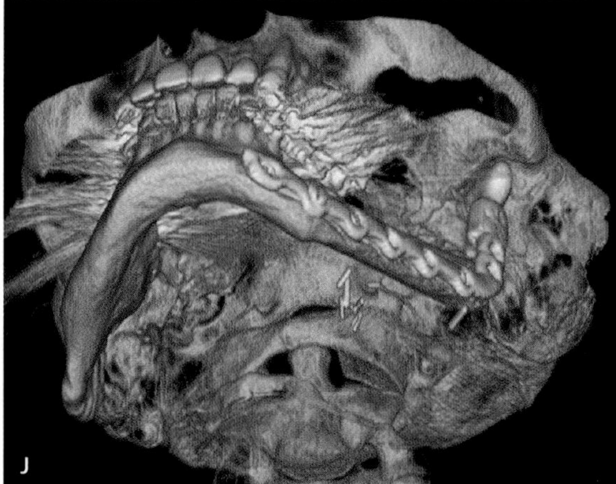

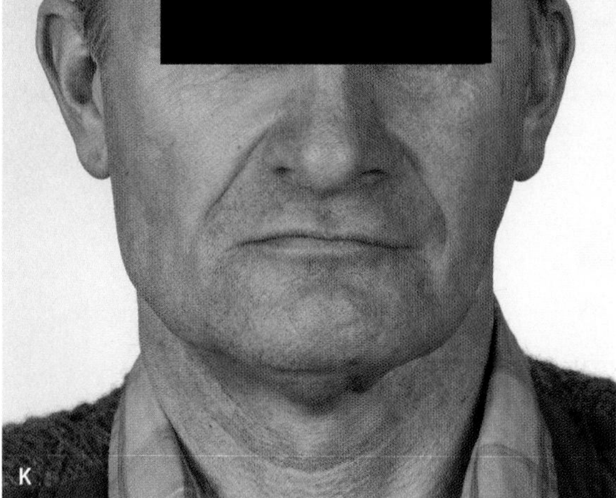

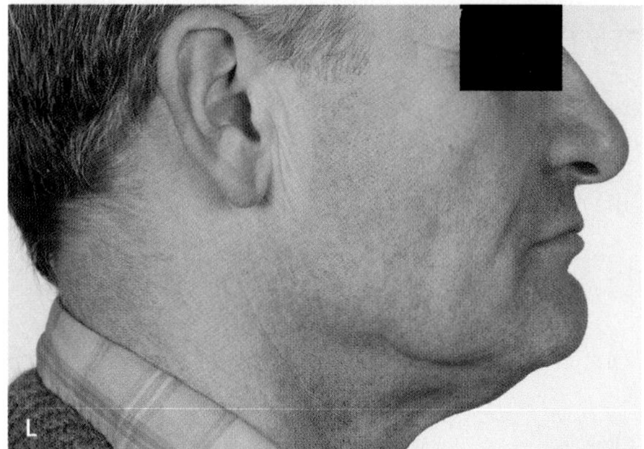

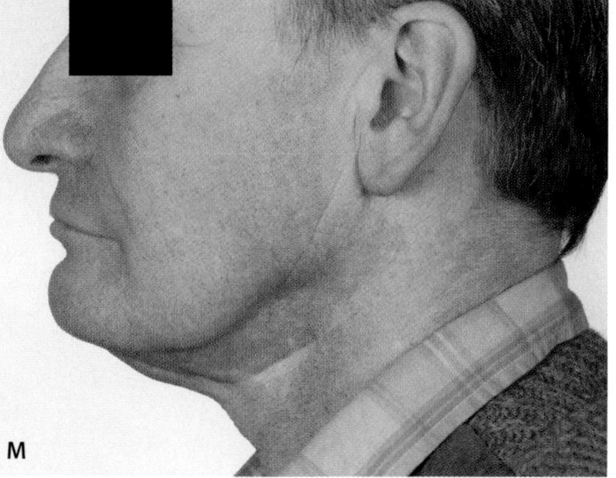

Figure 4.6

Mucoepidermoid carcinoma, mandible; 46-year-old male with incidental finding at routine dental radiography of impacted wisdom teeth. **A** Panoramic view shows multilocular radiolucency (*arrows*) with intact mandibular border (*arrowhead*), and impacted third molar. **B** Axial CT image shows multilocular radiolucency (*arrow*) with defect in lingual cortical bone. **C** Coronal CT image shows multilocular radiolucency (*arrow*). **D** Coronal CT image shows bone destruction lingually (*arrow*); note in particular at lower mandibular border (*arrowhead*). **E** Coronal T2-weighted MRI shows high signal in multilocular process (*arrow*). **F** Coronal T1-weighted post-Gd MRI shows contrast enhancement only in thin peripheral rim (*arrow*) except in a more solid component lingually at lower mandibular border (*arrowhead*). **G** Surgical specimen shows tumor lingually (*arrow*). **H** Vascular fibula graft. **I** Fibula graft in situ with titanium plate (**G**, **H**, and **I** courtesy of Dr. T. Bjornland, Rikshospitalet University Hospital, Oslo, Norway). **J** 3D CT image 5 years postoperatively shows excellent healing of graft and no tumor recurrence. **K**, **L**, and **M** Clinical photos en face, right and left (operated) side, respectively, 5 years after surgery show completely rehabilitated patient with normal mandibular function (mouth opening capacity more than 40 mm)

Adenoid Cystic Carcinoma

Definition

Infiltrative malignant tumor having various histologic features with three growth patterns: glandular (cribriform), tubular or solid. Tumor cells are of two types: duct-lining cells and myoepithelial cells. Perineural or perivascular spread without stromal reaction is very characteristic. All structural types of adenoid cystic carcinoma can be associated in same tumor (WHO).

Clinical Features

- Most commonly seen (although rare) in minor salivary glands of head and neck, usually palate
- Mostly as a painless mass, slowly growing
- Unlike most carcinomas, seldom metastasizes to regional lymph nodes
- Lung most common site of metastasis
- Perineural spread in more than 50%; frequent distant metastasis
- High survival rate after 5 years, low after 15 years
- Slight female predominance
- Fourth to sixth decades

Imaging Features

- Soft-tissue mass
- Radiolucency
- Border of bone destruction ill-defined
- Widened foramina such as major palatine foramen
- Perineural invasion of major nerves characteristically found; skip lesions

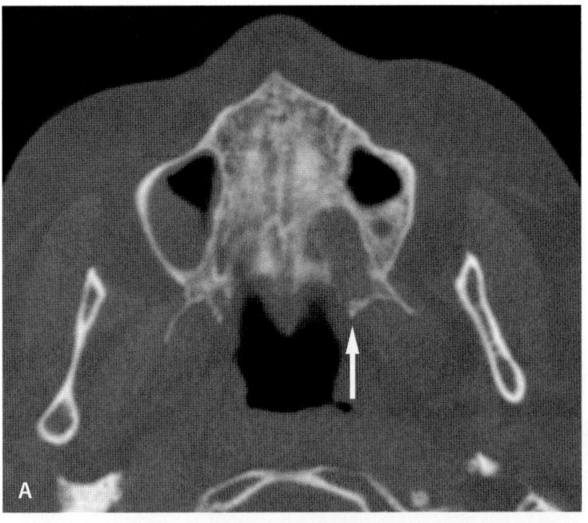

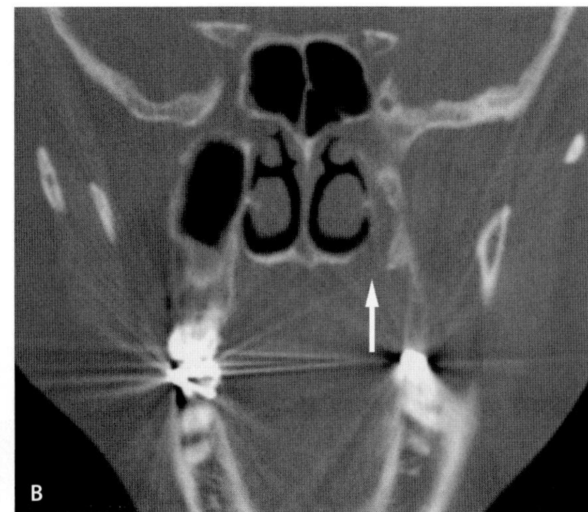

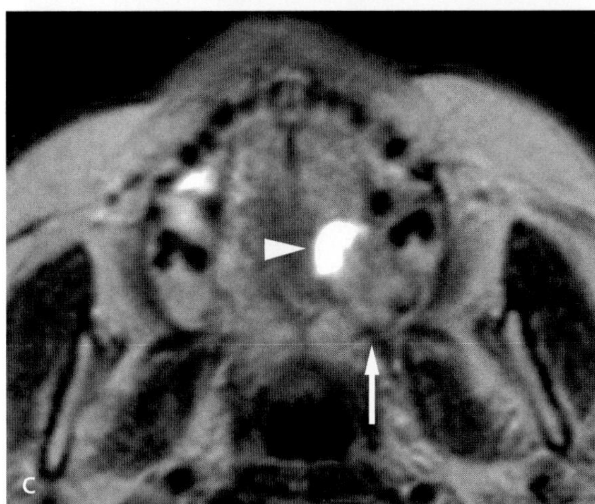

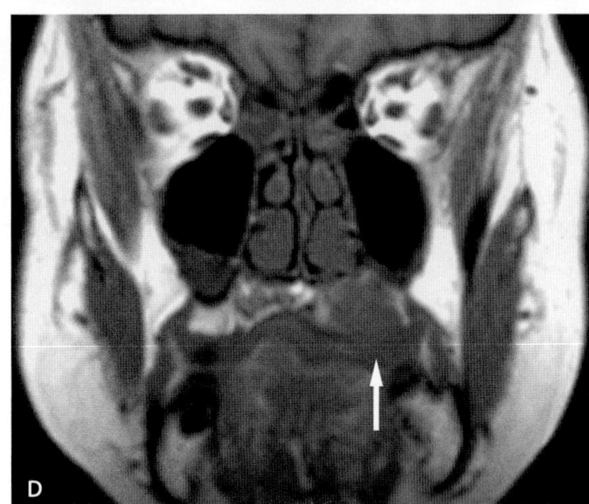

Figure 4.7

Adenoid cystic carcinoma, maxilla; 70-year-old female with painless swelling in hard palate; aspiration from soft part showed "fluid". A Axial CT image shows destruction in hard palate (*arrow*). B Coronal CT image shows widened major palatine foramen and pterygopalatine fissure (*arrow*). C Axial T2-weighted MRI shows high signal consistent with fluid (*arrowhead*) and tumor (*arrow*). D Coronal T1-weighted pre-Gd MRI shows reduced signal in bone marrow; intermediate–low signal of tumor (*arrow*). E Coronal T1-weighted post-Gd MRI shows contrast enhancement of tumor (*arrow*)

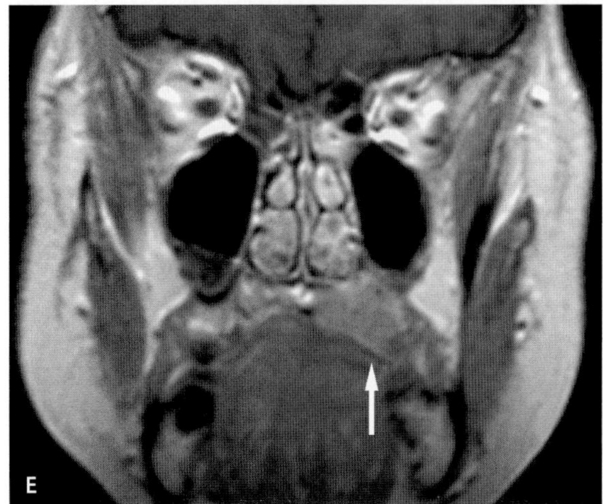

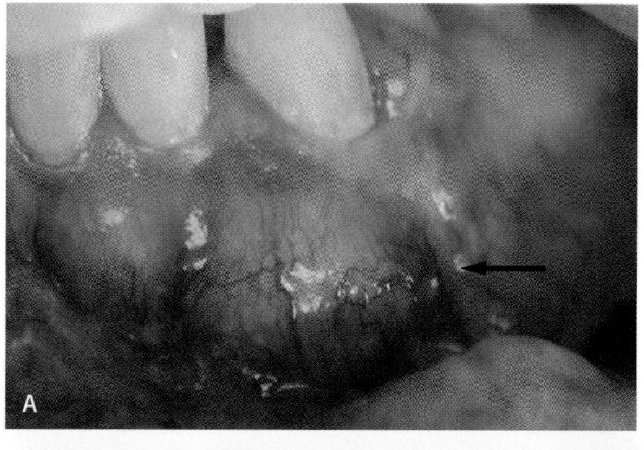
A

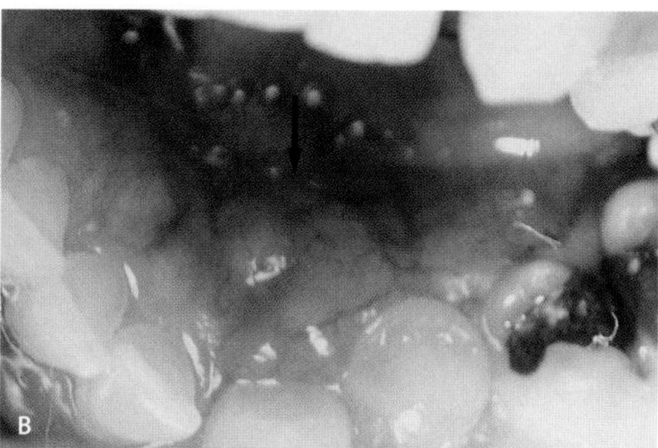
B

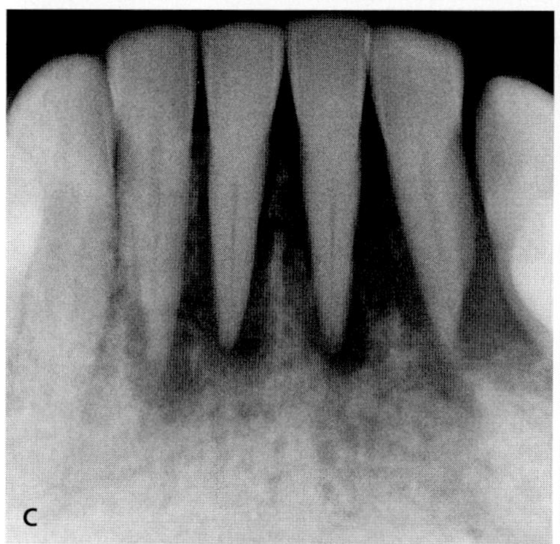
C

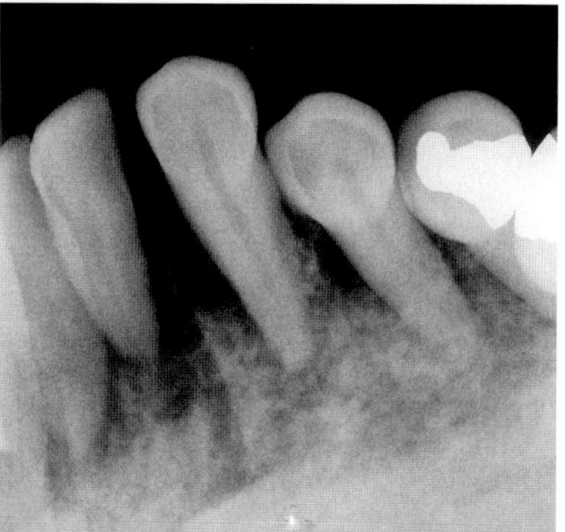

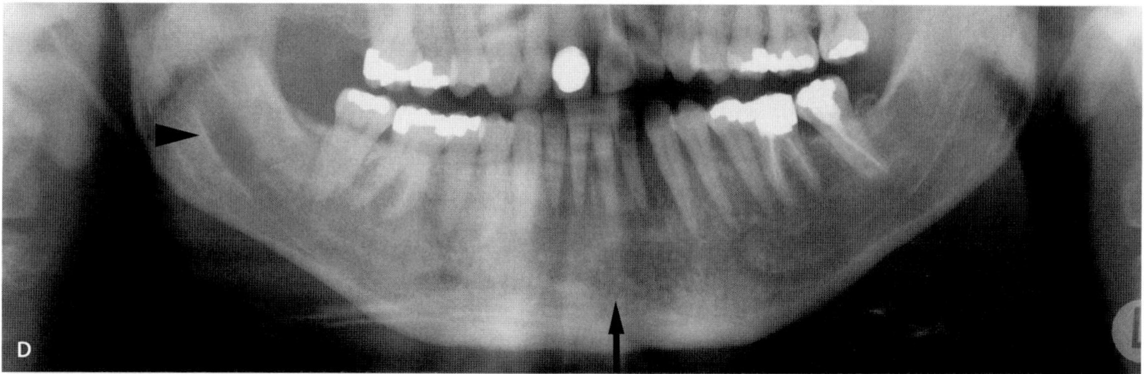
D

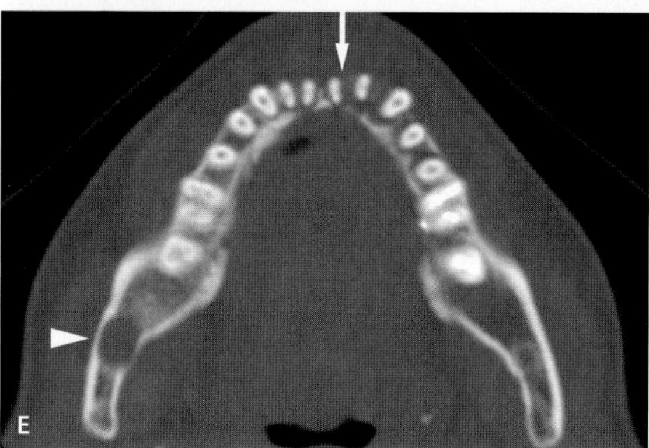
E

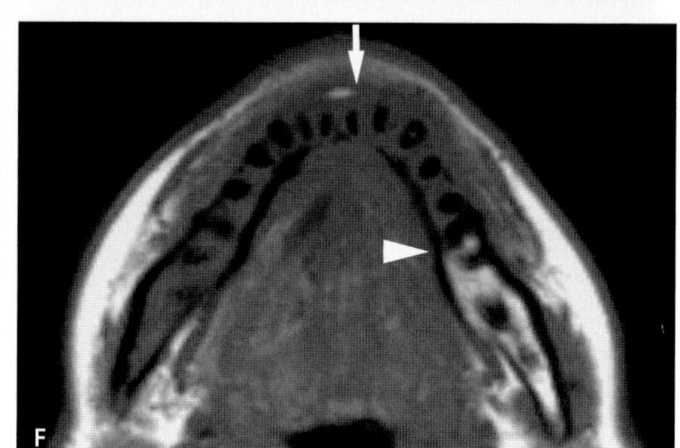
F

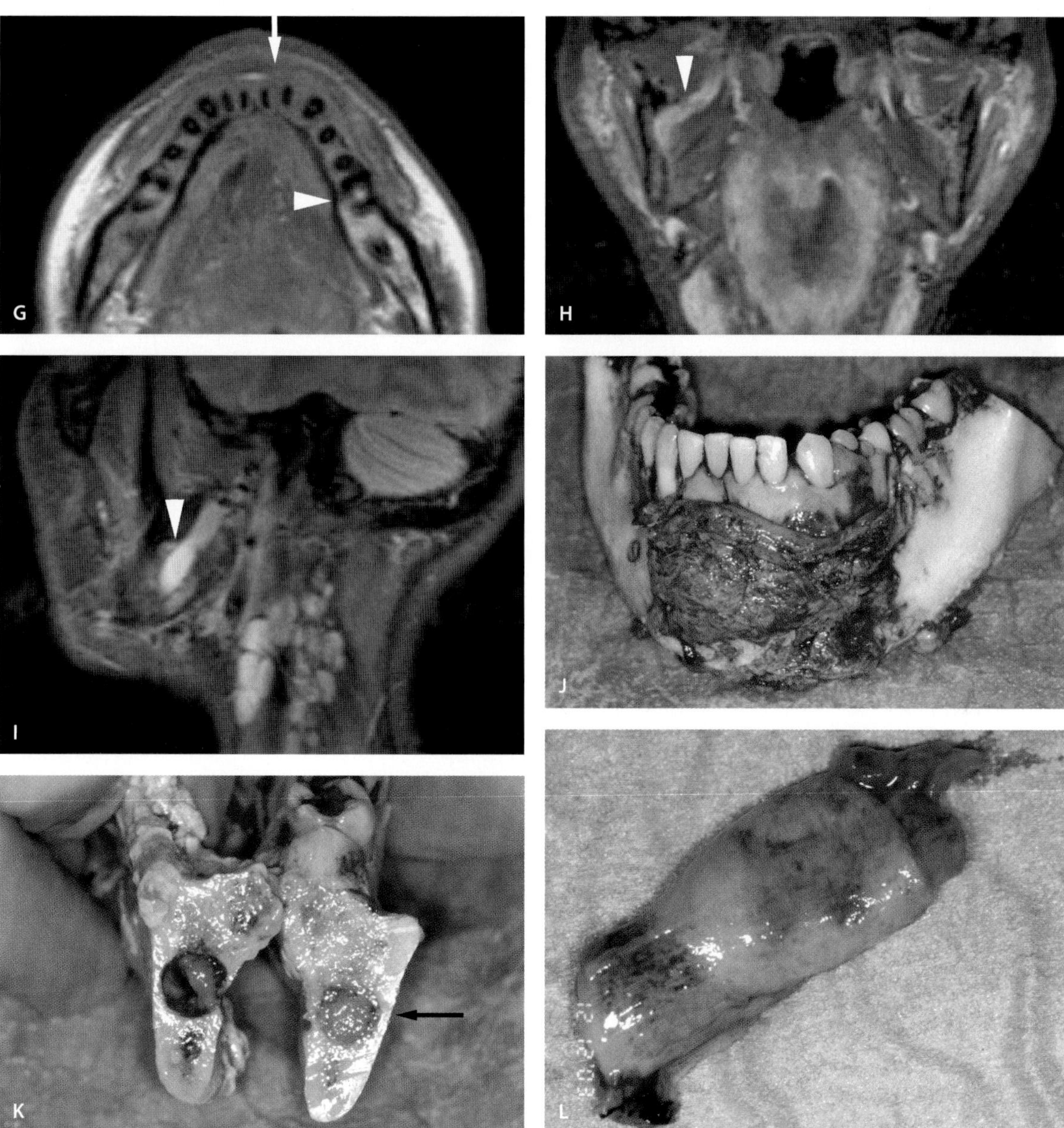

Figure 4.8

Adenoid cystic carcinoma, mandible; 43-year-old female with loose anterior teeth and hard gingival swelling. **A** Clinical photograph shows buccal swelling with normal mucosa (*arrow*). **B** Clinical photograph shows lingual swelling with normal mucosa (*arrow*). **C** Intraoral views show ill-defined bone destruction around several teeth. **D** Panoramic view shows destruction around anterior teeth (*arrow*) and widened mandibular canal (*arrowhead*). **E** Axial CT image shows bone destruction around anterior teeth (*arrow*) and widened mandibular canal (*arrowhead*). **F** Axial T1-weighted pre-Gd MRI shows cortical bone destruction (*arrow*) and reduced signal from marrow in entire mandible to molar region on left side (*arrowhead*). **G** Axial T-weighted post-Gd MRI shows tumor expansion in anterior region (*arrow*) and enhancement of entire mandibular marrow to molar region on left side (*arrowhead*). **H** Coronal STIR MRI shows enhancement of neurovascular tumor spread from mandibular foramen, approaching oval foramen (*arrowhead*). **I** Sagittal STIR MRI shows enhancement of neurovascular tumor spread from mandibular foramen (*arrowhead*). **J** Surgical specimen. **K** Surgical specimen, cut in two to show tumor invasion in mandibular canal (*arrow*). **L** Surgical specimen from neurovascular tumor spread from mandibular foramen (see I)

Non-Hodgkin's Lymphoma

Definition

Malignant neoplasm of cells from the lymphatic system.

Clinical Features

- Lymph node disease most common
- Non-Hodgkin's lymphoma of involves extranodal sites (as opposed to Hodgkin's lymphoma which is predominantly nodal)
- Extranodal involvement may include maxillary sinus and maxilla or, less frequently, mandible
- All age groups, adults in particular (except Burkitt's lymphoma)
- Burkitt's lymphoma was initially described as African jaw lymphoma; affects children; shows rapid growth and may involve one or both jaws

Imaging Features

- Soft-tissue mass
- Radiolucency
- Border of bone destruction ill-defined
- Non-Hodgkin's lymphoma, and rarely Hodkin's lymphoma, may present with necrofic lymph nodes
- However, it is not possible to definitely distinguish between non-Hodgkin's, Hodgkin's and metastatic lymph nodes based on CT and MRI
- T1-weighted MRI: intermediate–low signal
- T2-weighted and STIR MRI: intermediate signal
- T1-weighted MRI: contrast enhancement

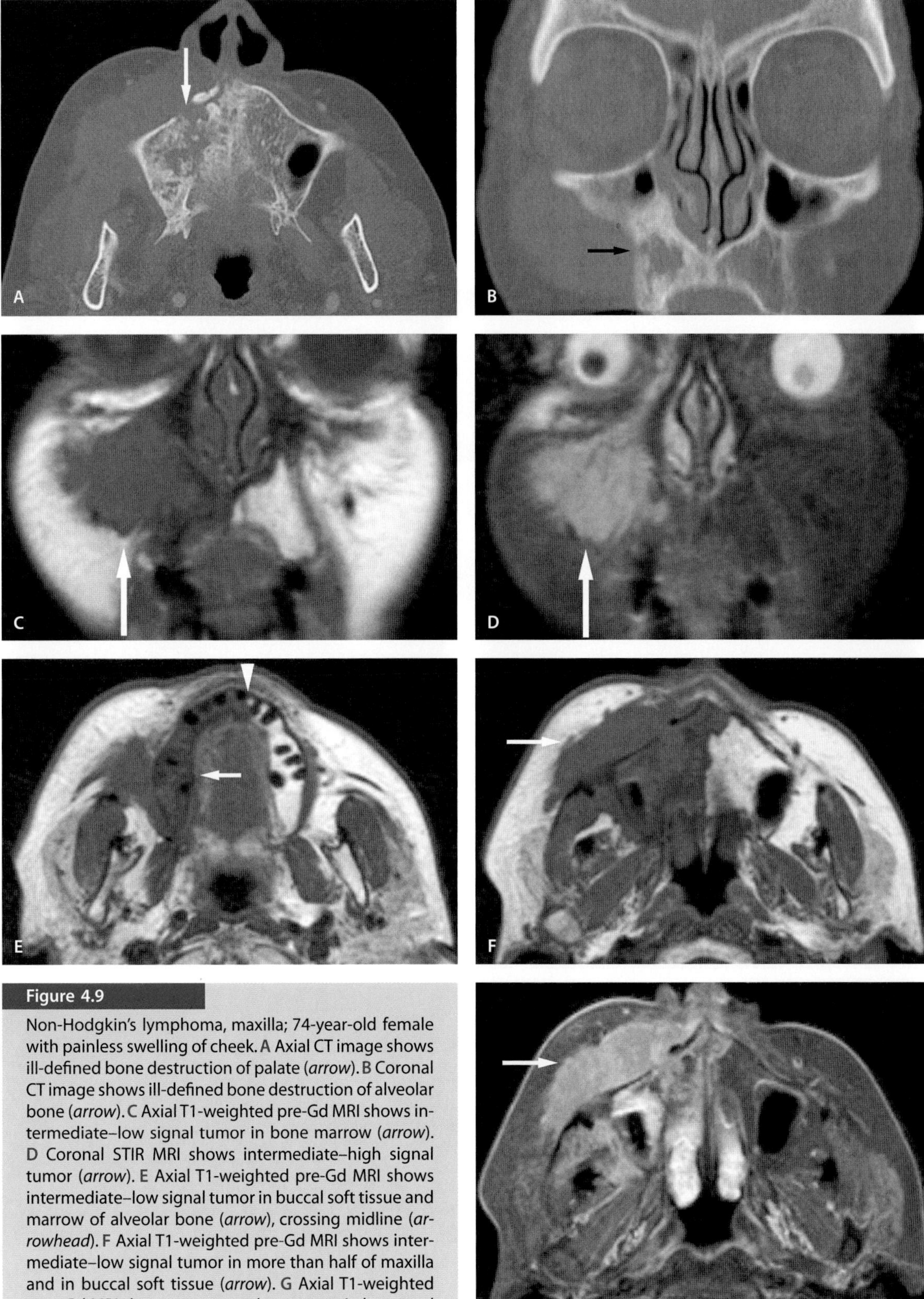

Figure 4.9

Non-Hodgkin's lymphoma, maxilla; 74-year-old female with painless swelling of cheek. A Axial CT image shows ill-defined bone destruction of palate (*arrow*). B Coronal CT image shows ill-defined bone destruction of alveolar bone (*arrow*). C Axial T1-weighted pre-Gd MRI shows intermediate–low signal tumor in bone marrow (*arrow*). D Coronal STIR MRI shows intermediate–high signal tumor (*arrow*). E Axial T1-weighted pre-Gd MRI shows intermediate–low signal tumor in buccal soft tissue and marrow of alveolar bone (*arrow*), crossing midline (*arrowhead*). F Axial T1-weighted pre-Gd MRI shows intermediate–low signal tumor in more than half of maxilla and in buccal soft tissue (*arrow*). G Axial T1-weighted post-Gd MRI shows contrast enhancement in bone and soft tissue (*arrow*)

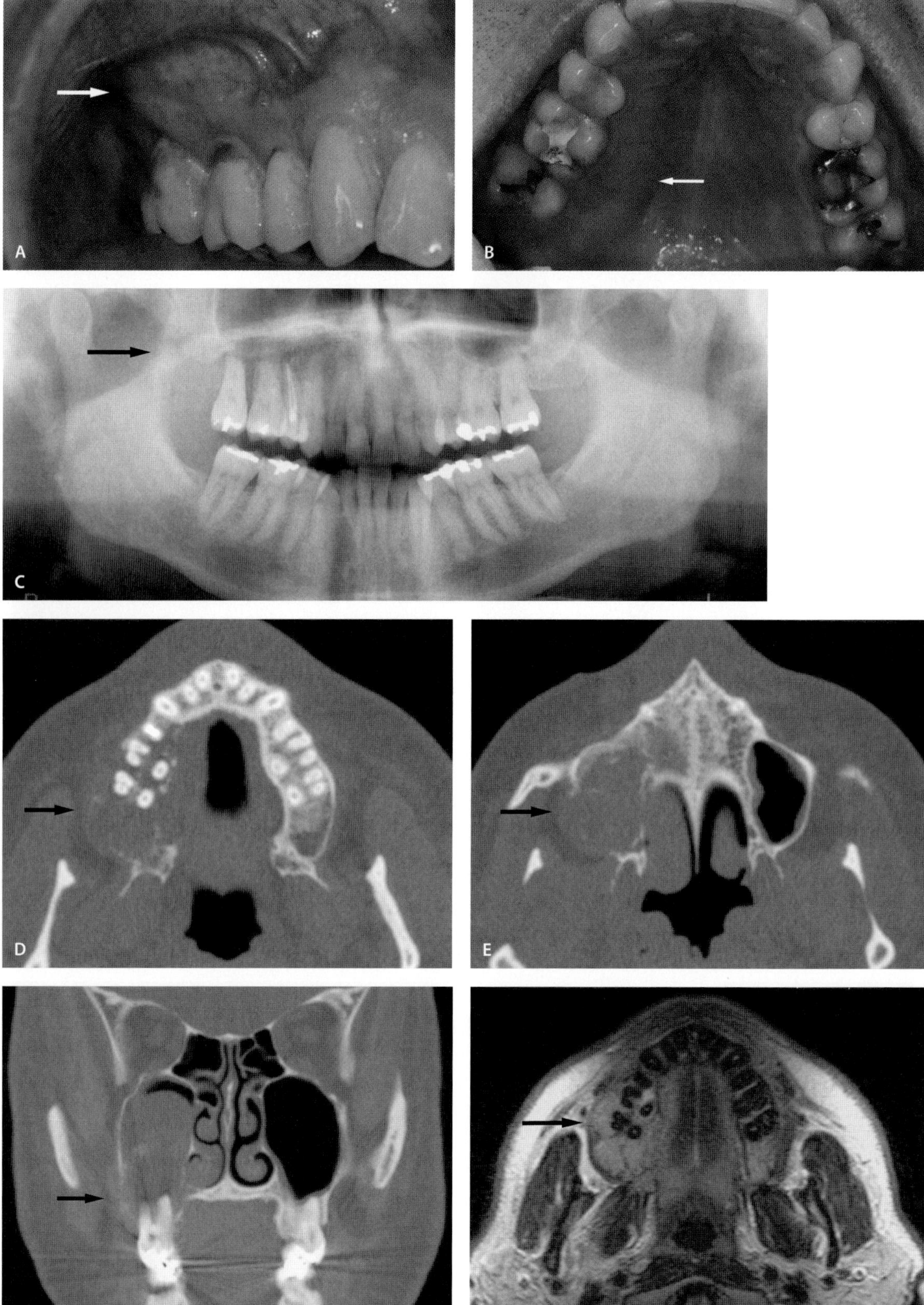

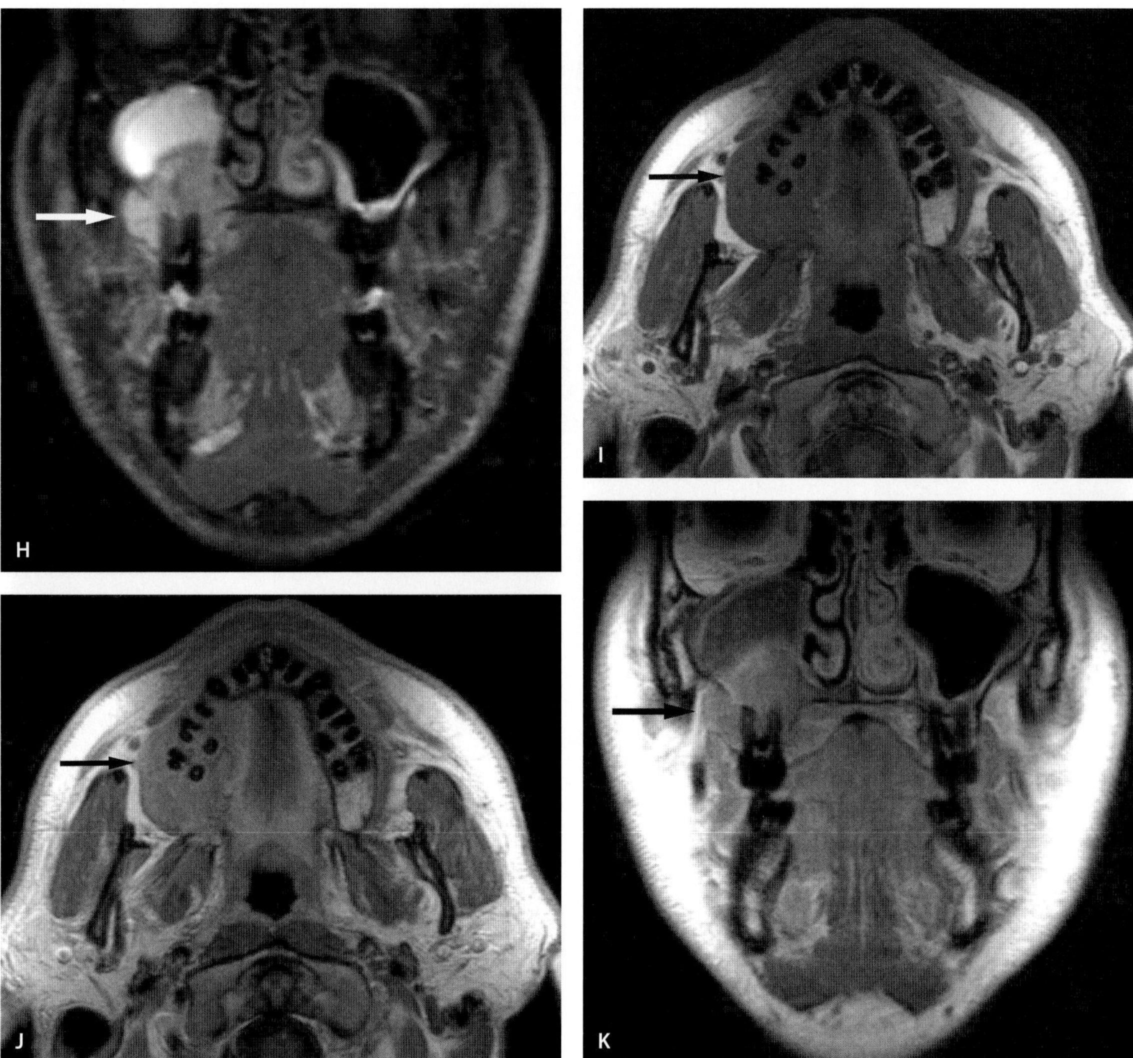

Figure 4.10

Non-Hodgkin's lymphoma, maxilla; 49-year-old male with slight, swelling, painless, but treated for apical periodontitis in right maxilla. **A** Clinical photograph shows buccal swelling with normal mucosa (*arrow*). **B** Clinical photograph shows palatal swelling with normal mucosa (*arrow*). **C** Panoramic view shows diffuse alveolar bone destruction (*arrow*). **D** Axial CT image shows ill-defined alveolar bone destruction (*arrow*). **E** Axial CT image shows ill-defined bone destruction of sinus walls (*arrow*). **F** Coronal CT image shows bone destruction and tumor in maxillary sinus (*arrow*). **G** Axial T2-weighted MRI shows expanded alveolar bone with intermediate–low signal (*arrow*). **H** Coronal STIR MRI shows intermediate signal of tumor (*arrow*) and high signal from mucosal thickening in maxillary sinus. **I** Axial T1-weighted pre-Gd MRI shows intermediate–low signal tumor in bone marrow of maxilla (*arrow*). **J** Axial T1-weighted post-Gd MRI shows contrast enhancement of tumor (*arrow*). **K** Coronal T1-weighted post-Gd MRI shows contrast enhancement of tumor (*arrow*)

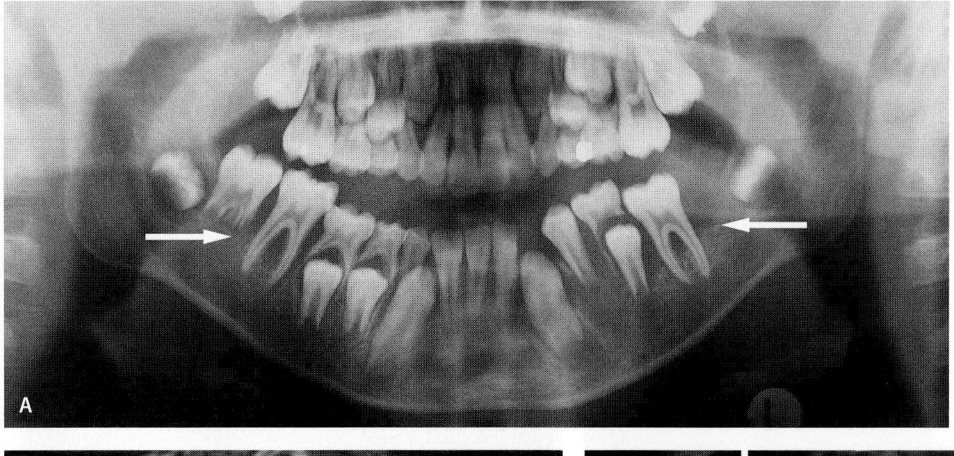
A

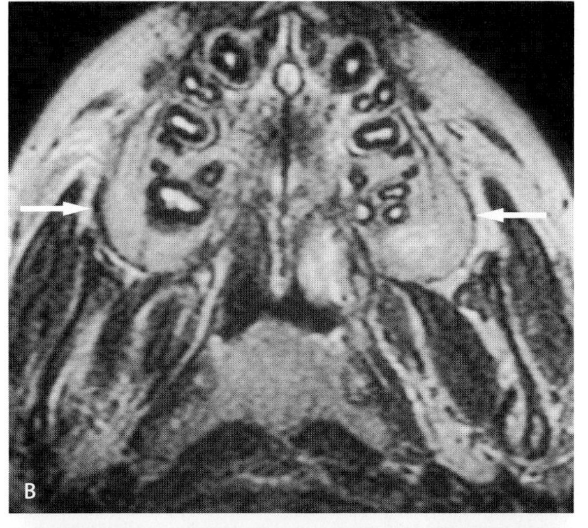
B

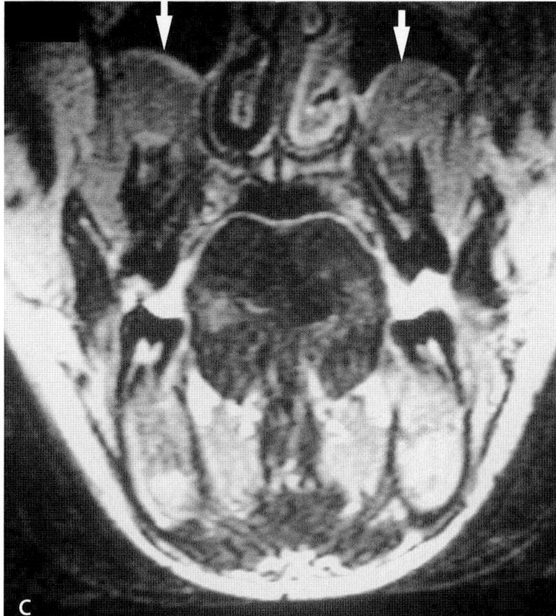
C

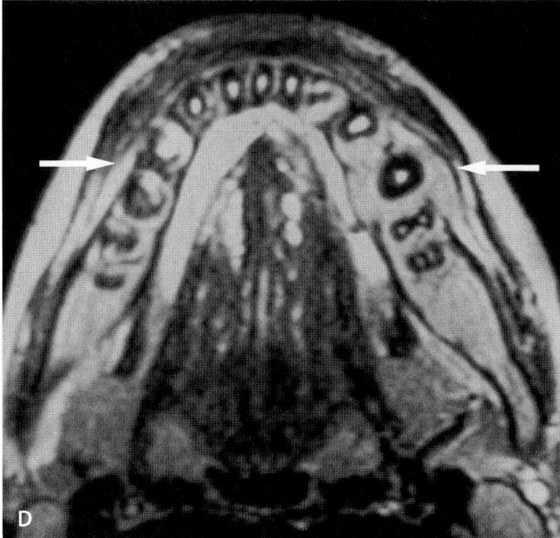
D

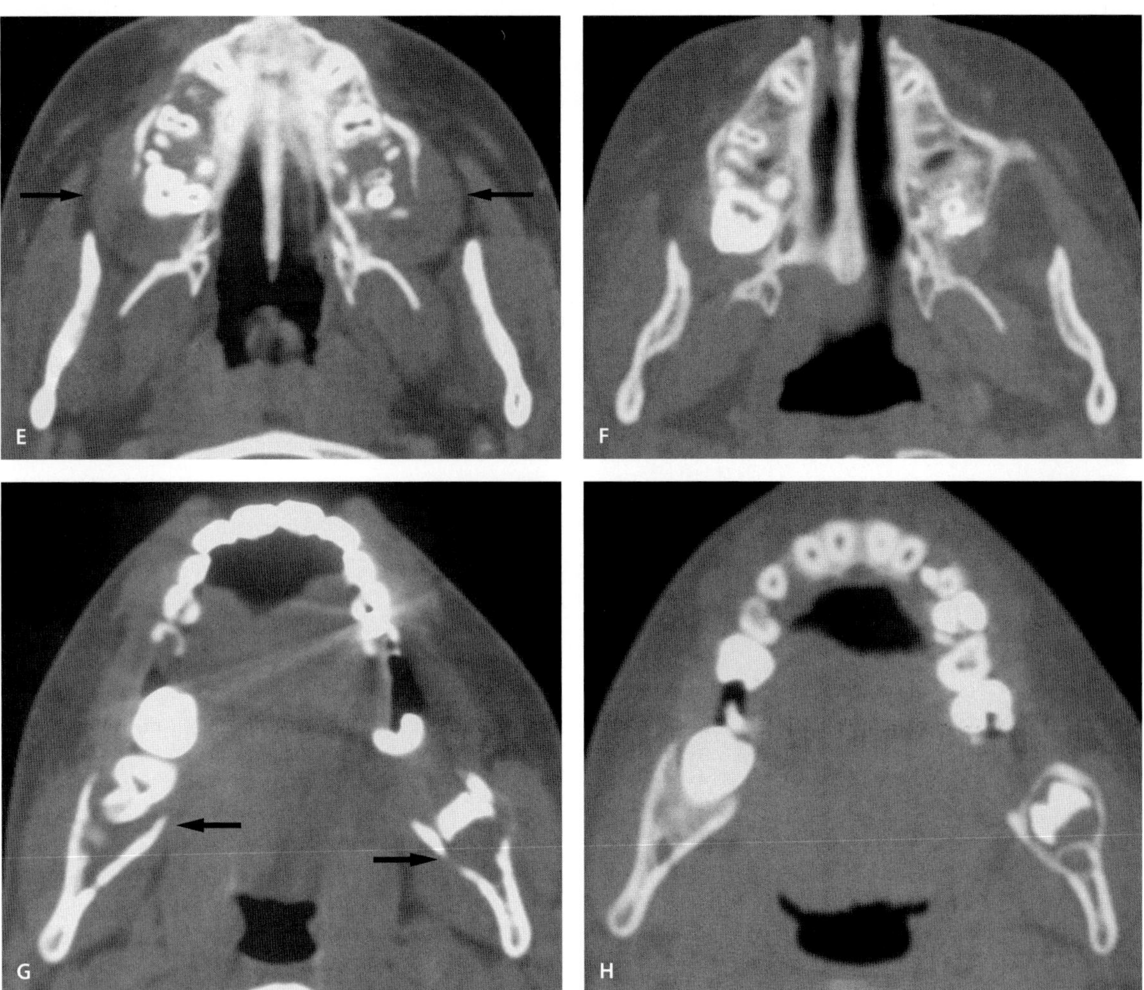

Figure 4.11

Burkitt's (non-Hodgkin's) lymphoma, mandible and maxilla; 11-year-old male with swelling of upper and lower jaw. A Panoramic view shows destruction of alveolar bone bilaterally in molar area (*arrows*). B Axial T2-weighted MRI shows expansion of alveolar processes bilaterally in maxilla (*arrows*). C Coronal T2-weighted MRI shows tumor in maxillary sinus bilaterally (*arrows*). D Axial T2-weighted MRI shows tumor expansion bilaterally in mandible (*arrows*). E Axial CT image shows expansion of maxilla with bone destruction bilaterally (*arrows*). F Axial CT image, 2 months posttreatment shows near normalization of maxilla. G Axial CT image shows bone destruction of mandible bilaterally (*arrows*). H Axial CT image, 2 months posttreatment shows near normalization of mandible

Myeloma

Synonyms: Multiple myeloma, myelomatosis

Definition

Malignant tumor, usually with multiple or diffuse bone involvement by neoplastic plasma cells showing varying degrees of immaturity, including atypical forms. Lesions are often associated with presence of abnormal proteins in blood and urine, and occasionally with presence of amyloid or para-amyloid in tumor tissue or other organs (WHO).

Plasmacytoma is solitary form of myeloma.

Clinical Features (Myeloma)

- Most common primary bone malignancy in adults
- Males more frequent than females
- Older age groups (50 years and older)
- Bone pain, malaise
- No curative treatment
- Jaw involvement seldom and usually asymptomatic

Imaging Features (Myeloma)

- Multiple radiolucencies, skull more often than jaws
- Mandible more often than maxilla
- Punched-out bone destruction

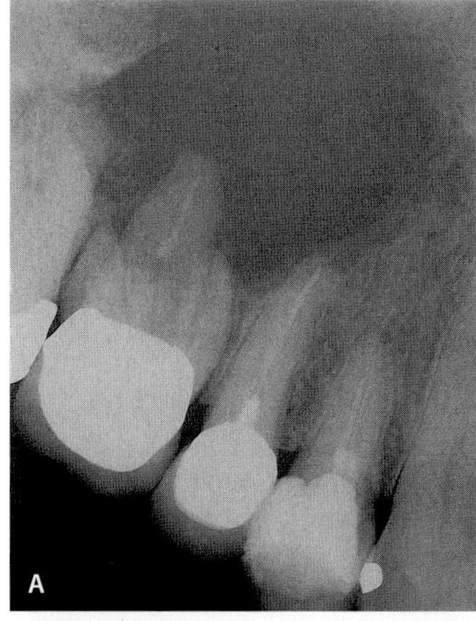

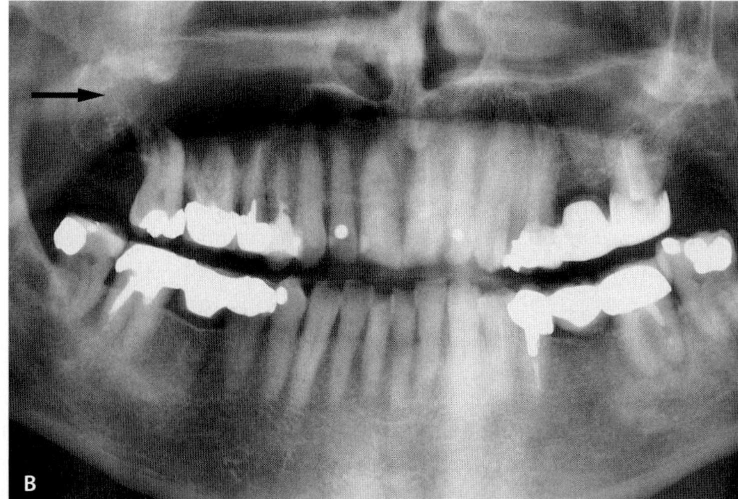

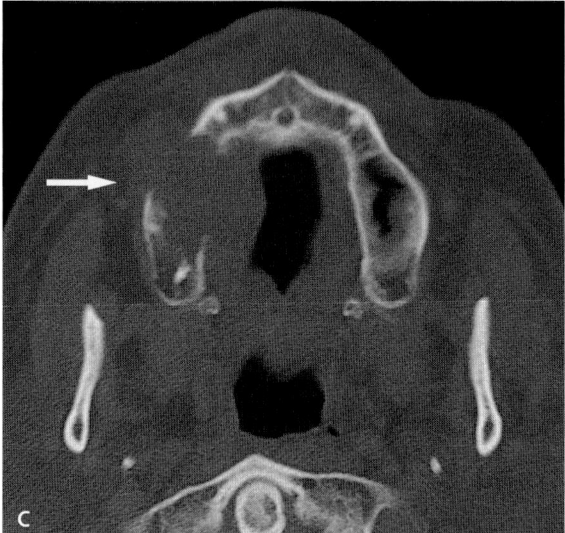

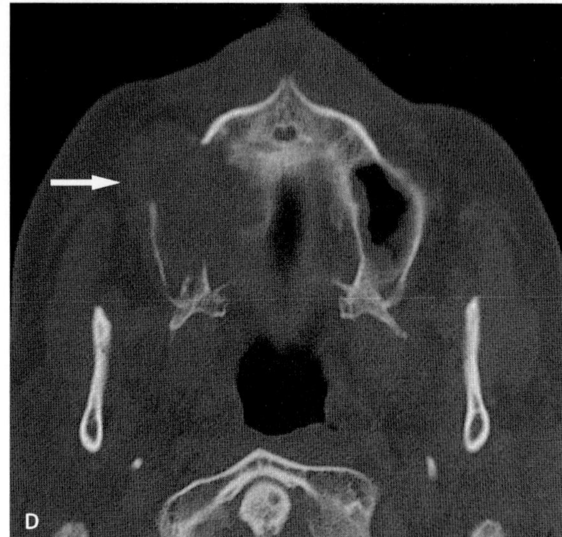

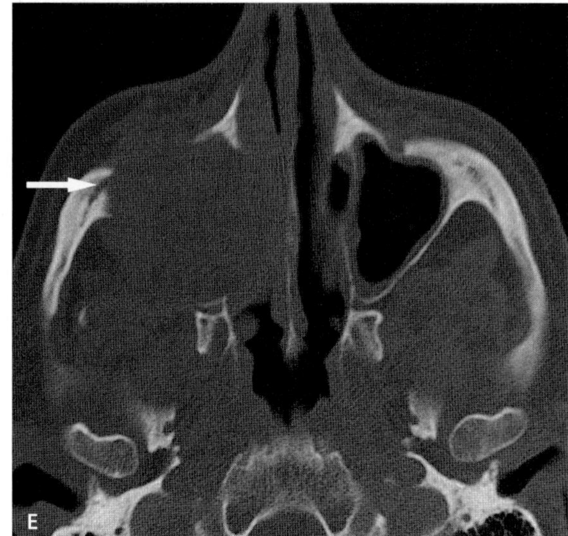

Figure 4.12

Plasmacytoma, maxilla; 76-year-old male with diffuse pain in right cheek, first treated for sinusitis and then endodontic treatment. A Intraoral view shows ill-defined bone destruction. B Panoramic view shows ill-defined demarcation of maxillary sinus (*arrow*). C Axial CT image shows destruction of alveolar process and soft-tissue mass (*arrow*). D Axial CT image shows destruction of hard palate (*arrow*). E Axial CT image shows destruction of all walls of maxillary sinus (*arrow*) (courtesy of Drs. Sahlstrom, Eriksson, Lindh, and Warfvinge, University Hospital, Malmo, Sweden)

Leukemia

Definition

Malignant neoplasm of hematopoietic stem cells often occurring in normal bone marrow.

Acute leukemias are accompanied by accumulation of immature, or blast, cells owing to defect in production of mature hemic cells; chronic leukemias are characterized by massive overgrowth of mature cells

Clinical Features

- Acute and chronic forms
- Acute: younger age groups, usually with severe general symptoms (such as bone pain, fever, lymphadenopathy, general fatigue and loss of appetite)
- Chronic: adults, usually with few or no symptoms
- Oral symptoms may include gingival inflammation and hyperplasia, ulceration, bleeding, petechiae, loose teeth

Imaging Features

- Radiolucency
- Border of bone destruction ill-defined
- Loss of lamina dura
- No bone expansion
- Jaw abnormalities reported in half of the patients or more
- One jaw, unilateral or bilateral, or both jaws
- MRI abnormalities with normal CT findings
- T1-weighted fat-suppressed post-Gd MRI: high signal from bone marrow and diffuse enhancement in surrounding soft tissue

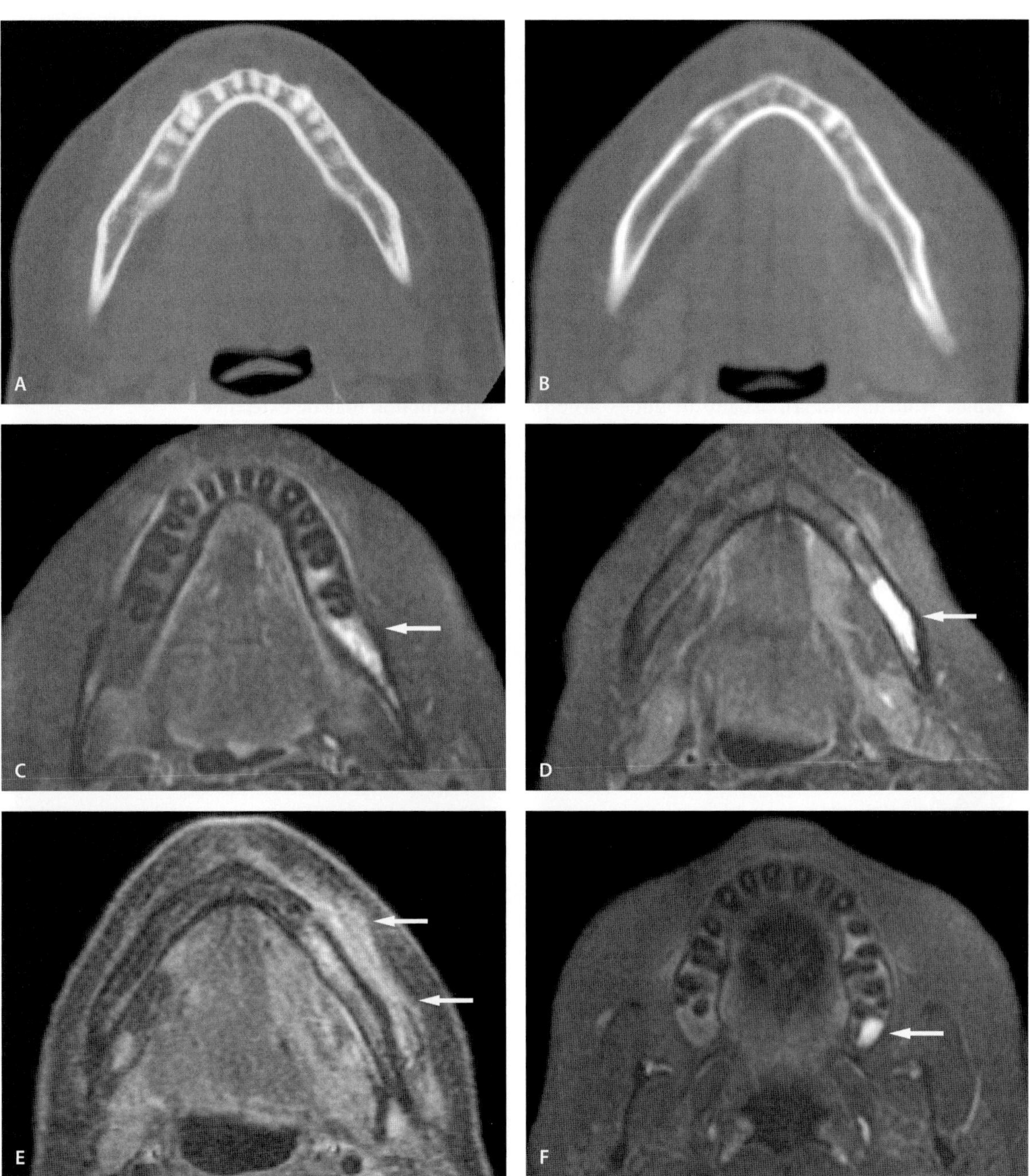

Figure 4.13

Leukemia, mandible and maxilla; 42-year-old female with numbness and weakness of left jaw. A Axial CT image shows normal bone of tooth-bearing areas. B Axial CT image shows normal bone caudad to teeth. C Axial T1-weighted fat-suppressed post-Gd MRI shows high signal in bone marrow of tooth-bearing area (*arrow*). D Axial T1-weighted fat-suppressed post-Gd MRI shows high signal from bone marrow caudad to teeth (*arrow*). E Axial T1-weighted fat-suppressed post-Gd MRI shows diffuse enhancement also in surrounding soft tissue, buccally in particular (*arrows*), but also lingually. F Axial T1-weighted fat-suppressed post-Gd MRI shows high signal in marrow of maxilla (*arrow*)

Bone-destructive and Bone-productive Tumors

Osteosarcoma

Synonym: Osteogenic sarcoma

Definition

Malignant tumor characterized by direct formation of bone or osteoid by tumor cells (WHO).

Clinical Features

- Most common primary malignancy in skeleton (apart from myeloma), usually in bones around the knee and primarily in children and adolescents; pain common
- Only 5–10% in head and neck; mostly in jaws
- Usually painless swelling in jaws, but also pain and mental nerve paresthesia
- Mandible slight predominance
- Males slight predominance
- May occur in any age group; peak in fourth decade
- Jaw osteosarcomas have tendency to occur in older patients than osteosarcomas in other bones and less likely to metastasize
- However, prognosis of jaw sarcoma is poor and does not seem to have improved with chemotherapy in a similar way to sarcomas in other bones
- Main cause of death is local recurrence

Imaging Features

- Soft-tissue mass, may grow aggressively and rapidly
- Radiolucent or most frequently, a combination of radiolucent and radiopaque appearance; bone production may be extensive
- Border of bone destruction ill-defined
- Bone production may typically have 'sunburst' appearance, best seen on CT images
- T1-weighted MRI: heterogeneous (intermediate–low) signal
- T2-weighted and STIR MRI: heterogeneous signal (variable high to intermediate–low) depending on bone production and cellular content
- T1-weighted post-Gd MRI: heterogeneous (intense to low) contrast enhancement

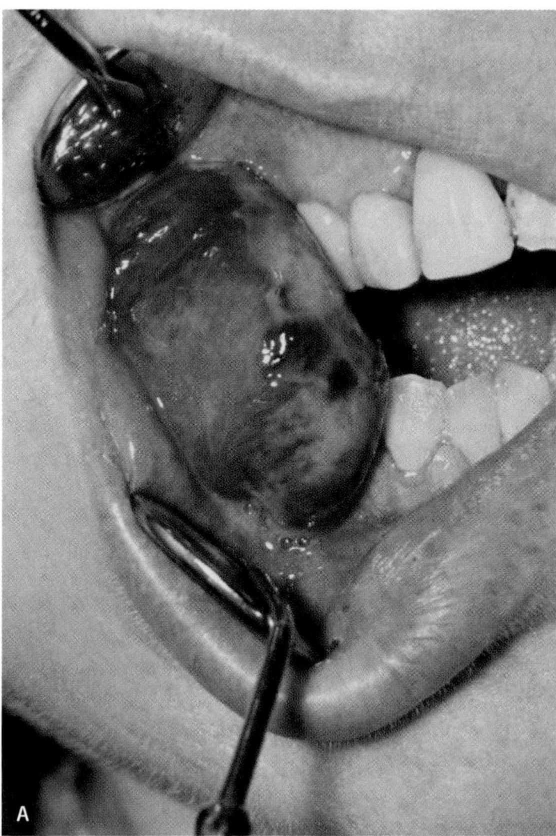

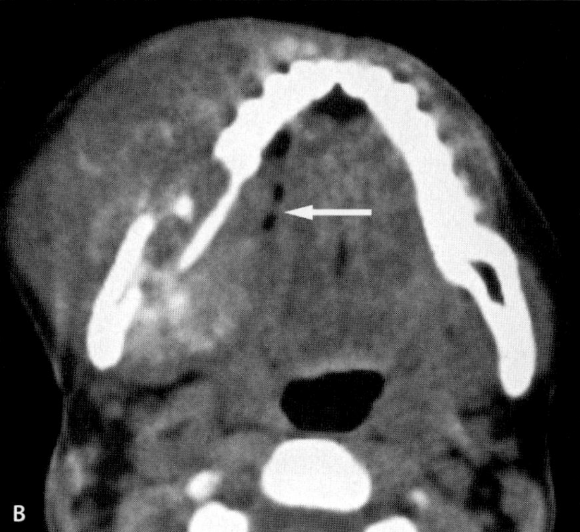

Figure 4.14

Osteosarcoma, mandible; 37-year-old female with aggressive tumor growth, which "exploded" after extraction of molar tooth in right mandible. **A** Clinical photograph show rapidly growing tumor mass. **B** Axial CT image shows bone destruction and aggressive tumor both buccally and lingually (*arrow*)

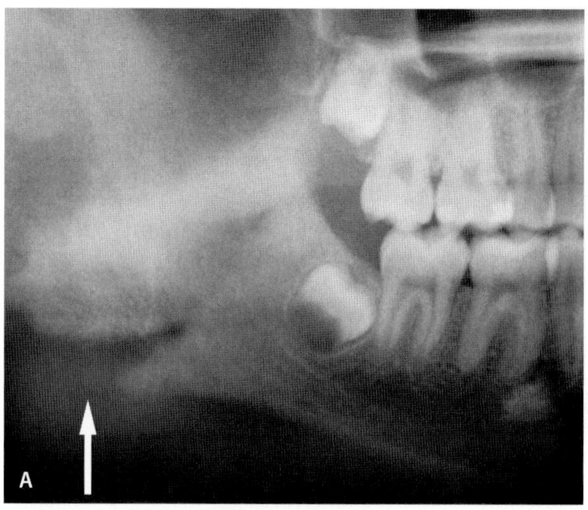

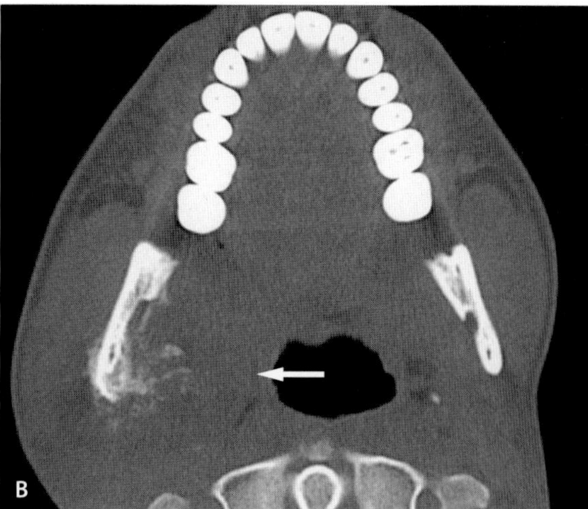

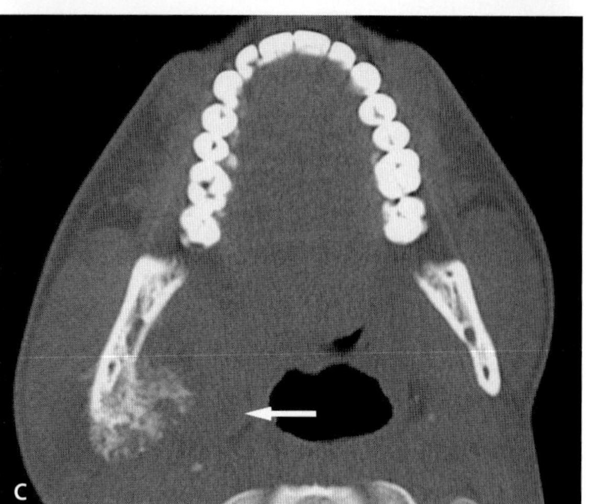

Figure 4.15

Osteosarcoma, mandible; 16-year-old male with painless buccal swelling at right mandibular angle. **A** Panoramic view shows diffuse bone mass (*arrow*). **B** Axial CT image shows bone destruction radiating from ramus, predominantly on lingual side (*arrow*). **C** Axial CT image shows more extensive bone production (*arrow*)

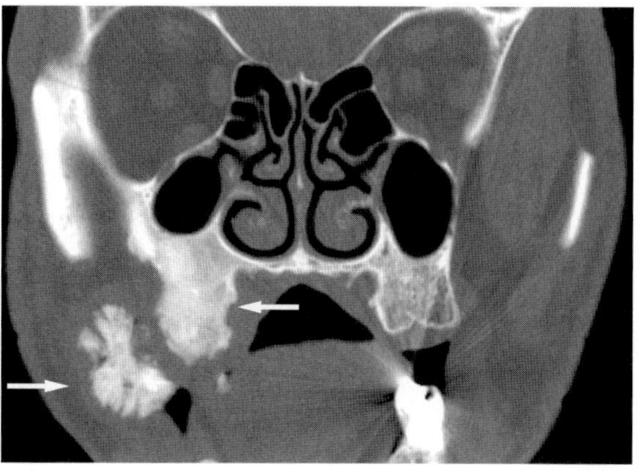

Figure 4.16

Osteosarcoma, maxilla; 43-year-old male after about 6 months of chemotherapy now presenting for presurgical evaluation. Coronal CT image shows expansive process with intense radiating bone production (*lateral arrow*) around intensively sclerotic alveolar bone (*arrow*)

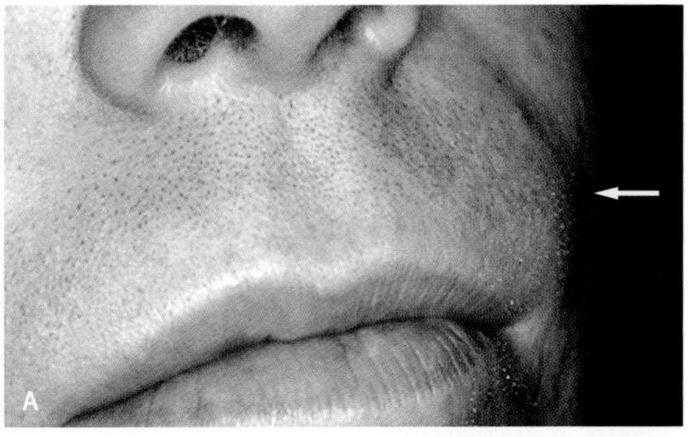

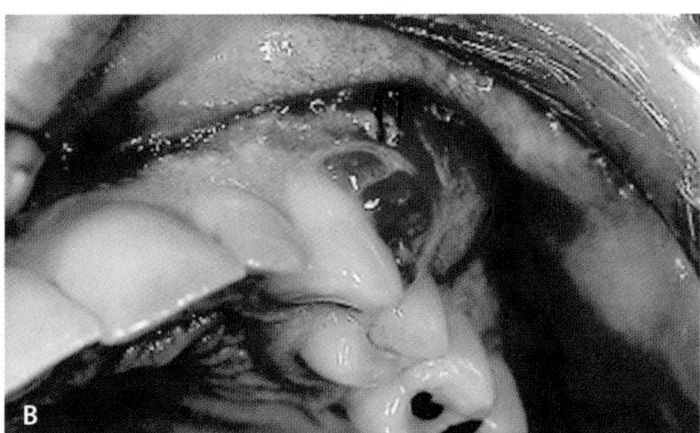

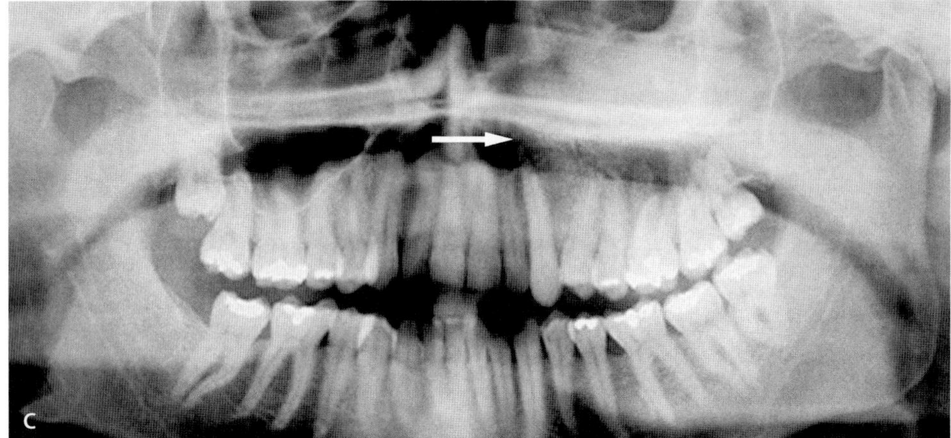

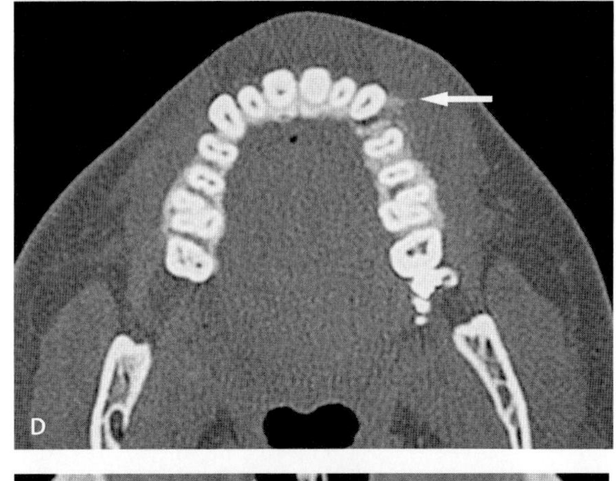

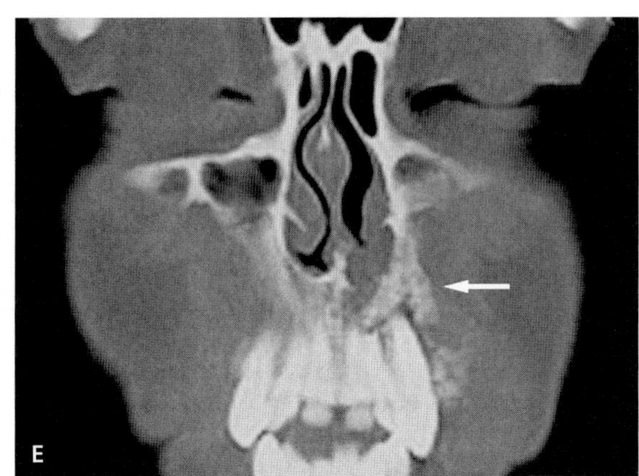

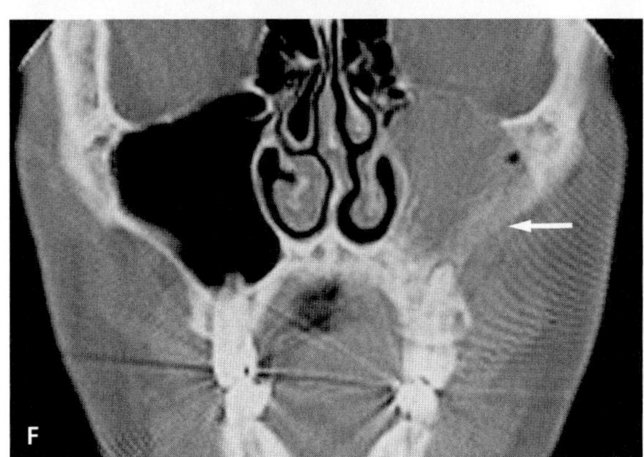

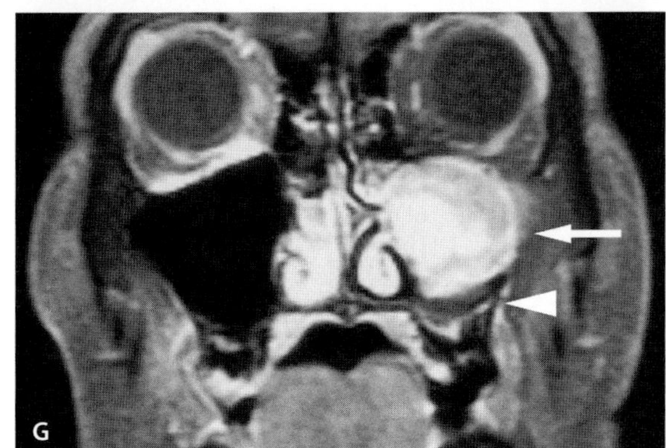

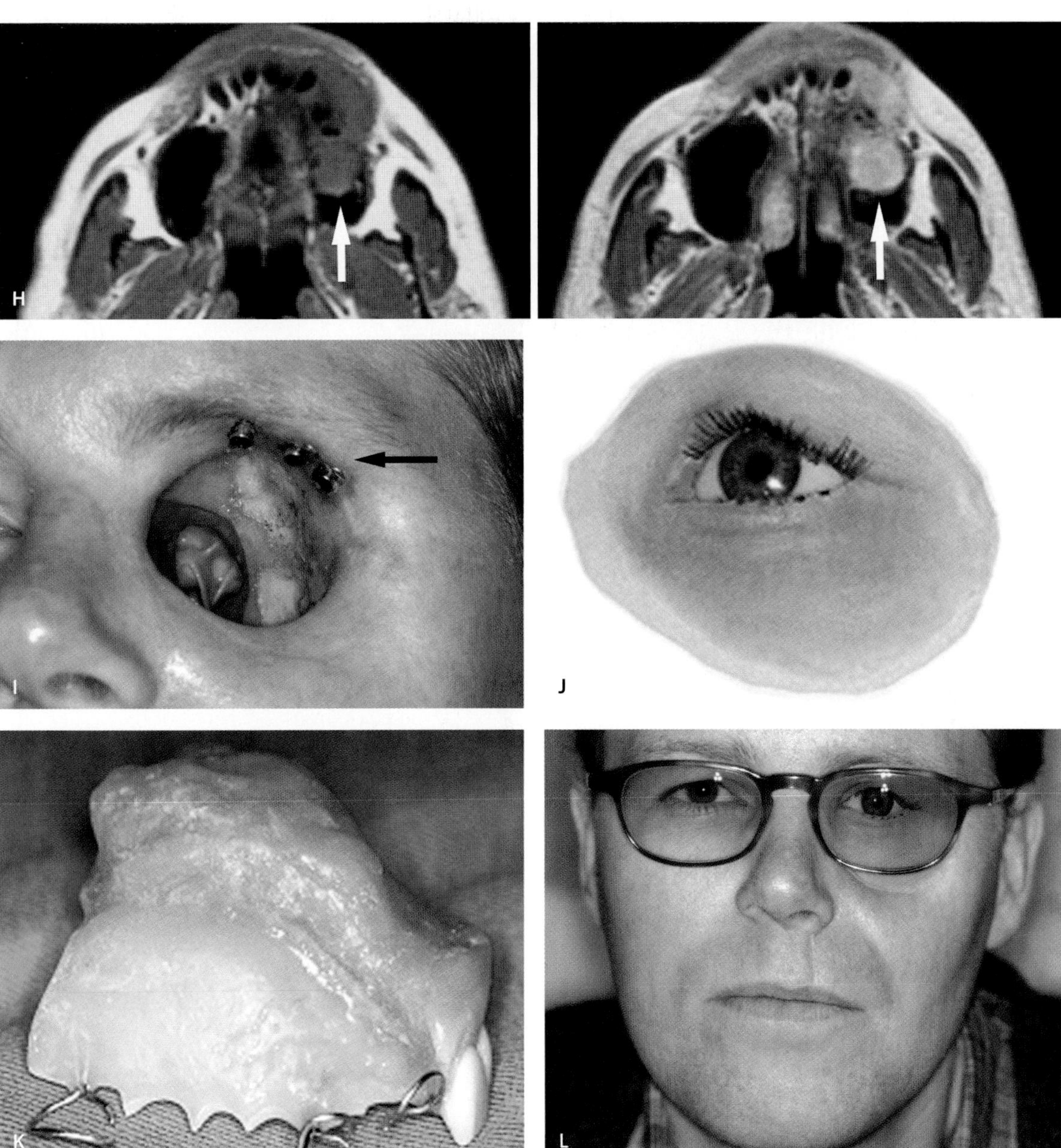

Figure 4.17

Osteosarcoma, maxilla; 28-year-old male with painless swelling of vestibulum. **A** Clinical photograph shows swelling of lip (*arrow*). **B** Clinical photograph shows swelling of gingiva (after biopsy). **C** Panoramic view shows opaque left maxillary sinus with absent alveolar sinus demarcation (*arrow*), and possible periapical bone destruction at first molar. **D** Axial CT image shows bone production with sunburst appearance (*arrow*). **E** Coronal CT image shows destruction of piriform aperture (*arrow*), and bone production at canine. **F** Coronal CT image shows left maxillary sinus opacity with expanded floor of orbit, and bone production in sinus walls (*arrow*). **G** Coronal T1-weighted fat suppressed post-Gd MRI shows intense contrast enhancement of tumor in maxillary sinus (arrow) with low signal bone production in alveolar part (arrow head). **H** Axial T1-weighted pre-Gd (left) and post-Gd (right) MRI shows contrast enhanced maxillary sinus tumor penetrating sinus wall and alveolar ridge (arrows). **I** Clinical photo of orbit with titanium implants (arrow) to fixate eye prosthesis. **J** Eye prosthesis. **K** Denture. **L** Clinical photo 10 years after surgical treatment; patient has no recurrence or metastases. (I, J, K, L: Courtesy of W. Widnes, C.D.T. anaplastologist, Rikshospitalet University Hospital, Oslo, Norway)

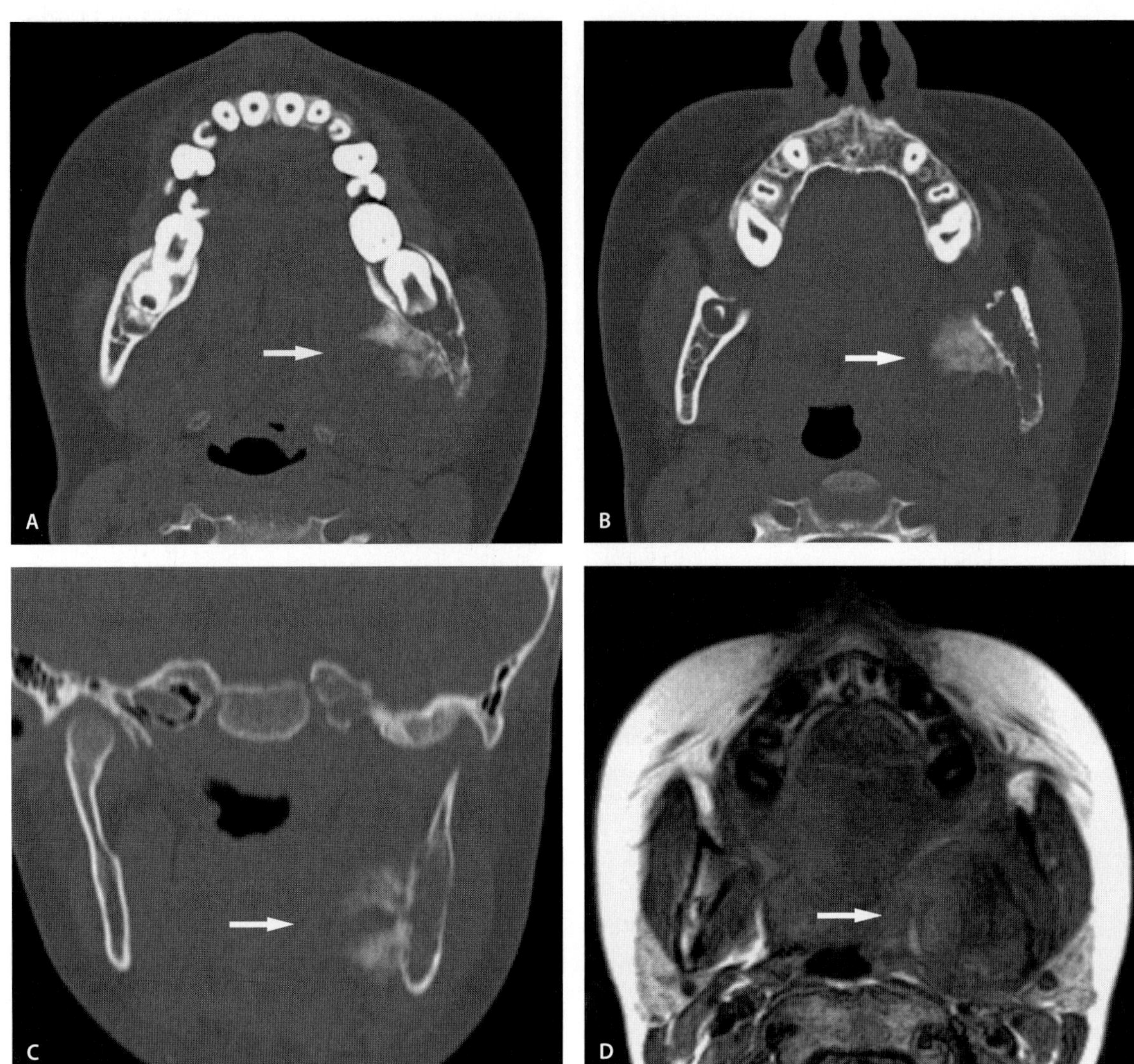
A
B
C
D

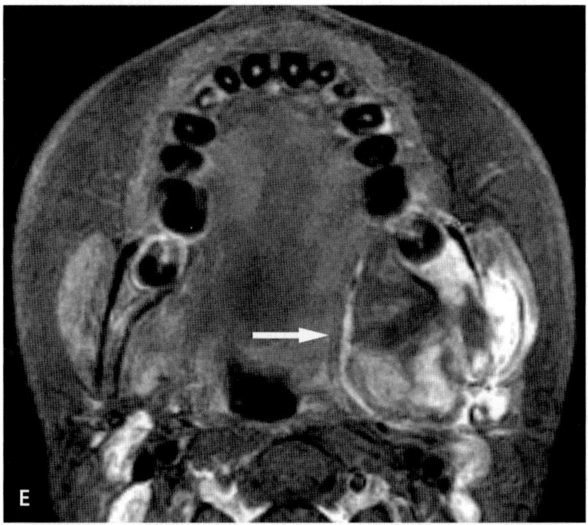

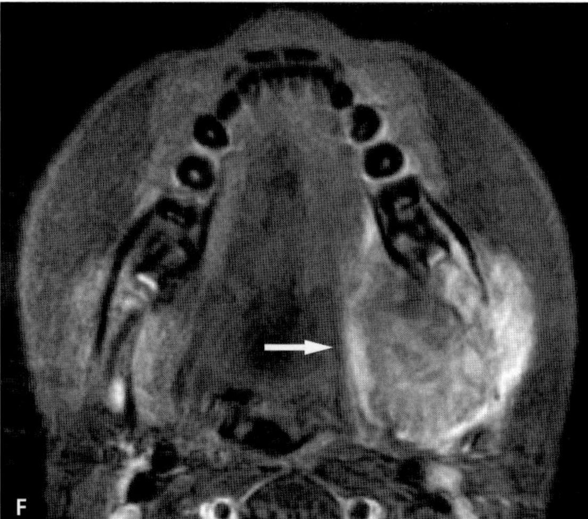

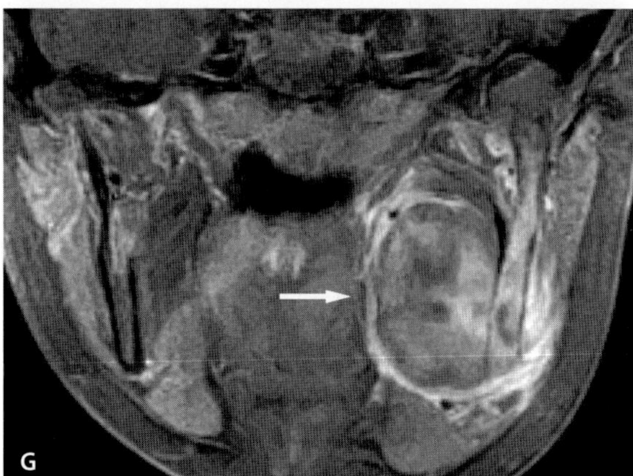

Figure 4.18

Osteosarcoma, mandible; 10-year-old female with painful mass in mandible and inability to open her mouth, and 3-year history of femur osteosarcoma. A Axial CT image shows radiating bone production on lingual aspect of mandible (*arrow*). B Axial CT image shows bone production and destruction of bone marrow and cortex (*arrow*). C Coronal CT image shows sunburst appearance (*arrow*). D Axial T1-weighted pre-Gd MRI shows intermediate–low signal tumor lingually and in bone marrow (*arrow*). E Axial T1-weighted post-Gd MRI shows intense contrast enhancement in masseter muscle and heterogeneous (intense to low) enhancement of large lingual tumor (*arrow*) with displacement of air way. F Axial T1-weighted post-Gd MRI shows another section of contrast enhancement (*arrow*), also in bone marrow. G Coronal T1-weighted post-Gd MRI shows tumor predominantly on lingual side (*arrow*)

Chondrosarcoma

Definition

Malignant tumor characterized by formation of cartilage, but not of bone, by tumor cells. It is distinguished from chondroma by its higher cellularity, greater pleomorphism and appreciable numbers of plump cells with large or double nuclei. Mitotic cells are infrequent (WHO).

May arise from a pre-existing cartilaginous neoplasm.

Clinical Features

- Rather common
- Wide variation of clinical features
- Mostly in adults in fourth to sixth decades
- Less aggressive, more slowly growing than osteosarcoma
- Better prognosis; metastasizes more seldom than osteosarcoma
- Mandible and maxilla, but rare

Imaging Features

- Round soft-tissue mass with ring or crescent calcification characteristic, but may also show sunburst appearance
- MRI: heterogeneous (high to low) signal, see Osteosarcoma

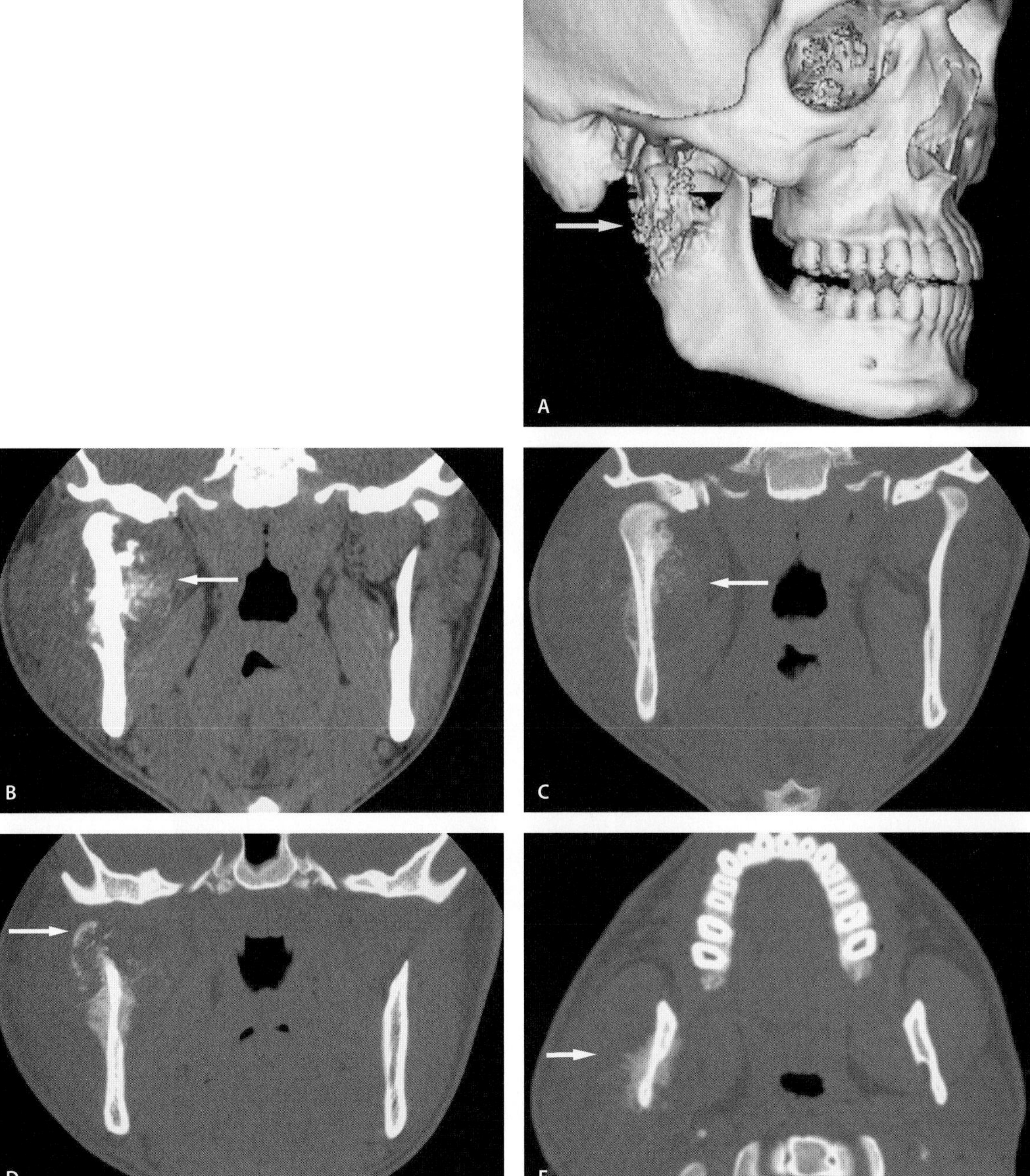

Figure 4.19

Chondrosarcoma, mandible; 19-year-old male with facial swelling, no pain. **A** 3D CT image shows tumor in right mandibular collum (*arrow*). **B** Coronal CT image, soft-tissue window, shows soft-tissue mass around ramus (*arrow*). **C** Coronal CT image shows radiating bone production (*arrow*). **D** Coronal CT image shows crescent calcification and dense sunburst appearance (*arrow*). **E** Axial CT image shows dense sunburst appearance (*arrow*)

Ewing Sarcoma

Definition

Malignant tumor with rather uniform histologic appearance composed of densely packed, glycogen-rich small cells with round nuclei but without prominent nucleoli or distinct cytoplasmic outlines. Tumor tissue is typically divided into irregular strands or lobules by fibrous septa, but intercellular network of reticulin fibers, which is a feature of malignant lymphoma, is not seen. Mitoses are generally infrequent. Hemorrhage and extensive areas of necrosis are common (WHO).

Clinical Features

- Only 1–4% in head and neck area; most commonly mandible
- Hard swelling, pain or pain-free
- Males more frequent than females
- Usually first and second decades, but may occur at any age

Imaging Features

- Soft-tissue mass
- 'Moth-eaten' bone destruction
- Bone production characteristic; periosteal 'onion skin' reaction (usually in long bones), but not so typical in jaws

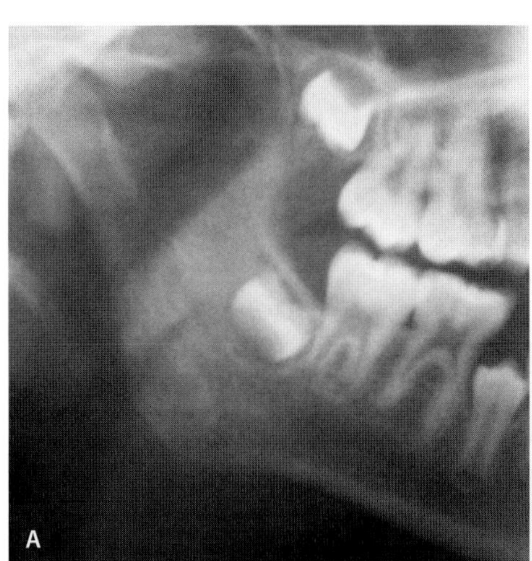

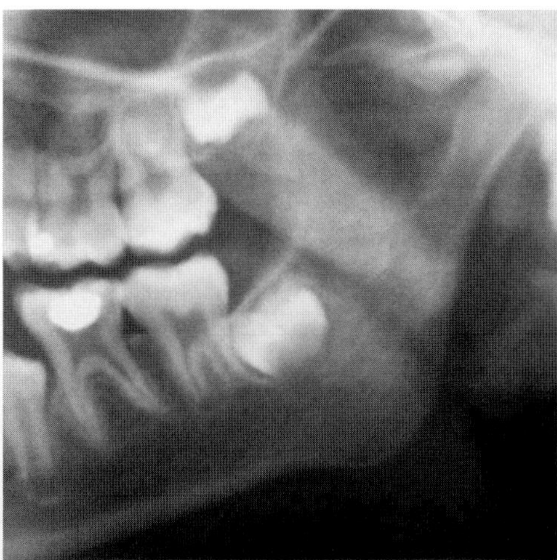

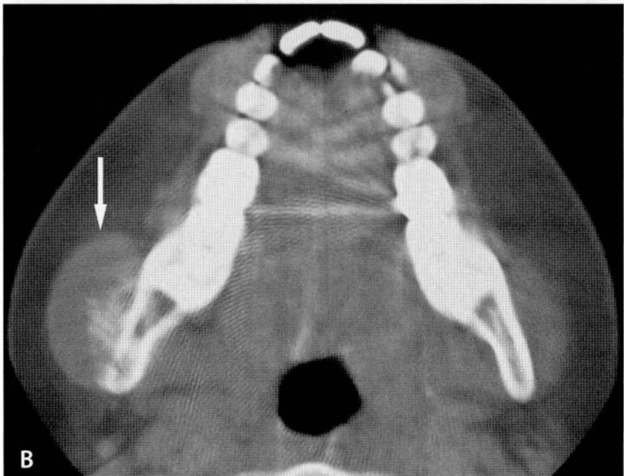

Figure 4.20

Ewing sarcoma, mandible; 10-year-old male with painless swelling at right mandibular angle. **A** Panoramic view shows no abnormality. **B** Axial CT image shows soft-tissue mass and radiating bone production on buccal aspect (*arrow*)

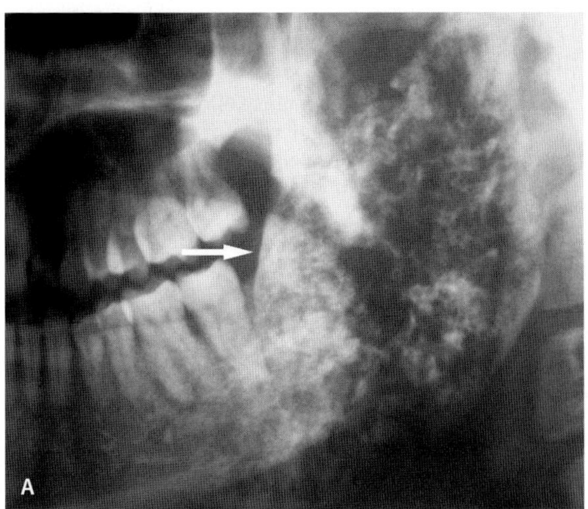

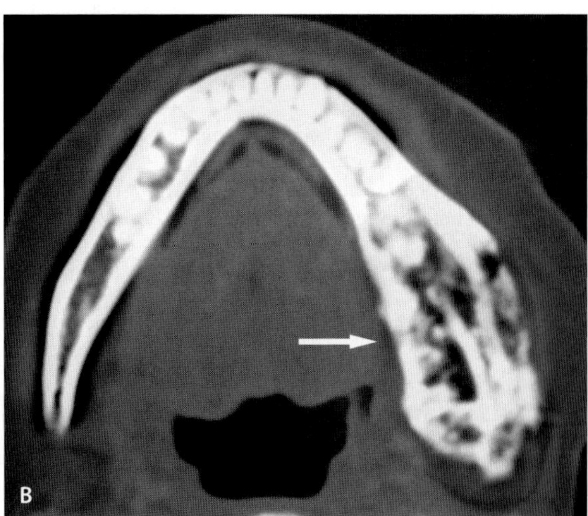

Figure 4.21

Ewing sarcoma, mandible; 24-year-old female with 10-year history of Ewing sarcoma treated with radiotherapy and chemotherapy, and a rather unchanged condition; now with pain and swelling and new soft-tissue mass, possibly due to infection. **A** Panoramic view shows bone production in entire half of mandible (*arrow*). **B** Axial CT image shows bone production both buccally and lingually (*arrow*)

Suggested Reading

Ator GA, Abemayor E, Lufkin RB, Hanafee WN, Ward PH (1990) Evaluation of mandibular tumor invasion with magnetic resonance imaging. Arch Otolaryngol Head Neck Surg 116:454–459

Bianchi SD, Boccardi A (1999) Radiological aspects of osteosarcoma of the jaws. Dentomaxillofac Radiol 28:42–47

Bredesen K, Aalokken TM, Kolbenstvedt A (2001) CT of the oral vestibule with distended cheeks. Acta Radiol 42:84–87

Browand BC, Waldron CA (1975) Central mucoepidermoid tumors of the jaws. Report of nine cases and review of the literature. Oral Surg Oral Med Oral Pathol 40:631–643

Brown JS, Griffith JF, Phelps PD, Browne RM (1994) A comparison of different imaging modalities and direct inspection after periosteal stripping in predicting the invasion of the mandible by oral squamous cell carcinoma. Br J Oral Maxillofac Surg 32:347–359

Deepti S, Somanathan T, Ramdas K, Pandey M (2003) Central mucodermoid carcinoma of mandible. A case report and review of literature. World J Surg Oncol 1:1–5

Eversole LR, Sabes WR, Rovin S (1975) Aggressive growth and neoplastic potential of odontogenic cysts: with special reference to central epidermoid and mucoepidermoid carcinomas. Cancer 35:270–282

Farman AG, Nortje C, Wood RE (1993) Malignancies affecting the jaws In: Oral and maxillofacial diagnostic imaging. Mosby, St. Louis, pp 280–316

Fordice J, Kershaw C, El-Nagger A, Goepfert H (1999) Adenoid cystic carcinoma of the head and neck: predictors of morbidity and mortality. Arch Otolaryngol Head Neck Surg 125:149–152

Kimura Y, Sumi M, Sumi T, Ariji Y, Ariji E, Nakamura T (2002) Deep extension from carcinoma arising from the gingiva: CT and MR imaging features. AJNR Am J Roentgenol 23:468–472

Laine FJ, Braun IF, Jensen ME, Nadel L, Som PM (1990) Perineural tumor extension through the foramen ovale: evaluation with MR imaging. Radiology 174:65–71

Larheim TA, Kolbenstvedt A, Lien HH (1984) Carcinoma of maxillary sinus, palate and maxillary gingiva: occurrence of jaw destruction. Scand J Dent Res 92:235–240

Larheim TA, Kolbenstvedt A, Lien HH (1984) Bony destruction from intraoral carcinomas. Dentomaxillofac Radiol 13:33–37

Lovas JGL (1991) Malignant neoplasms In: Miles DA, Van Dis M, Kaugers GE, Lovas JGL (eds) Oral and maxillofacial radiology. Radiologic/pathologic correlations. Saunders, Philadelphia, pp 97–124

Mardinger O, Givol N, Talmi YP, Taicher S (2001) Osteosarcoma of the jaw. The Chaim Sheba Medical Center experience. Oral Surg Oral Med Oral Pathol Oral Radiol Endod 91:445–451

Nakayama E, Yoshiura K, Ozeki S, Nakayama H, Yamaguchi T, Yoshikawa H, Kanda S, Ohishi M, Shirasuna K (2003) The correlation of histologic features with a panoramic radiography pattern and a computed tomography pattern of bone destruction in carcinoma of the mandibular gingiva. Oral Surg Oral Med Oral Pathol Oral Radiol Endod 96:774–782

Pindborg JJ, Reichart PA, Smith CJ, van der Waal I (1997) World Health Organisation. Histological typing of cancer and precancer of the oral mucosa, 2nd edn. Springer, Berlin, p 11

Resnick D (1996) Bone and joint imaging, 2nd edn. Saunders, Philadelphia, p 625

Schajowicz F (1993) World Health Organisation. Histological typing of bone tumors, 2nd edn. Springer, Berlin, pp 10, 17, 22, 25

Scheer M, Koch AM, Drebber U, Kubler AC (2004) Primary intraosseous carcinoma of the jaws arising from an odontogenic cyst – a case report. J Craniomaxillofac Surg 32:166–169

Seifert G (1991) World Health Organisation. Histological typing of salivary gland tumors, 2nd edn. Springer, Berlin, pp 20, 21

Sigal R, Monnet O, de Baere T, Micheau C, Shapeero LG, Julieron M, Bosq J, Vanel D, Piekarski JD, Luboinski B (1992) Adenoid cystic carcinoma of the head and neck: evaluation with MR imaging and clinical-pathologic correlation in 27 patients. Radiology 184:95–101

Thomas G, Pandey M, Mathew A, Abraham EK, Francis A, Somanathan T, Iype M, Sebastian P, Nair MK (2001) Primary intraosseous carcinoma of the jaw: pooled analysis of the world literature and report of two new cases. Int J Oral Maxillofac Surg 30:349–355

Vrielinck LJ, Ostyn F, van Damme B, van den Bogaert W, Fossion E (1988) The significance of perineural spread in adenoid cystic carcinoma of the major and minor salivary glands. Int J Oral Maxillofac Surg 17:190–193

Waldron CA, Mustoe TA (1989) Primary intraosseous carcinoma of the mandible with probable origin in an odontogenic cyst. Oral Surg Oral Med Oral Pathol 67:716–724

Weber AL, Kaneda T, Scrivani SJ, Aziz S (2003) Jaw: cysts, tumors, and nontumorous lesions. In: Som PM, Curtin HD (eds) Head and neck imaging, 4th edn. Mosby, St. Louis, pp 930–994

Wood RE (2004) Malignant diseases of the jaws. In: White SW, Pharoah MJ (eds) Oral radiology. Principles and interpretation, 5th edn. Saunders, Philadelphia, pp 458–484

Wood RE, Nortje CJ, Hesseling P, Grotepass F (1990) Ewing's tumor of the jaw. Oral Surg Oral Med Oral Pathol 69:120–127

Jaw Infections

Introduction

Dental caries, periodontal disease and apical periodontitis (periapical granuloma, abscess, or cyst) are common pathologic conditions and usually restricted to the region of the teeth and adjacent bone. These conditions are most often adequately assessed by intraoral or panoramic radiography. Infection also appears as condensing or sclerosing osteitis frequently defined as a localized form of osteomyelitis but usually limited to the periapical region of the mandibular molars. However, other and larger areas of jaw bone may become infected as a direct extension from a common odontogenic infection, or as a result trauma, large doses of therapeutic radiation, and hematogenous spread from a distant site. Most cases of jaw osteomyelitis are nonspecific infections (in contrast to osteomyelitis in other parts of skeleton), but specific types such as tuberculosis and actinomycosis may occur.

When infection develops in jaw bone marrow as an osteomyelitis or in surrounding soft tissues as an abscess, advanced imaging in particular CT, may be of great diagnostic value as a supplement to projectional (conventional or digital) radiography.

Osteomyelitis

Definition

Inflammatory process accompanied by bone destruction and caused by infecting microorganisms.

The infection can be limited to a single portion of bone or can involve several regions including marrow, cortex, periosteum, and surrounding soft tissue.

Clinical Features

- Mandible far more often than maxilla
- Acute form presents with severe symptoms, chronic form with vague or no symptoms, but episodes of exacerbation
- Pain and swelling, may be variable
- Regional lymphadenopathy, fever, malaise
- Mobile teeth sensitive to percussion
- Fistula draining of pus
- Paresthesia in lower lip (mental nerve)
- Trismus if masticatory muscles are infiltrated
- Enlargement of mandible; jaw asymmetry
- Usually odontogenic infectious etiology, but idiopathic, chronic, nonsuppurative forms may occur in adults, children or adolescents

Imaging Features

- Initial blurring of bone trabeculae
- Ill-defined ('moth-eaten') osteolytic areas, apparently interspersed by normal bone
- Sequestrum; fragment of necrotic bone
- Involucrum; sequestrum surrounded by viable bone
- Periosteal bone formation; 'onion skin' appearance
- Mixture of ill-defined osteolytic and ill-defined osteosclerotic areas
- Completely radiopaque areas
- T1-weighted MRI: reduced signal from bone marrow
- T2-weighted and STIR MRI: high signal from bone marrow
- T1-weighted post-Gd MRI: contrast enhancement of bone marrow and adjacent soft tissue
- T1-weighted, T2-weighted, and STIR MRI: low signal from sequestra

Comment

From a radiologic point of view, three types of osteomyelitis may be distinguished: rarefying or destructive (suppurative) osteomyelitis, diffuse sclerosing osteomyelitis, and osteomyelitis with periostitis. A mixture of these types is common

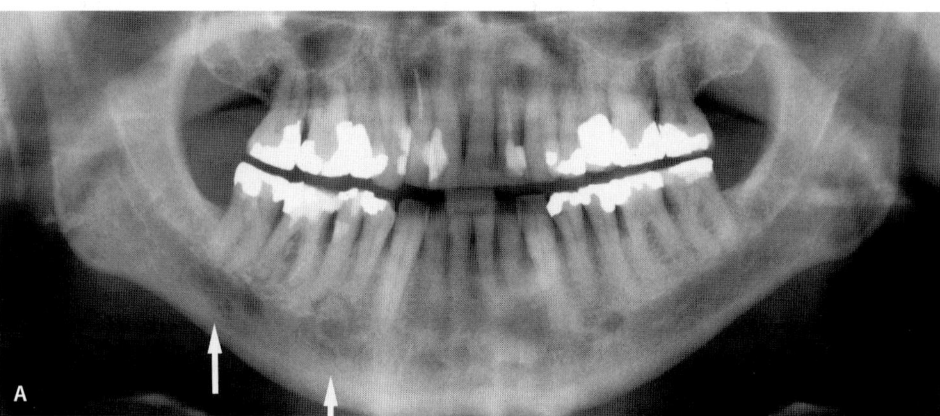

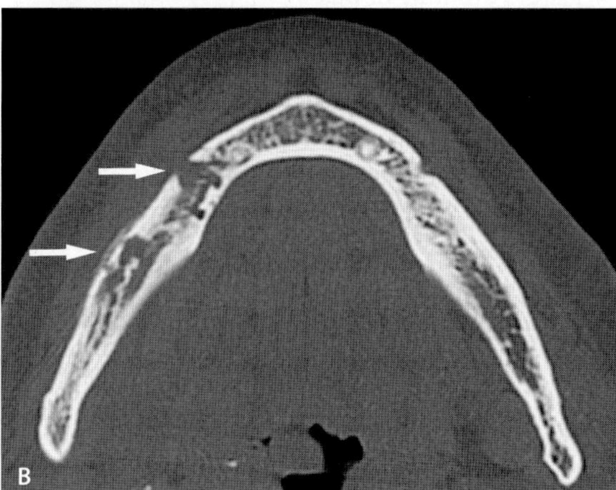

Figure 5.1

Osteomyelitis, mandible; 58-year-old male with pain and perimandibular swelling. **A** Panoramic view shows diffuse bone destruction caudad to molars (*arrow*), and suspected sequestrum caudad to premolars (*arrow*). **B** Axial CT image shows destruction from widened mental foramen (*upper arrow*) to molar area and defects in lingual cortical bone, but no sequestrum. Note small buccal periosteal reaction in molar region (*arrow*)

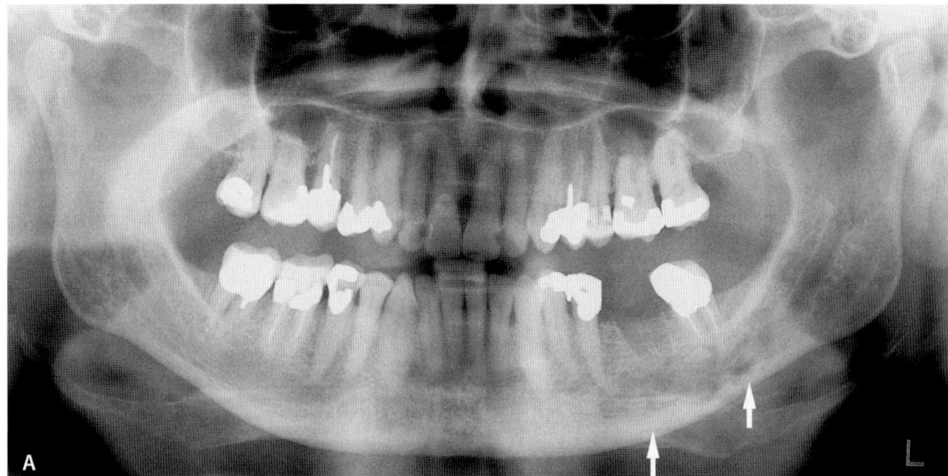

Figure 5.2

Osteomyelitis, mandible; 46-year-old female with previous pain from molar that was extracted, but still pain and additionally, perimandibular swelling. A Panoramic view shows diffuse bone destruction (*arrows*). B Axial CT image shows diffuse destruction of buccal cortical bone (*arrow*) and sequestrum (*arrowhead*)

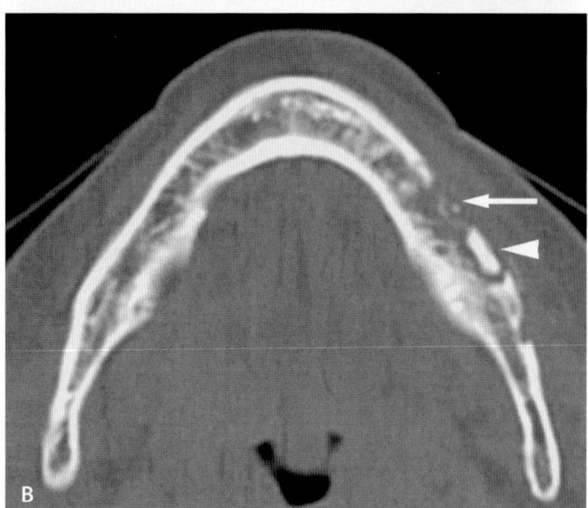

Figure 5.3

Osteomyelitis, mandible; 68-year-old female with pain, mandibular cellulitis, and diffuse swelling in neck. Axial CT image shows 'moth-eaten' and extensive infection bilaterally (*arrows*)

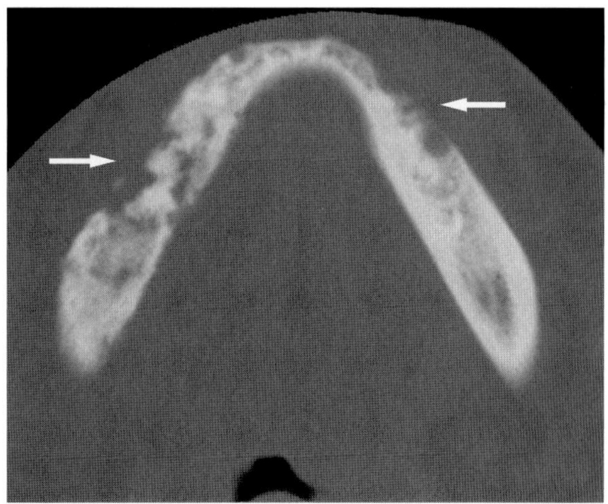

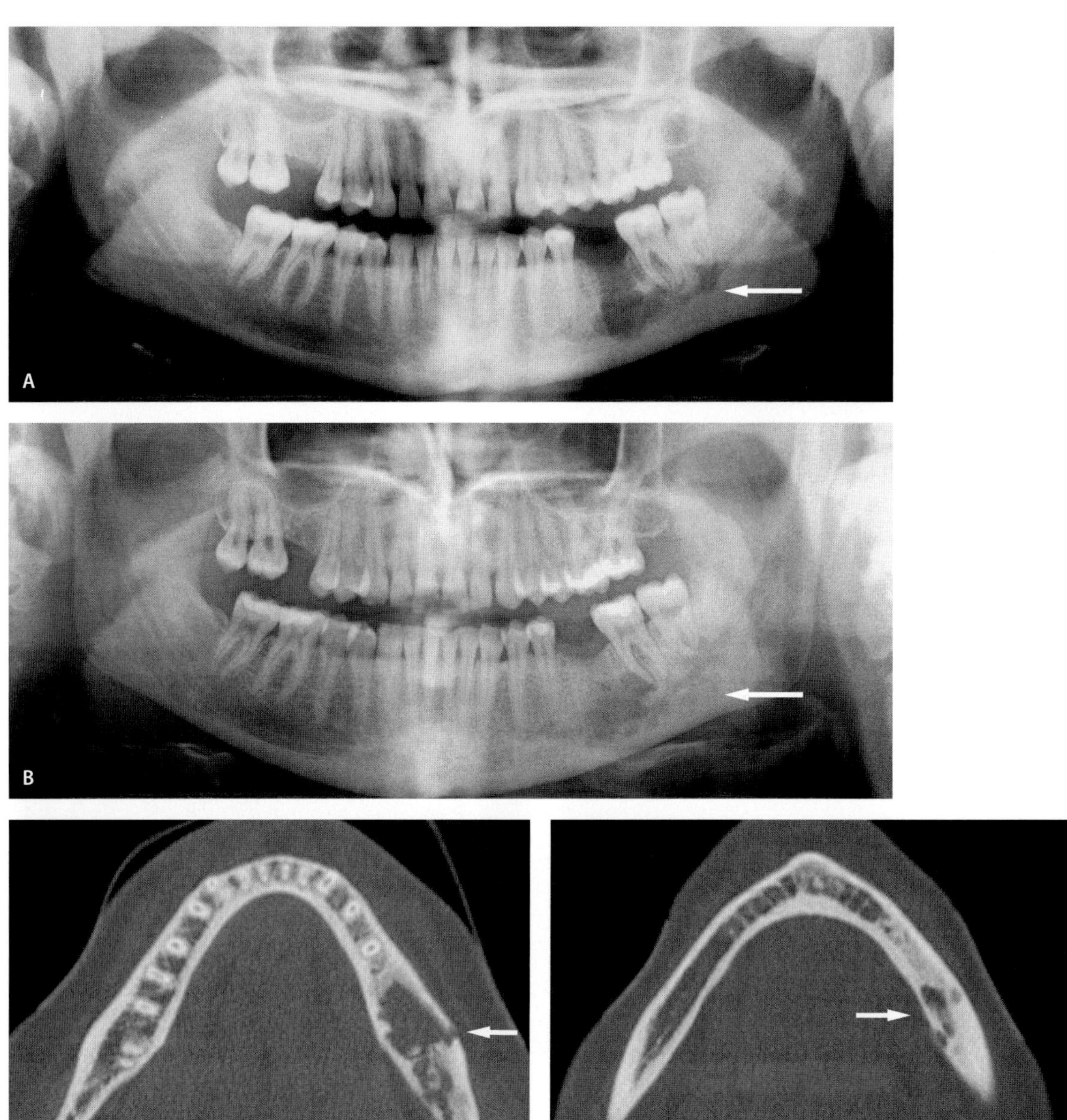
A
B
C
D

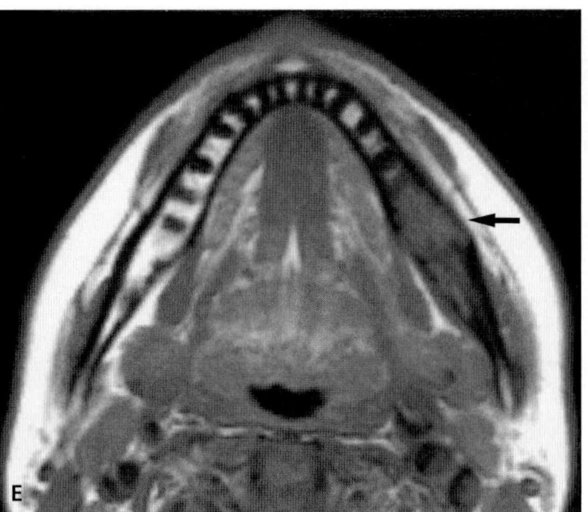

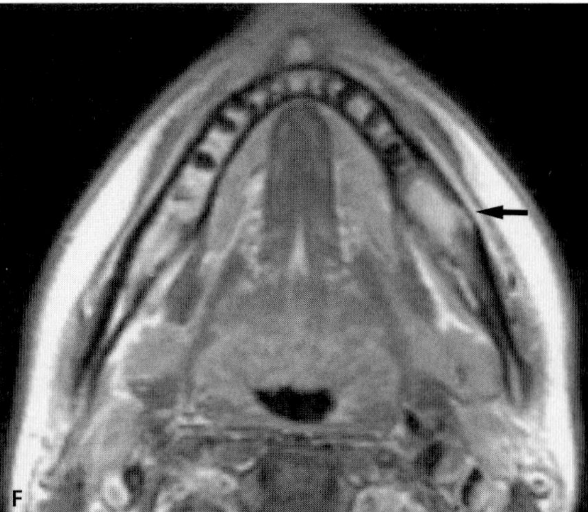

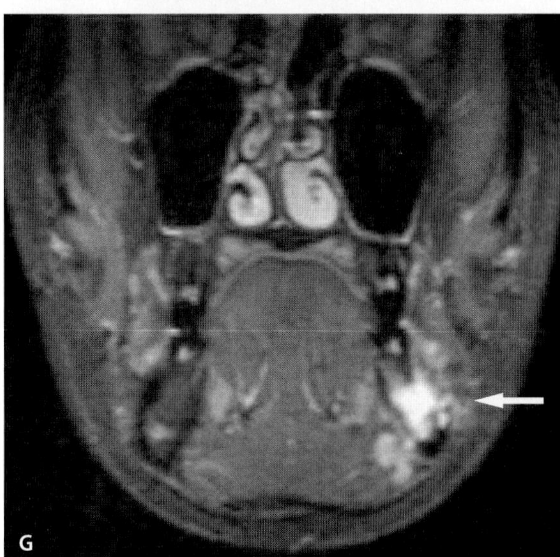

Figure 5.4

Osteomyelitis, mandible; 25-year-old female with molar extracted after unsuccessful endodontic therapy, but progression of mandibular infection despite antibiotic therapy, little pain. **A** Panoramic view shows bone destruction in molar area with diffuse sclerotic bone (*arrow*). **B** Panoramic view about 1 year later shows healing in alveolar bone, but progression of bone destruction in caudad areas (*arrow*), with 'honey-bobble' appearance that required a tumor diagnosis to be ruled out. **C** Axial CT image shows severe bone destruction, with cortical defect (*arrow*), but no periosteal reaction. **D** Axial CT image shows multilocular appearance in lower mandibular border and sclerosis (*arrow*). **E** Axial T1-weighted pre-Gd MRI shows reduced signal in bone marrow (*arrow*). **F** Axial T1-weighted post-Gd MRI shows contrast enhancement (*arrow*). **G** Coronal STIR MRI shows intense signal in bone marrow (*arrow*). Surgical decortication confirmed osteomyelitis and no tumor

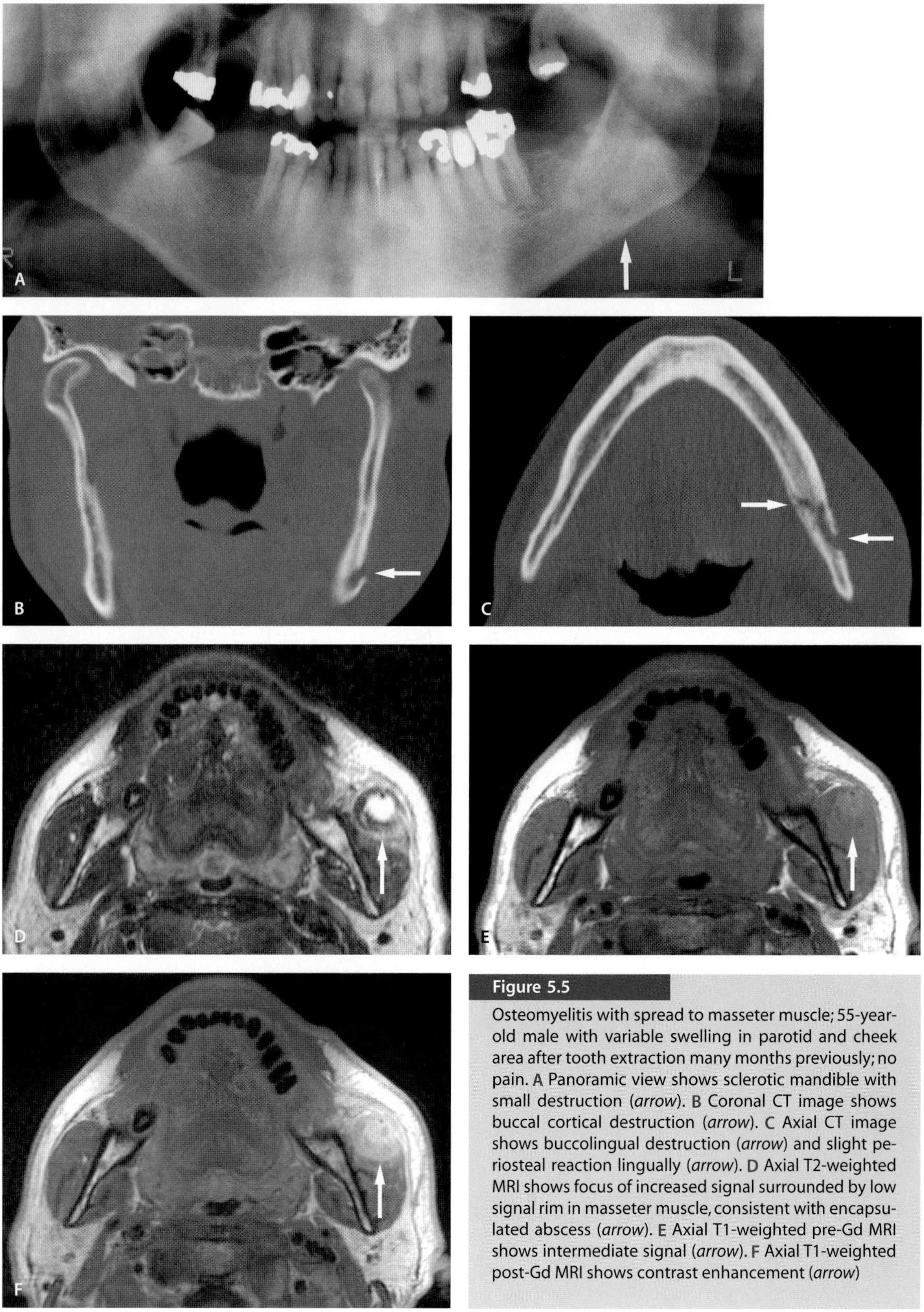

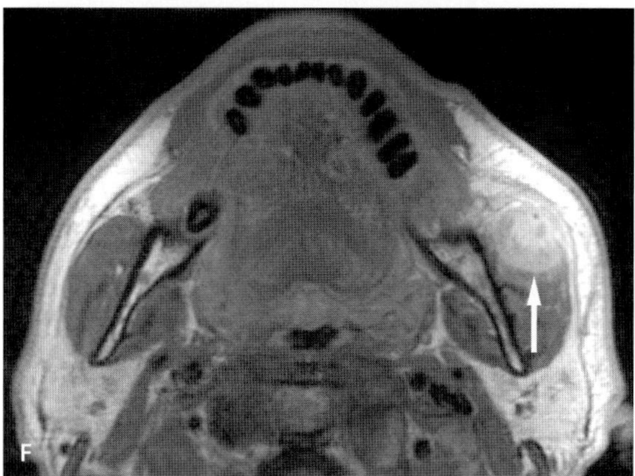

Figure 5.5

Osteomyelitis with spread to masseter muscle; 55-year-old male with variable swelling in parotid and cheek area after tooth extraction many months previously; no pain. A Panoramic view shows sclerotic mandible with small destruction (*arrow*). B Coronal CT image shows buccal cortical destruction (*arrow*). C Axial CT image shows buccolingual destruction (*arrow*) and slight periosteal reaction lingually (*arrow*). D Axial T2-weighted MRI shows focus of increased signal surrounded by low signal rim in masseter muscle, consistent with encapsulated abscess (*arrow*). E Axial T1-weighted pre-Gd MRI shows intermediate signal (*arrow*). F Axial T1-weighted post-Gd MRI shows contrast enhancement (*arrow*)

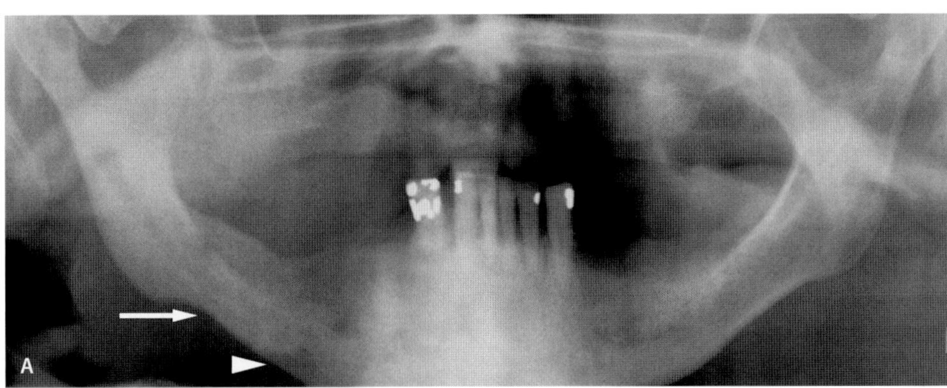

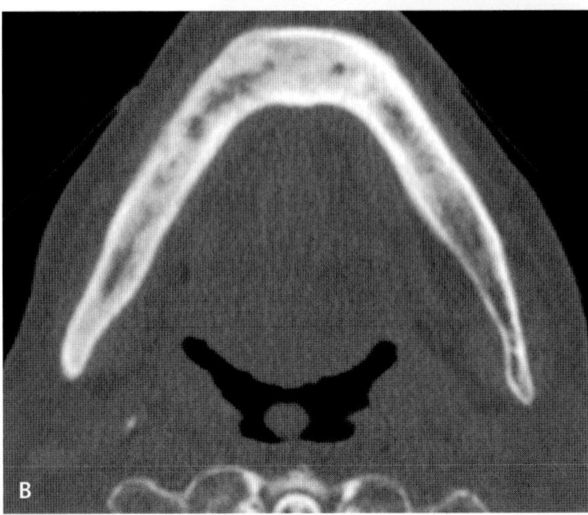

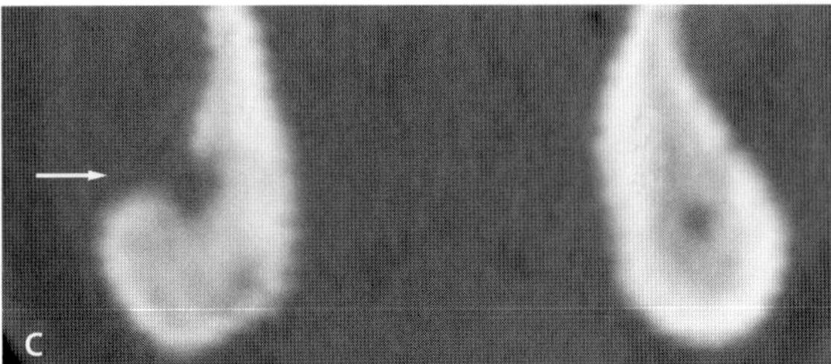

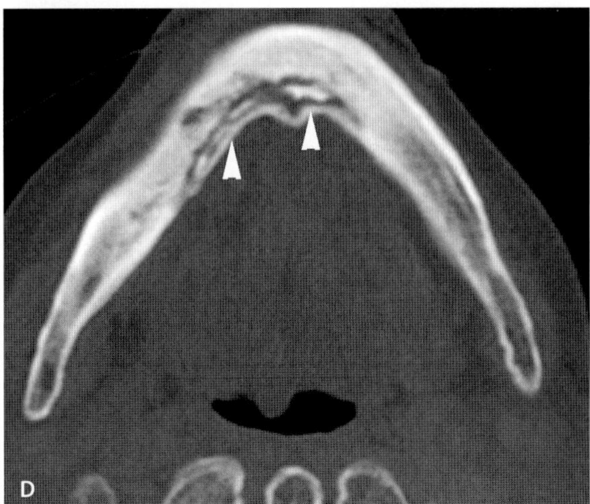

Figure 5.6

Osteomyelitis, mandible; 72-year-old female with variable, but little pain and variable swelling 3 years after teeth extraction, now with mental nerve paresthesia. A Panoramic view shows diffuse sclerotic changes (*arrow*), and small focus of bone destruction (*arrowhead*). B Axial CT image shows diffuse, extensive sclerotic changes in right mandible, crossing midline. C Coronal CT through mental foramina shows severe bone destruction on right side (*arrow*), explaining paresthesia. D Axial CT 7 years later still shows sclerotic osteomyelitis, now with exacerbation and sequestration (*arrowheads*)

Osteomyelitis with Periostitis

Synonyms: Periostitis ossificans, proliferative periostitis

Definition

Osteomyelitis with dominating periosteal new bone formation.

Clinical Features

- Mostly in children and young adults
- Unilateral hard swelling of jaw, asymmetry
- May be bilateral
- Symptoms usually vague
- Predominantly in mandible

Imaging Features

- Cortical expansion by periosteal bone formation; buccal, lingual, inferior aspects
- Characteristic 'onion skin' appearance
- Usually also bone destruction

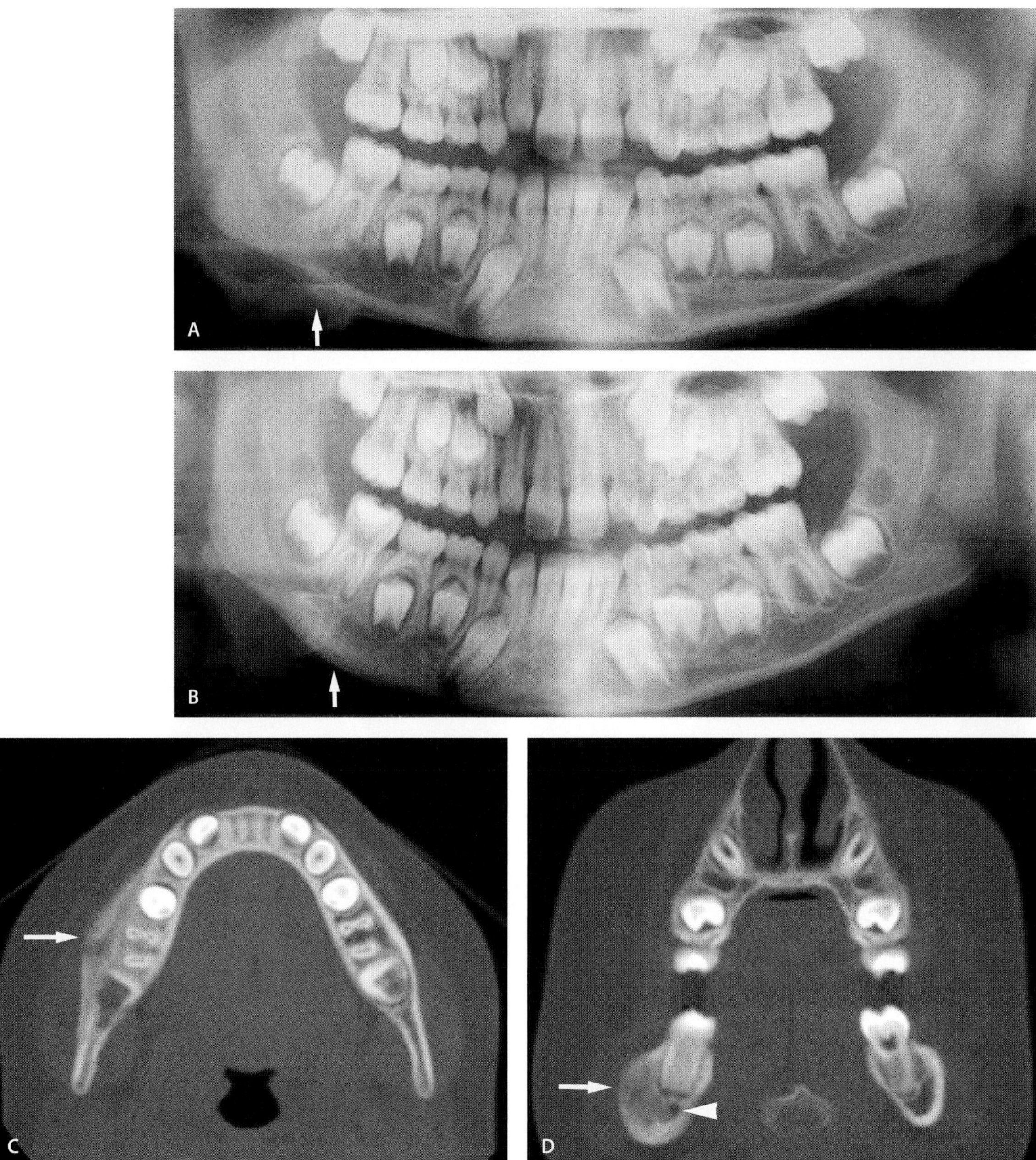

Figure 5.7

Osteomyelitis with periostitis, mandible; 7-year-old female with variable perimandibular swelling, painless, probably caused by trauma against mandible 1 month before. **A** Panoramic view shows no abnormalities except slight periosteal reaction (*arrow*) (not noted until later examinations were performed). **B** Panoramic view 2 months after trauma shows more clearly periosteal reaction (*arrow*). **C** Axial CT image shows severe periosteal reaction buccally (*arrow*). **D** Coronal CT image shows sclerotic mandible with thickness almost twice normal (*arrow*), with radiolucent mandibular canal (*arrowhead*)

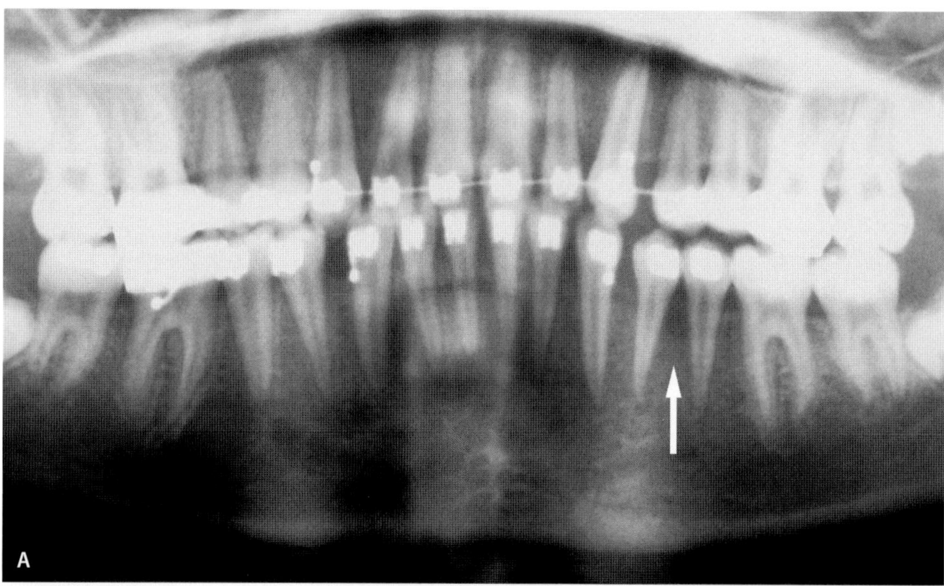

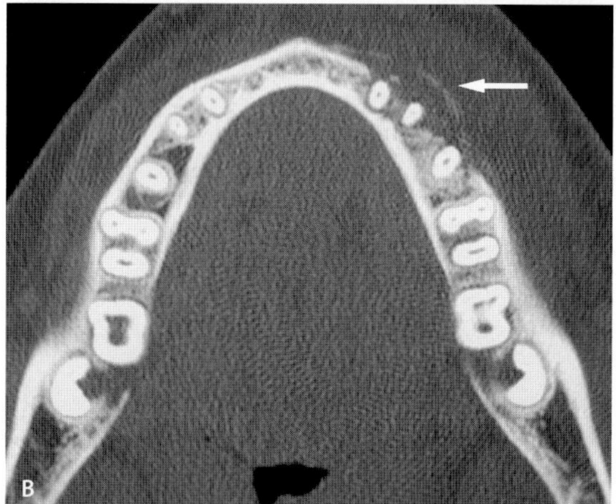

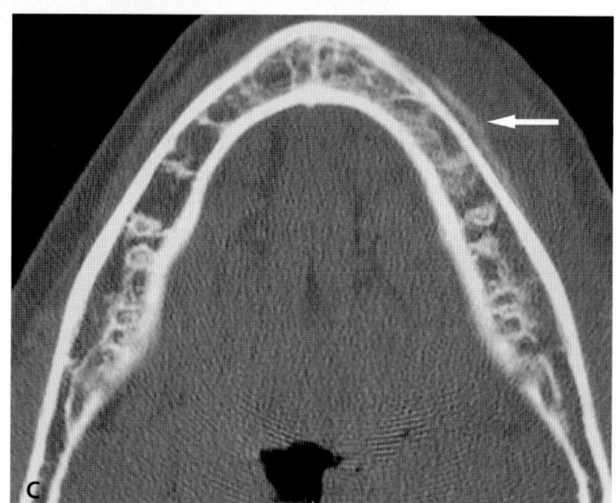

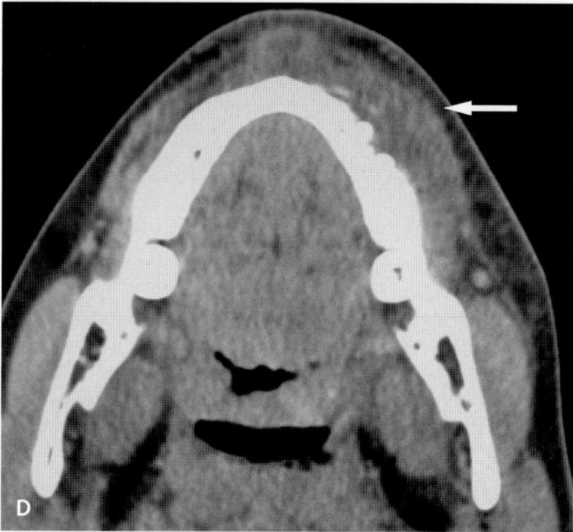

Figure 5.8

Osteomyelitis with periostitis, mandible; 12-year-old female with three weeks history of gingival swelling that begun less than a week after orthodontic adjustment of braces. **A** Panoramic view shows diffuse destruction in premolar area (*arrow*). **B** Axial CT image shows bone destruction and periosteal reaction in premolar area (*arrow*). **C** Axial CT image shows periosteal reaction caudad to teeth (*arrow*). **D** Axial CT, soft tissue window, shows diffuse soft tissue swelling consistent with inflammatory infiltrate (*arrow*)

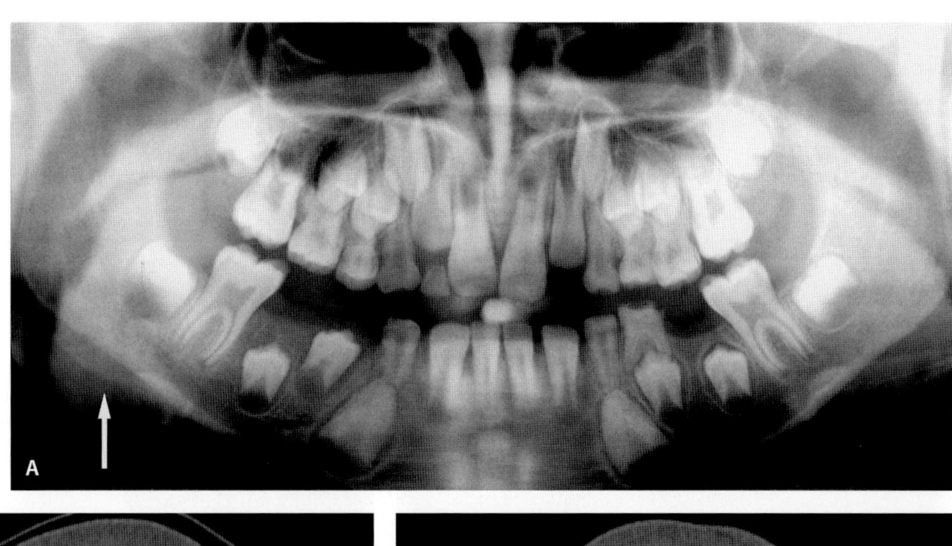

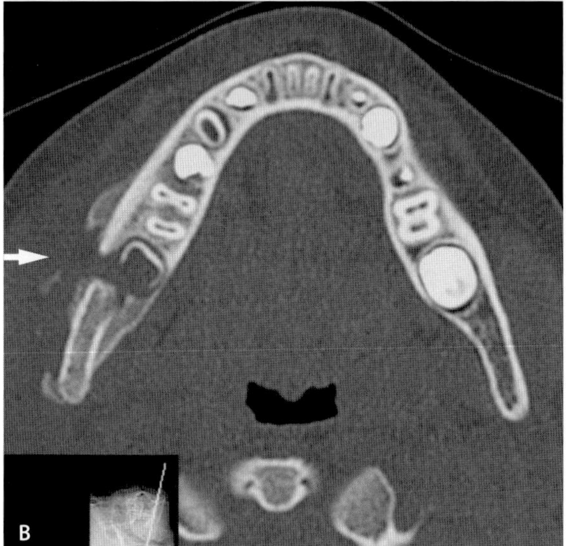

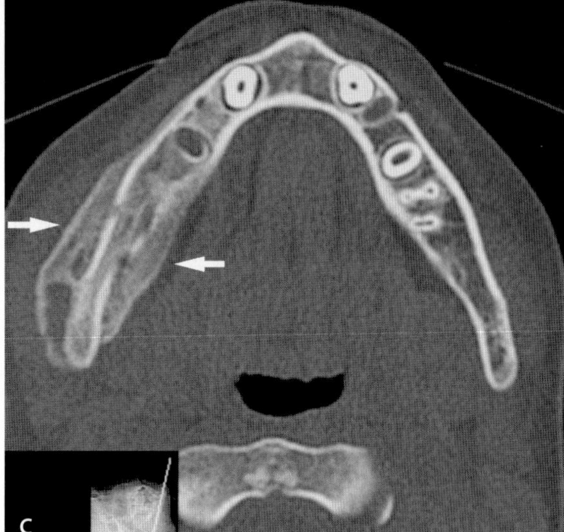

Figure 5.9

Osteomyelitis with periostitis, mandible; 8-year-old male with variable right perimandibular swelling and pain for some months. **A** Panoramic view shows periosteal reaction (*arrow*). **B** Axial CT image shows destruction of buccal bone at second molar germ (*arrow*). **C** Axial CT image shows extensive periosteal bone, buccally and lingually (*arrows*)

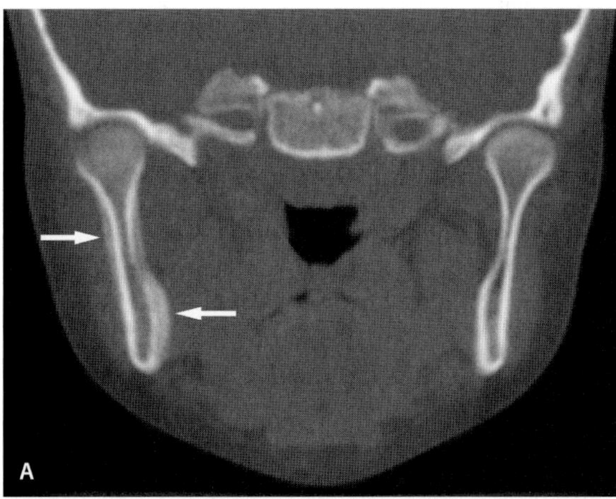

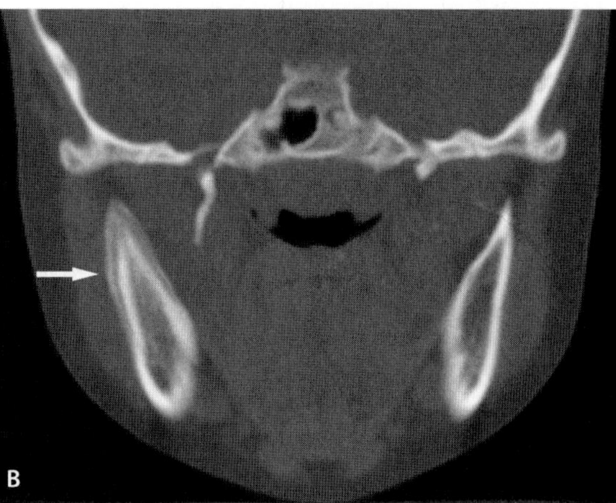

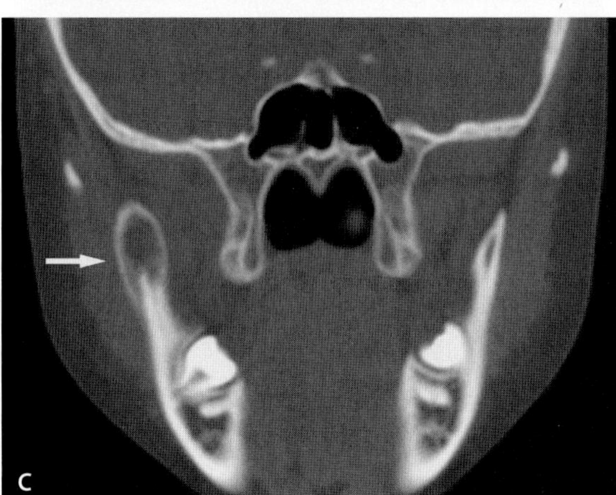

Figure 5.10

Osteomyelitis with periostitis, mandible; 10-year-old female with variable facial swelling and restricted mouth opening capacity. **A** Coronal CT image shows periosteal reaction buccally and lingually (*arrows*). **B** Coronal CT image shows periosteal reaction caudad for semilunar incisure (*arrow*). **C** Coronal CT show extensive reaction in coronoid process (*arrow*)

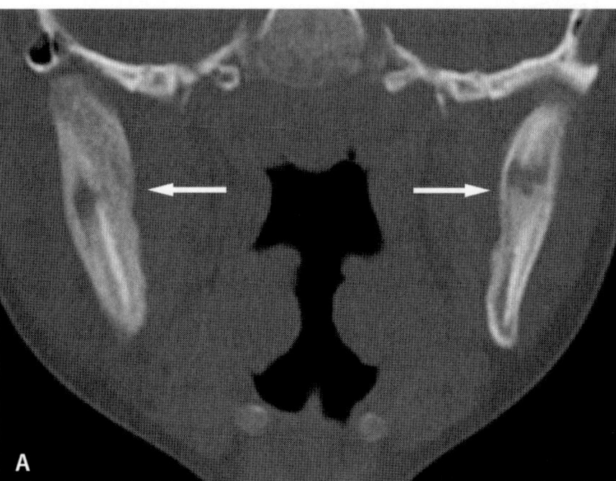

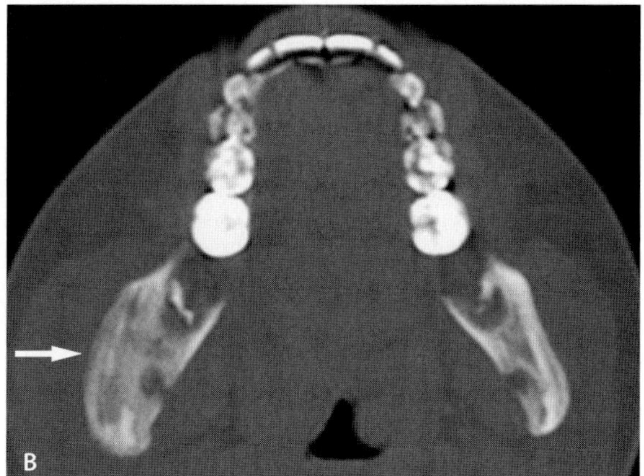

Figure 5.11

Osteomyelitis with bilateral periostitis, mandible; 11-year-old female with variable pain and mouth opening capacity for about 6 months, believed to be caused by juvenile arthritis. **A** Coronal CT image shows extensive periosteal bone bilaterally in ramus (*arrows*). **B** Axial CT image shows characteristic 'onion skin' periosteal bone (*arrow*)

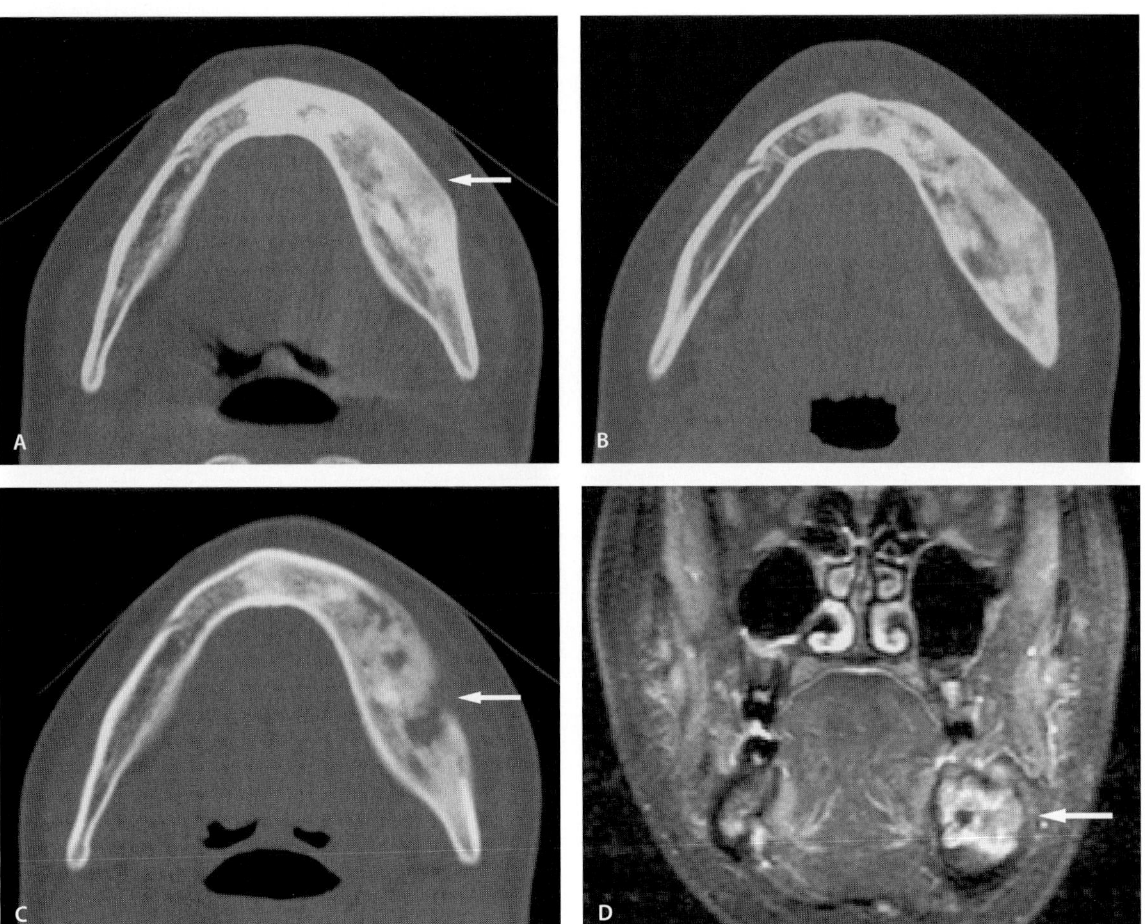

Figure 5.12

Osteomyelitis with periostitis, mandible; 16-year-old female with a 2-year history of infection, with development of facial asymmetry after unsuccessful endodontic treatment of first and second molars that eventually were extracted. **A** Axial CT image shows sclerotic and thickened mandibular bone (*arrow*). **B** Axial CT image, 1-year follow-up, shows smaller areas of bone destruction. **C** Axial CT image, 2-year follow-up, shows larger areas of bone destruction (*arrow*). **D** Coronal STIR MRI, 2-year follow-up, shows high signal consistent with active inflammation (*arrow*)

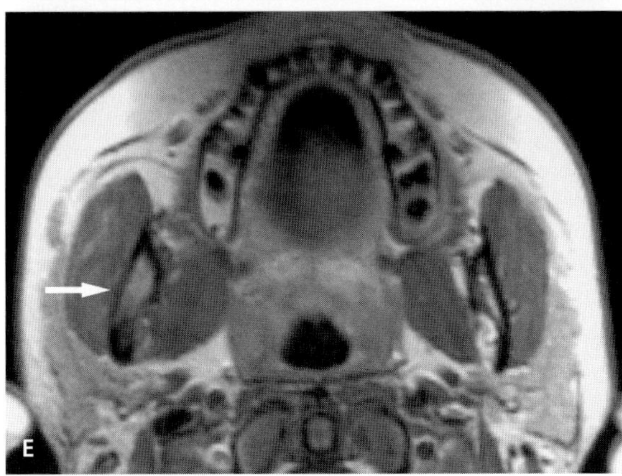

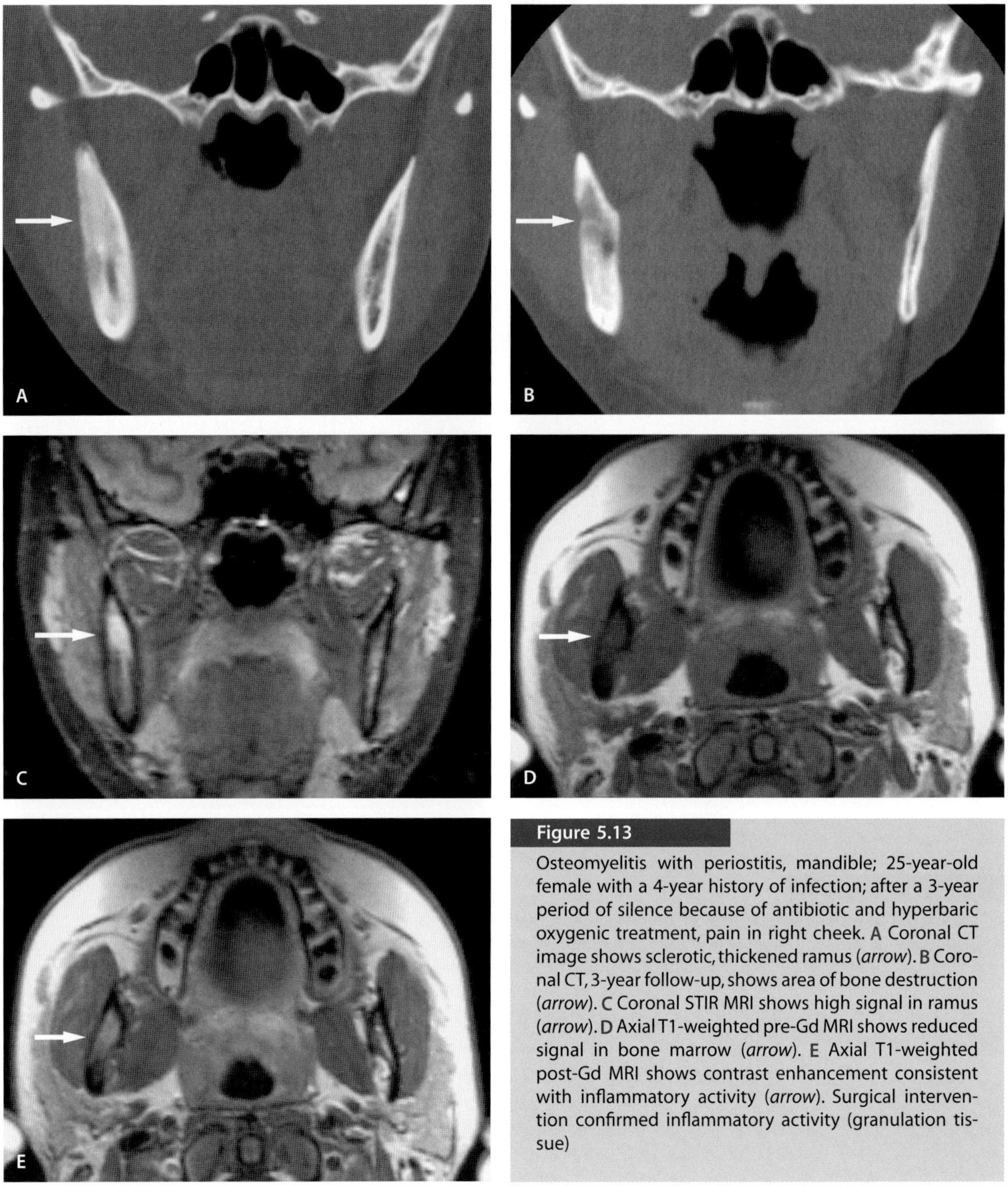

Figure 5.13

Osteomyelitis with periostitis, mandible; 25-year-old female with a 4-year history of infection; after a 3-year period of silence because of antibiotic and hyperbaric oxygenic treatment, pain in right cheek. A Coronal CT image shows sclerotic, thickened ramus (*arrow*). B Coronal CT, 3-year follow-up, shows area of bone destruction (*arrow*). C Coronal STIR MRI shows high signal in ramus (*arrow*). D Axial T1-weighted pre-Gd MRI shows reduced signal in bone marrow (*arrow*). E Axial T1-weighted post-Gd MRI shows contrast enhancement consistent with inflammatory activity (*arrow*). Surgical intervention confirmed inflammatory activity (granulation tissue)

Osteosclerosis, idiopathic

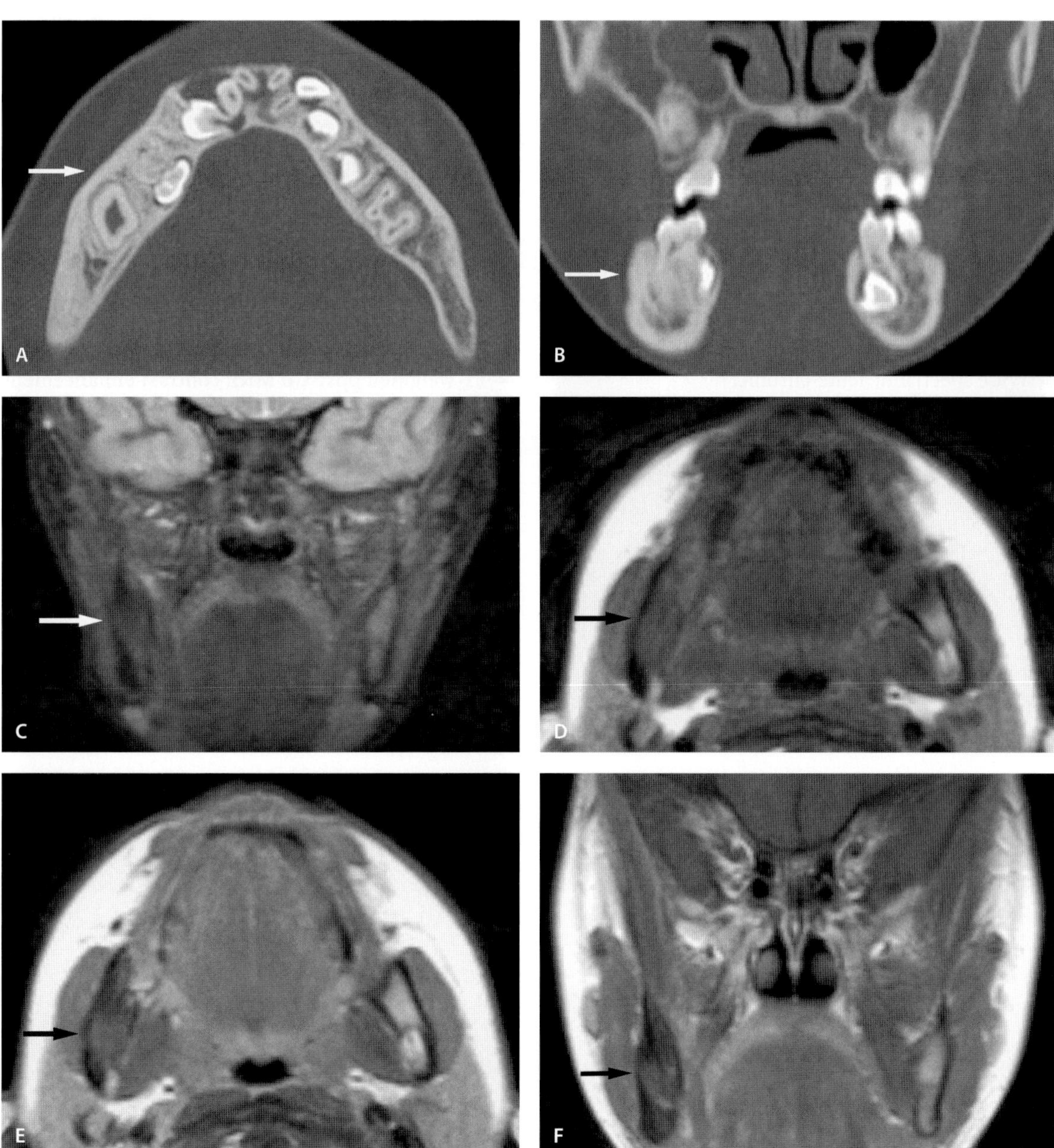

Figure 5.14

Osteosclerosis, idiopathic, mandible; 11-year-old female with perimandibular pain after extraction of a tooth germ, and suspected osteomyelitis. Patient had an unclassified congenital anomaly with generalized osteosclerosis. **A** Axial CT image shows thick, sclerotic mandibular body but no foci of bone destruction (*arrow*). **B** Coronal CT image shows thick cortical bone but no periosteal bone (*arrow*). **C** Coronal STIR MRI shows intermediate–low signal in ramus (*arrow*). **D** Axial T1-weighted pre-Gd MRI shows reduced signal in marrow (*arrow*). **E** Axial T1-weighted post-Gd MRI shows no contrast enhancement (*arrow*). **F** Coronal T1-weighted post-Gd MRI shows no contrast enhancement (*arrow*). Extraction wound eventually healed, and patient was asymptomatic with a thick, dense mandible consistent with idiopathic osteosclerosis

Osteoradionecrosis

Definition

Several proposed. One most frequently used is 'area of exposed bone larger than 1 cm in field of irradiation that has failed to show any evidence of healing for at least 6 months'.

An alternative is 'radiologic evidence of bone necrosis within radiation field where tumor recurrence has been excluded', also including cases with intact oral mucosa.

Clinical Features

- Mandible far more often than maxilla
- Wide spectrum; acute/chronic, nonsuppurative/suppurative
- Pain or no pain
- Exposed bone frequent, but also soft tissue cover
- In advanced stage: trismus, fistula, pathologic fracture
- Similar condition has been reported after bisphosphonate therapy in patients who are not irradiated

Imaging Features

- Mainly destructive; cancellous and/or cortical bone
- Mixture of radiolucent and radiopaque appearance
- Unilateral or bilateral
- Usually without periosteal reaction
- Advanced stage: sequestration, pathologic fracture
- T1-weighted MRI: reduced signal in bone marrow
- T2-weighted and STIR MRI: high signal in marrow
- T1-weighted post-Gd MRI: contrast enhancement
- T1-weighted, T2-weighted, and STIR MRI: low signal from sequestra

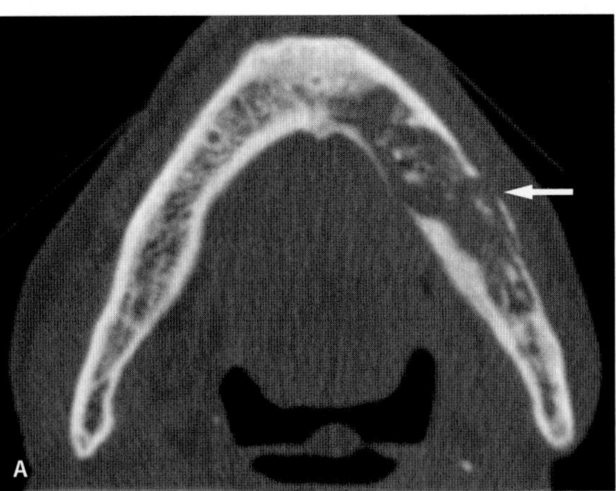

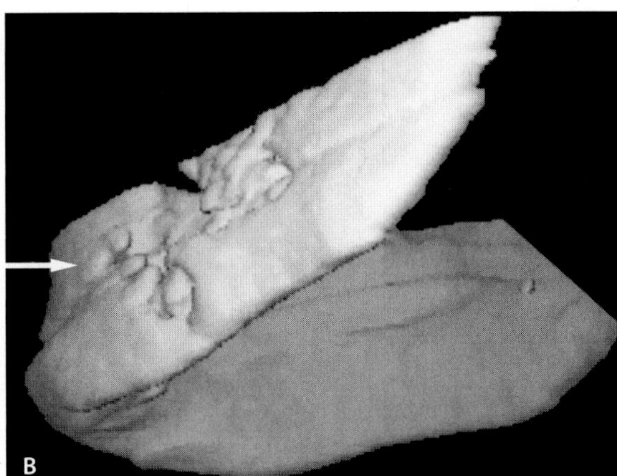

Figure 5.15

Osteoradionecrosis, mandible; 79-year-old male with hemimandible resection due to extensive abnormalities and severe symptoms. **A** Axial CT image shows severe destruction of left mandibular body (*arrow*). **B** 3D CT image shows severe destruction of buccal cortical bone (*arrow*). **C** Surgical specimen with destruction (*arrow*) corresponding to 3D CT image presentation (courtesy of Dr. G. Støre, Rikshospitalet University Hospital, Oslo, Norway)

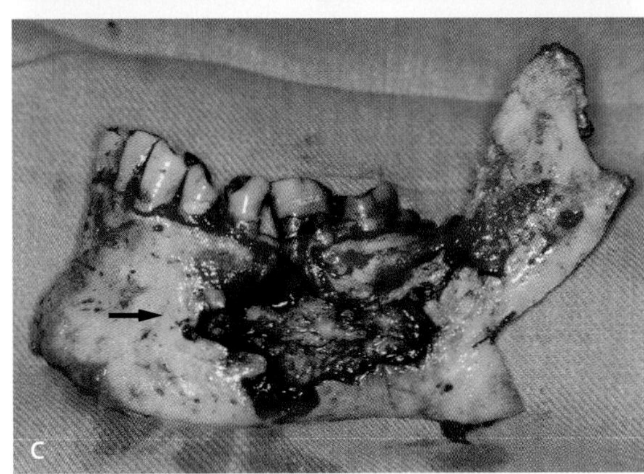

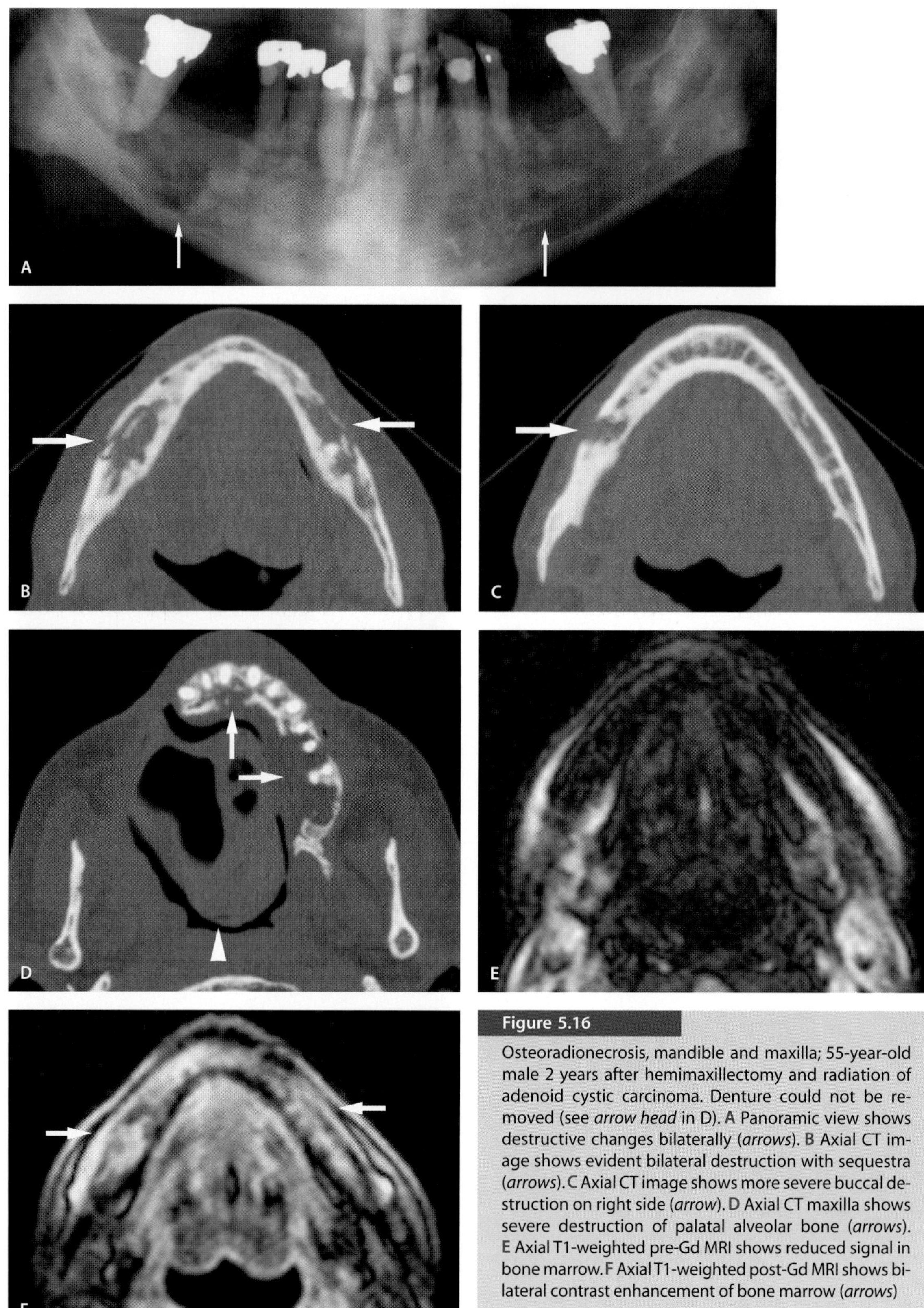

Figure 5.16

Osteoradionecrosis, mandible and maxilla; 55-year-old male 2 years after hemimaxillectomy and radiation of adenoid cystic carcinoma. Denture could not be removed (see *arrow head* in D). **A** Panoramic view shows destructive changes bilaterally (*arrows*). **B** Axial CT image shows evident bilateral destruction with sequestra (*arrows*). **C** Axial CT image shows more severe buccal destruction on right side (*arrow*). **D** Axial CT maxilla shows severe destruction of palatal alveolar bone (*arrows*). **E** Axial T1-weighted pre-Gd MRI shows reduced signal in bone marrow. **F** Axial T1-weighted post-Gd MRI shows bilateral contrast enhancement of bone marrow (*arrows*)

Abscess

Definition
Collection of pus in bone or soft tissue.

Clinical Features
- Swelling, pain
- Redness, warmth
- Trismus
- Fever, malaise
- Swallowing problems
- Breath problems

Imaging Features
- Bone destruction if infection is in bone
- Round or lobulated soft-tissue structure with enhancing peripheral rim and hypodense (necrotic) center
- T2-weighted MRI and STIR: high-signal center surrounded by low-signal periphery
- T1-weighted pre-Gd MRI: intermediate signal
- T1-weighted post-Gd MRI: no contrast enhancement except periphery
- A phlegmon or cellulitis will enhance diffusely and entirely

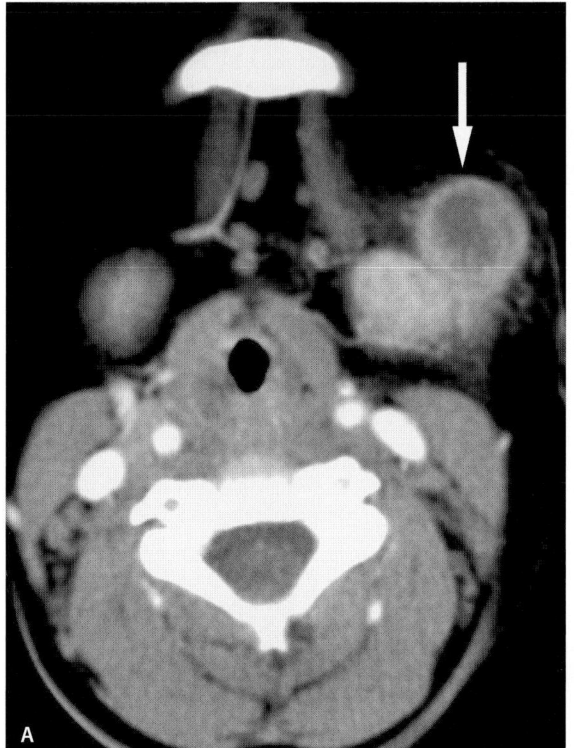

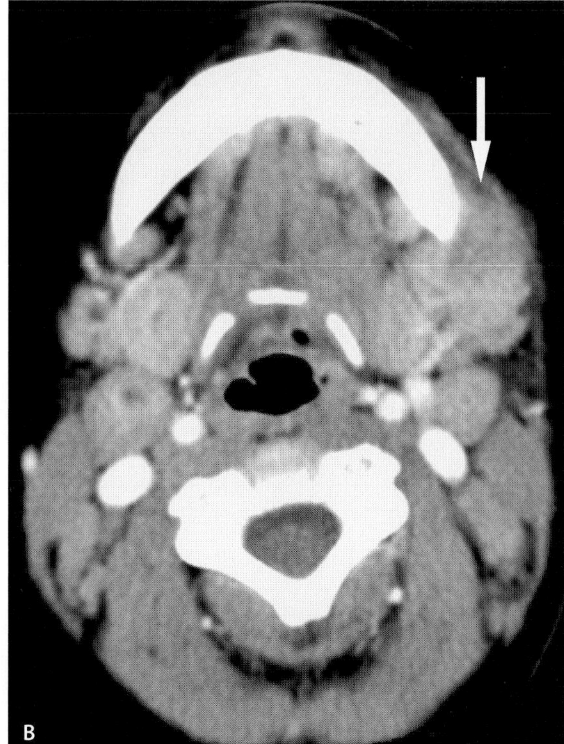

Figure 5.17

Abscess, submandibular; 22-month old male with history of left neck mass, strep throat, and fever. **A** Axial CT image, soft-tissue window, shows anterior and lateral to left submandibular gland a hypodense nodular, circular structure surrounded by hyperintense rim (*arrow*). **B** Axial CT image, soft-tissue window, shows abscess (*arrow*) surrounded by diffuse infiltration in fat planes, and scattered cervical lymphadenopathy. Normal bone structures were seen.

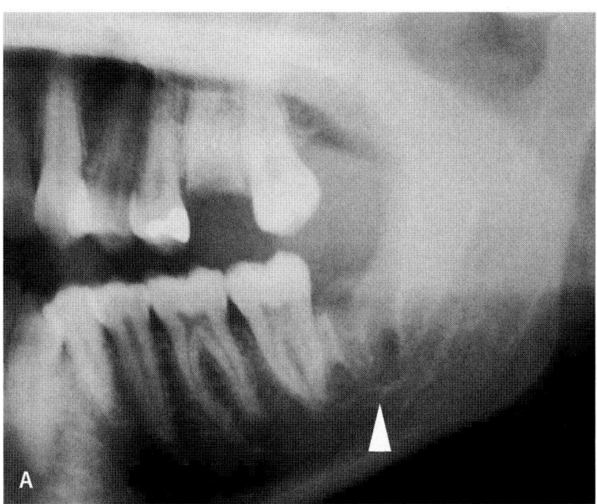

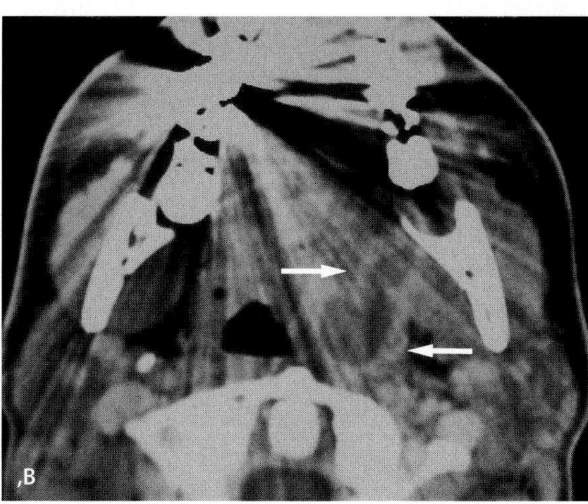

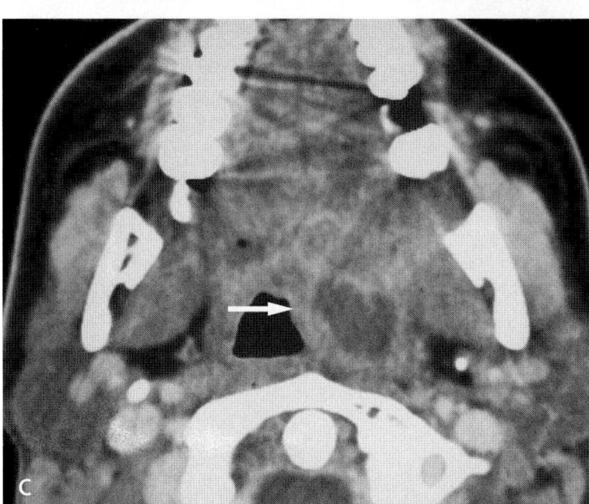

Figure 5.18

Abscess, parapharyngeal; 24-year-old female with pharyngeal swelling after extraction of infected third molar. **A** Panoramic view shows tooth socket (*arrowhead*) and infectious first molar in maxilla. **B** Axial CT image, soft-tissue window, shows abscess from tooth socket, extending parapharyngeally (*arrows*). **C** Axial CT image, soft-tissue window, shows parapharyngeal abscess narrowing air space (*arrow*)

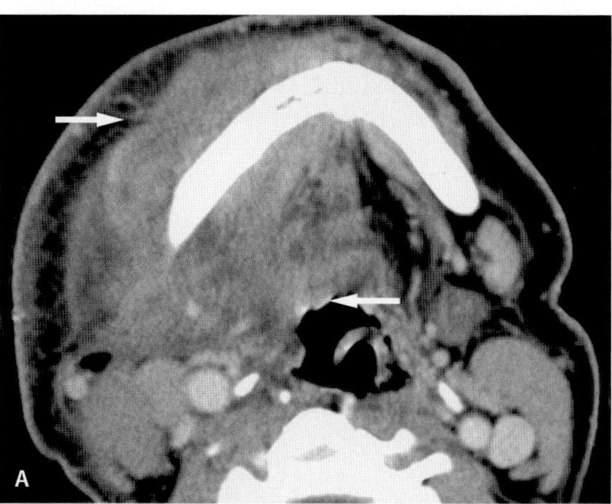

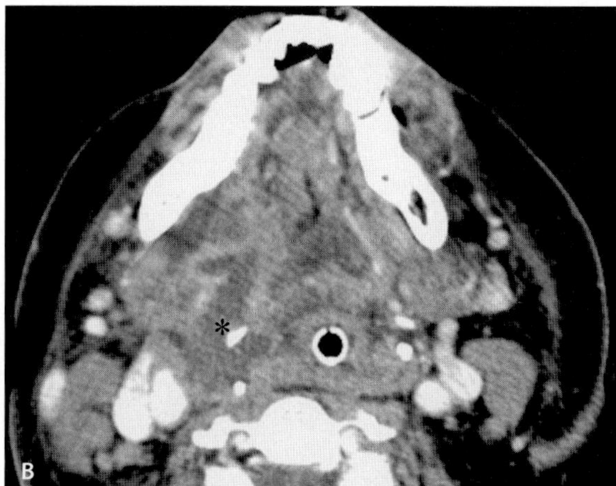

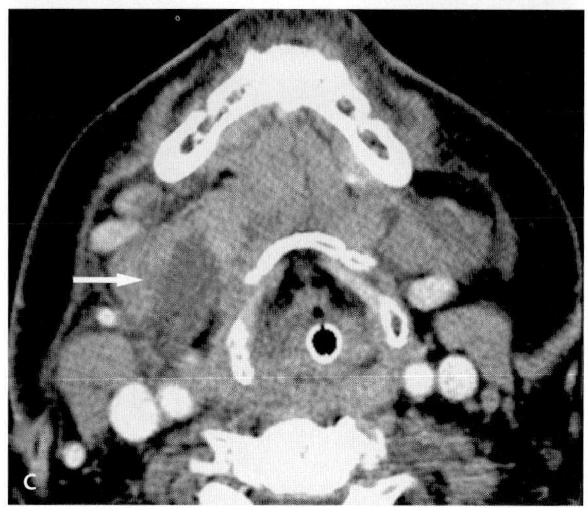

Figure 5.19

Abscess, parapharyngeal; 36-year-old male with swelling of face from orbit to neck from mandibular osteomyelitis. **A** Axial CT image shows soft-tissue swelling in masticator, submandibular, submental, and parapharyngeal spaces, as well as tonsillar region (*arrows*). **B** Axial CT image, soft-tissue window, shows parapharyngeal abscess (*asterisk*) and edema in floor of mouth and around pharynx (note canula in place), which is displaced. **C** Axial CT image, soft-tissue window, shows abscess at level of hyoid bone (*arrow*)

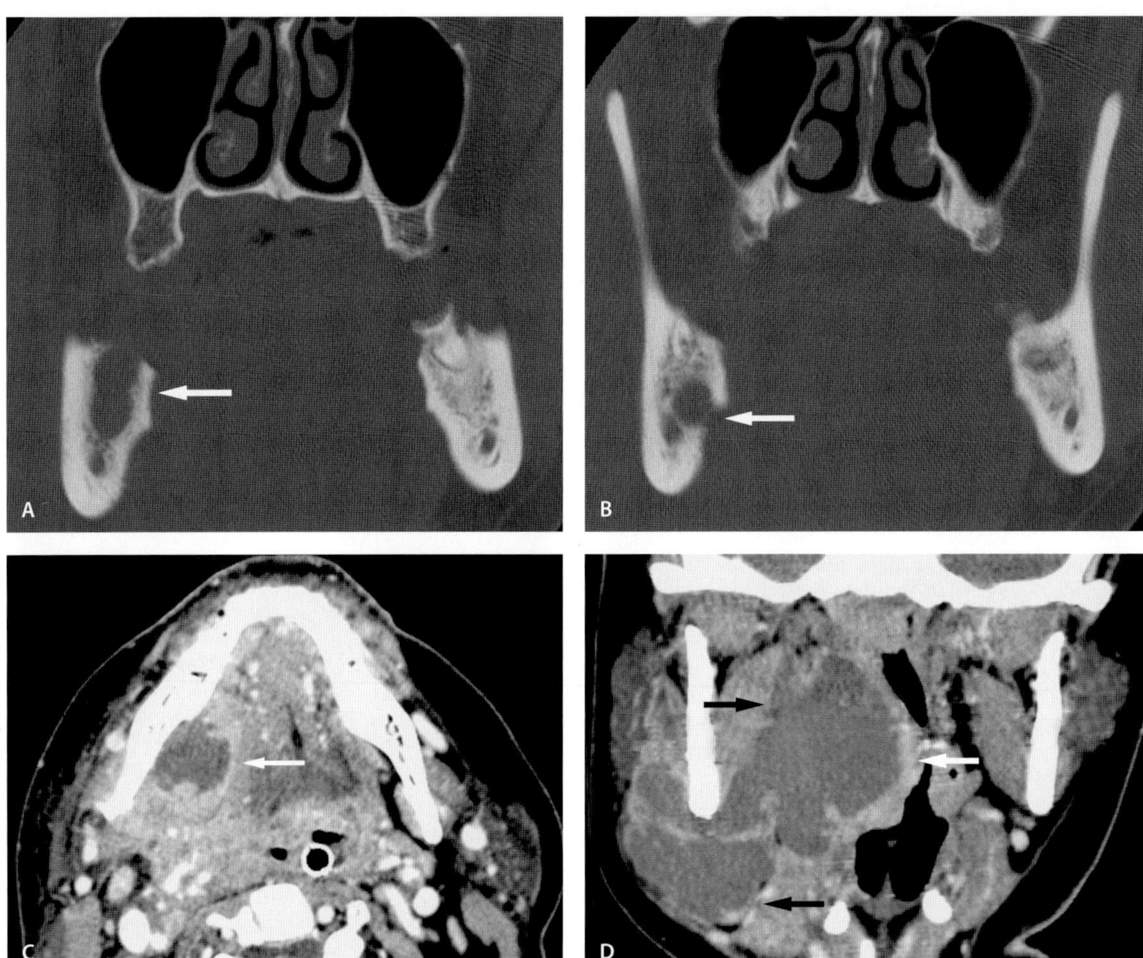

Figure 5.20

Abscess, parapharyngeal; 29-year-old female with infected third molar in mandible extracted 1 week previously and history of lateral pharyngeal wall infection, large perimandibular swelling, swelling in floor of mouth, and air breathing problems. A Coronal CT image shows tooth socket (*arrow*) and infectious root also on contralateral side. B Coronal CT image shows destruction of lingual cortical plate below attachment of mylohyoid muscle (*arrow*). C Axial CT, soft-tissue window, shows abscess lingual to tooth socket (*arrow*) and diffuse edema in entire floor of mouth, closure of airspace and canula in place. D Coronal CT image, soft-tissue window, shows large abscess in masticator, submandibular and parapharyngeal spaces with closure of airspace (*arrows*). Enlarged lymph nodes (more than 1 cm) were seen

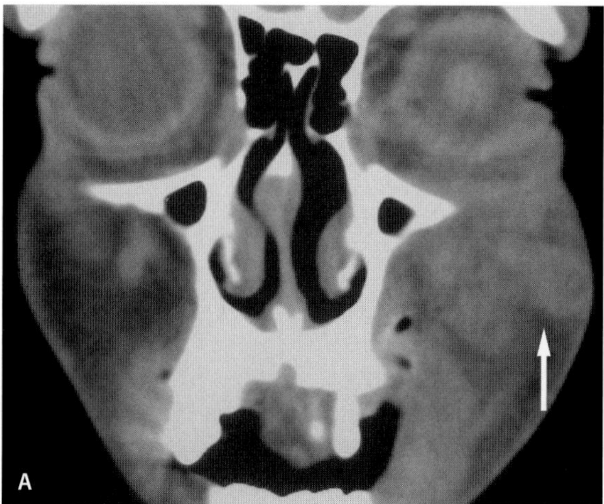

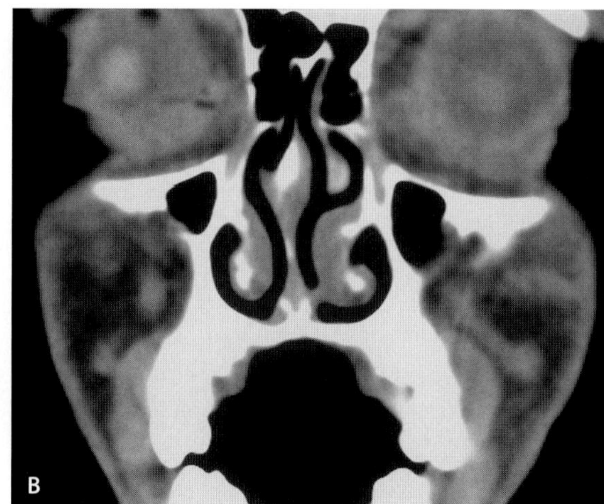

Figure 5.21

Abscess in cheek; 31-year-old female with dental infection with pain and swelling in palate and cheek (history of multiple dental abscesses). **A** Coronal CT image shows soft-tissue swelling in the palate, small gas collections close to alveolar process and abscess in cheek (*arrow*). **B** Coronal CT image 4 years later shows normal cheek (possibly some scar tissue)

Suggested Reading

Baltensperger M, Gratz K, Bruder E, Lebeda, R, Makek M, Eyrich G (2004) Is primary chronic osteomyelitis a uniform disease? Proposal of a classification based on a retrospective analysis of patients treated in the past 30 years. J Craniomaxillofac Surg 32:43–50

Eyrich GK, Baltensperger MM, Bruder E, Graetz KW (2003) Primary chronic osteomyelitis in childhood and adolescence: a retrospective analysis of 11 cases and review of the literature. J Oral Maxillofac Surg 61:561–573

Farman AG, Nortje C, Wood RE (1993) Infections of the teeth and jaws. In: Oral and maxillofacial diagnostic imaging. Mosby, St. Louis, pp 181–209

Hermans R, Fossion E, Ioannides C, Van den Bogaert W, Ghekiere J, Baert AL (1996) CT findings in osteoradionecrosis of the mandible. Skeletal Radiol 25:31–36

Kaneda T, Minami M, Ozawa Y, Akimoto T, Utsunomiya T, Yamamoto H, Suzuki H, Sasaki Y (1995) Magnetic resonance imaging of osteomyelitis. Comparative study with other radiologic modalities. Oral Surg Oral Med Oral Pathol Oral Radiol Endod 79:634–640

Larheim TA, Aspestrand F, Trebo S (1993) Periostitis ossificans of the mandible. The value of computed tomography. Dentomaxillofac Radiol 22:93–96

Lee K, Kaneda T, Mori, S, Minami M, Motohashi J, Yamashiro M (2003) Magnetic resonance imaging of normal and osteomyelitis in the mandible: assessment of short inversion time inversion recovery sequence. Oral Surg Oral Med Oral Pathol Oral Radiol Endod 96:499–507

Lee L (2004) Inflammatory lesions of the jaws. In: White SW, Pharoah MJ (eds) Oral radiology. Principles and interpretation, 5th edn. Saunders, Philadelphia, pp 373–383

Lew DP, Waldvogel FA (2004) Osteomyelitis. Lancet 364:369–379

Lovas JGL (1991) Infection/inflammation. In: Miles DA, Van Dis M, Kaugars GE, Lovas JGL (eds) Oral and maxillofacial radiology. Radiologic/pathologic correlations. Saunders, Philadelphia, pp 7–20

Marx RE (1983) Osteoradionecrosis: a new concept of its pathophysiology. J Oral Maxillofac Surg 41:283–288

Nortje CJ, Wood RE, Grotepass F (1988) Periostitis ossificans versus Garre's osteomyelitis. Part II: Radiographic analysis of 93 cases in the jaws. Oral Surg Oral Med Oral Pathol 66:249–260

Notani K, Yamazaki Y, Kitada H, Sakakibara N, Fukuda H, Omori K, Nakamura M (2003) Management of mandibular osteoradionecrosis corresponding to the severity of osteoradionecrosis and the method of radiotherapy. Head Neck 25:181–186

Ruggiero SL, Mehrotra B, Rosenberg TJ, Engroff SL (2004) Osteonecrosis of the jaws associated with the use of bisphosphonates: a review of 63 cases. J Oral Maxillofac Surg 62:527–534

Seabold JE, Simonson TM, Weber PC, Thompson BH, Harris KG, Rezai K, Madsen MT, Hoffman HT (1995) Cranial osteomyelitis: diagnosis and follow-up with In-111 white blood stem and Tc-99m methylene diphosphonate bone SPECT, CT, and MR imaging. Radiology 196:779–788

Støre G, Larheim TA (1999) Mandibular osteoradionecrosis: a comparison of computed tomography with panoramic radiography. Dentomaxillofac Radiol 28:295–300

Støre G, Smith H-J, Larheim TA (2000) Dynamic MR imaging of mandibular osteoradionecrosis. Acta Radiol 41:31–37

Støre G, Boysen M (2000) Mandibular osteoradionecrosis: clinical behaviour and diagnostic aspects. Clin Otolaryngol 25:378–384

Støre G, Evensen J, Larheim TA (2001) Osteoradionecrosis of the mandible. Comparison of the effects of external beam irradiation and brachytherapy. Dentomaxillofac Radiol 30:114–119

Thorn JJ, Hansen HS, Specht L, Bastholt L (2000) Osteoradionecrosis of the jaws: clinical characteristics and relation to the field of irradiation. J Oral Maxillofacial Surg 58:1088–1093

Weber AL, Kaneda T, Scrivani SJ, Aziz S (2003) Jaw: cysts, tumors, and nontumorous lesions. In: Som PM, Curtin HD (eds) Head and neck imaging, 4th edn. Mosby, St. Louis, pp 930–994

Temporomandibular Joint

Introduction

Patients with temporomandibular disorders constitute a heterogeneous group. Many have symptoms that are not directly related to the joints proper. Although the clinical assessment of the temporomandibular joint (TMJ) provides limited information with respect to its status, imaging should only be performed if a thorough physical examination indicates the need for more information and for patient management.

A number of imaging modalities have been used in the past and are still used to examine patients with TMJ problems. In this chapter we focus on magnetic resonance imaging (MRI), which is an appropriate imaging modality for most patient categories. The imaging protocol consists of oblique sagittal and oblique coronal images that are obtained perpendicular or parallel to the long axis of the mandibular condyle. The diagnostic accuracy of MRI on fresh autopsy material using this protocol has been found to be nearly 95% in determining disc position and cortical bone status.

When appropriate, other imaging modalities are presented. In selected cases clinical photos, histologic evidence, and surgical specimens are shown. In addition, a series of illustrations from autopsy specimens supplement the MR images.

If not specifically mentioned in the legends, all images in this chapter are proton density (intermediate-weighted) or T1-weighted MR images at closed mouth, obtained perpendicular to the long axis of the mandibular condyle. In most images the posterior band of the disc is indicated by an *arrow*

MRI findings in healthy asymptomatic volunteers are shown in Chap. 1, Maxillofacial Imaging Anatomy.

Internal Derangements

Definition

General orthopedic term implying a mechanical fault that interferes with the smooth action of a joint; internal arrangement is thus a functional diagnosis and for the TMJ far the most common internal derangement is displacement of the articular disc.

Clinical Features

- Clicking sounds from joint(s)
- Earlier clicking sounds that have disappeared
- Restricted or normal mouth opening capacity
- Deviation or other irregular jaw motion on opening
- Pain or no pain in joint areas and/or masticatory muscles
- Occasionally, joints may show inflammatory signs
- A variety of other symptoms such as headache
- Women more frequent than men
- Also younger age groups

Imaging Features

- Anterior disc displacement: posterior band of the disc located anterior to the superior portion of the condyle at closed mouth on oblique sagittal images
- Disc may have normal (biconcave) or deformed morphology
- In opened mouth position disc may be in a normal position ("with reduction") or continue to be displaced ("without reduction")
- Anterior disc displacement without or with lateral or medial disc displacement most common
- Lateral or medial disc displacement best seen on oblique coronal images
- Pure lateral or medial or posterior disc displacement uncommon
- Disc may be in normal position at closed mouth, but not move at opened mouth
- Effusion, typically located in upper compartment of anterior recess, may be seen
- Bone marrow edema in the condyle may be seen
- Cortical bone is normal

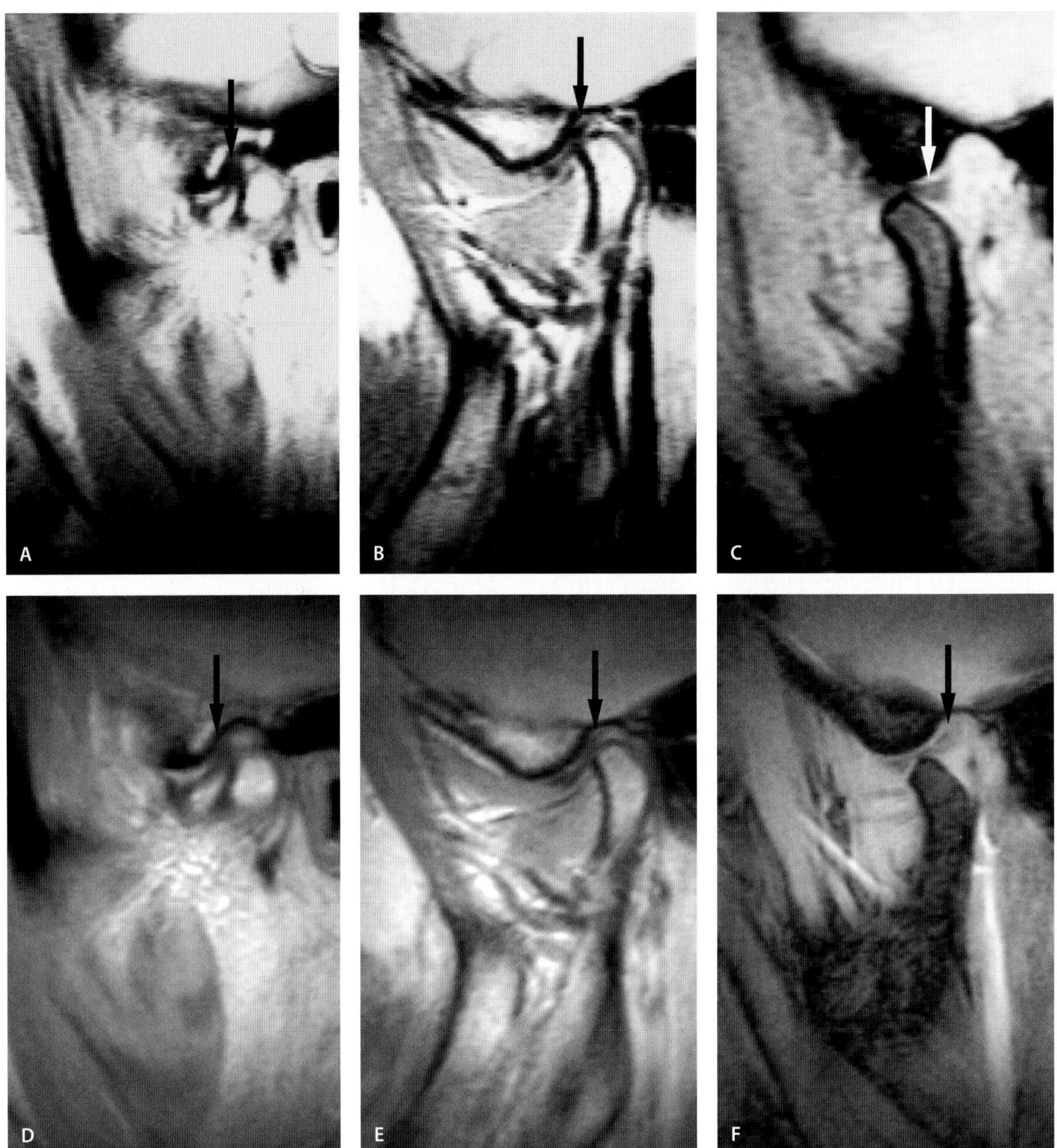

Figure 6.1

Partial anterior disc displacement at baseline (A, B, C) and at 8-year follow up (D, E, F), with normal bone; identical joint status (except function) at both examinations. A, D MRI shows slightly displaced disc (*arrow*) in lateral sections. B, E MRI shows normal position of disc (*arrow*) in central sections. C, F MRI shows normal position of disc (*arrow*) in open-mouth images; condylar translation is somewhat reduced at follow-up compared to baseline

Figure 6.2

Complete anterior disc displacement and normal bone. **A, B, C** MRI shows displaced and deformed disc (*arrow*) in lateral (**A**), central (**B**), and medial section (**C**). **D** Open-mouth MRI shows anteriorly displaced disc (*arrow*). **E, F, G** Autopsy specimen shows anteriorly displaced disc (*arrow*) in lateral (**E**), central (**F**), and medial (**G**) sections. A–D reproduced with permission from Larheim et al. (2001)

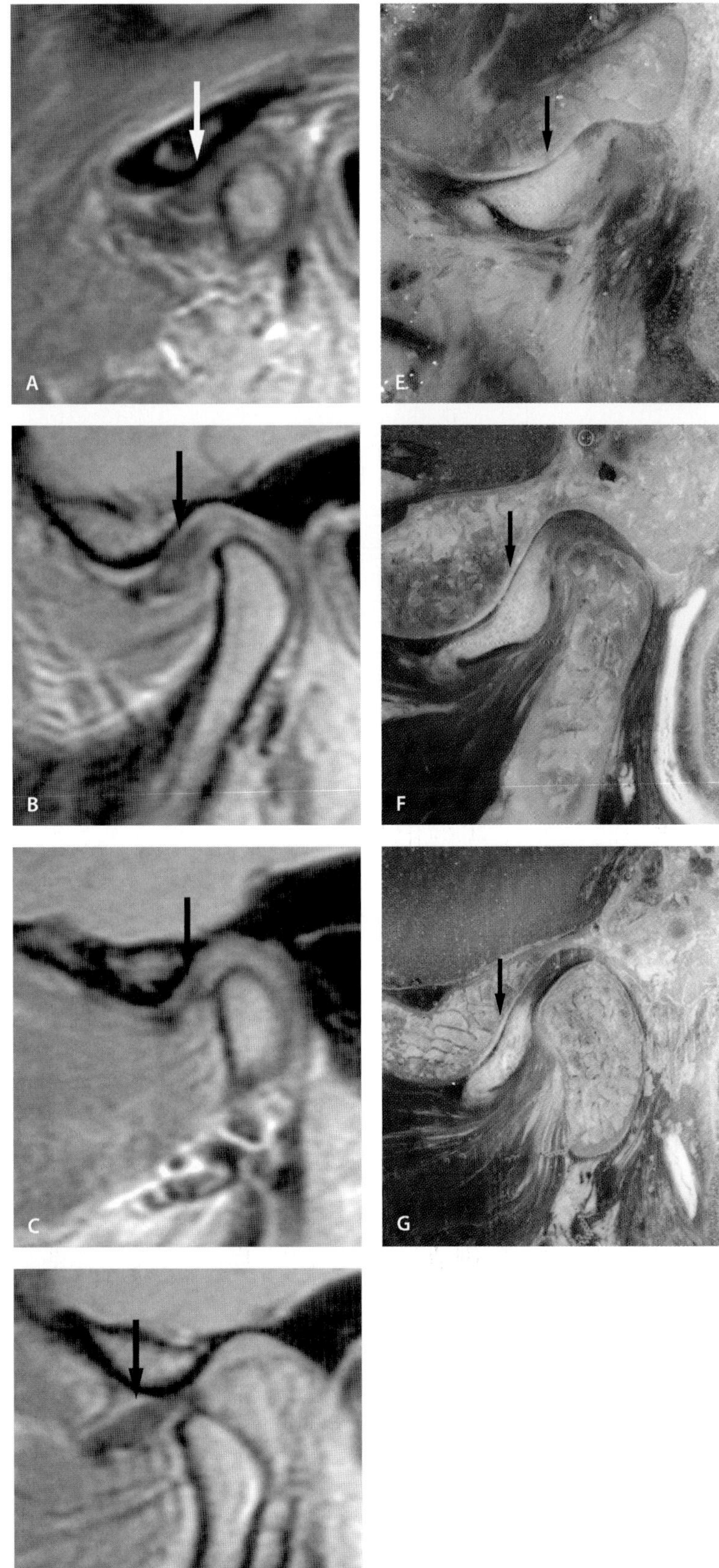

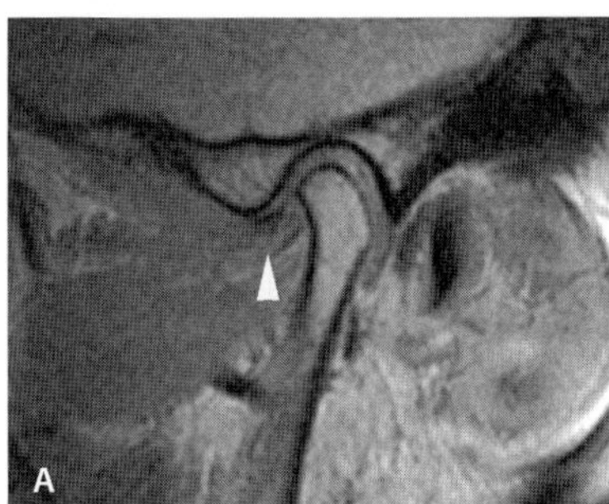

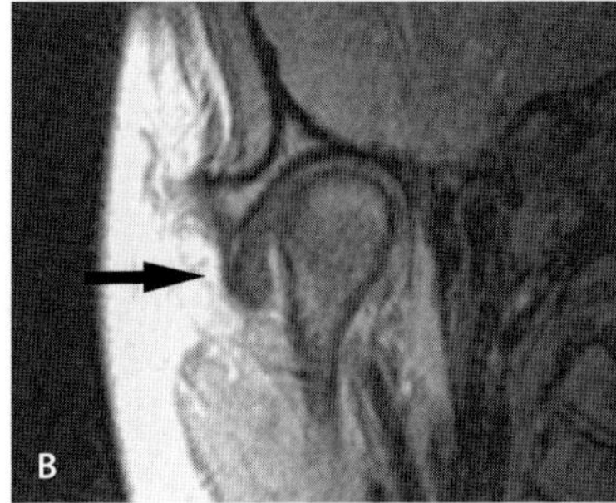

Figure 6.3

Lateral disc displacement and normal bone. A MRI shows no disc structure, but tendon to lateral pterygoid muscle (*arrowhead*). B Oblique coronal MRI shows disc (*arrow*) completely displaced in lateral direction

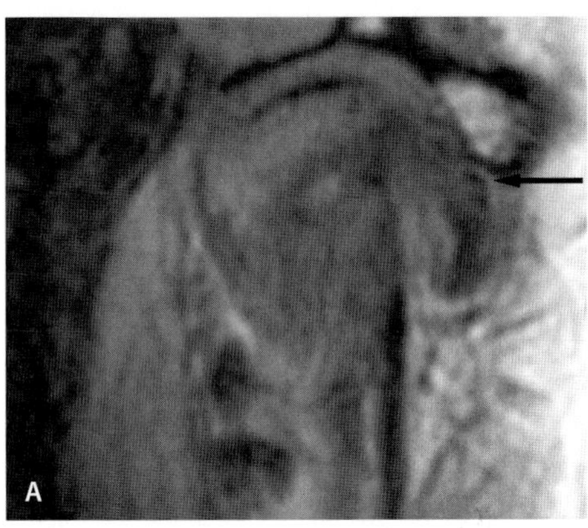

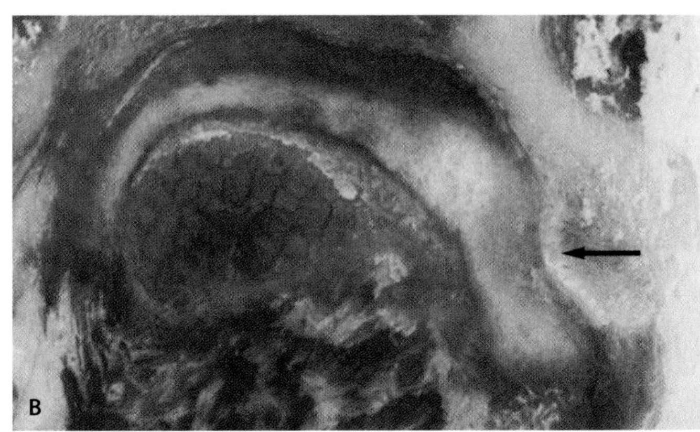

Figure 6.4

Lateral disc displacement and normal bone. A Oblique coronal MRI shows laterally displaced disc (*arrow*). B Autopsy specimen shows laterally displaced disc (*arrow*). Reproduced with permission from Tasaki et al. (1996)

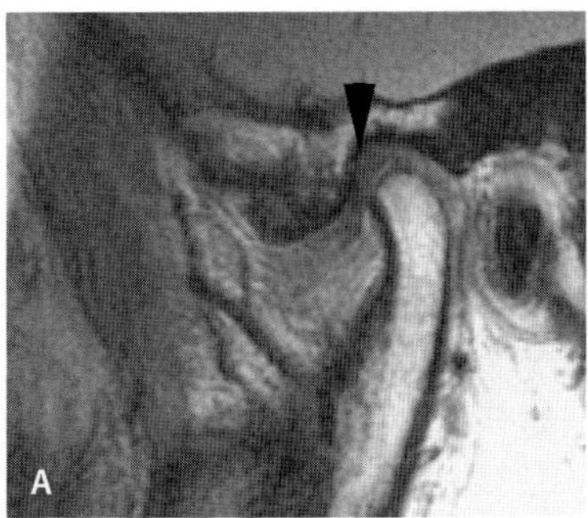

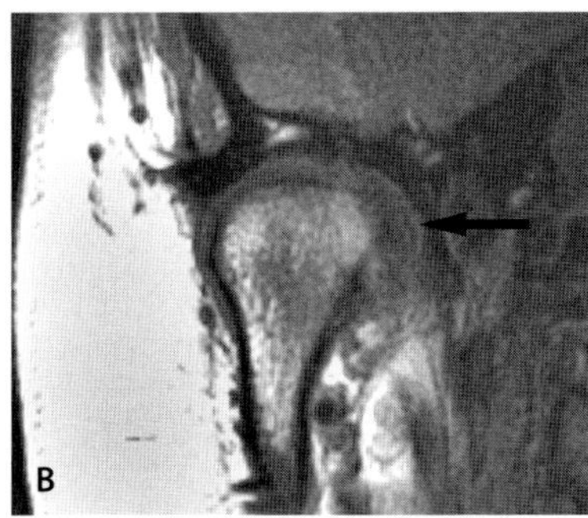

Figure 6.5

Medial disc displacement and normal bone. A MRI shows normal position of disc (*arrowhead*). B Oblique coronal MRI shows medially displaced disc (*arrow*)

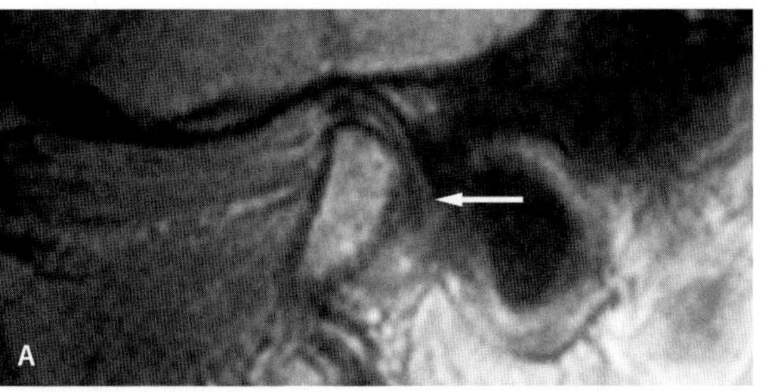

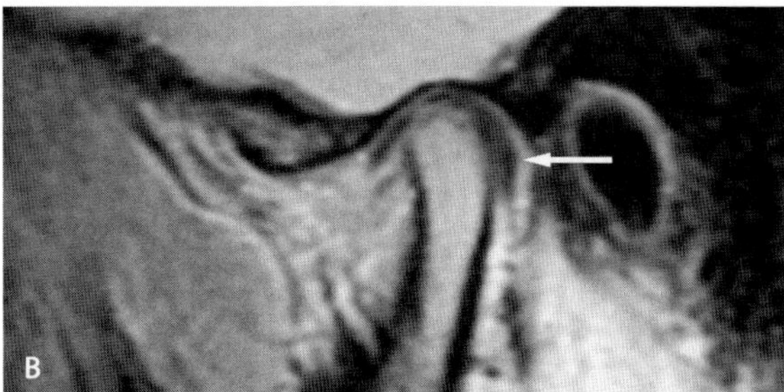

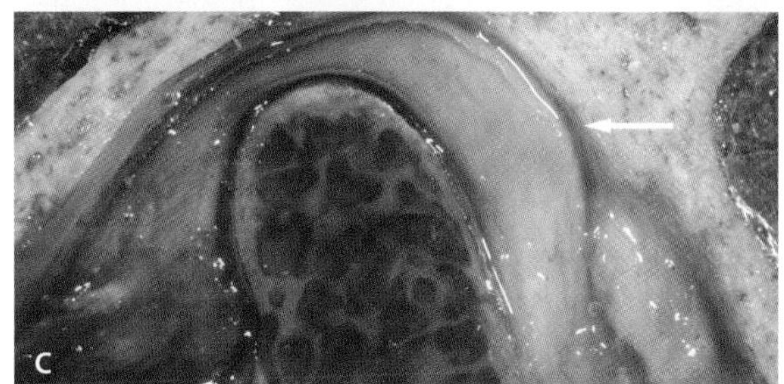

Figure 6.6

Posterior disc displacement and normal bone. A, B Posteriorly displaced disc (*arrow*) in patients. C Autopsy specimen shows posteriorly displaced disc (*arrow*). Reproduced with permission from Westesson et al. (1998)

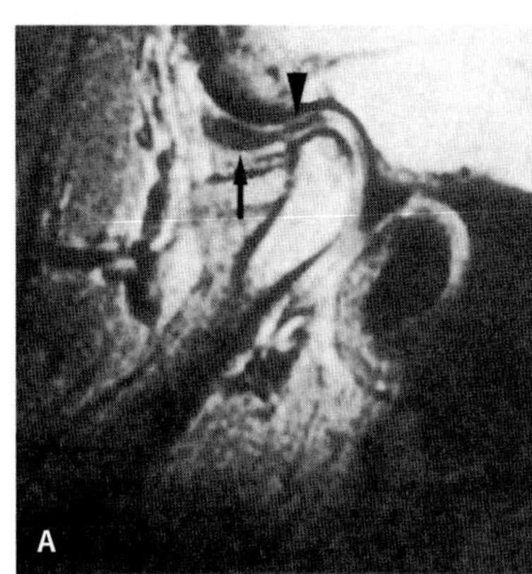

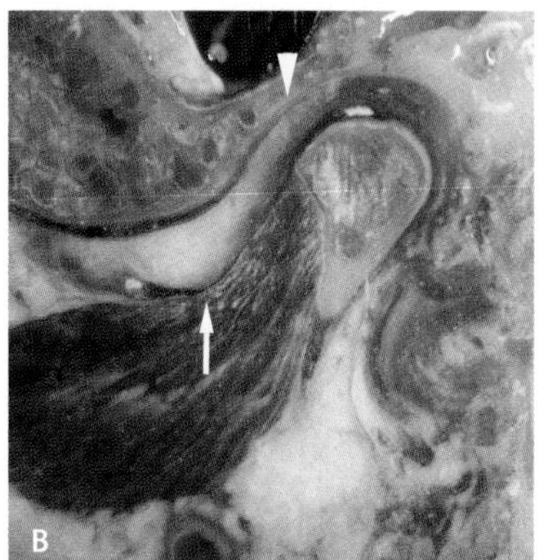

Figure 6.7

Anterior disc displacement and fibrous posterior attachment (pseudodisc), and normal bone. A MRI shows anteriorly displaced disc (*arrow*) and thin, low-signal posterior attachment (*arrowhead*). B Autopsy specimen shows anteriorly displaced disc (*arrow*) and elongated, thin and fibrotic posterior attachment (*arrowhead*). Reproduced with permission from Westesson et al. (2003)

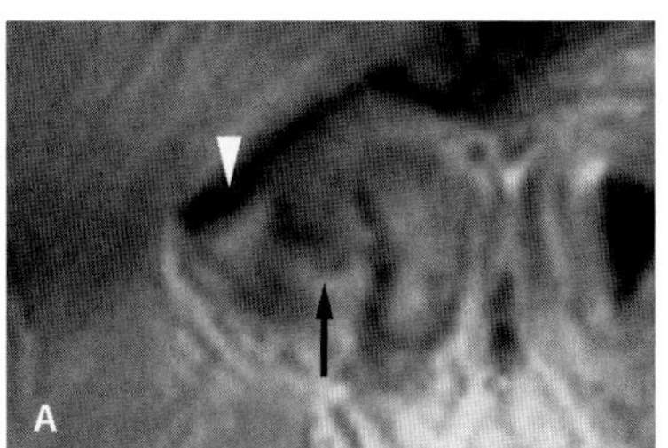

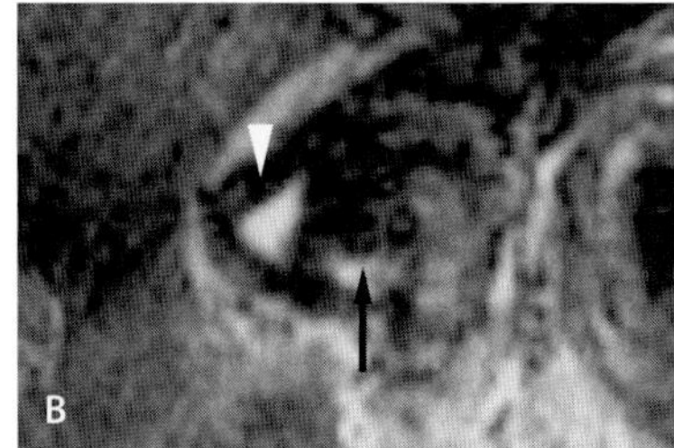

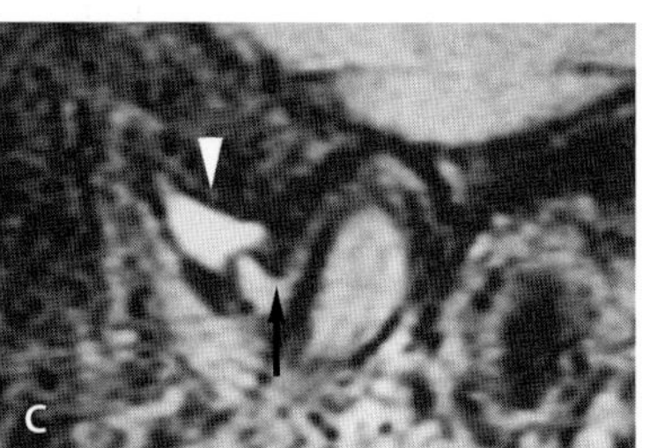

Figure 6.8

Anterior disc displacement with joint effusion, and normal cortical bone, without or with bone marrow edema in condyle. A MRI shows anteriorly displaced and deformed disc (*arrow*) and intermediate signal from upper compartment (*arrowhead*). B T2-weighted MRI shows increased signal from upper (*arrowhead*) and lower compartment but normal condyle marrow (*arrow* indicates disc) (A and B have been used as reference images for the definition of joint effusion, and are reproduced with permission from Larheim et al. 2001). C T2-weighted MRI of another patient shows anteriorly displaced, deformed disc (*arrow*), more extensive fluid in upper compartment (*arrowhead*), and increased signal in condyle marrow indicating marrow edema

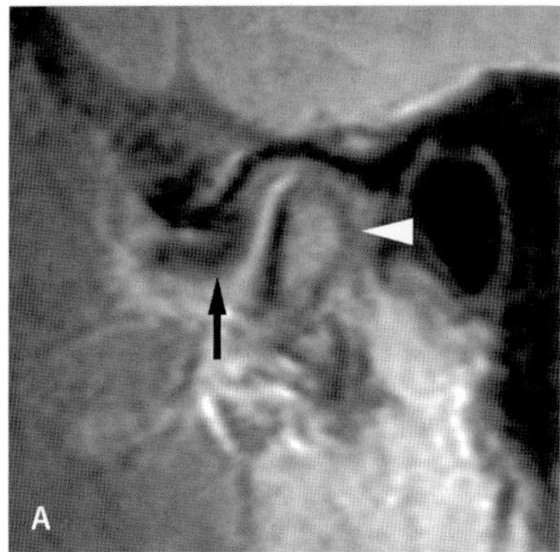

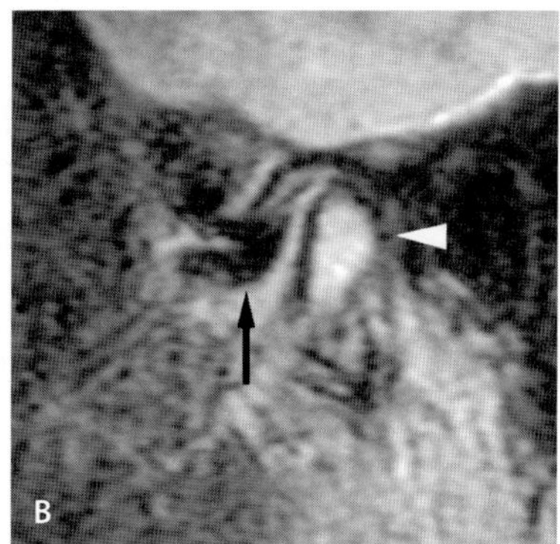

Figure 6.9

Anterior disc displacement and bone marrow edema, with normal cortical bone. **A** MRI shows anteriorly displaced disc (*arrow*) and intermediate signal in condyle marrow (*arrowhead*). **B** T2-weighted MRI shows increased signal in condyle marrow; *arrowhead* edema, *arrow* displaced disc. Reproduced with permission from Larheim et al. (2001)

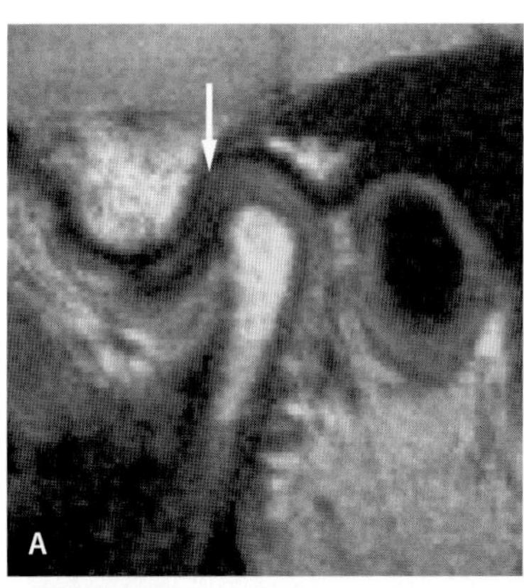

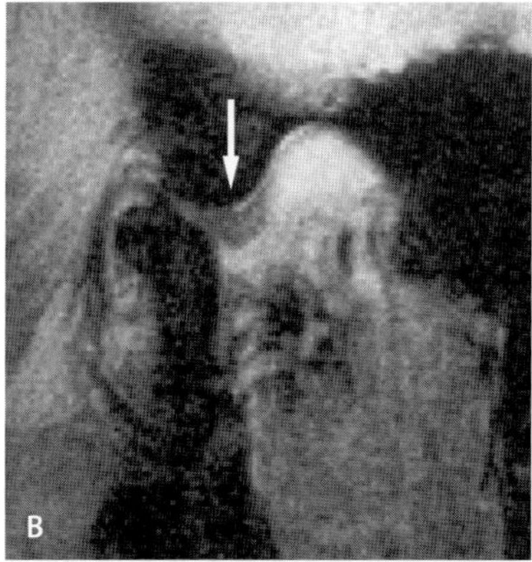

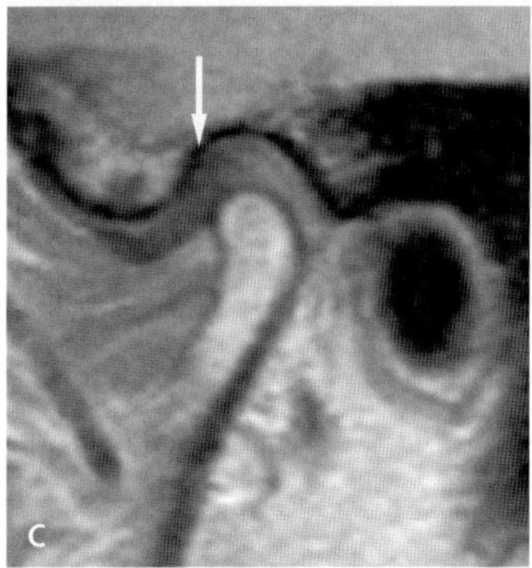

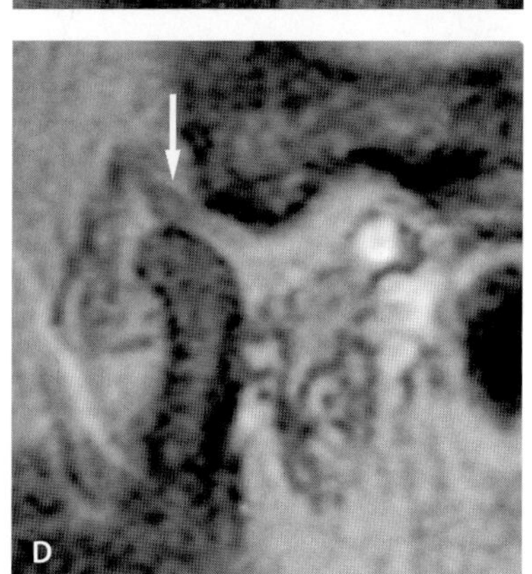

Figure 6.10

Reducing disc displacement progressing to non-reducing disc displacement, with normal bone, during a 10-year period. **A, B** MRI at baseline shows anteriorly displaced disc (*arrow*), reducing (normalizing) in open-mouth image (**B**). **C, D** MRI at follow-up shows anteriorly displaced disc (*arrow*), also in open-mouth image (**D**)

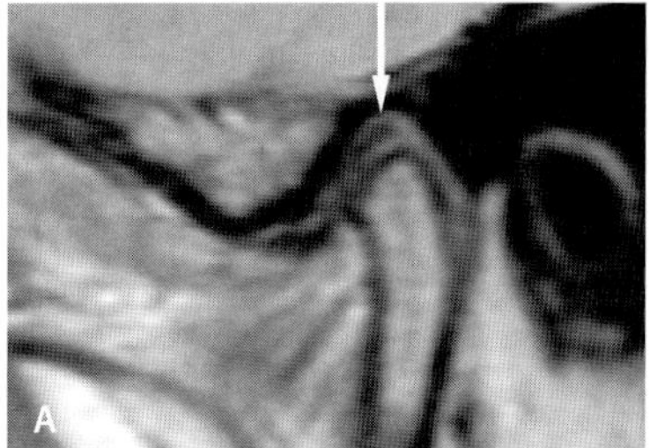

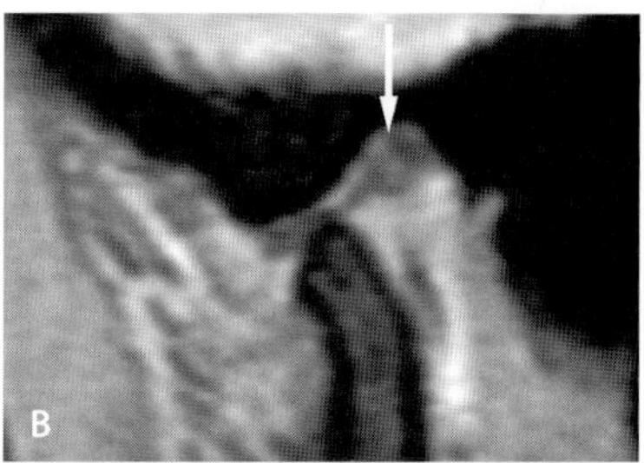

Figure 6.11

Stuck disc and normal bone. **A** MRI shows disc (*arrow*) in normal position. **B** Open-mouth MRI also shows normal position of disc (*arrow*); no motion of disc with condyle, probably due to fibrous adhesions

Osteoarthritis

Synonyms: osteoarthrosis, degenerative joint disease

Definition

Non-inflammatory focal degenerative disorder of synovial joints, primarily affecting articular cartilage and sub-condylar bone; initiated by deterioration of articular soft-tissue cover and exposure of bone.

Cases with evident inflammatory signs on MRI could be characterized as osteoarthritis, whereas joints without such signs could be characterized as osteoarthrosis.

Clinical Features

- Crepitation sounds from joint(s)
- Restricted or normal mouth opening capacity
- Pain or no pain from joint areas and/or of mastication muscles
- Occasionally, joints may show inflammatory signs
- A variety of other symptoms such as headache
- Women more frequent than men
- Older age groups more frequent than younger age groups
- Arthrosis deformans juveniles in young patients

Imaging Features

- Disc displacement, degenerated or absent disc very frequent
- Abnormal cortical bone; both joint components; most evident in condyle
- Early stage: cortical erosion
- Advanced stage: joint space reduction, bone production; osteophytosis, sclerosis
- Joint effusion may be seen, either in early or advanced stage
- Bone marrow edema or bone marrow sclerosis, or in combination, may be seen, either in early or advanced stage
- Usually intravenous contrast injection is not applied but occasionally osteoarthritis may be clearly inflammatory and thus demonstrate contrast enhancement of thickened synovium
- Osteoarthritis secondary to trauma or arthritides, usually with normal disc position

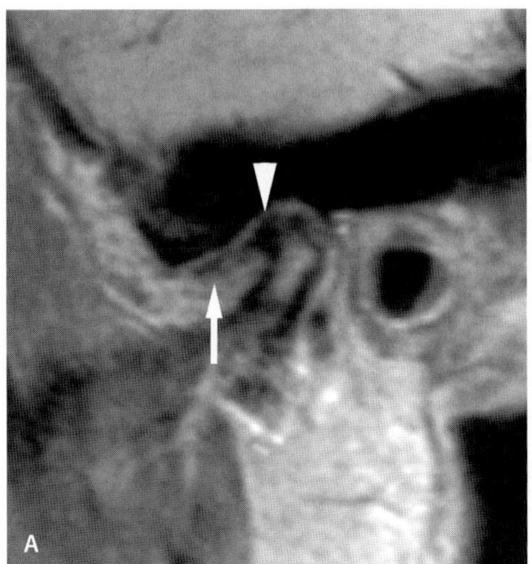

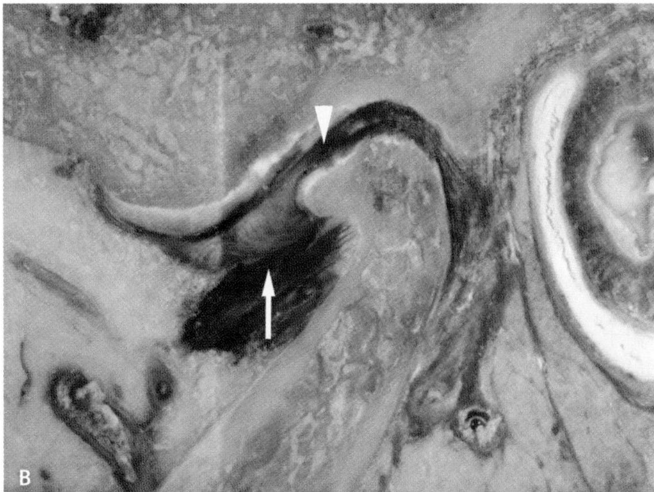

Figure 6.12

Osteoarthritis and anterior disc displacement. **A** MRI shows anteriorly displaced and deformed, degenerated disc (*arrow*) and irregular cortical outline with osteophytosis and sclerosis of condyle (*arrowhead*). **B** Autopsy specimen shows anteriorly displaced and deformed disc (*arrow*) and osteophytosis and sclerosis of condyle (*arrowhead*)

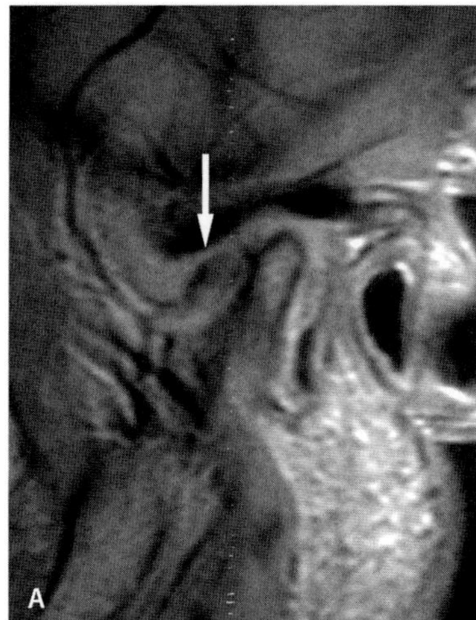

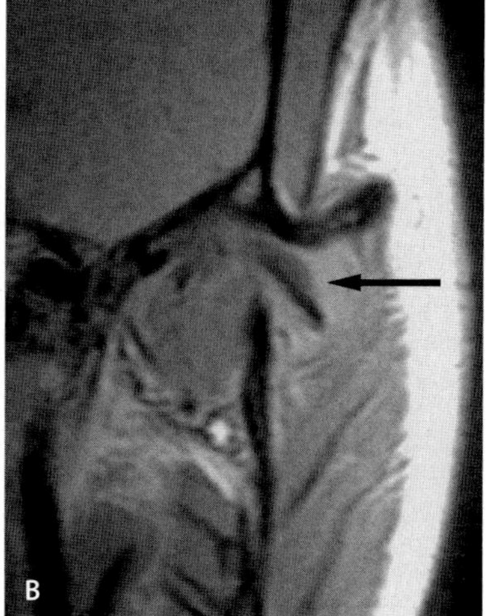

Figure 6.13

Osteoarthritis and anterolateral disc displacement. A MRI shows anteriorly displaced, deformed disc (*arrow*), and cortical irregularities and flattening of condyle. B Oblique coronal MRI shows laterally displaced disc (*arrow*)

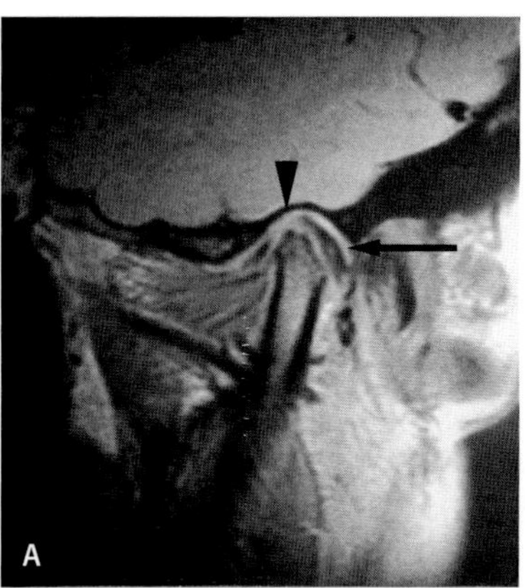

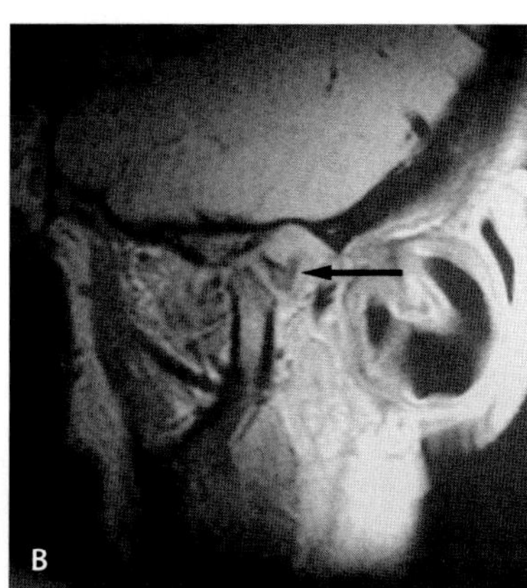

Figure 6.14

Osteoarthritis and posterior disc displacement. A MRI shows disc perforation and cortical irregularities of condyle (*arrowhead*), and posteriorly displaced disc (*arrow*). B Open-mouth MRI shows disc (*arrow*) adherent to condyle. Reproduced with permission from Westesson et al. (1998)

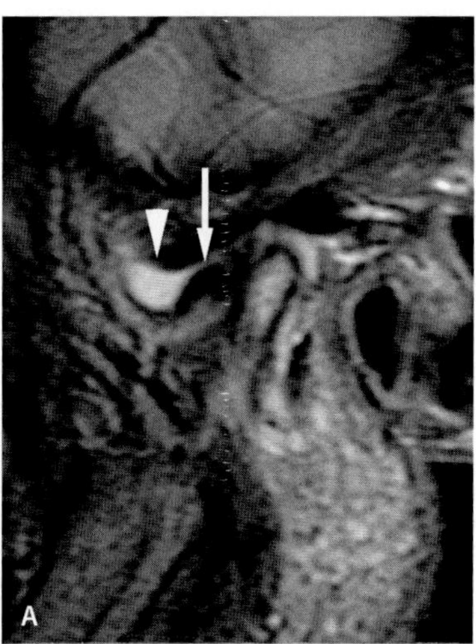

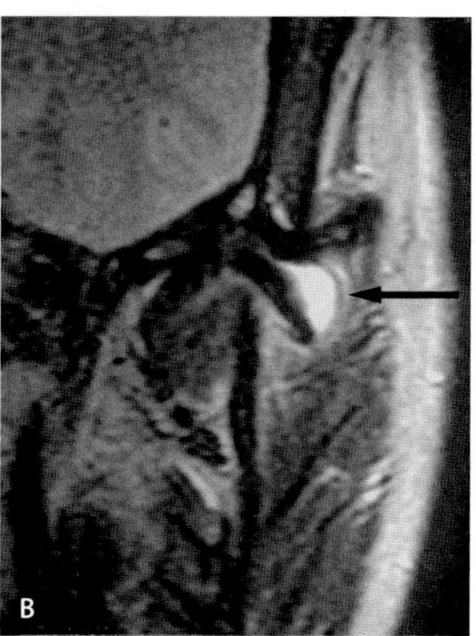

Figure 6.15

Osteoarthritis and anterolateral disc displacement, with joint effusion. A T2-weighted MRI shows anteriorly displaced disc (*arrow*), flattened condyle and joint effusion in upper compartment of anterior recess (*arrowhead*). B Oblique coronal T2-weighted MRI shows joint effusion in lateral part of joint above laterally displaced disc (*arrow*)

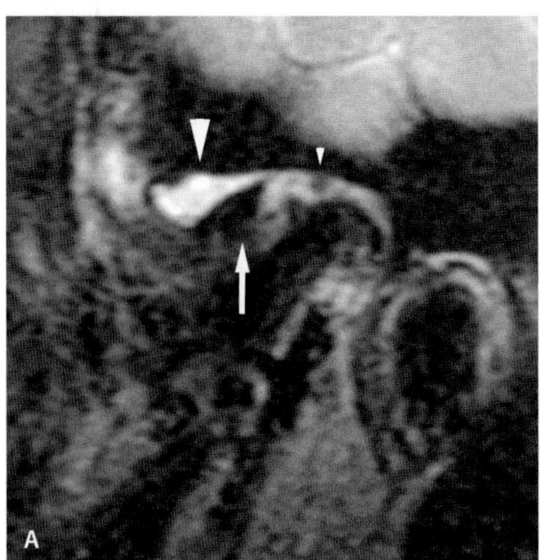

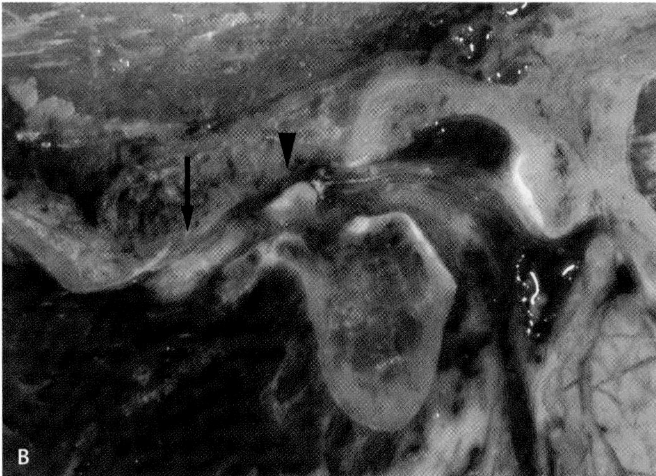

Figure 6.16

Advanced osteoarthritis and anterior disc displacement, with joint effusion. **A** T2-weighted MRI shows anteriorly displaced, deformed disc (*arrow*), large joint effusion (*large arrowhead*), and possible bone fragment (*small arrowhead*) superior to condyle, which has cortical irregularities and is completely sclerotic. Reproduced with permission from Larheim et al. (2001). **B** Autopsy specimen shows anteriorly displaced, deformed disc (*arrow*), osteophytosis and cortical irregularities of condyle, and bone fragment in joint space (*arrowhead*) suggesting osteochondritis dissecans. Reproduced with permission from Westesson et al. (2003)

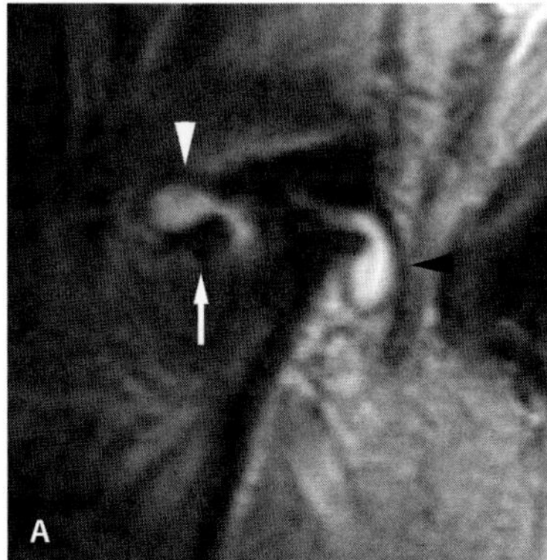

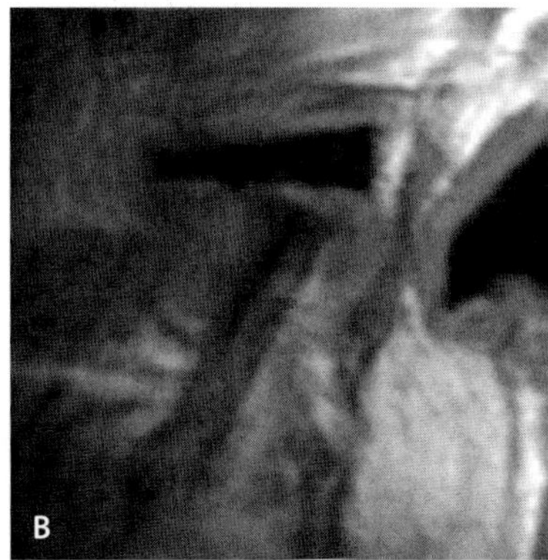

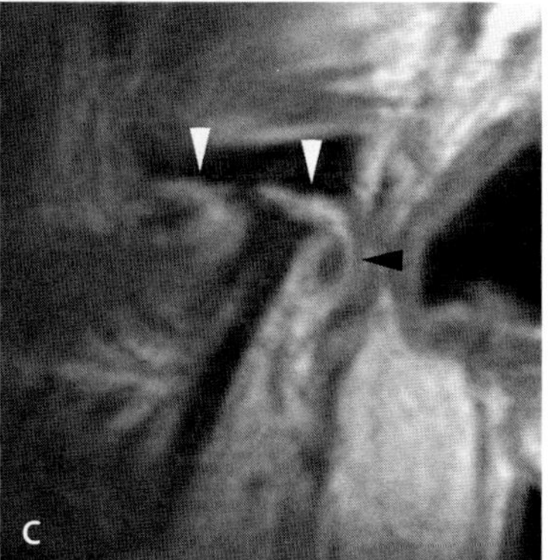

Figure 6.17

Advanced osteoarthritis and anterior disc displacement, with joint effusion and synovitis. **A** T2-weighted MRI shows anteriorly displaced, deformed disc (*arrow*), deformed condyle with osteophytosis and sclerosis, and large joint effusion in anterior (*white arrowhead*) and posterior (*black arrowhead*) compartments. **B, C** T1-weighted pre-Gd (**B**) and T1-weighted post-Gd (**C**) MRI show contrast enhancement in periphery of joint effusion in anterior (*left arrowhead*) and posterior (*black arrowhead*) compartments, and in joint space (*central arrowhead*), consistent with thickened (inflamed) synovium

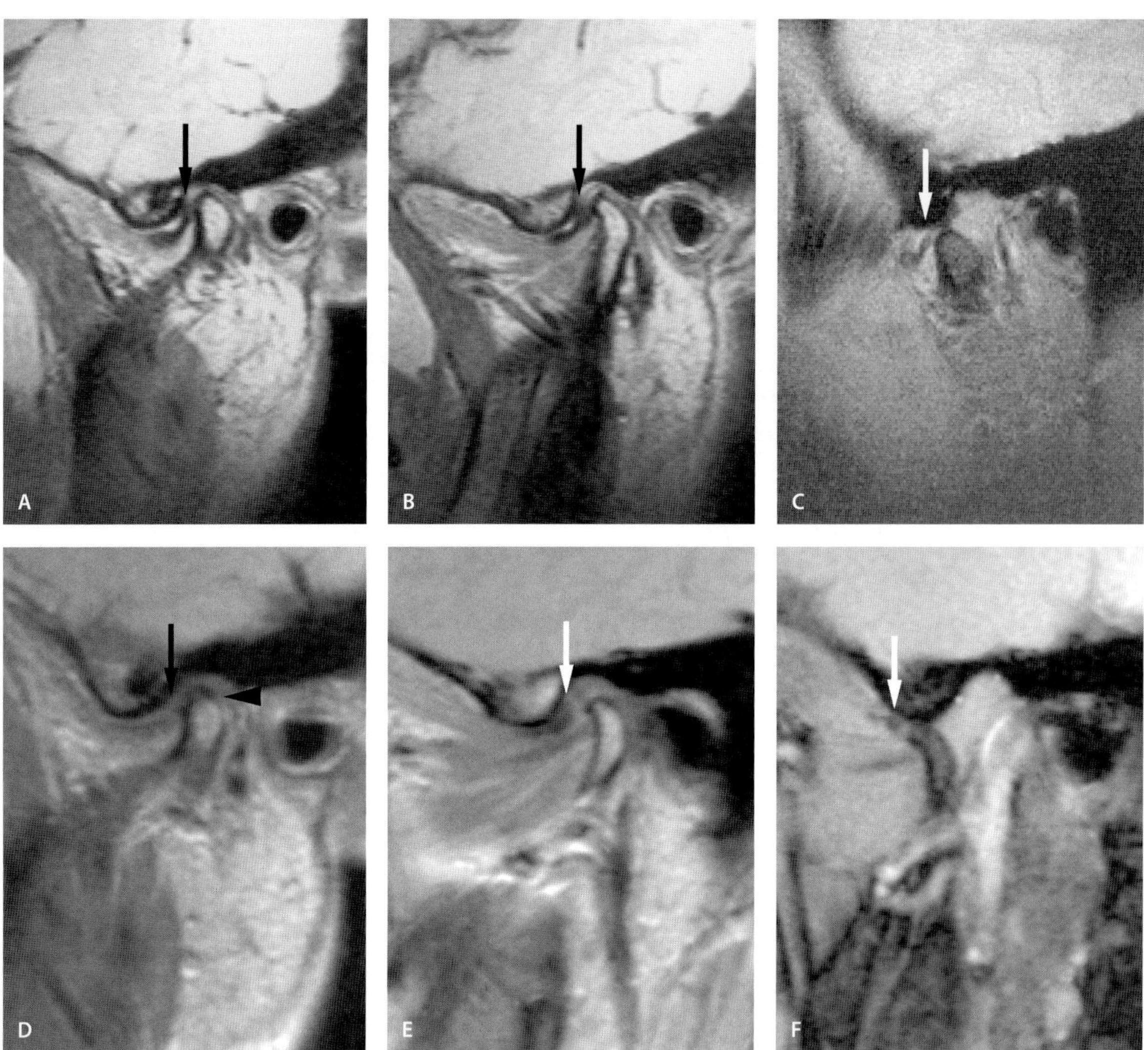

Figure 6.18

Osteoarthritis developed during a 15-year period from non-reducing disc displacement with normal bone. A, B, C MRI at baseline shows anteriorly displaced disc (*arrow*) in lateral (A) and central (B) sections, and in open-mouth image (C), with normal cortical bone. D, E, F MRI at follow-up shows anteriorly displaced disc (*arrow*) in lateral (D) and central-medial (E) sections, and in open-mouth image (F), with abnormal bone; condyle has developed irregular, flattened, sclerotic surface laterally (*arrowhead*) (D). Note better condylar translation in osteoarthritic joint (F)

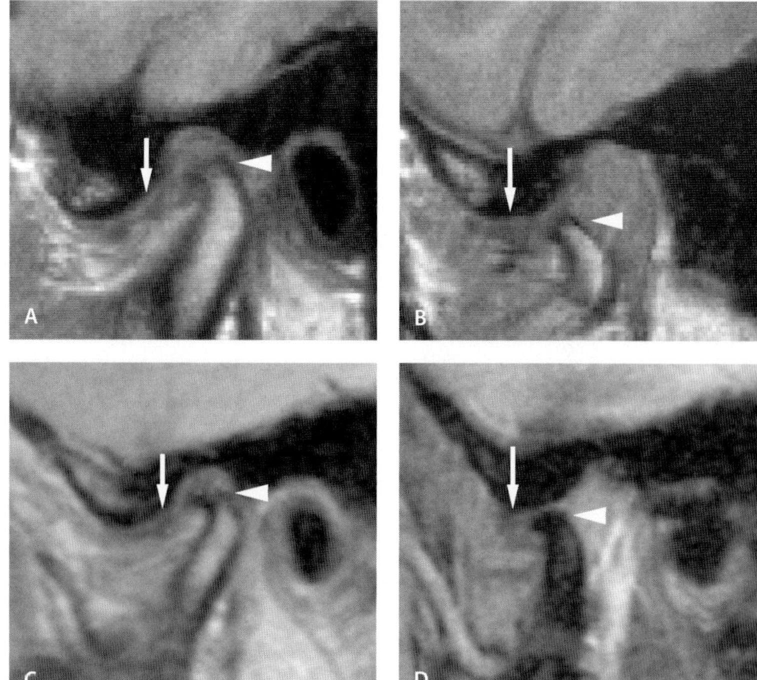

Figure 6.19

Osteoarthritis progression, contralateral joint of patient in Fig. 6.18, with non-reducing disc displacement at baseline (A, B) and at follow-up (C, D). A, B MRI shows anteriorly displaced disc (*arrow*), also in open-mouth image (B), and flattened condyle (*arrowhead*). C, D MRI shows anteriorly displaced disc (*arrow*), also in open-mouth image (D), and condyle has become evidently osteoarthritic (*arrowhead*). Osteoarthritis is even more evident in a more lateral section of the same joint (see A in Fig. 6.12)

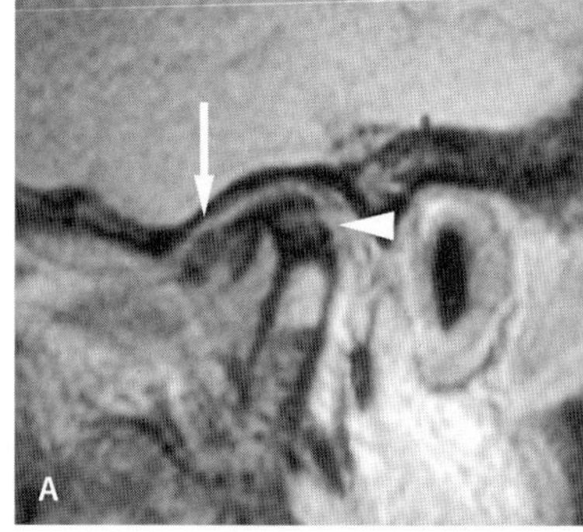

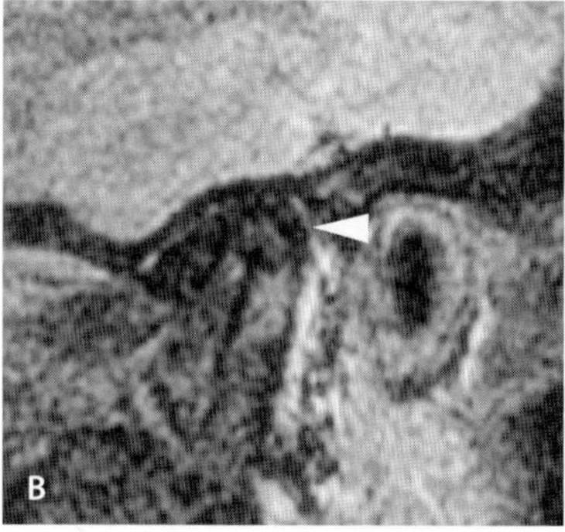

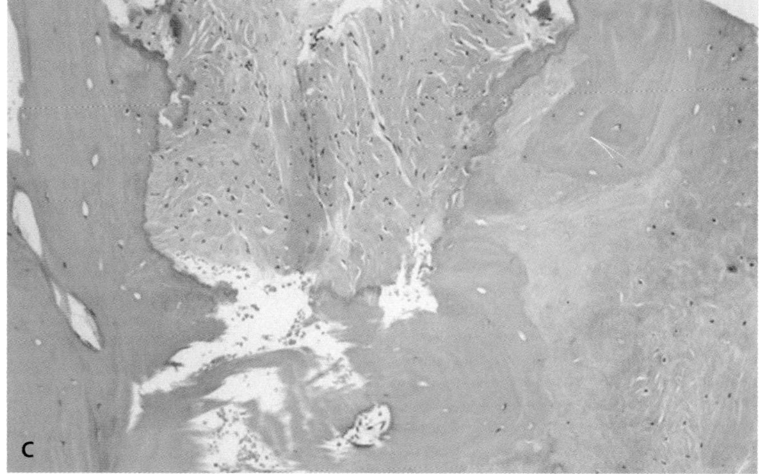

Figure 6.20

Advanced osteoarthritis and anterior disc displacement. A MRI shows anteriorly displaced disc (*arrow*) and flattened condyle with osteophytosis and extensive marrow sclerosis or fibrosis (*arrowhead*). B T2-weighted MRI shows reduced signal in condyle marrow confirming marrow sclerosis or fibrosis (*arrowhead*). C Histologic section from condyle marrow shows replacement of marrow by dense, sclerotic bone and fibrous tissue, suggesting a reparative process (hematoxylin eosin; original magnification ×50). Reproduced with permission from Larheim et al. (1999)

Bone Marrow Abnormalities

Definition

Bone marrow edema: serum proteins within marrow interstitium surrounded by normal hematopoietic marrow.

Osteonecrosis: complete loss of hematopoietic marrow.

Clinical Features

- More pain from joints with internal derangement and abnormal bone marrow than from joints with internal derangement and normal bone marrow is reported
- Otherwise there are no specific features compared to internal derangement or osteoarthritis

Imaging Features

- Abnormal signal on T2-weighted image from condyle marrow: increased signal indicates marrow edema; reduced signal indicates marrow sclerosis or fibrosis
- Combination of marrow edema signal and marrow sclerosis signal in condyle most reliable sign for histologic diagnosis of osteonecrosis
- Marrow sclerosis signal may indicate advanced osteoarthritis without osteonecrosis, or osteonecrosis
- Abnormal bone marrow signal is frequently associated with joint effusion
- Marrow edema or osteonecrosis is occasionally seen in joints with normal cortical bone and disc displacement, but more frequently in joints with osteoarthritis

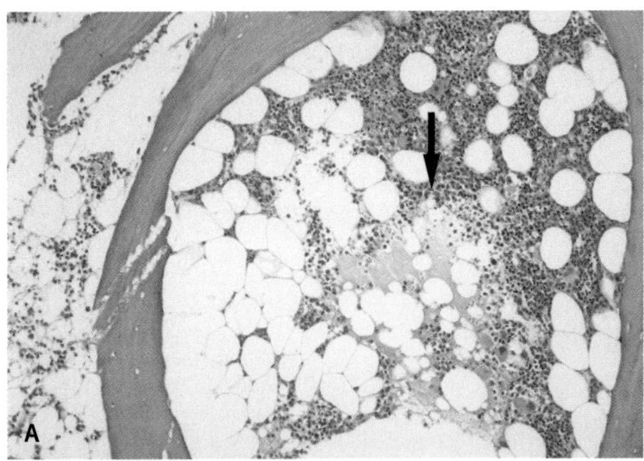

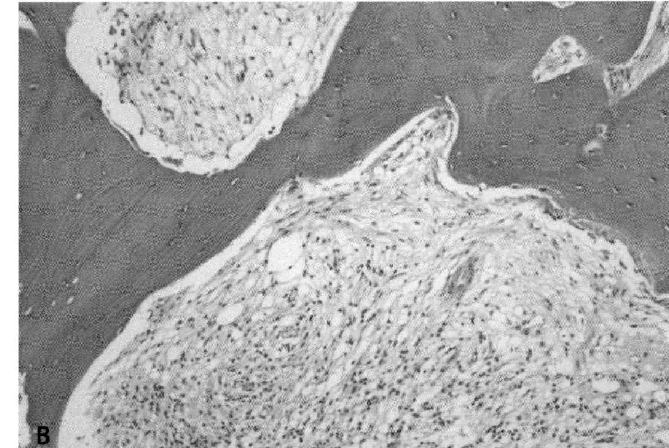

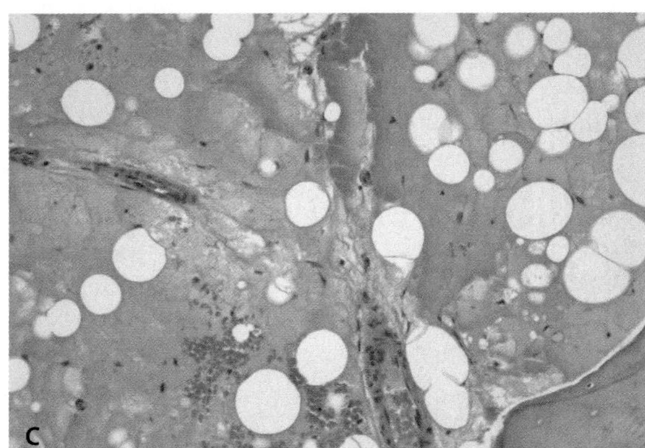

Figure 6.21

Bone marrow edema and osteonecrosis. A Histologic section from mandibular condyle marrow shows early marrow edema (*arrow*); a patchy focus of serum proteins surrounded by normal marrow. B Histologic section from mandibular condyle marrow shows osteonecrosis; complete loss of hematopoietic marrow with evidence of inflammatory cell infiltrate. C Histologic section from femoral head marrow shows complete loss of hematopoietic marrow (avascular necrosis) (hematoxylin eosin; original magnification ×50). A and B are reproduced with permission from Larheim et al. (1999)

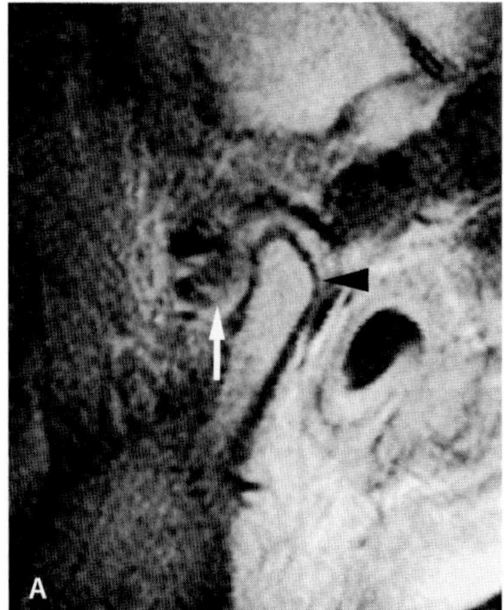

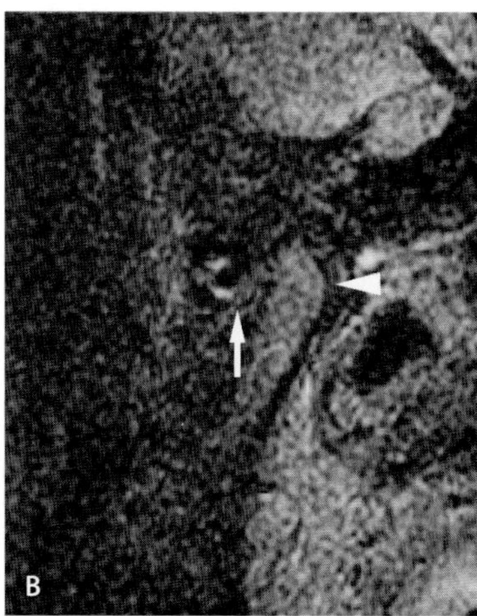

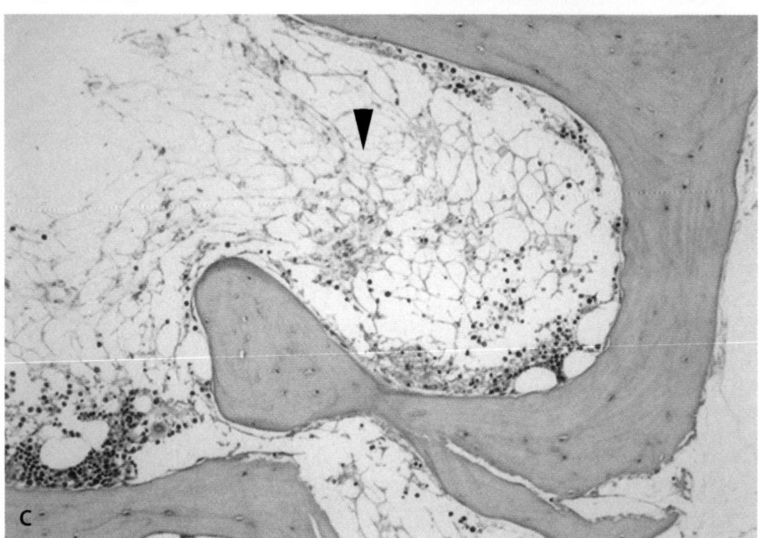

Figure 6.22

Osteonecrosis and anterior disc displacement, apparently with normal cortical bone. A MRI shows anteriorly displaced, deformed disc (*arrow*), and normal bone; cortex and marrow (*arrowhead*). B T2-weighted MRI shows displaced disc (*arrow*) with minimal fluid in upper and lower compartment and normal, low signal from bone marrow (*arrowhead*). C Histologic section of same patient shows focus of marrow necrosis; loss of hematopoietic elements (*arrowhead*) with break down of marrow fat (hematoxylin eosin, original magnification ×50). Reproduced with permission from Larheim et al. (1999)

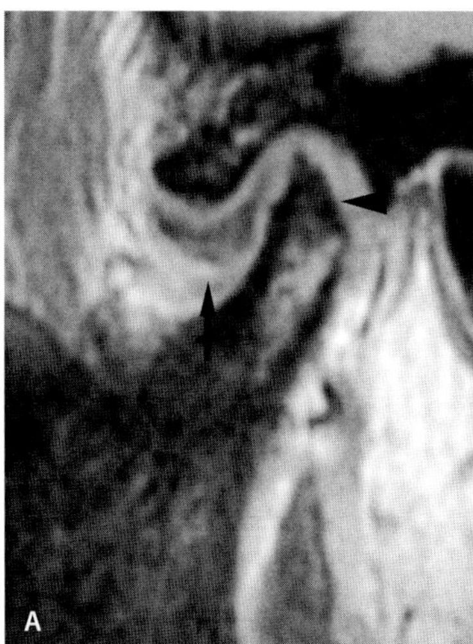

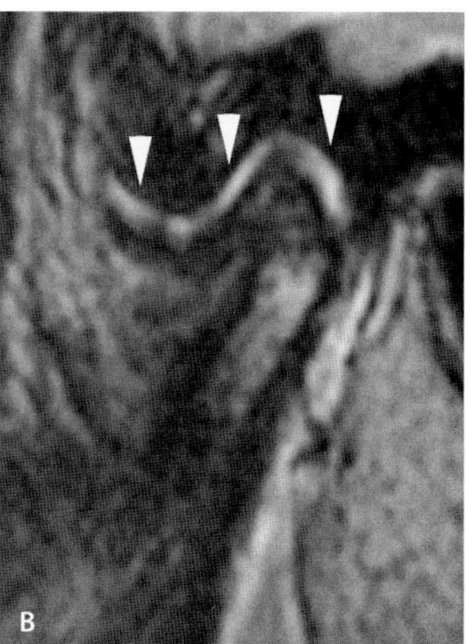

Figure 6.23

Osteonecrosis and anterior disc displacement, with osteoarthritis and joint effusion. A MRI shows anteriorly displaced, deformed disc (*arrow*), cortical irregularities of condyle with reduced signal from condyle marrow (*arrowhead*). B T2-weighted MRI shows joint effusion in entire upper compartment (*arrowheads*), and marrow sclerosis or fibrosis in condyle, but no marrow edema. Histologic section from condyle marrow (not shown) demonstrated osteonecrosis. Reproduced with permission from Larheim et al. (1999)

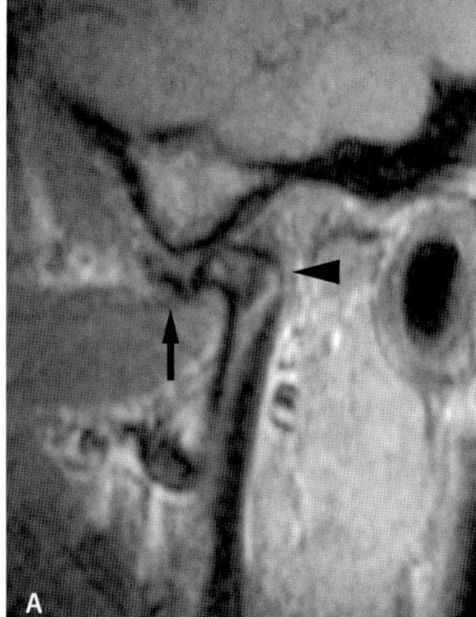

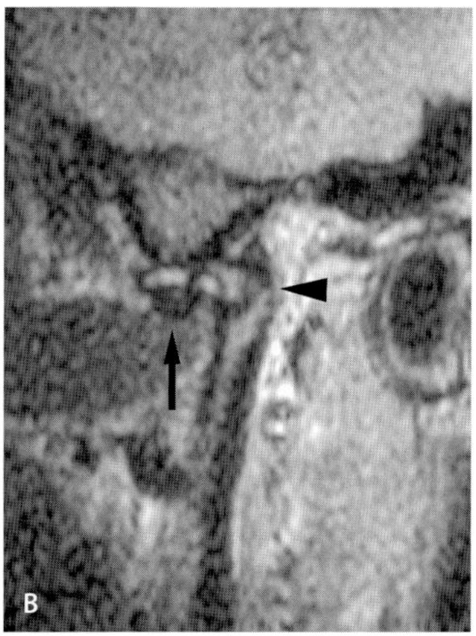

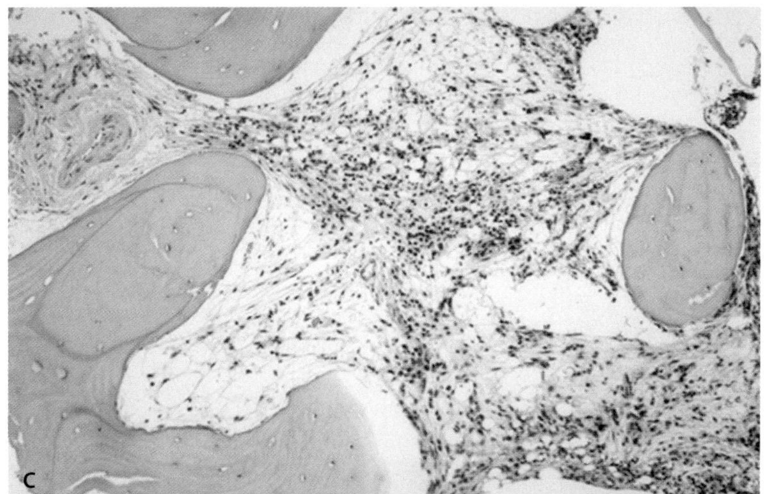

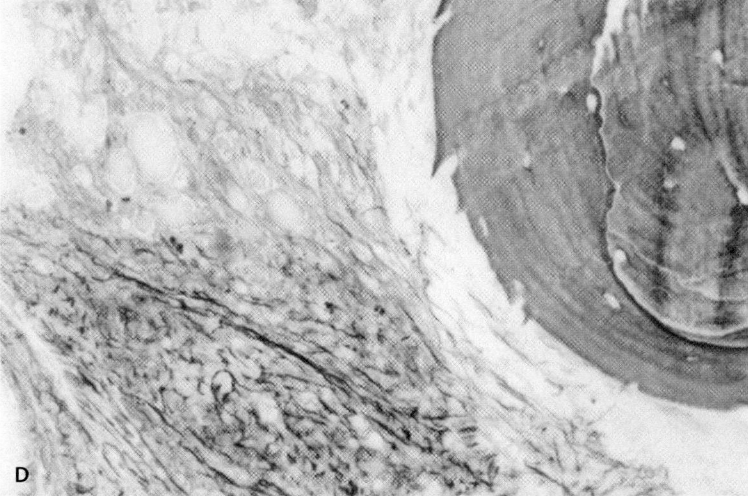

Figure 6.24

Osteonecrosis (characteristic MRI findings) and anterior disc displacement, with osteoarthritis. **A** Open-mouth MRI shows anteriorly displaced, deformed disc (*arrow*), condyle osteophytosis, and reduced signal in condyle marrow (*arrowhead*), consistent with sclerosis or fibrosis. **B** Open-mouth T2-weighted MRI shows fluid in anterior recess of upper compartment above disc (*arrow*), and increased signal in condyle marrow; marrow edema, and reduced signal in condyle marrow; marrow sclerosis or fibrosis (*arrowhead*). **C** Histologic section of condyle marrow shows complete loss of hematopoietic marrow, with evidence of inflammatory cell infiltrate (hematoxylin eosin; original magnification ×50). **D** Histologic section of condyle marrow shows marked increase of reticulin fiber deposition (reticulin fiber stain; original magnification ×50). Reproduced with permission from Larheim et al. (1999)

Arthritides

Definition

Inflammation of synovial membrane characterized by edema, cellular accumulation, and synovial proliferation (villous formation).

Clinical Features

- Swelling of joint area, not frequently seen in TMJ
- Pain (in active disease) from joints
- Restricted mouth opening capacity
- Morning stiffness, in particular stiff neck
- Dental occlusion problems; "my bite doesn't fit"
- Anterior bite opening, contact only on molars at closed mouth
- Crepitation due to secondary osteoarthritis
- Symptoms may be similar to those of common TMJ disorders
- Clicking sounds uncommon
- Disc displacement may occur in a rheumatic joint

Imaging Features

- Cortical punched-out erosions
- Abnormal disc (flattened, elongated), most frequently in normal position
- Disc fragments, or completely destroyed disc may be found
- Active disease: marrow edema and/or joint effusion
- Active disease: enhancement of synovial membrane, pannus after intravenous contrast injection
- Fibro-osseous ankylosis may be 'end-stage' of inflammatory disease
- Secondary osteoarthritis
- No principal difference in TMJ imaging signs of rheumatoid arthritis, ankylosing spondylitis, or psoriatic arthropathy
- Disc displacement may occur in joints with inflammatory arthritis

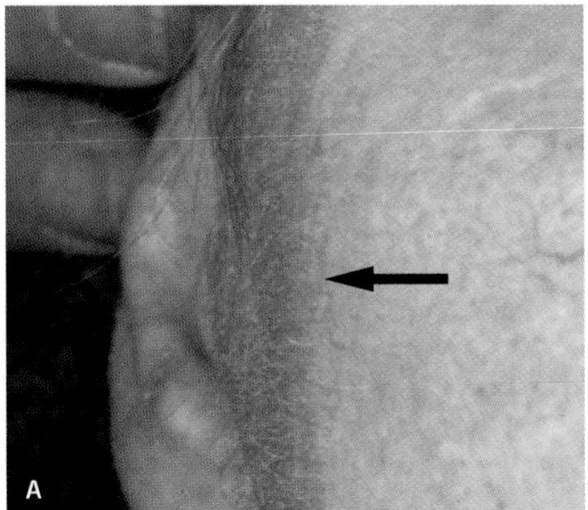

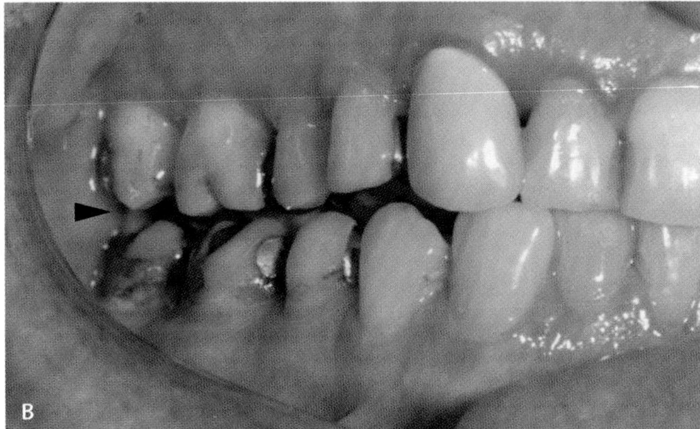

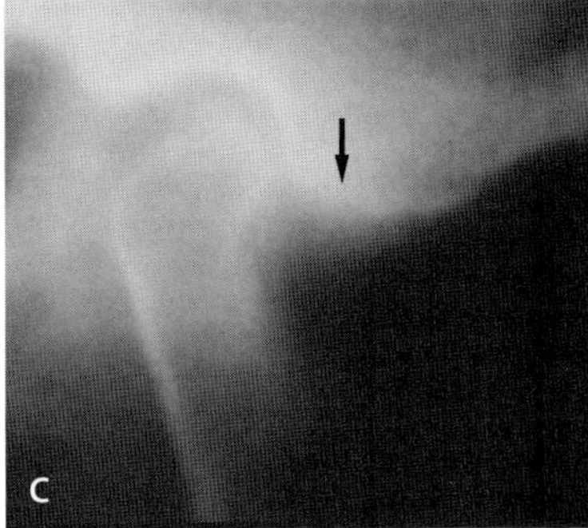

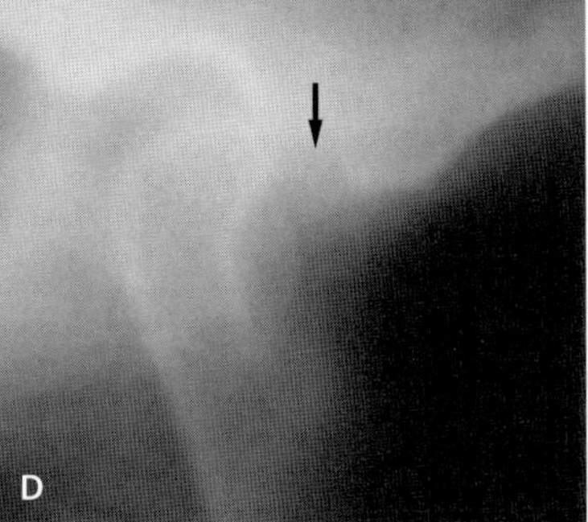

Figure 6.25

Rheumatoid arthritis. **A** Clinical photograph shows swelling over joint area (*arrow*). **B** Dental occlusion does not fit properly (*arrowhead*). **C** Conventional tomography 1 year previously showed normal position of condyle in fossa and normal bone; note in particular the eminence (*arrow*). **D** Tomography now shows condyle displaced anteriorly (probably due to joint effusion) and erosion in articular eminence (*arrow*)

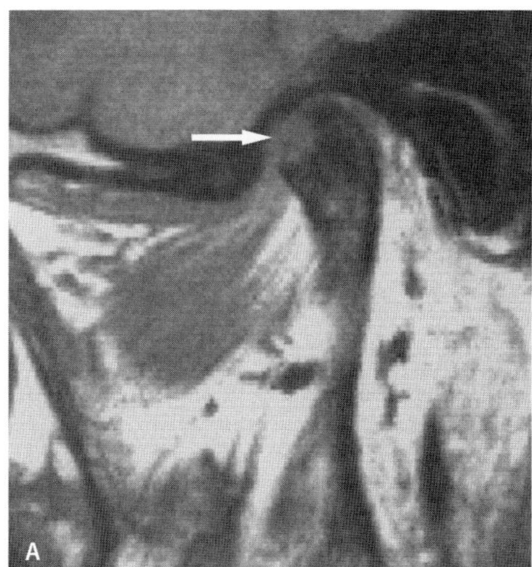

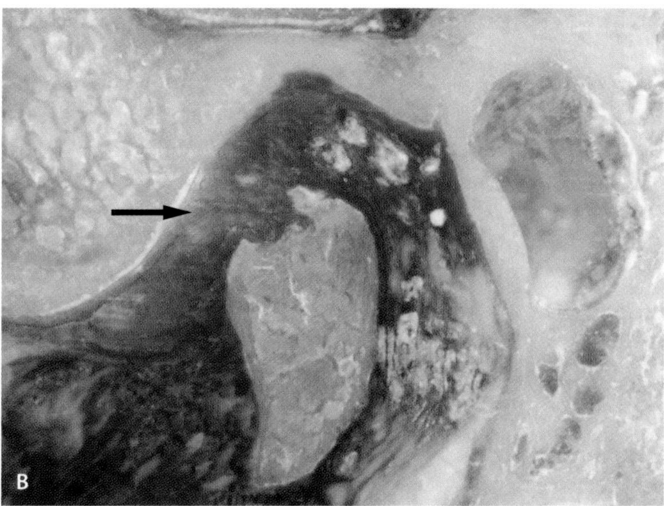

Figure 6.26

Rheumatoid arthritis. A MRI shows completely destroyed disc, replaced by fibrous or vascular pannus and cortical punched-out erosion (*arrow*) with sclerosis (shown by CT) in condyle. B Autopsy specimen shows no disc structure but pannus, and erosion in condyle (*arrow*) from patient with known long-standing rheumatoid arthritis (B is reproduced with permission from Westesson et al. 2003)

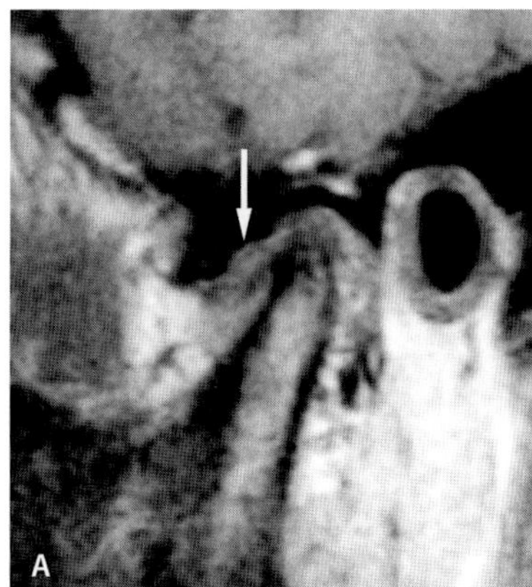

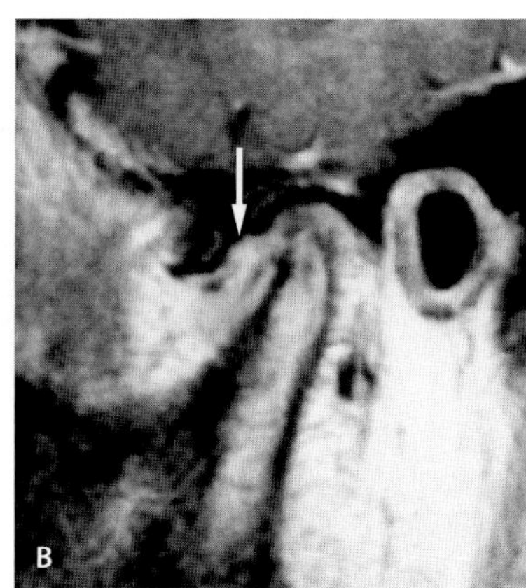

Figure 6.27

Rheumatoid arthritis. A, B T1-weighted pre-Gd (A) and T1-weighted post-Gd (B) MRI shows contrast enhancement of pannus that has replaced disc structure (*arrow*), and cortical erosions in condyle and temporal bone. Note contrast enhancement also in condyle

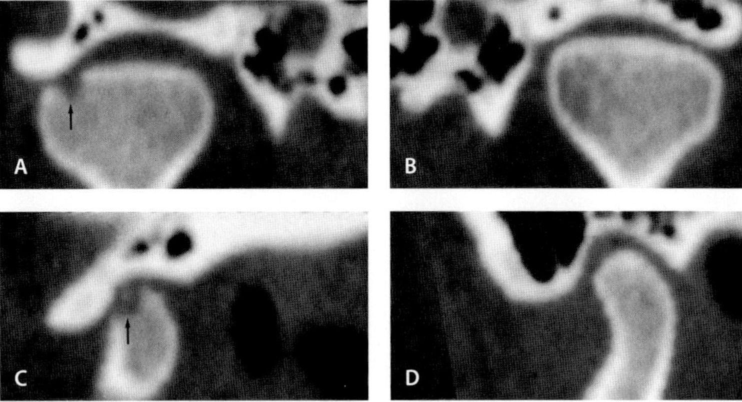

Figure 6.28

Psoriatic arthropathy. A, C Oblique coronal (A) and oblique sagittal (C) CT images show punched-out erosion in lateral part of condyle (*arrow*). B, D Similar CT sections of contralateral joint show normal bone

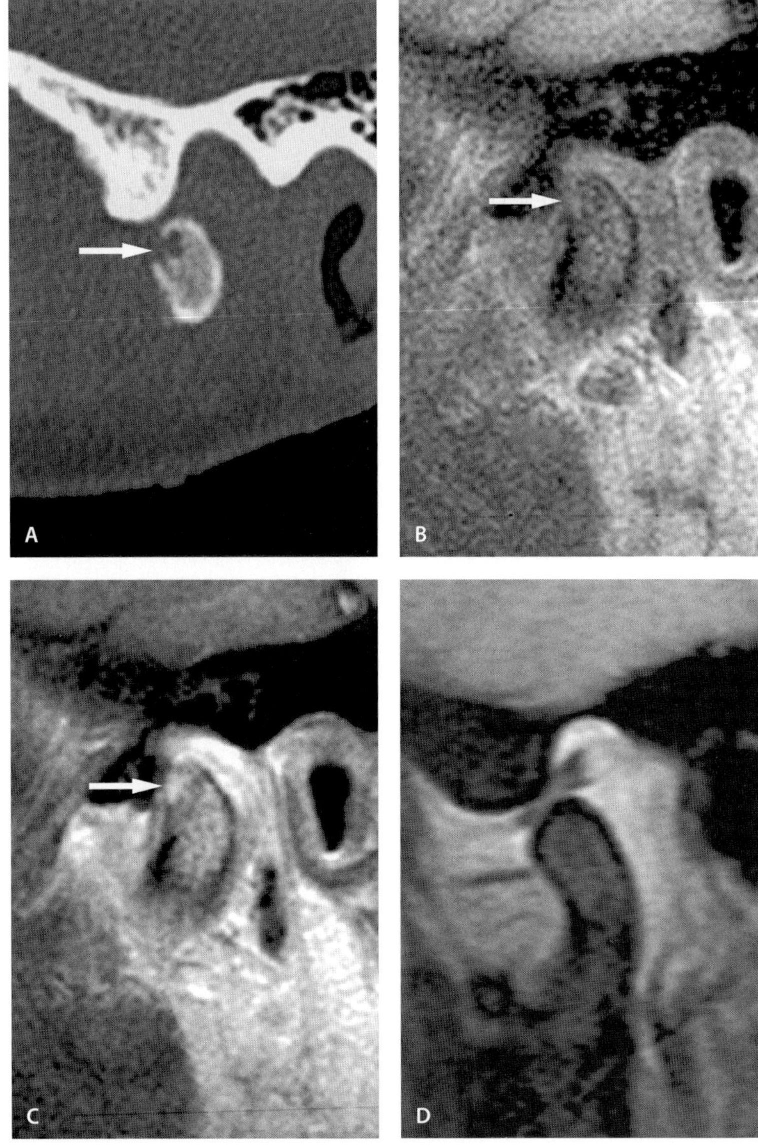

Figure 6.29

Psoriatic arthropathy (same patient as in Fig. 6.28). A Direct sagittal CT image shows punched-out erosion (*arrow*). B, C T1-weighted pre-Gd (B) and T1-weighted post-Gd (C) MRI shows contrast enhancement within bone erosion (*arrow*) and in joint space, consistent with thickened synovium/pannus formation. D Open-mouth MRI shows reduced condylar translation but normally located disc (and normal bone in this section)

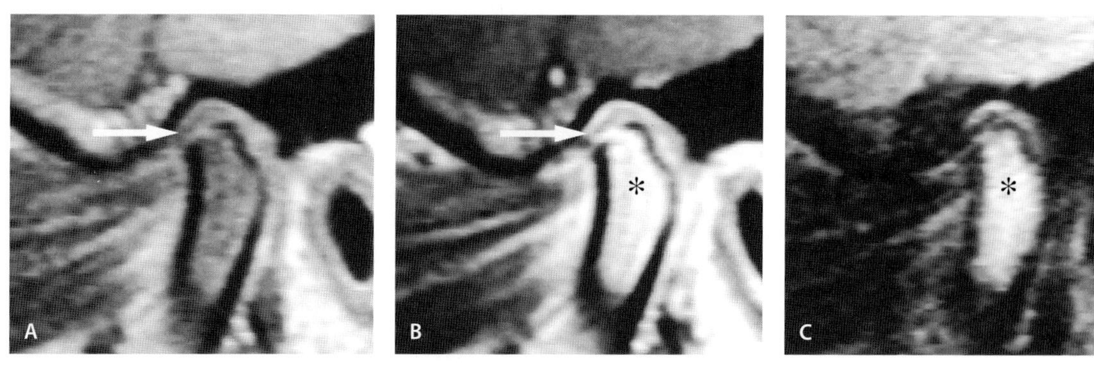

Figure 6.30

Ankylosing spondylitis. **A, B** T1-weighted pre-Gd (**A**) and T1-weighted post-Gd (**B**) MRI shows cortical erosion, deformed, thin disc in normal position (*arrow*) and contrast enhancement in upper and lower compartment and within condyle marrow (*asterisk*). **C** T2-weighted MRI shows bone marrow edema in entire condyle (*asterisk*)

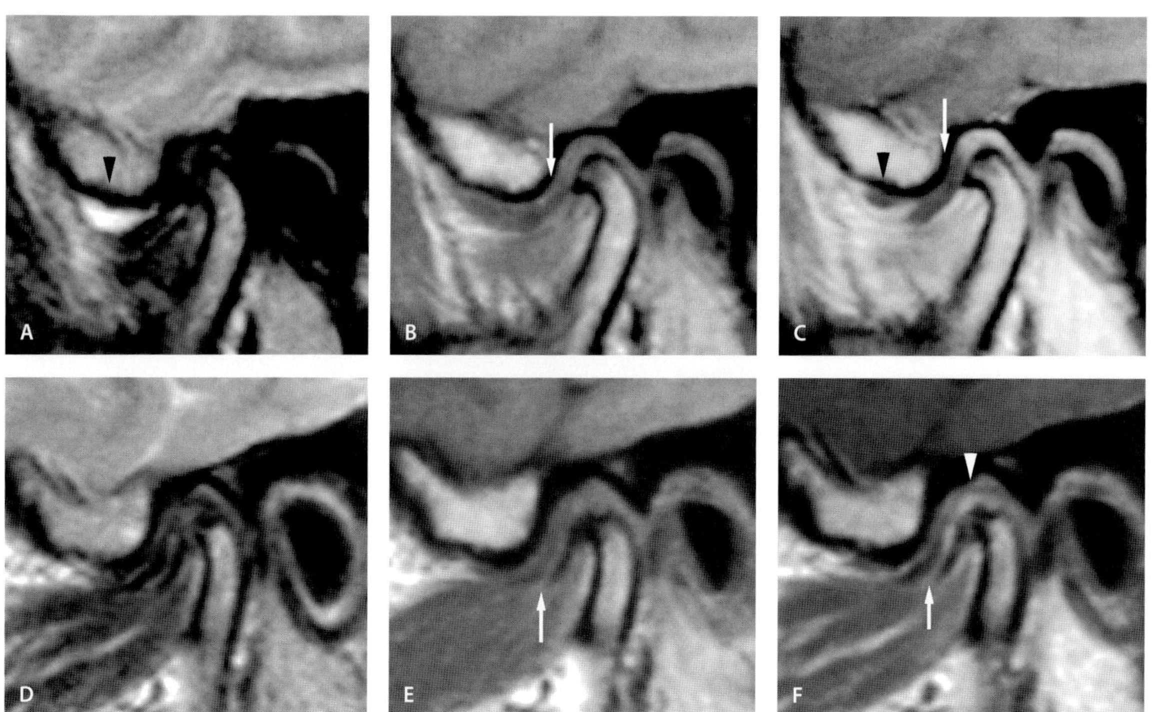

Figure 6.31

Rheumatoid arthritis and disc displacement of right (**A, B, C**) and left (**D, E, F**) joint. **A** T2-weighted MRI shows joint effusion in upper compartment of anterior recess (*arrowhead*). **B, C** T1-weighted pre-Gd (**B**) and T1-weighted post-Gd (**C**) MRI shows anteriorly displaced disc (*arrow*) and contrast enhancement in peripheral rim of joint effusion (*arrowhead*) and in posterior attachment, consistent with thickened synovium. Secondary osteoarthritis. **D** T2-weighted MRI shows no effusion. **E, F** T1-weighted pre-Gd (**E**) and T1-weighted post-Gd (**F**) MRI shows anteriorly displaced disk (*arrow*) and slight contrast enhancement around disc and in joint space (*arrowhead*), consistent with thickened synovium. Secondary osteoarthritis

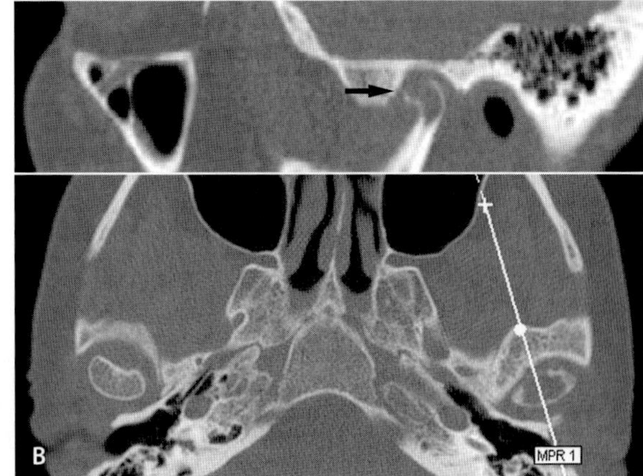

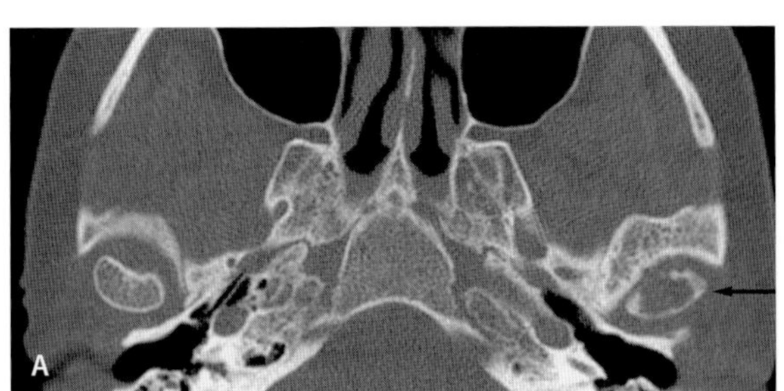

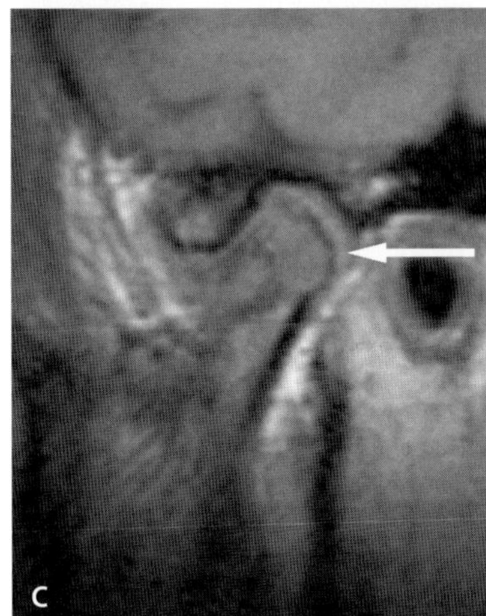

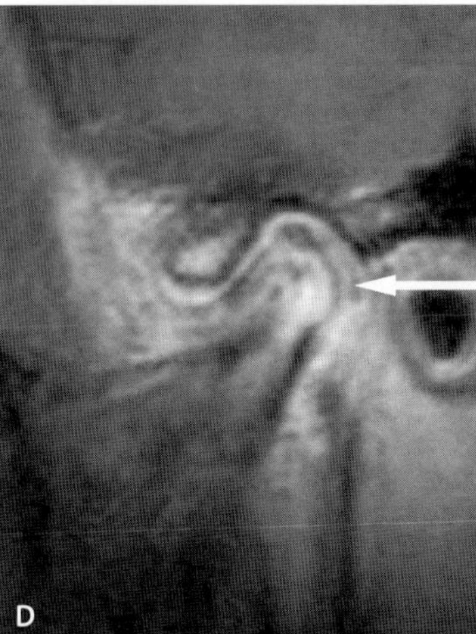

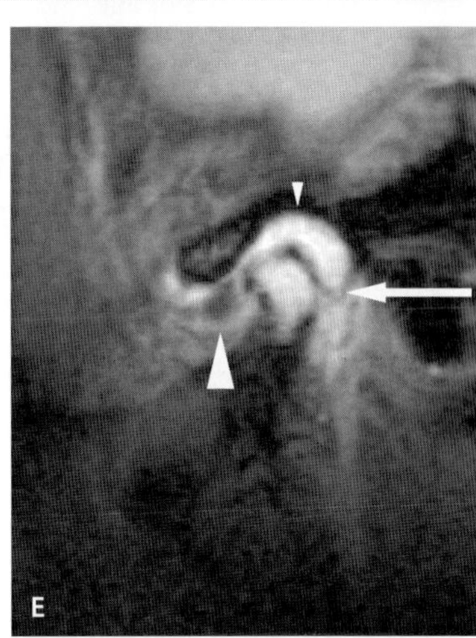

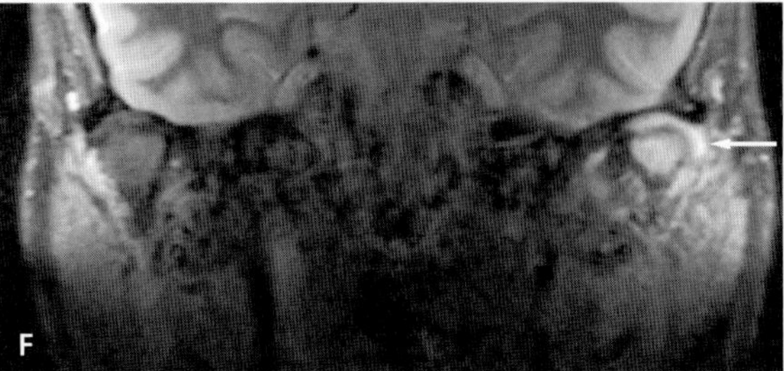

Figure 6.32

Inflammatory arthritis in patient without known generalized joint disease. **A** Axial CT image shows severe destruction of cortical bone in mandibular condyle. **B** Oblique sagittal CT image (perpendicular to long axis of condyle) shows destruction of entire condyle (*arrow*). **C, D** T1-weighted pre-Gd (**C**) and T1-weighted post-Gd (**D**) MRI shows contrast enhancement, particularly in upper compartment and in condyle (*arrow*), and thin, elongated disc, apparently in normal disc position. **E** Oblique sagittal (post-Gd) open-mouth MRI shows increased signal from condyle marrow (*arrow*) and increased signal from joint space (*small arrowhead*). Disc is anteriorly displaced and deformed (*large arrowhead*). **F** Coronal STIR image shows marrow edema or vascular pannus in condyle and vascular pannus in joint space, particularly in lateral region (*arrow*). Surgery (by Dr. T. Bjørnland, Rikshospitalet University Hospital, Oslo, Norway) confirmed severe condyle destruction and inflammatory pannus within and around condyle, particularly in lateral part of joint (patient was referred for rheumatologic evaluation due to family history of rheumatic disease, but had no symptoms from other joints)

Juvenile Idiopathic Arthritis

Definition

Rheumatoid arthritis (see definition) with onset before 16 years of age.

Clinical Features

- Juvenile arthritis differs in many respects from rheumatoid arthritis in adults
- Heterogeneous disease with different subgroup classifications
- Rheumatoid factor seropositivity not common
- Two peaks of onset, between 1 and 3 years of age and around 9 years of age
- More girls than boys
- Large joints (knees, wrists, and ankles) are more prominently involved than small peripheral joints
- Bony ankylosis in cervical spine is characteristic
- Underdeveloped mandible, micrognathia, is characteristic
- Restricted mouth-opening capacity
- Pain from TMJs not so common

Imaging Features

- Bony joint components abnormal, frequently without cortical erosions
- Flat fossa, underdeveloped eminence
- Condyle deformed: short, thick, flat, round
- Condyle located anteriorly in fossa at closed mouth
- Restricted condylar translation at opened mouth
- Soft-tissue abnormalities: flat, thin, elongated, or destroyed disc
- Active disease: bone marrow edema and/or joint effusion
- Active disease: enhancement of synovial membrane, pannus after intravenous contrast injection
- Secondary osteoarthritis, remodeling

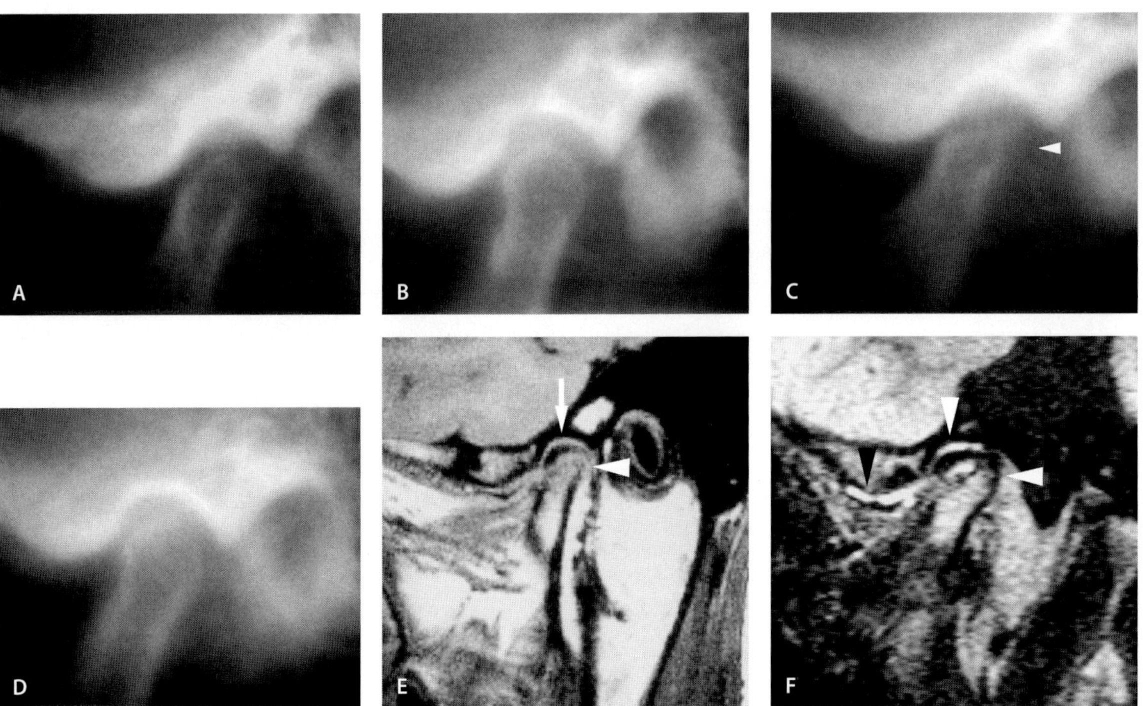

Figure 6.33

Juvenile idiopathic arthritis in a 14-year-old female. Oblique lateral tomography at baseline (A, B) and at 4 months follow-up (C, D), with supplementary MRI at follow-up (E, F). A, C Tomography shows resorption of condyle (*arrowhead*) during a 4-month period (with high disease activity) compared to normal contralateral joint (B, D). E T1-weighted MRI shows normally positioned disc (*arrow*), flat, deformed condyle with lack of cortical outline, and reduced signal from condyle marrow (*arrowhead*). F T2-weighted MRI shows extensive effusion in upper and lower compartments (*vertical arrowheads*) and bone marrow edema in condyle (*horizontal arrowhead*)

Figure 6.34

Juvenile idiopathic arthritis in a 12-year-old female with no history of generalized joint disease. A Panoramic view shows flattened condyles bilaterally (*arrows*). B Lateral cephalography shows anterior bite opening at orthodontic consultation. C Oblique coronal and sagittal CT of right joint (similar changes in left joint) shows deformed condyle: flat, short and small in mediolateral direction (*left image*), and condyle located at eminence at closed mouth, with abnormal flat fossa (*right image*). D, E, F, T1-weighted pre-Gd (D, E) and T1-weighted post-Gd (F) MRI of left joint (similar changes in right joint) shows normally positioned disc (*arrow*) and contrast enhancement of upper and lower joint compartment (F), consistent with thickened synovium. Patient was referred for rheumatologic examination which confirmed diagnosis of juvenile idiopathic arthritis.

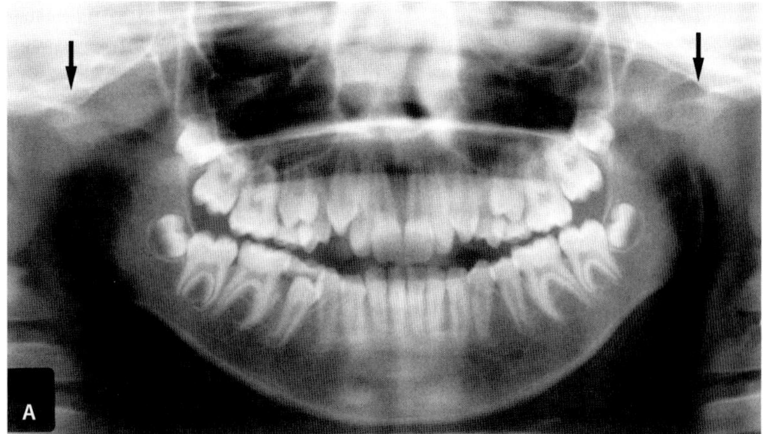

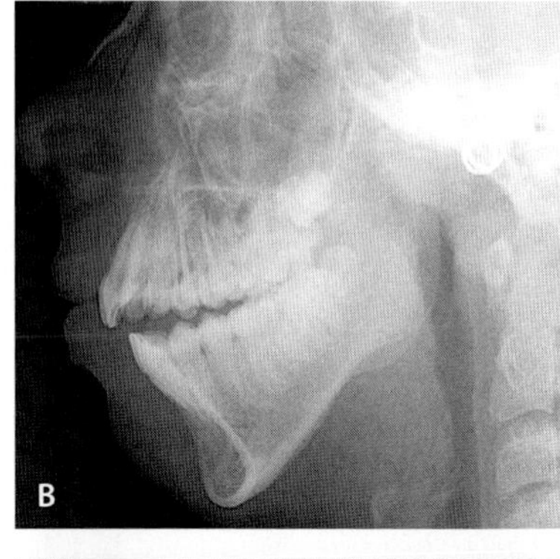

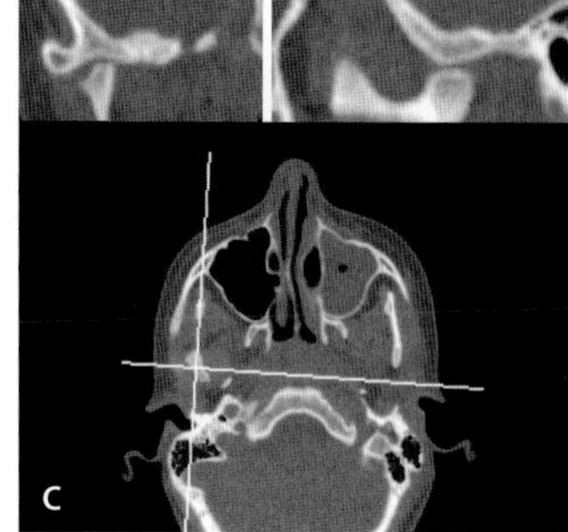

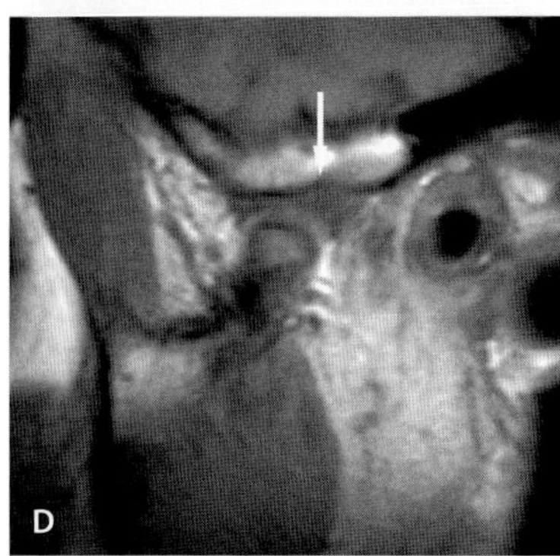

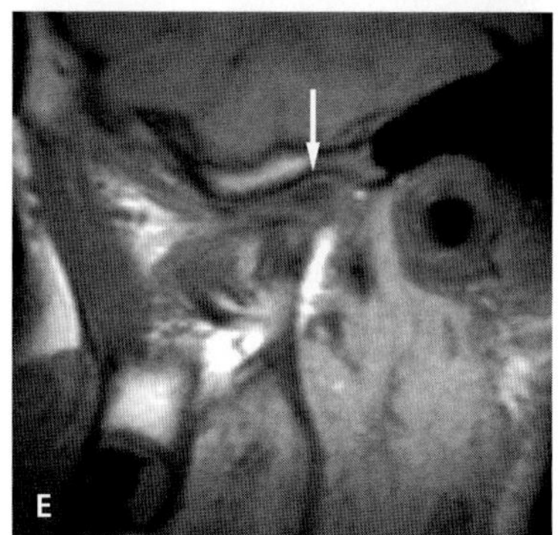

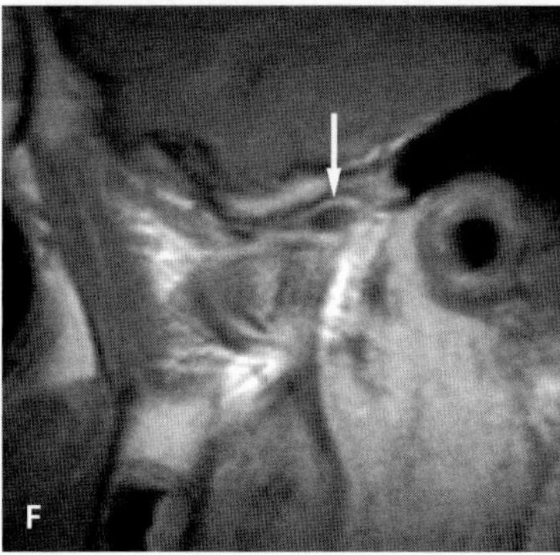

Ankyloses

Definition

Fibrous or bony union between joint components.

Clinical Features

- Severely limited mouth-opening capacity, gradually
- Usually no pain
- No joint sounds
- Secondary to arthritides, in particularly ankylosis spondylosis
- Secondary to trauma, fracture
- Idiopathic

Imaging Features

- Fibrous ankylosis; joint space visible
- Bony ankylosis; no joint space (at least in parts of joint) visible
- Joint space better seen on CT than on MRI
- No clear definition of any joint structures
- No joint effusion or contrast enhancement
- No or very limited condylar translation at (very restricted) mouth-opening capacity

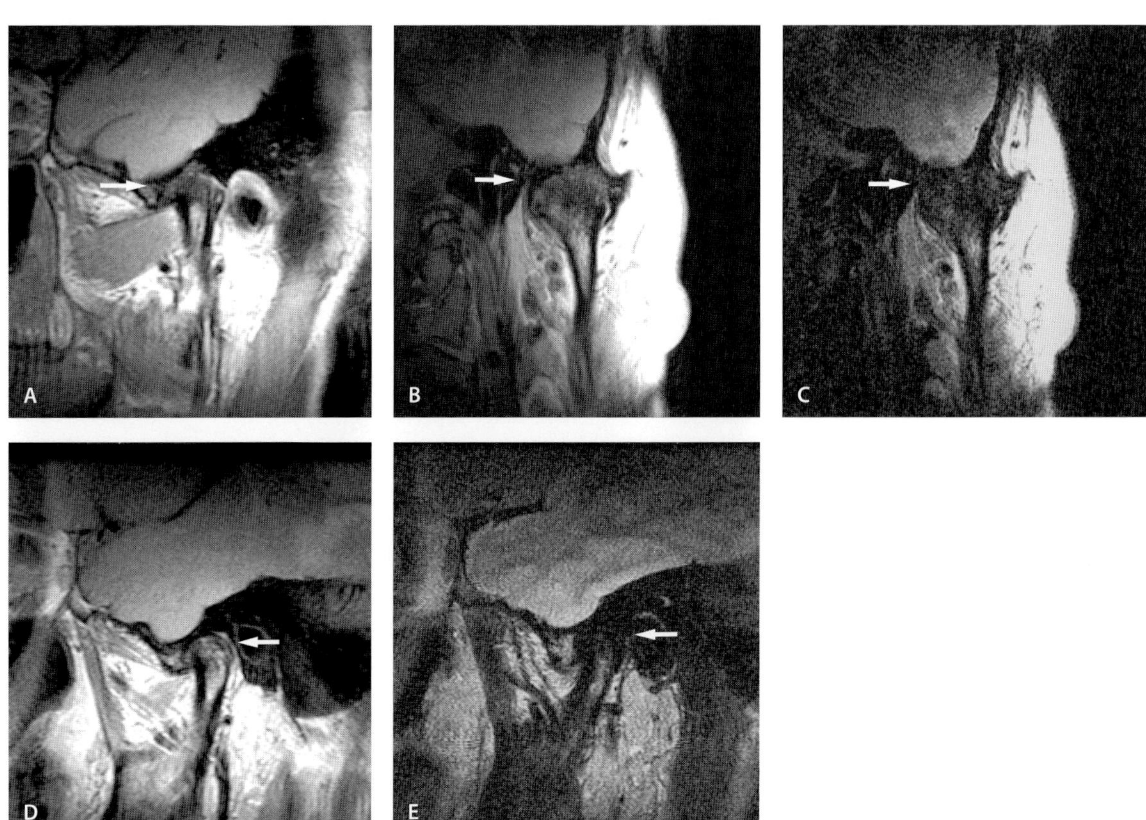

Figure 6.35

Ankylosis. **A** T1-weighted MRI of right joint shows no delineation of disc, fossa or condyle (*arrow*). **B** Oblique coronal T1-weighted MRI of right joint confirms loss of structures (*arrow*). **C** Oblique coronal T2-weighted MRI of right joint shows no structures or effusion (*arrow*). **D** T1-weighted MRI of left joint shows poor delineation of structures (*arrow*). **E** T2-weighted MRI of left joint shows no structures or effusion (*arrow*). Condylar translation is absent in open-mouth images (**A, D**). Fibrous or osseous union cannot be determined

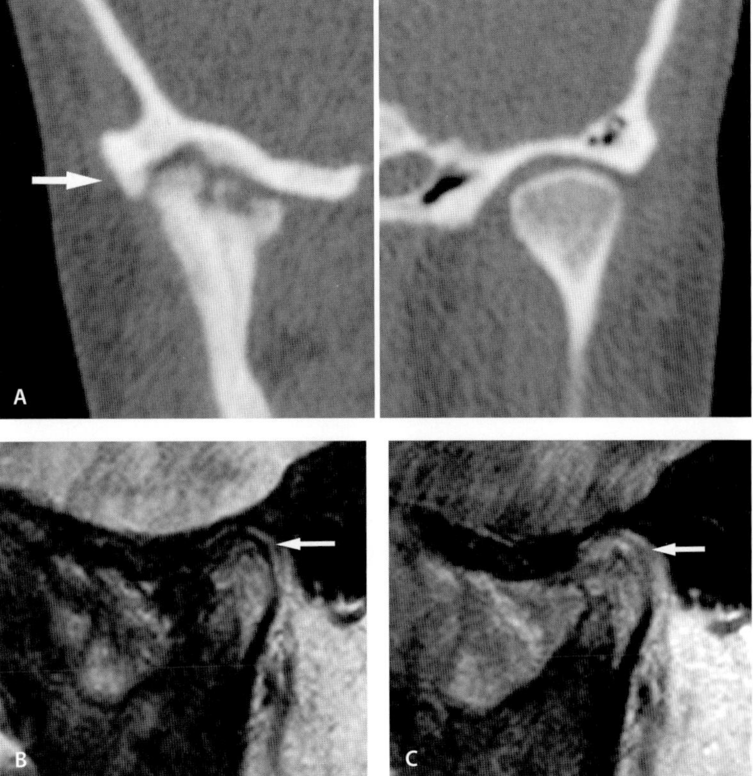

Figure 6.36

Fibrous ankylosis. A Coronal CT image shows severe cortical irregularities, particularly in mandibular condyle, and joint space through entire joint (*arrow*). B T2-weighted MRI shows no joint structures or effusion (*arrow*). C T1-weighted post-Gd MRI shows no contrast enhancement (*arrow*)

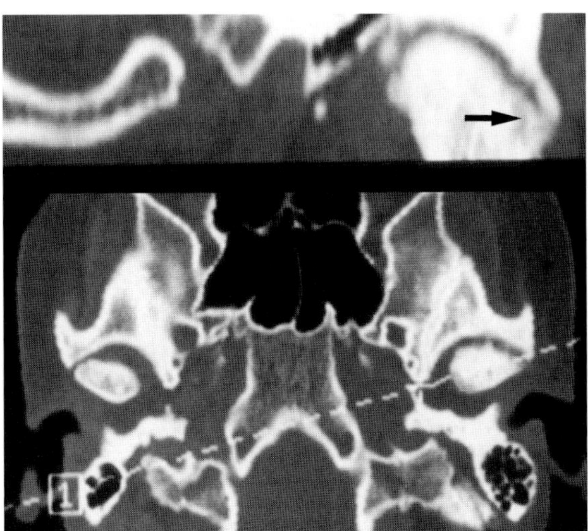

Figure 6.37

Bony ankylosis in patient with ankylosing spondylitis. Oblique coronal CT image (parallel with long axis of condyle) shows bony union in lateral part of joint (*arrow*)

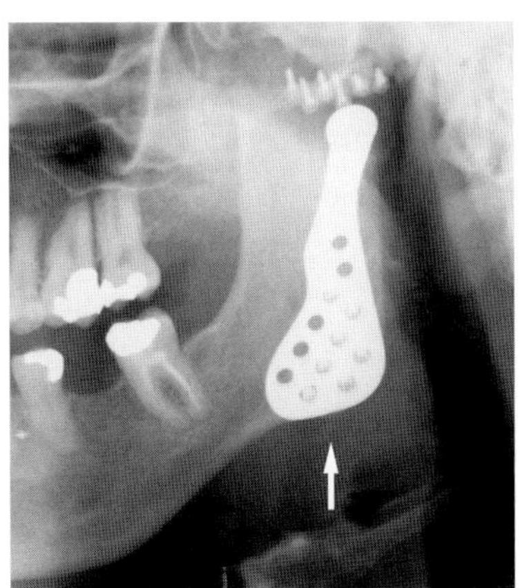

Figure 6.38

Ankylosis treated with total joint prosthesis (Lorenz). Panoramic view shows prosthesis (*arrow*), consisting of artificial fossa (fixed with six titanium screws in temporal bone), and artificial condylar process (fixed with seven titanium screws to mandibular ramus) (courtesy of Dr. G. Støre, Rikshospitalet University Hospital, Oslo, Norway)

Growth Disturbances (Anomalies)

Definition

Abnormal growth of mandibular condyle; overgrowth, undergrowth, or bifid appearance.

Clinical Features

- Facial (mandibular) asymmetry
- Mandibular overgrowth
- Mandibular undergrowth

Imaging Features

- Unilateral hyperplastic condyle
- Usually not enlarged in mediolateral direction
- Normal bone structure
- Normal disc position
- Hypoplastic condyle, unilateral or bilaterally
- Anterior disc displacement or normal disc position
- Condyle remodeling (flattened, deformed)
- Arthrosis deformans juveniles
- Bifid or split condyle

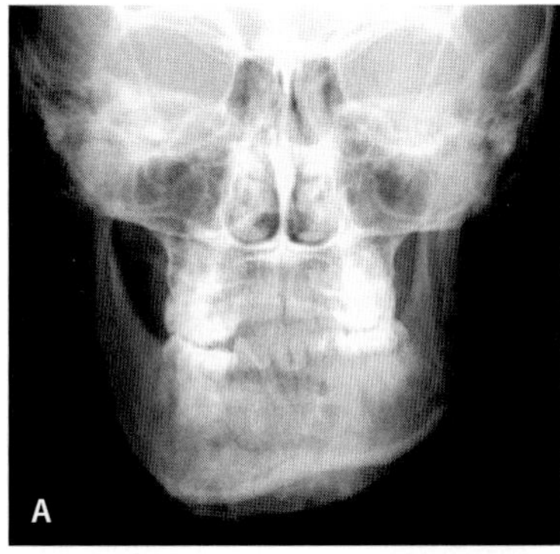
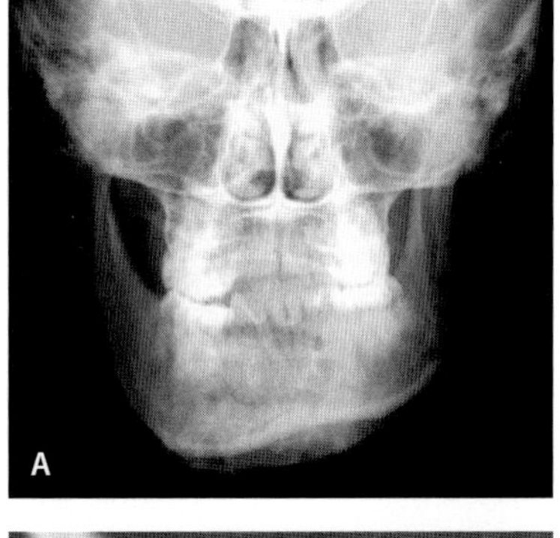

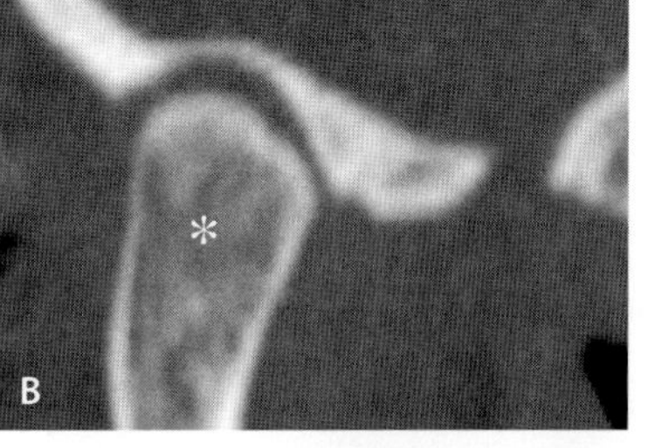

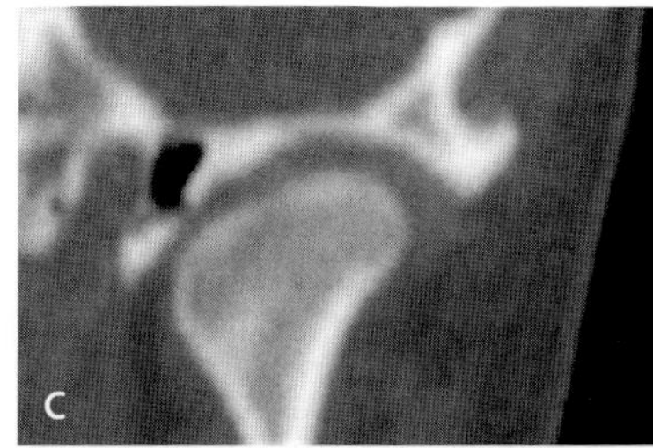

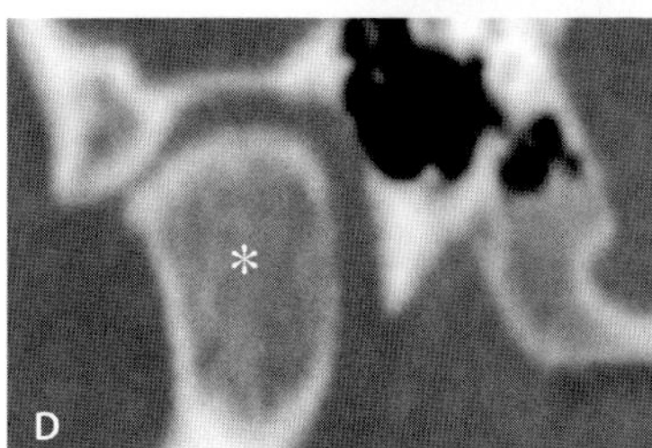

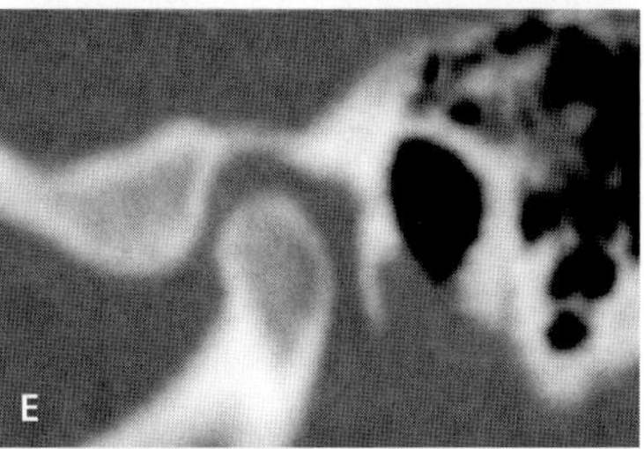

Figure 6.39

Condylar hyperplasia and facial asymmetry; 23-year-old female. A Posteroanterior facial view shows jaw asymmetry due to unilateral mandibular overgrowth (right side). B, D Oblique coronal CT (B) and sagittal (D) CT images show mandibular condyle (*asterisk*) with abnormal shape and size; enlarged but not in mediolateral dimension, and widened fossa in anteroposterior dimension. C, E Oblique coronal (C) and sagittal (E) CT images show normal contralateral joint

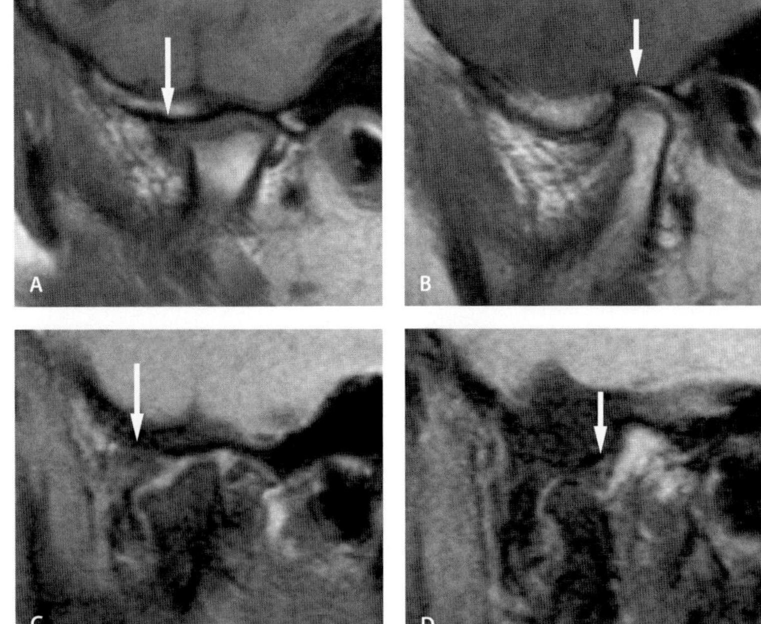

Figure 6.40

Condylar hypoplasia and facial asymmetry (underdeveloped right side) of 12-year-old female with 4-year history of trauma, but no confirmed fracture. A, C MRI shows abnormal right joint with displaced disc (*arrow*), also in open-mouth image (C). Condyle is deformed, flat and enlarged in anteroposterior direction, and fossa is flattened. B, D MRI of left joint shows normal bone and normal disc (*arrow*), also in open-mouth image (D)

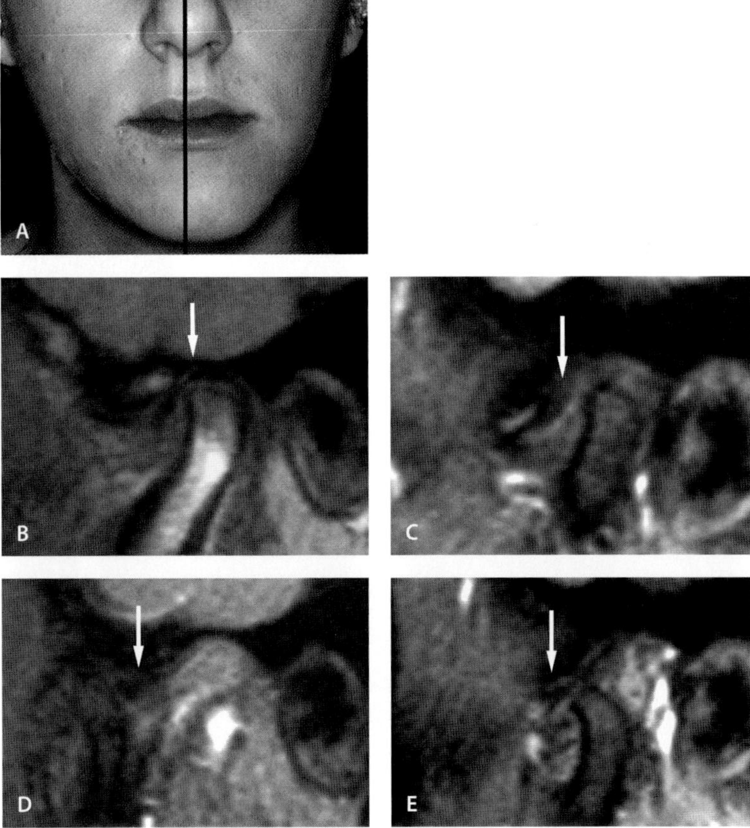

Figure 6.41

Condylar hypoplasia and facial asymmetry without history of trauma. A Clinical photograph shows mandible deviating to patient's left side. B, D MRI of right joint shows normal disc (*arrow*) and normal bone, also in open-mouth image (D). C, E MRI of left joint shows anteriorly displaced disc (*arrow*), also in open-mouth image (E). Left condyle is small but otherwise normal and condylar translation is restricted compared to contralateral joint (courtesy of Drs. A. Isberg and P.E. Legrell, Umea University, Sweden)

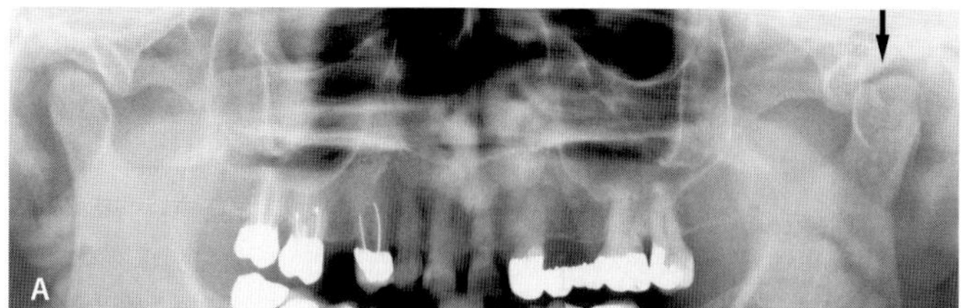

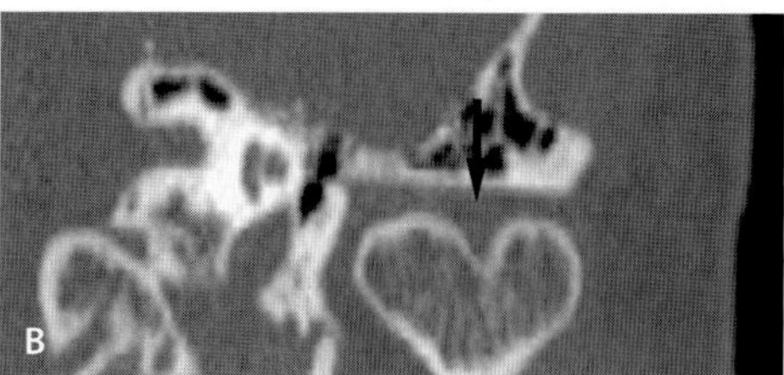

Figure 6.42

Bifid condyle. **A** Panoramic view shows abnormal left condyle (*arrow*) as an incidental finding. **B** Oblique coronal CT image (parallel with long axis of condyle) shows split condyle (*arrow*), but otherwise normal bone structure

Inflammatory or Tumor-like Conditions

Calcium Pyrophosphate Dehydrate Crystal Deposition Disease (Pseudogout)

Definition

Gout-like joint inflammation with subtle or severe calcium crystal deposits (chondrocalcinosis), not uric acid as in gout.

Clinical Features

- Joint pain and swelling
- Symptoms may be similar to those of common TMJ disorders

Imaging Features

- Calcifications within joint space
- Subtle or massive calcifications
- Both condyle and glenoid fossa may be eroded and actually simulate malignancy

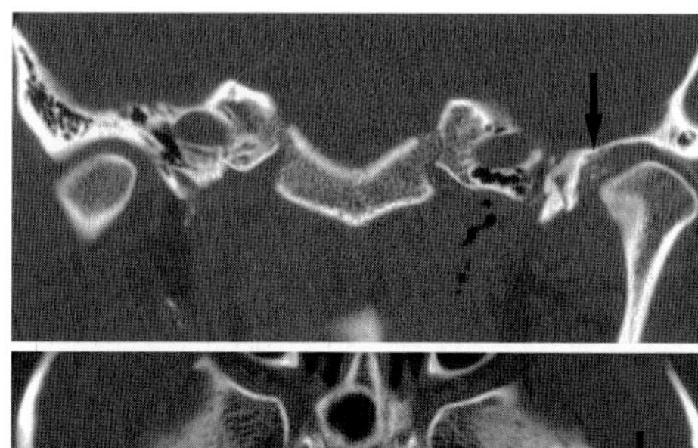

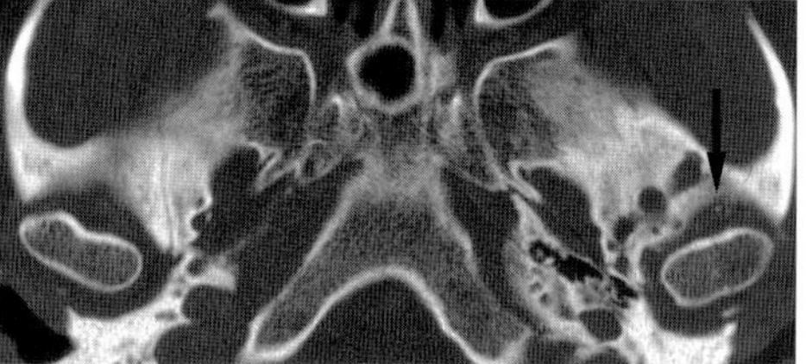

Figure 6.43

Pseudogout. Coronal and axial CT images show subtle calcifications within joint space (*arrows*) consistent with early stage

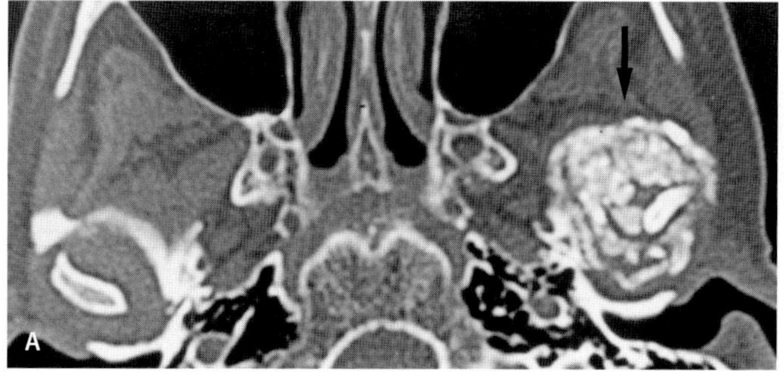

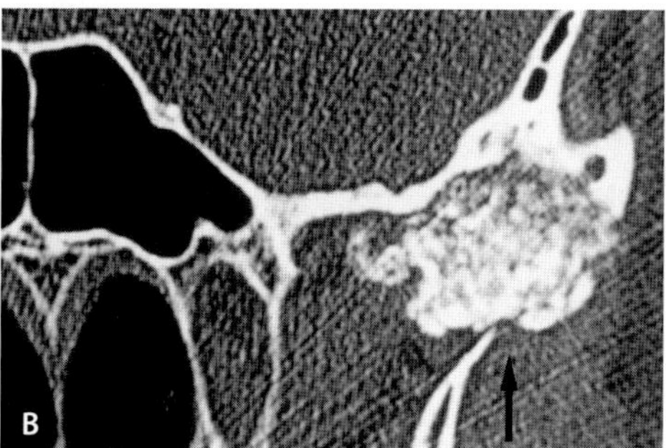

Figure 6.44

Pseudogout. **A**, **B** Axial (**A**) and coronal (**B**) CT images show extensive calcifications (*arrow*) consistent with advanced stage

Pigmented Villonodular Synovitis

Definition

Joint inflammation, or benign neoplastic process, characterized by synovial proliferation, joint effusion, hemosiderin deposition, histiocytes, giant cells, and occasionally, bone erosions.

Clinical Features

- Joint swelling and swelling, but symptoms may be vague
- Symptoms may be similar to those of common TMJ disorders

Imaging Features

- Condyle may show erosions
- Glenoid fossa may show erosions, with intracranial extension
- Periarticular soft tissue density may be seen
- T1-weighted and T2-weighted MRI shows characteristic (almost pathognomonic) low signal because of hemorrhage by-products

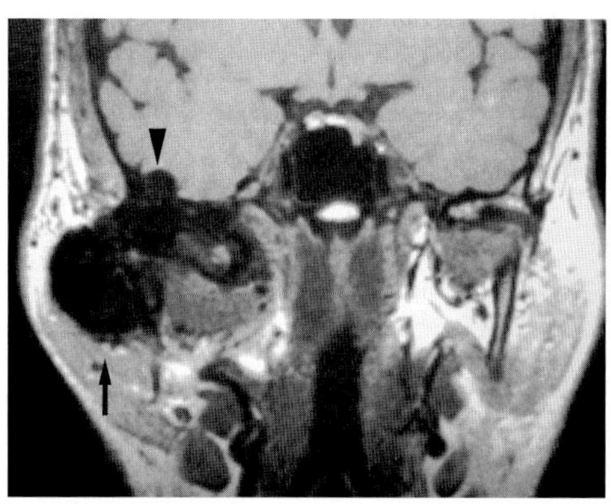

Figure 6.45

Pigmented villonodular synovitis. Coronal T1-weighted MRI shows large mass of very low signal (*arrow*), penetrating skull base (*arrowhead*). Very low signal also characteristic on T2-weighted and post-Gd MRI (not shown) (courtesy of Dr. T. Larsson, Seattle, Washington)

Traumatic Bone Cyst

Definition

Cavity within bone, empty or partially filled with sanguinous fluid, without epithelial lining, with or without expansion of bone.

Clinical Features

- Incidental finding; asymptomatic

Imaging Features

- Enlarged condyle
- Expanded, thin but intact cortical bone
- Other joint components normal

Figure 6.46

Traumatic bone cyst. A MRI shows enlarged mandibular condyle (*arrow*), with normal disc and temporal bone. B Coronal CT image shows enlarged condyle with intact cortical bone (*arrow*)

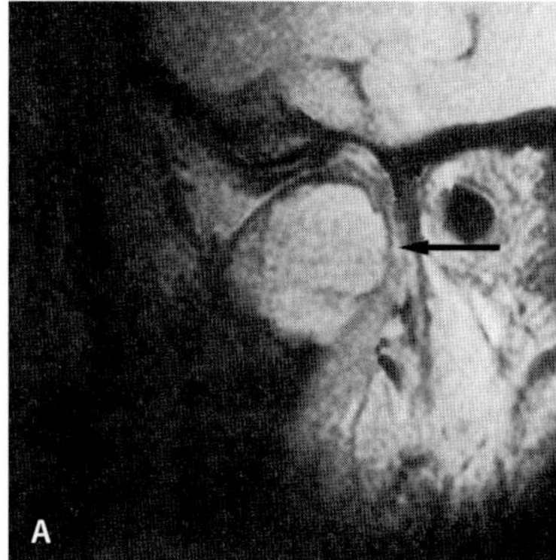

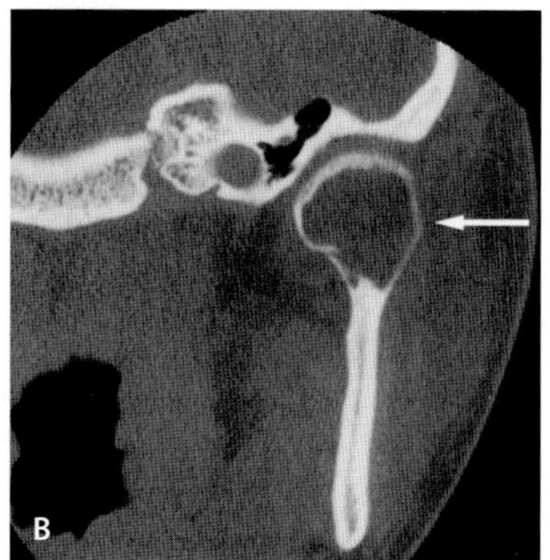

Benign Tumors

Synovial Chondromatosis

Definition

Benign tumor characterized by cartilaginous metaplasia of synovial membrane, usually in knee, producing small nodules of cartilage, which essentially separate from membrane to become loose bodies that may ossify.

Clinical Features

- Joint pain and swelling, but symptoms may be vague
- Facial asymmetry
- Dental occlusion problems; "my bite doesn't fit"
- Symptoms may be similar to those of common TMJ disorders

Imaging Features

- Calcifications within joint space
- Large or small calcifications, usually multiple
- Joint effusion, synovitis
- Condyle normal or osteoarthritis
- May be locally aggressive with destruction of fossa
- Intracranial extension has been reported

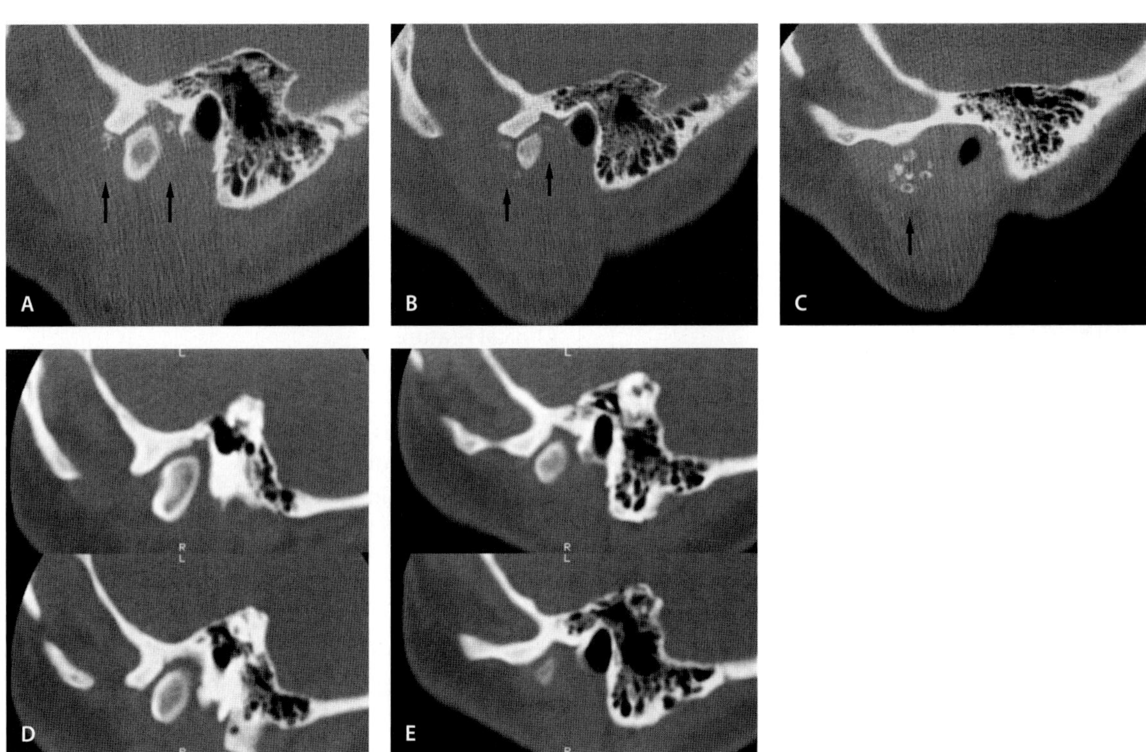

Figure 6.47

Synovial chondromatosis. A, B, C Sagittal CT images show multiple soft-tissue calcifications (*arrows*) anterior, posterior and lateral to condyle Also osteoarthritis. D, E Four sagittal CT images from an examination 4 years previously do not show calcifications when patient was referred for TMJ disorder

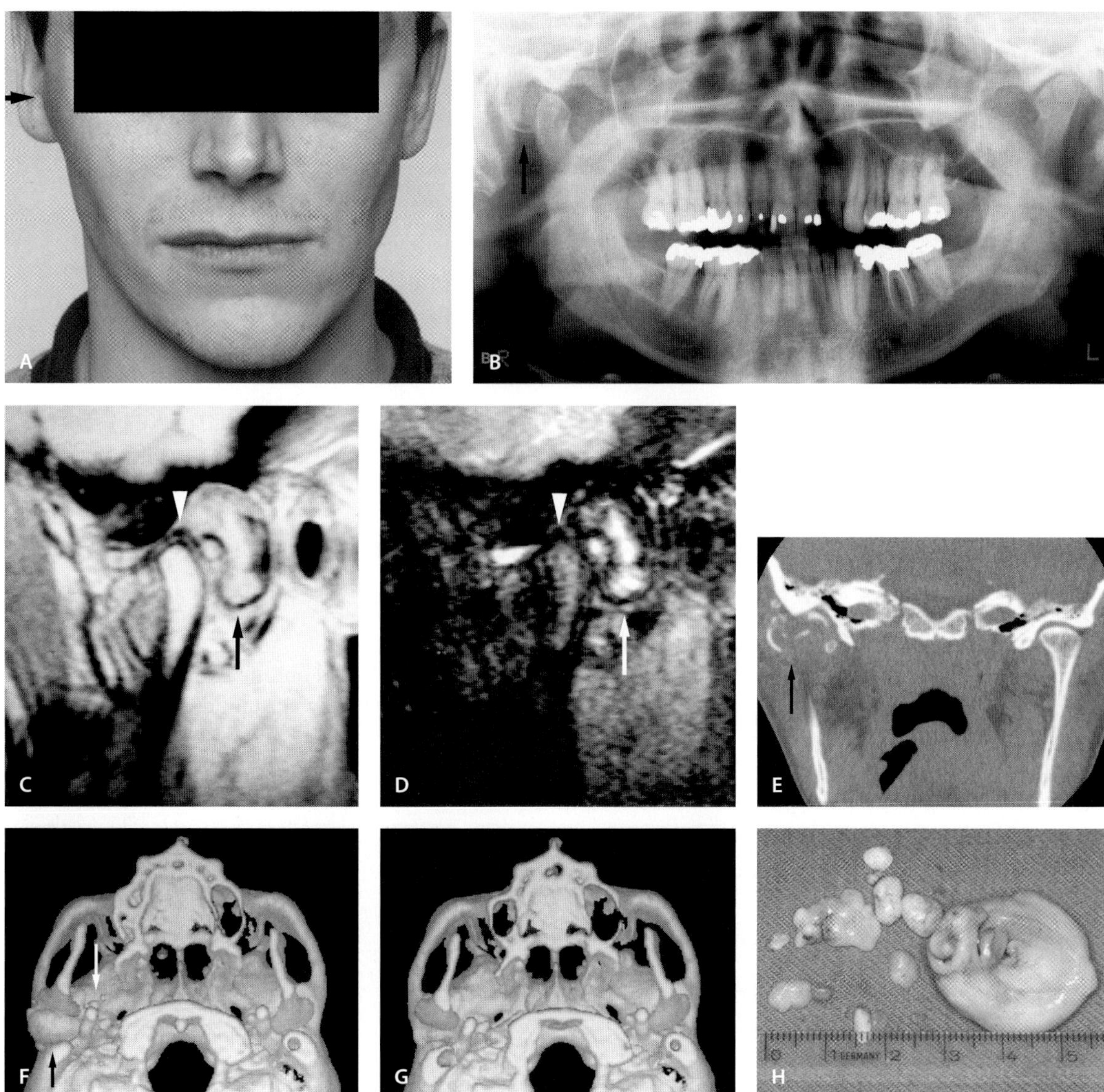

Figure 6.48

Synovial chondromatosis. A Clinical photograph shows facial asymmetry and swelling over right joint (*arrow*). B Panoramic view shows large calcification (*arrow*) posterior to condyle. C T1-weighted MRI shows large structure (*arrow*) posterior to condyle, which is normal but displaced anteriorly with normal disc (*arrowhead*) at closed mouth. D T2-weighted MRI shows increased signal from expansive process (*arrow*) and effusion in upper joint space; *arrowhead* condyle. E Coronal CT image confirms calcifications posterior to condyle (*arrow*). F Axial 3D CT image before surgery shows large calcification (*black arrow*) and smaller ones (*white arrow*). G Axial 3D CT image after surgery for comparison. H One large and a number of smaller calcifications were removed (H courtesy of Drs. G. Støre and T. Bjørnland, Rikshospitalet University Hospital, Oslo, Norway)

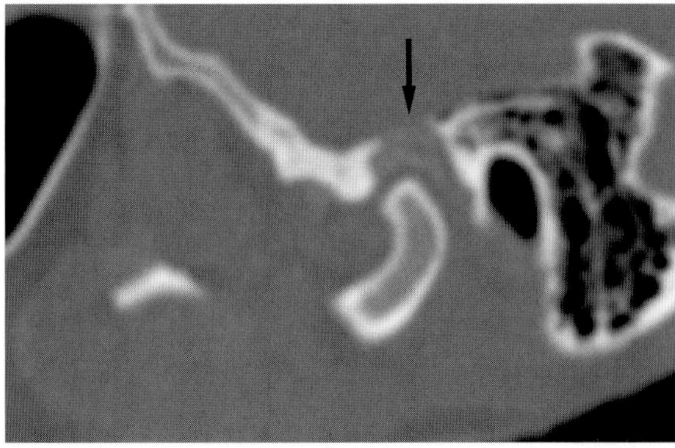

Figure 6.49

Synovial chondromatosis. Sagittal CT image shows destruction of fossa and slightly calcified tissue in joint space (*arrow*). Surgery confirmed destruction of fossa and calcified tissue, but no intracranial tumor growth

Osteochondroma

Synonym: Osteocartilaginous exostosis

Definition

Benign tumor characterized by normal bone and cartilage, near growth zones.

Clinical Features

- Asymptomatic
- Facial, mandibular asymmetry

Imaging Features

- Enlarged condyle
- Irregular in cortical outline and internal structure
- Cortical outline may be smooth

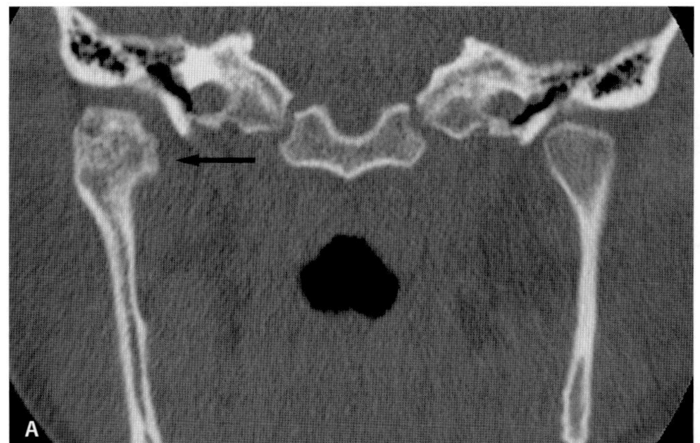

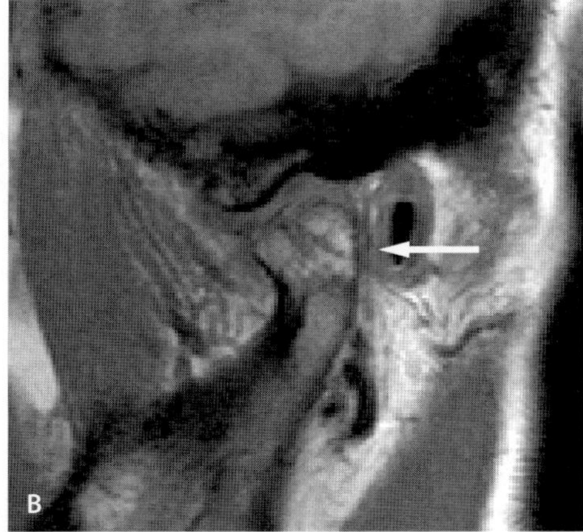

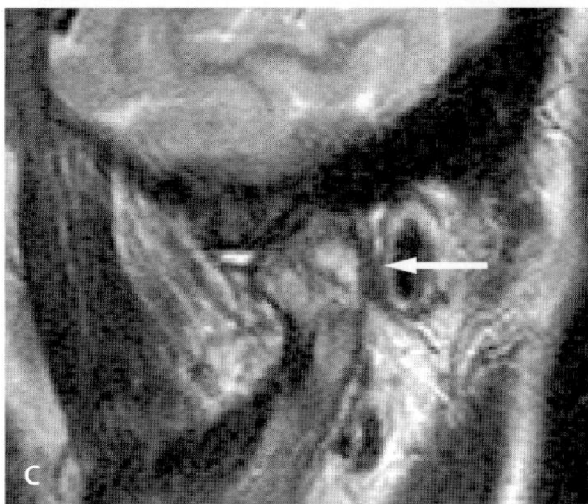

Figure 6.50

Osteochondroma. **A** Coronal CT shows enlarged condyle with irregular outline and mineralization (*arrow*). **B, C** T1-weighted (**B**) and T2-weighted (**C**) MRI shows heterogeneous signal from condyle (*arrow*), and normal disc in normal position, with minimal fluid

Osteoma

See also Chapter 3.

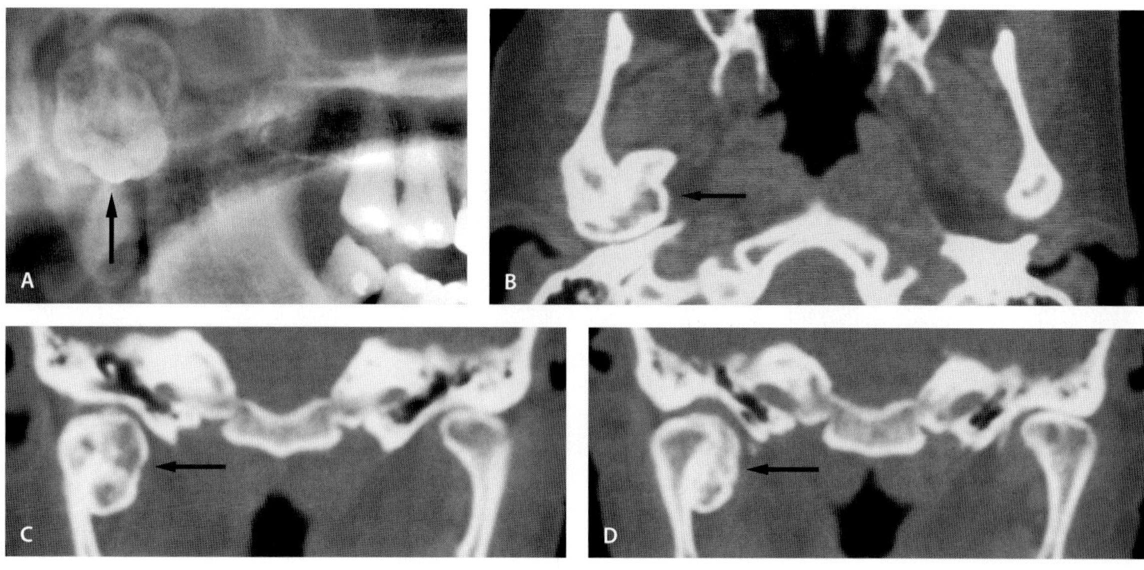

Figure 6.51

Osteoma, incidental finding at routine panoramic radiography. A Panoramic view shows bone structure (*arrow*) partially superimposed on mandibular condyle. B, C, D Axial (B) and coronal (C, D) CT images show bony outgrowth (*arrow*) of medial aspect of condyle

Sphenoid Meningioma

Definition

Benign brain tumor (meninges) from greater wing of sphenoid.

Clinical Features

- Restricted mouth-opening capacity
- No pain or other symptoms

Imaging Features

- Normal bone structures except destruction of fossa

Figure 6.52

Sphenoid meningioma; restricted mouth-opening capacity as only TMJ symptom. A, C Oblique coronal (A) and oblique sagittal (C) CT images parallel and perpendicular to long axis of condyle show destruction of fossa (*arrow*). B, D CT images of normal contralateral joint for comparison

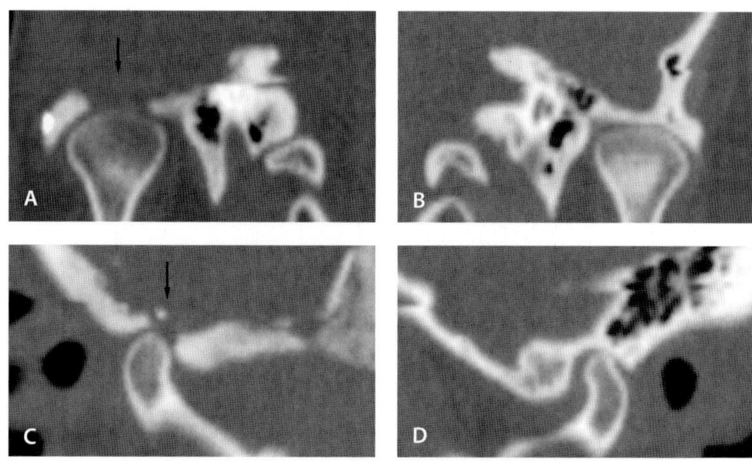

Malignant Tumors

Malignant tumors rarely affect the TMJ but should never be forgotten in differential diagnosis; two cases of metastases are presented.

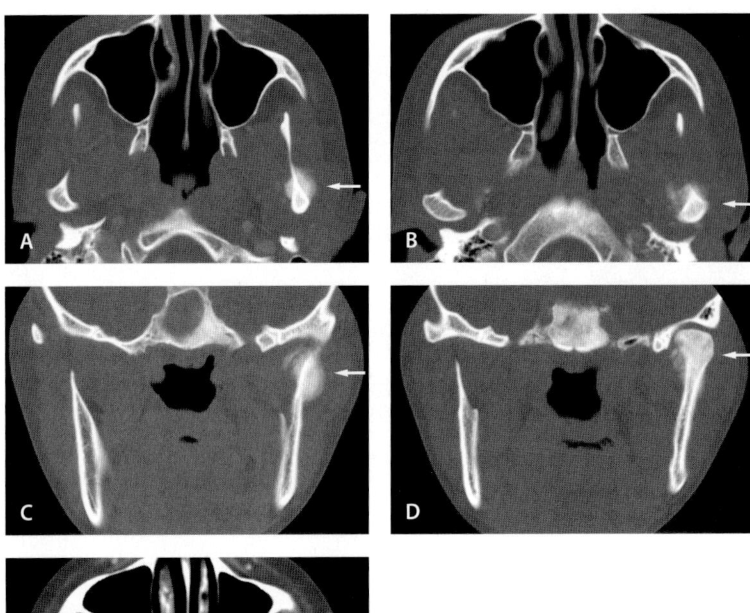

Figure 6.53

Osteosarcoma, mandible; 18-year-old female with terminal widespread osteosarcoma (2.5-year history) and recent metastasis to mandible. **A** Axial CT image shows intense bone production in ramus (*arrow*). **B** Axial CT image shows more irregular bone production in condyle (*arrow*). **C** Coronal CT image shows irregular bone production, but no evident bone destruction of ramus (*arrow*). **D** Coronal CT image shows well-defined bone production (*arrow*). **E** Axial CT image, soft-tissue window, shows contrast-enhancing tumor surrounding and encasing the condyle. There is peripheral contrast enhancement suggesting central necrosis

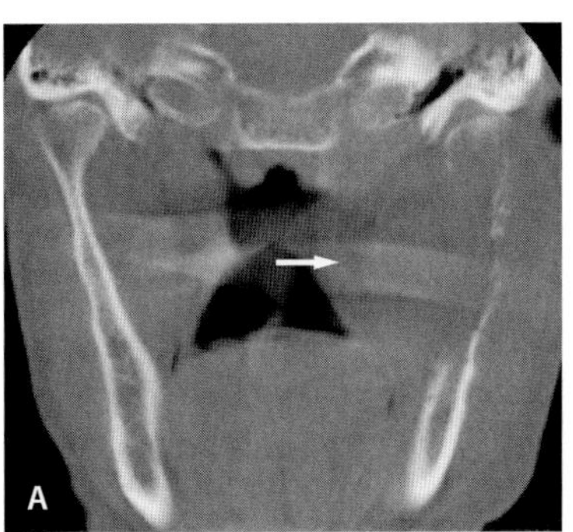

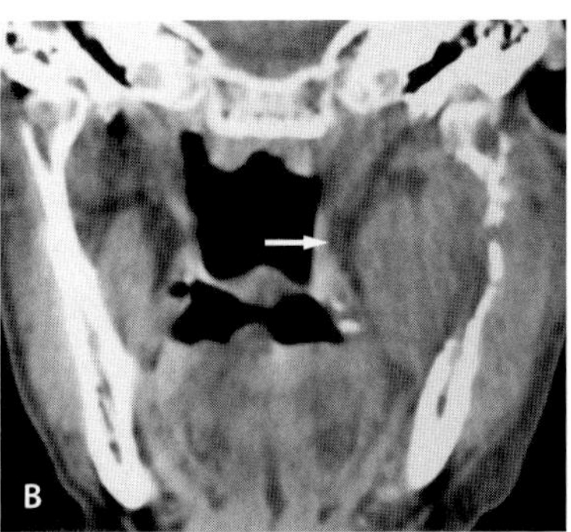

Figure 6.54

Malignant tumor, mandible; 70-year-old male with metastasis from lung cancer and restricted mouth-opening capacity as only TMJ symptom. **A** Coronal CT image shows destruction of ramus and condyle (*arrow*). **B** Coronal CT image, soft-tissue window, shows soft-tissue mass in masticator space infiltrating mandible (*arrow*)

Osteoradionecrosis

See also Chapter 5.

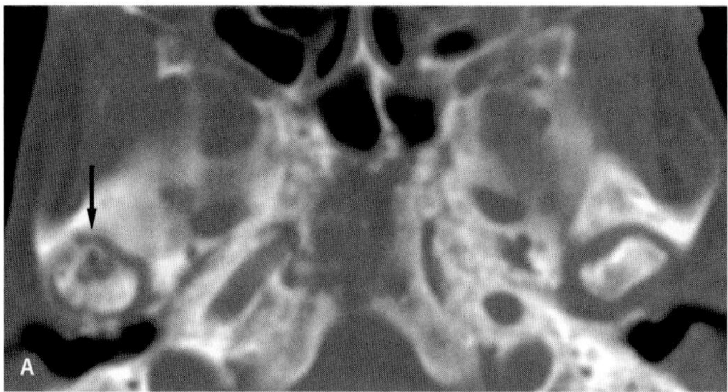

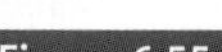

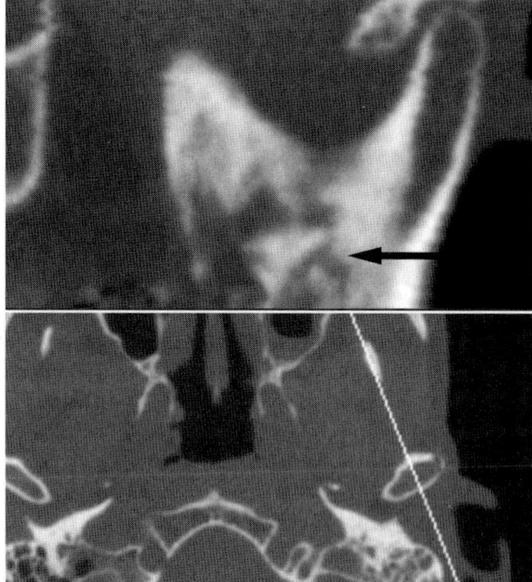

Figure 6.55

Osteoradionecrosis. A Axial CT image shows destruction of condyle in one patient (*arrow*), also note destruction in clivus. B Oblique sagittal CT image of mandibular ramus of another patient (with axial reference image) shows destruction of coronoid process (*arrow*)

Coronoid Hyperplasia

Definition

Enlarged coronoid process, unilaterally or bilaterally (1 cm above zygomatic arch has been mentioned as a definition)

Clinical Features

- Restricted mouth-opening capacity over time
- No pain

Imaging Features

- Enlarged coronoid process, otherwise normal
- Interfering with mouth opening; coronoid process is not allowed to move freely

Figure 6.56

Coronoid hyperplasia. A, B 3D CT images at closed (A) and opened mouth (B) show enlarged coronoid process (*arrow*) which does not allow normal motion of mandible

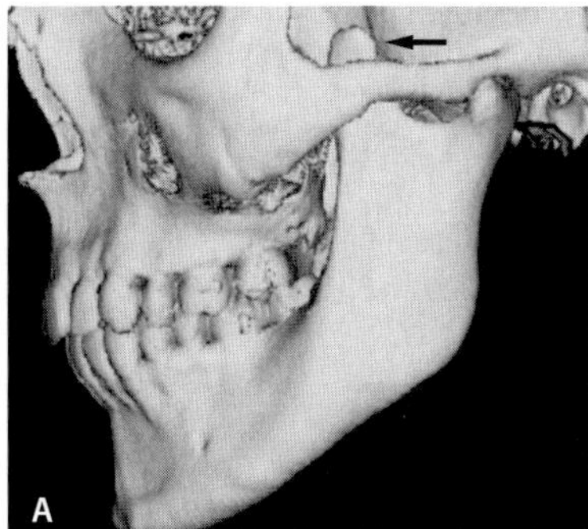

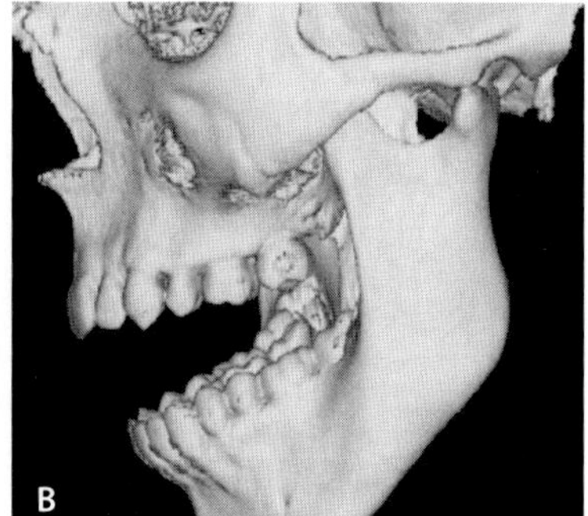

Suggested Reading

Adams JC, Hamblen DL (2001) Outline of orthopedics, 13th edn. Churchill Livingstone, London, p 135

De Bont LG, Dijkgraaf LC, Stegenga B (1997) Epidemiology and natural progression of articular temporomandibular disorders. Oral Surg Oral Med Oral Pathol Oral Radiol Endod 83:72–76

De Leeuw R, Boering G, Stegenga B, de Bont LG (1995) TMJ articular disc position and configuration 30 years after initial diagnosis of internal derangement. J Oral Maxillofac Surg 53:234–241

Emshoff R, Brandlmaier I, Schmid C, Bertram S, Rudisch A (2003) Bone marrow edema of the mandibular condyle related to internal derangement, osteoarthrosis, and joint effusion. J Oral Maxillofac Surg 61:35–40

Eriksson L, Westesson P-L (1983) Clinical and radiological study of patients with anterior disk displacement of the temporomandibular joint. Swed Dent J 7:55–64

Isberg A, Isacsson G, Nah K-S (1987) Mandibular coronoid process locking: a prospective study of frequency and association with internal derangement of the temporomandibular joint. Oral Surg Oral Med Oral Pathol 63:275–279

Katzberg RW, Keith DA, Guralnick WC, Manzione JV Jr, Ten Eick WR (1983) Internal derangements and arthritis of the temporomandibular joint. Radiology 146:107–112

Katzberg RW, Tallents RH, Hayakawa K, Miller TL, Goske MJ, Wood BP (1985) Internal derangements of the temporomandibular joint: findings in the pediatric age group. Radiology 154:125–127

Katzberg RW, Westesson P-L, Tallents RH, Drake CM (1996) Anatomic disorders of the temporomandibular joint disc in asymptomatic subjects. J Oral Maxillofac Surg 54:147–153

Kuseler A, Pedersen TK, Herlin T, Gelineck J (1998) Contrast enhanced magnetic resonance imaging as a method to diagnose early inflammatory changes in the temporomandibular joint in children with juvenile chronic arthritis. J Rheumatol 25:1406–1412

Larheim TA (1981) Radiographic appearance of the normal temporomandibular joint in newborns and small children. Acta Radiol 22:593–599

Larheim TA (1991) Imaging of the temporomandibular joint in juvenile rheumatoid arthritis. In: Westesson P-L, Katzberg RW (eds) Imaging of the temporomandibular joint, vol. 1. Cranio Clinics International. Williams and Wilkins, Baltimore, pp 155–172

Larheim TA (1993) Rheumatoid arthritis and related joint diseases. In: Katzberg RW, Westesson P-L (eds) Diagnosis of the temporomandibular joint. Saunders, Philadelphia, pp 303–326

Larheim TA (1995) Current trends in temporomandibular joint imaging. Oral Surg Oral Med Oral Pathol Oral Radiol Endod 80:555–576

Larheim TA, Katzberg RW, Westesson P-L, Tallents RH, Moss ME (2001) MR evidence of temporomandibular joint fluid and condyle marrow alterations: occurrence in asymptomatic volunteers and symptomatic patients. Int J Oral Maxillofac Surg 30:113–117

Larheim TA, Smith H-J, Aspestrand F (1990) Rheumatic disease of the temporomandibular joint: MR imaging and tomographic manifestations. Radiology 175:527–531

Larheim TA, Westesson P-L, Hicks, DG, Eriksson L, Brown DA (1999) Osteonecrosis of the temporomandibular joint: correlation of magnetic resonance imaging and histology. J Oral Maxillofac Surg 57:888–898

Larheim TA, Westesson P-L, Sano T (2001) Temporomandibular joint disk displacement: comparison in asymptomatic volunteers and patients. Radiology 218:428–432

Larheim, TA, Westesson P-L, Sano T (2001) MR grading of temporomandibular joint fluid: association with disk displacement categories, condyle marrow abnormalities and pain. Int J Oral Maxillofac Surg 30:104–112

Lieberman JM, Gardner CL, Milgram JW (1990) Osteonecrosis due to traumatic and idiopathic causes in radiologic and histologic pathology of non-tumorous diseases of bone and joints. Northbrook Publishing Company, Northbrook, pp 959

Lieberman JM, Gardner CL, Motta AO, Schwartz RD (1996) Prevalence of bone marrow signal abnormalities observed in the temporomandibular joint using magnetic resonance imaging. J Oral Maxillofac Surg 54:434–439

Mitchell DG, Steinberg ME, Dalinka MK, Rao VM, Fallon M, Kressel HY (1989) Magnetic resonance imaging of the ischemic hip: alterations within the osteonecrotic, viable, and reactive zones. Clin Orthop Relat Res 244:60–77

Nebbe B, Major PW, Prasad NG (1999) Male adolescent facial pattern associated with TMJ disk displacement and reduction in disk length: part II. Am J Orthod Dentofacial Orthop 116:301–307

Paesani D, Salas E, Martinez A, Isberg A (1999) Prevalence of temporomandibular joint disk displacement in infants and young children. Oral Surg Oral Med Oral Pathol Oral Radiol Endod 87:15–19

Peyron JG, Altman RD (1992) The epidemiology of osteoarthritis. In: Moskowitz RW, Howell DS, Goldberg VM, Mankin HJ (eds) Osteoarthritis: diagnosis and medical/surgical management, 2nd edn. Saunders, Philadelphia, pp 15–37

Rao VM, Liem MD, Farole A, Razek AA (1993) Elusive "stuck" disk in the temporomandibular joint: diagnosis with MR imaging. Radiology 189:823–827

Resnick D (1988) Common disorders of synovium-lined joints: pathogenesis, imaging abnormalities, and complications. AJR Am J Roentgenol 151:1079–1093

Sano T, Westesson P-L, Larheim TA, Takagi R (2000) The association of temporomandibular joint pain with abnormal bone marrow in the mandibular condyle. J Oral Maxillofac Surg 58:254–257

Schellhas KP, Wilkes CH (1989) Temporomandibular joint inflammation: comparison of MR fast scanning with T1- and T2-weighted imaging techniques. AJR Am J Roentgenol 153:93–98

Schellhas KP, Wilkes CH, Fritts HM, Omlie MR, Lagrotteria LB (1989) MR of osteochondritis dissecans and avascular necrosis of the mandibular condyle. AJR Am J Roentgenol 152:551–560

Smith HJ, Larheim TA, Aspestrand F (1992) Rheumatic and nonrheumatic disease in the temporomandibular joint: gadolinium-enhanced MR imaging. Radiology 185:229–234

Sokoloff L (1980) The pathology of osteoarthrosis and the role of aging. In: Nuki G (ed) The etiopathogenesis of osteoarthrosis. Pitman Medical, London, pp 1–15

Stegenga B, de Bont LG, Boering G, Van Willigen JD (1991) Tissue responses to degenerative changes in the temporomandibular joint: a review. J Oral Maxillofac Surg 49:1079–1088

Sweet DE, Madewell JE (1988) Pathogenesis of osteonecrosis. In: Resnick D, Niwayama G (eds) Diagnosis of bone and joint disorders. Saunders, Philadelphia, p 3188

Tasaki MM, Westesson P-L (1993) Temporomandibular joint: diagnostic accuracy with sagittal and coronal MR imaging. Radiology 186:723–729

Tasaki MM, Westesson P-L, Isberg AM, Ren Y-F, Tallents RH (1996) Classification and prevalence of temporomandibular joint disk displacement in patients and symptom-free volunteers. Am J Orthod Dentofacial Orthop 109:249–262

Westesson P-L, Brooks SL (1992) Temporomandibular joint: relationship between MR evidence of effusion and the presence of pain and disk displacement. AJR Am J Roentgenol 159:559–563

Westesson P-L, Larheim TA, Tanaka H (1998) Posterior disc displacement in the temporomandibular joint. J Oral Maxillofac Surg 56:1266–1273

Westesson P-L, Yamamoto M, Sano T, Okano T (2003) Temporomandibular joint. In: Som PM, Curtin HD (eds) Head and neck imaging, 4th edn. Mosby, St. Louis, pp 995–1053

Wilkes CH (1989) Internal derangements of the temporomandibular joint. Pathological variations. Arch Otolaryngol Head Neck Surg 115:469–477

Yamamoto M, Sano T, Okano T (2003) Magnetic resonance evidence of joint fluid with temporomandibular joint disorders. J Comput Assist Tomogr 27:694–698

Dentoalveolar Structures and Implants

In collaboration with N. Kakimoto

Introduction

Intraoral film or digital radiography is the mainstay of imaging teeth and surrounding structures such as lamina dura and alveolar bone. However, advanced imaging in particular CT, may be a supplementary diagnostic tool in selected cases. With multidetector CT scanners, virtually any desired section may be of high quality. It should be remembered that the patient dose with conventional CT can be significantly lowered when imaging dentoalveolar hard tissues, compared to the routine use including soft tissue imaging.

Cone beam CT, specifically developed for imaging dentoalveolar structures with a smaller radiation field than conventional CT, has a better spatial resolution and a lower radiation dose. However, the contrast resolution is much better with conventional CT. The pioneering cone beam CT systems were developed for application in angiography. After being introduced in the late 1990s for dental imaging, research is in progress on different aspects of this application. Both image-intensifying and flat-panel detectors are under investigation as well as different fields of view. This type of CT equipment may possibly be more important than any other advanced imaging modality for evaluation of dentoalveolar structures in the near future.

In this short chapter we present patients to illustrate the potential of CT for imaging dentoalveolar structures, including a few cases of cone beam CT. In some of these patients, CT imaging changed the diagnosis and thus had a significant impact on patient management.

CT has in particular proved valuable in the evaluation of the dental implant patient, to measure edentulous alveolar process dimensions preoperatively. Dental CT reformatting programs have been available since the late 1980s. More recently it has been shown that an even better accuracy of linear measurements can be obtained with cone beam CT.

Finally we demonstrate that CT can also visualize complications to dental implant treatment.

Tooth Anatomy, Tooth Pathology and Adjacent Structures

CT scanning in direct axial, coronal or oblique coronal planes, or with reformatted images perpendicular or parallel to the alveolar process, tooth or anatomic structure such as the mandibular canal.

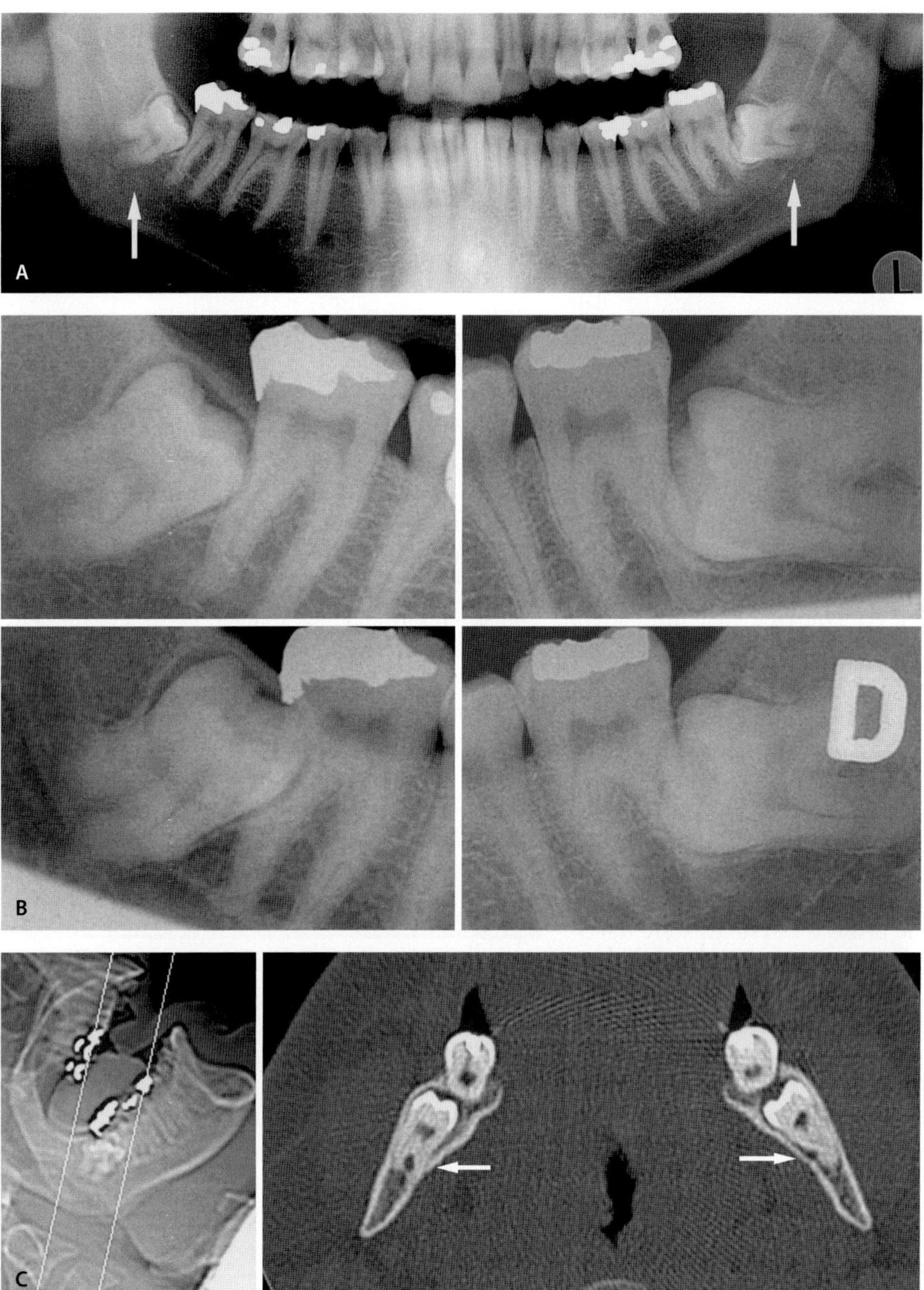

Figure 7.1

Tooth anatomy (mandibular wisdom tooth); 28-year-old patient with impacted, asymptomatic mandibular third molars. **A** Panoramic view suggests a possible intimate relationship between wisdom tooth roots and mandibular canal bilaterally (*arrows*) that needs to be assessed before surgery. **B** Intraoral radiography with different projections of both wisdom teeth is inconclusive, but indicates an intimate relation to mandibular canal bilaterally. **C** CT image approximately parallel to long axis of wisdom teeth and perpendicular to mandibular canals (as shown in scout view) demonstrates that the mandibular canal penetrates the right molar root and makes a lingual groove of the left molar root (*arrows*)

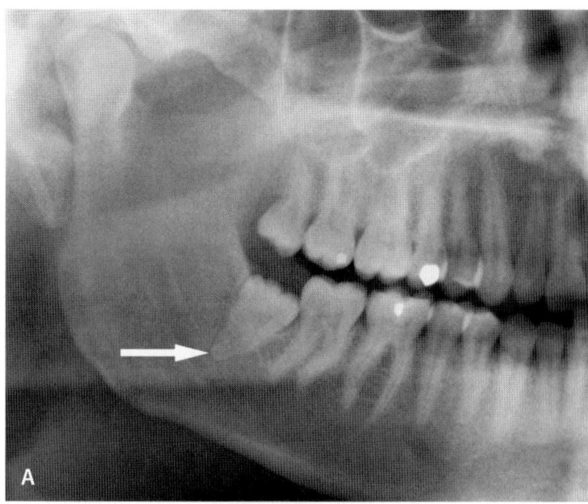

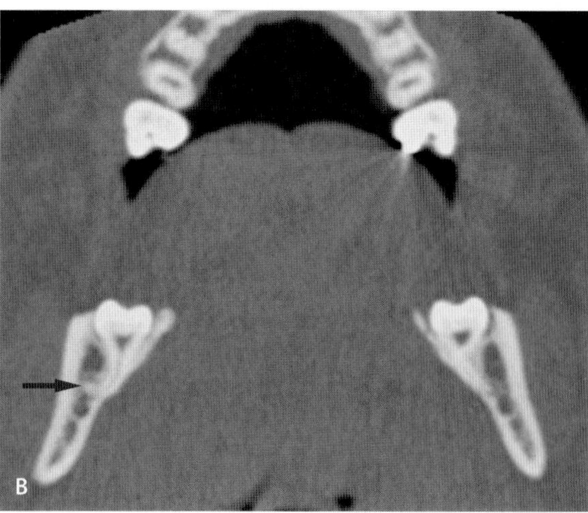

Figure 7.2

Tooth anatomy (mandibular wisdom tooth); 20-year-old patient with clinical symptoms of mandibular third molar pericoronitis. **A** Panoramic view shows apparently a smooth root complex of impacted wisdom tooth, but note apex anatomy (*arrow*). **B** CT image parallel to long axis of wisdom tooth (similar scout view as shown in Fig. 7.1C) demonstrates that the root has a 90° angulation in the buccal direction (*arrow*)

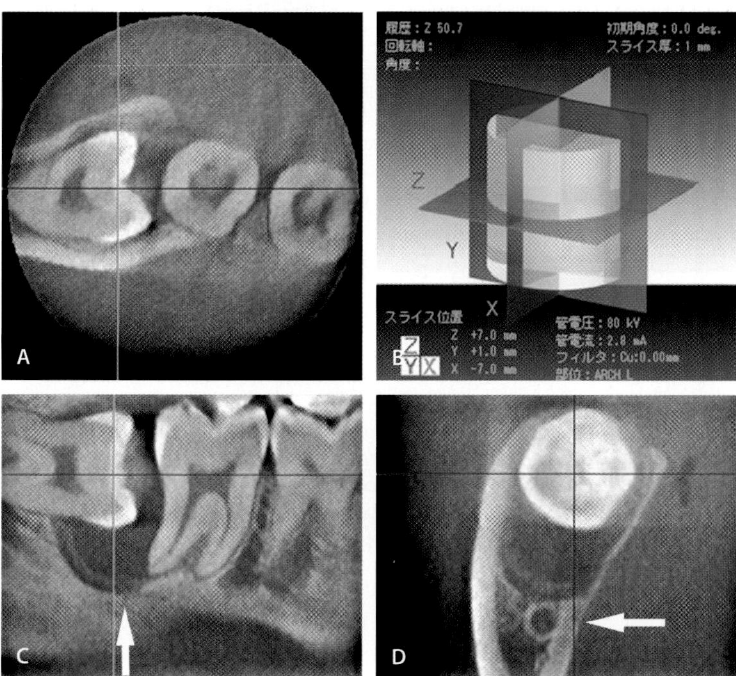

Figure 7.3

Follicular cyst (mandibular wisdom tooth); 38-year-old patient with incidental finding of impacted mandibular third molar with pathology; cone beam CT examination. **A** Axial section shows radiolucency around crown of horizontally impacted mandibular wisdom tooth with thinning of lingual cortical plate but no bone expansion. **B** Three image planes indicated by different colors. **C** Sagittal view shows typical follicular cyst around wisdom tooth crown (*arrow*). **D** Coronal view shows follicular cyst close to mandibular canal (*arrow*) and thinning of entire lingual cortical plate but no expansion (courtesy of Dr. K. Honda, Nihon University School of dentistry, Tokyo, Japan)

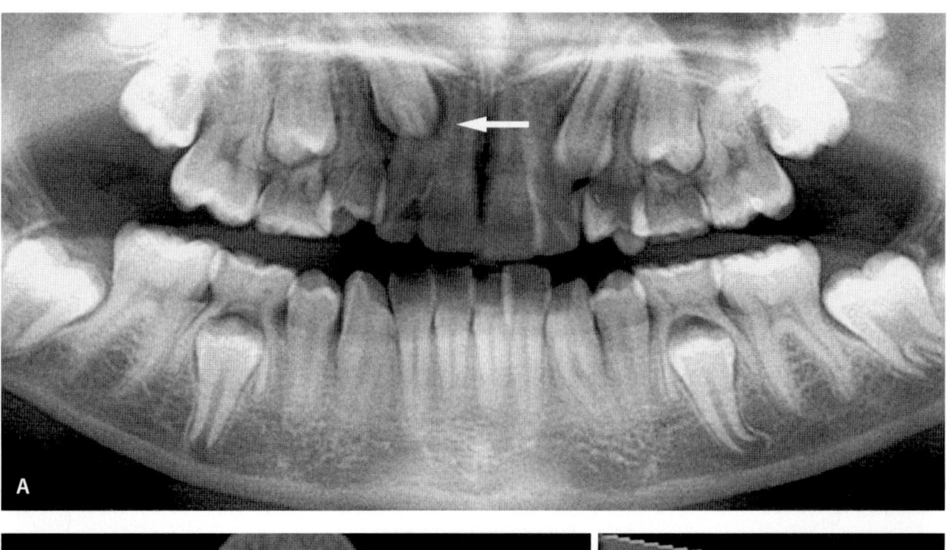

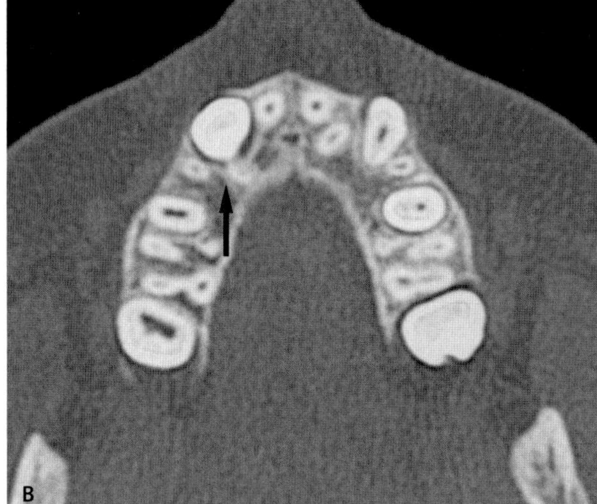

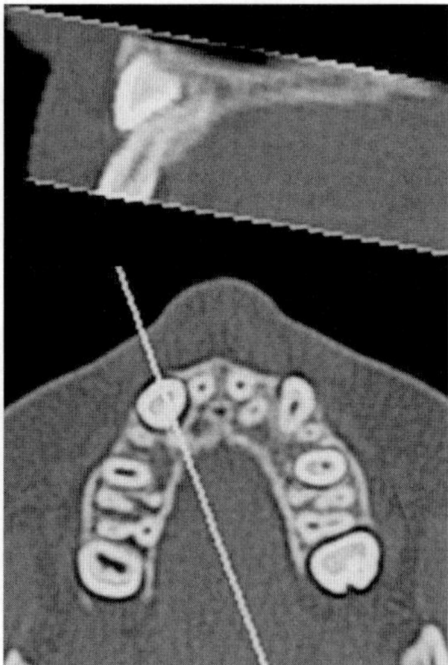

Figure 7.4

Tooth anatomy (lateral incisor); 10-year-old patient with curved maxillary lateral incisor. **A** Panoramic view shows that relationship between lateral incisor root and erupting canine (*arrow*) needs to be evaluated before orthodontic treatment. **B** Axial CT image with reformatted section perpendicular to alveolar process according to reference image, demonstrates close relationship between lateral incisor and buccally erupting canine (*arrow*) but no injury to incisor root

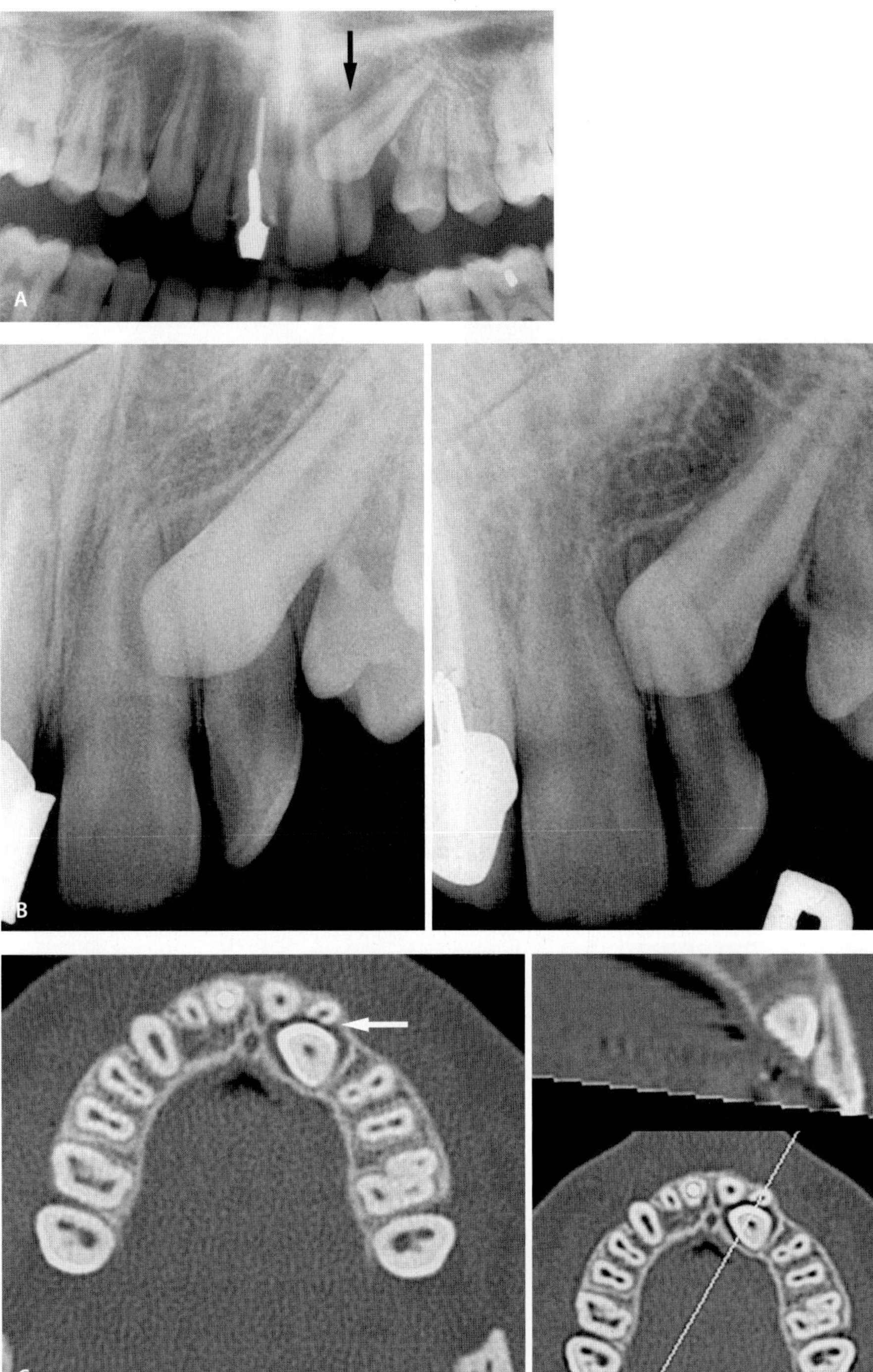

Figure 7.5

Tooth resorption (lateral incisor); 16-year-old patient with impacted canine and previous injury to central incisor, with subsequent endodontic therapy. **A** Panoramic view shows that relationship between canine and lateral incisor (*arrow*) needs to be assessed before treatment, leading to removal of either impacted canine or lateral incisor. **B** Intraoral radiography with different projections indicates no injury to lateral incisor root. **C** Axial CT image with reformatted section perpendicular to alveolar process according to reference image demonstrates intimate relationship between lateral incisor and palatally erupting canine with evident resorption of incisor root (*arrow*)

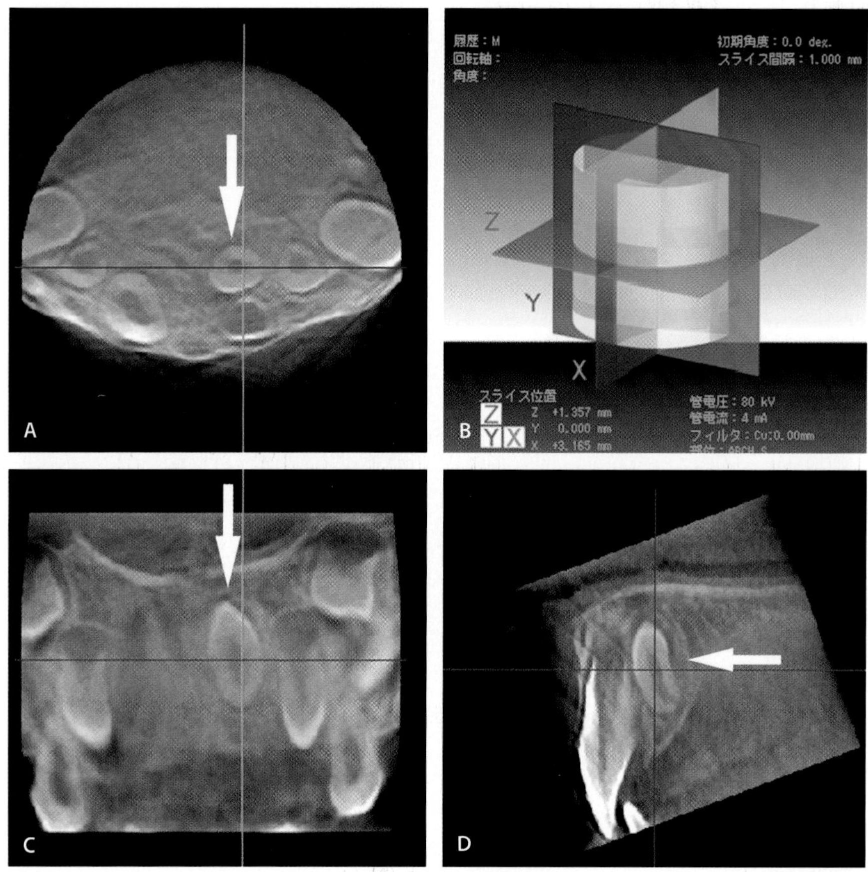

Figure 7.6

Supernumerary tooth (mesiodens) in anterior maxilla; 8-year-old male with incidental finding; cone beam CT examination. **A** Axial section shows mesiodens in palatal position and close to but not in contact with permanent incisor (*arrow*). **B** Three image planes indicated by different colors. **C** Coronal section shows inverted mesiodens (*arrow*). **D** Sagittal view shows mesiodens at apex level of permanent incisor (*arrow*) (courtesy of Dr. K. Honda, Nihon University School of Dentistry, Tokyo, Japan)

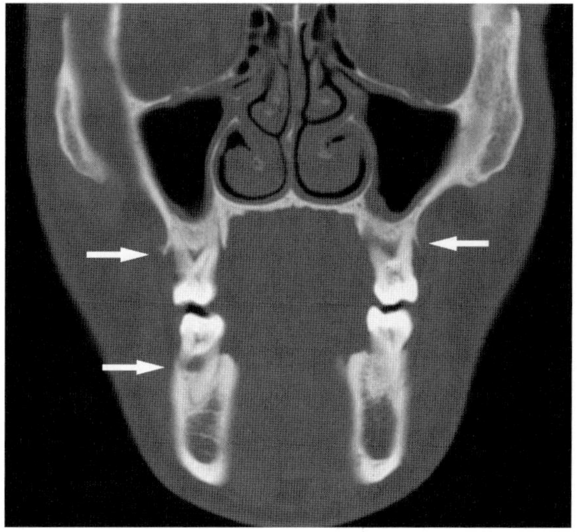

Figure 7.7

Periodontal disease; 35-year-old male with incidental finding. Coronal CT image shows destruction of alveolar bone both in maxilla and mandible with loss of periodontal bone support in bifurcation of mandibular molar roots and trifurcation of maxillary molar roots (*arrows*); left maxillary molar has no remaining bone support of palatal "floating" root

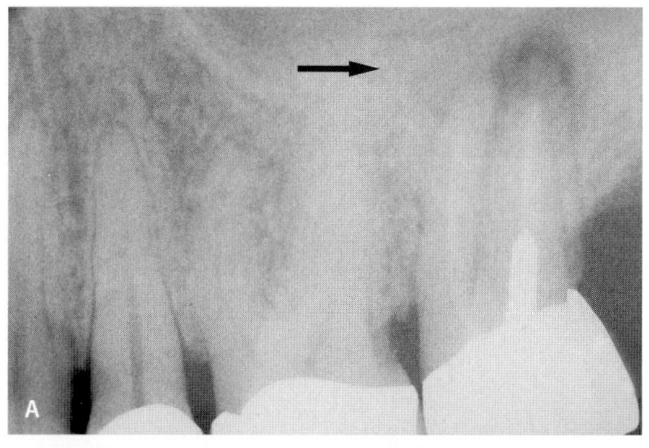

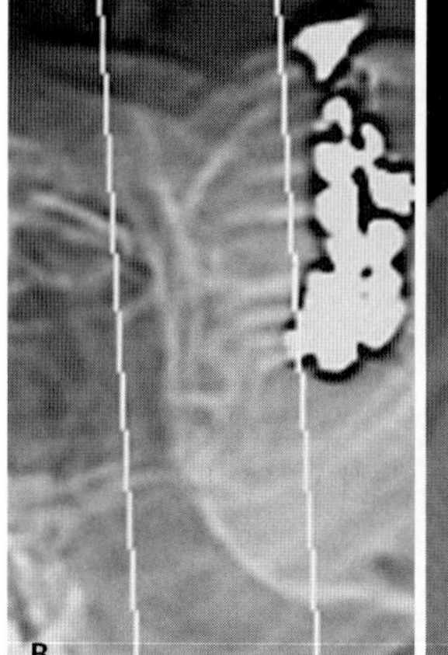

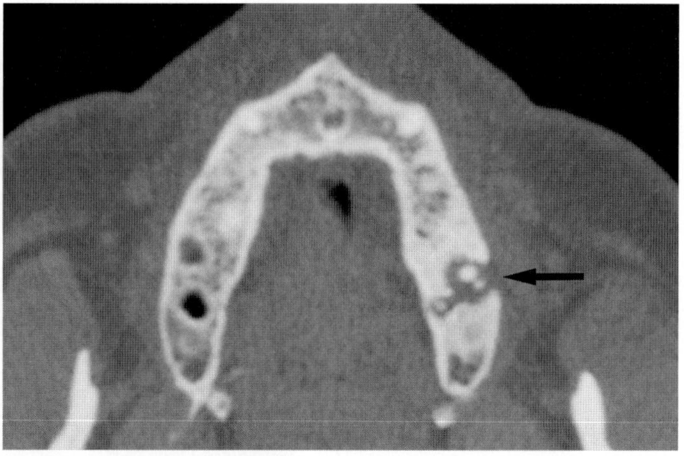

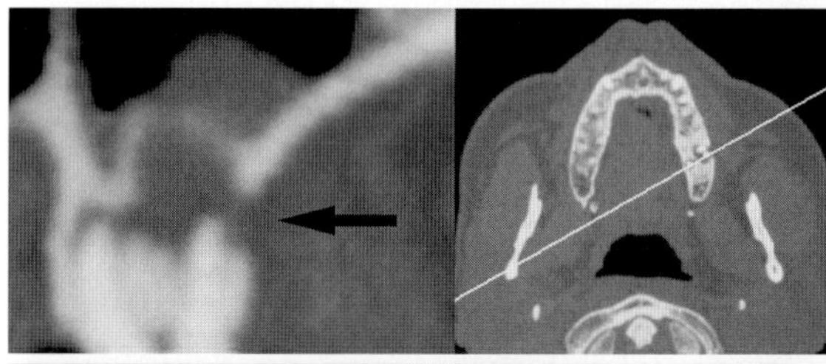

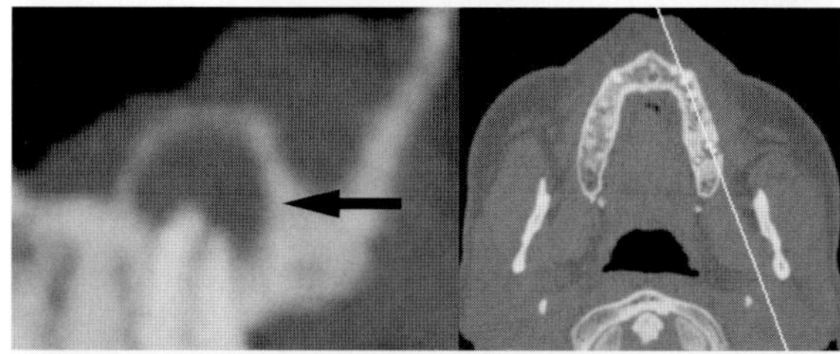

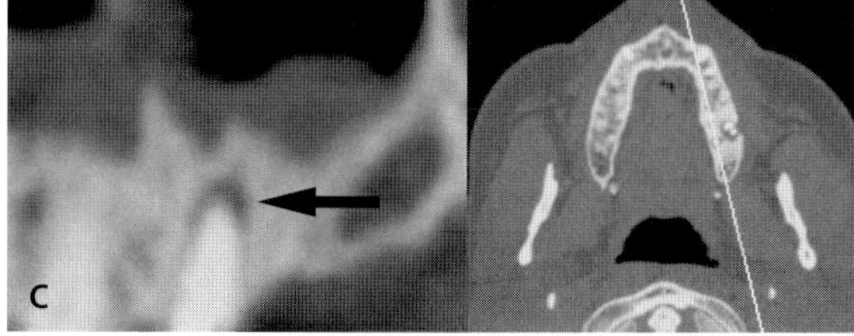

Figure 7.8

Apical periodontitis; 50-year-old male with variable pain from left maxilla. A Intraoral radiography shows apical periodontitis of second molar, apparently at palatal root (*arrow*). Involvement of different roots needs to be assessed to decide whether or not an apicoectomy can be performed successfully. B Axial CT image (with scout view and cursor lines to avoid amalgam artifacts from teeth) shows a larger radiolucency at buccal roots than at palatal root of second molar and bone destruction in trifurcation of roots (*arrow*), with surrounding bone sclerosis. C *upper row* Coronal CT image perpendicular to maxillary alveolar process through distobuccal and palatal roots of second molar according to reference image, shows cystic process with destroyed buccal cortex (*arrow*). C *middle row* Sagittal CT image parallel with maxillary alveolar process through buccal roots of second molar according to reference image, shows cystic process with intact cortical outline (*arrow*) and with some antral mucosal thickening. C *lower row* Sagittal CT image parallel to alveolar process through palatal root of second molar according to reference image, shows small radiolucency (widened periodontal space) at palatal root (*arrow*), with surrounding sclerotic bone

Dental Implant Imaging, Pre- and Postoperative CT Scanning

- Single reformatted scans perpendicular to alveolar process
- Dental reformatting programs with multiple cross-sectional views perpendicular to entire alveolar process and panoramic reconstructions "parallel" to alveolar process

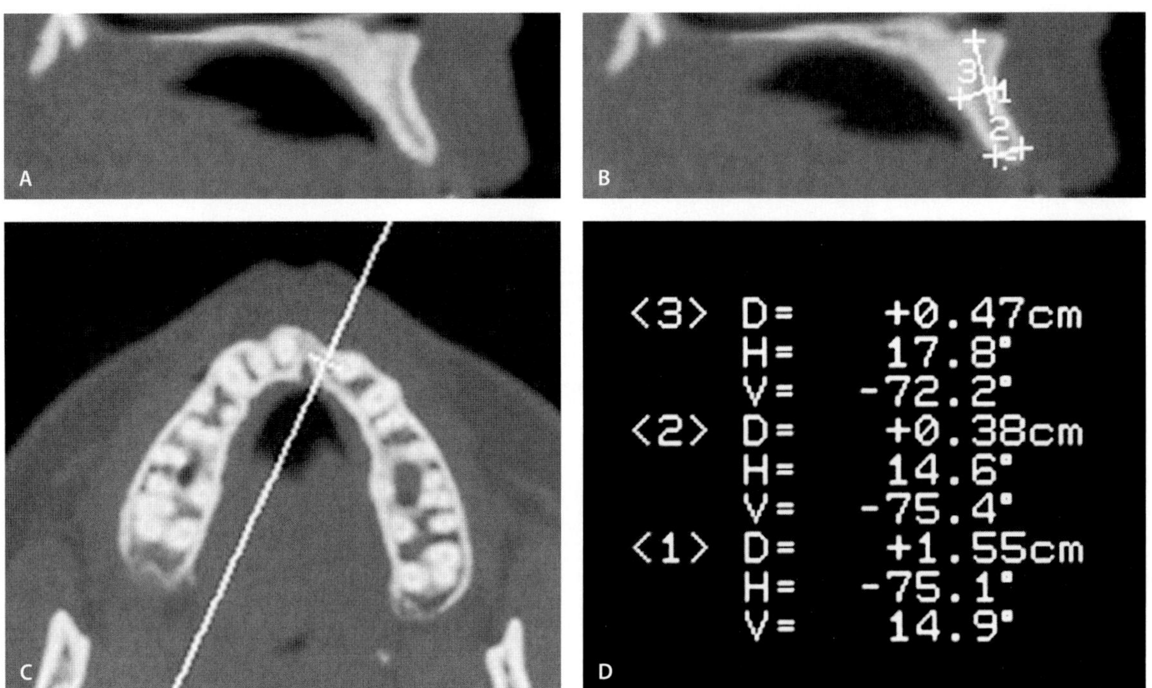

Figure 7.9

Alveolar process examination before dental implant surgery; 20-year-old male with loss of incisor due to trauma many years previously. **A** Reformatted CT image perpendicular to edentulous alveolar process of maxilla according to reference image (**C**). **B** Same image as in **A** with measured distances indicated. **D** Alveolar process dimensions from **B**: Height of alveolar process just above 15 mm; width of alveolar process from just below 4 to almost 5 mm

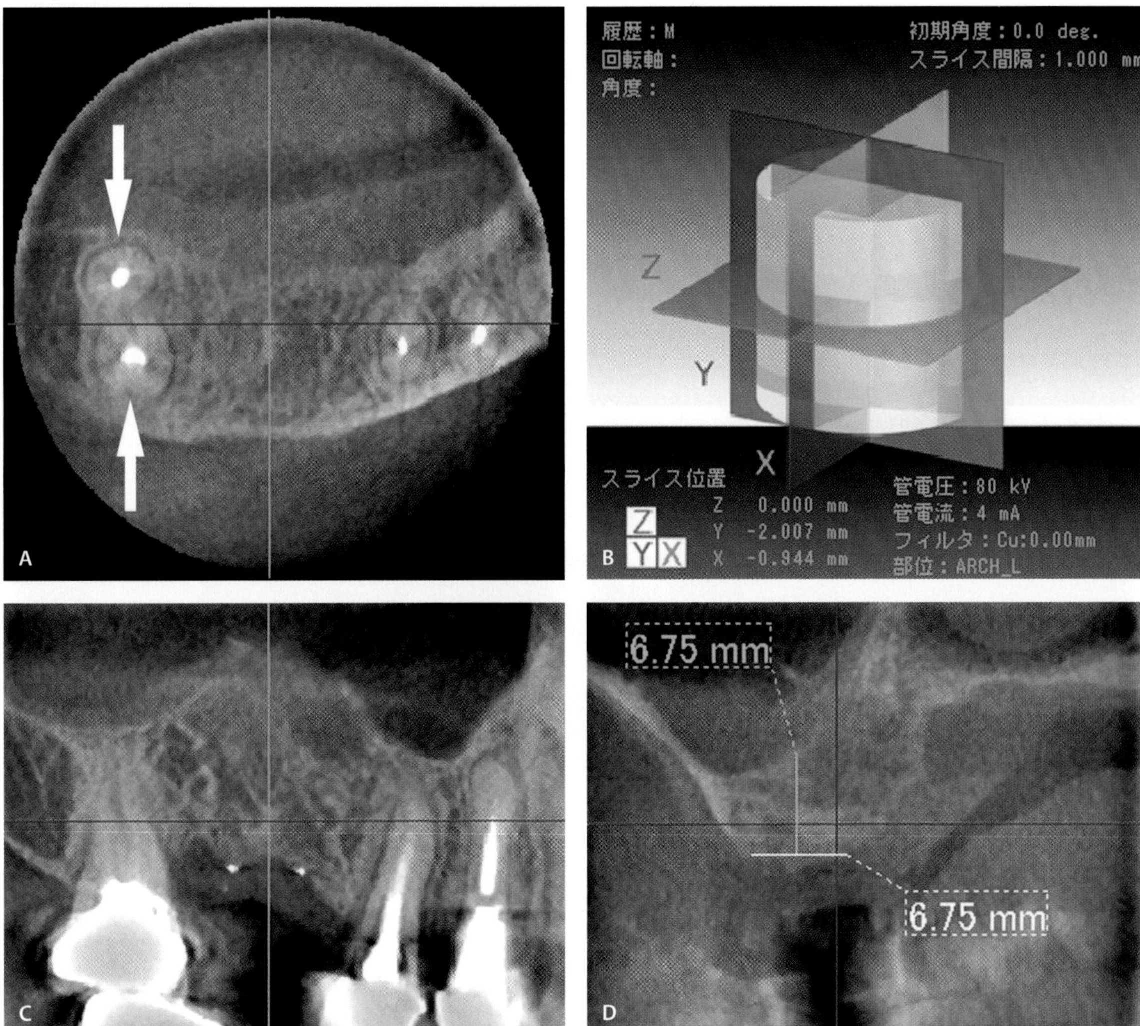

Figure 7.10

Alveolar process examination before dental implant surgery; 50-year-old female; cone beam CT examination. **A** Axial section shows acceptable width of edentulous alveolar process of maxilla, and good bone quality. Note two roots of molar tooth (*arrows*) and one root each of premolar teeth; all with root filling material and normal periodontal membrane. **B** Three image planes indicated by different colors. **C** Sagittal section shows acceptable height and bone quality of edentulous alveolar process, and rather normal periodontal membranes of teeth. **D** Edentulous alveolar process dimensions: same height and width (courtesy of Dr. K. Honda, Nihon University School of Dentistry, Tokyo, Japan)

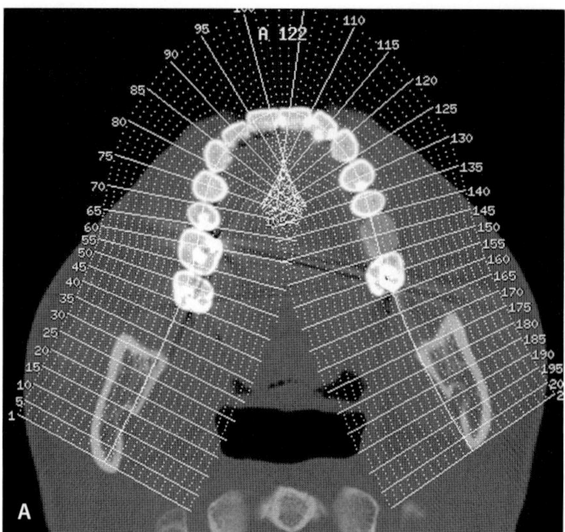

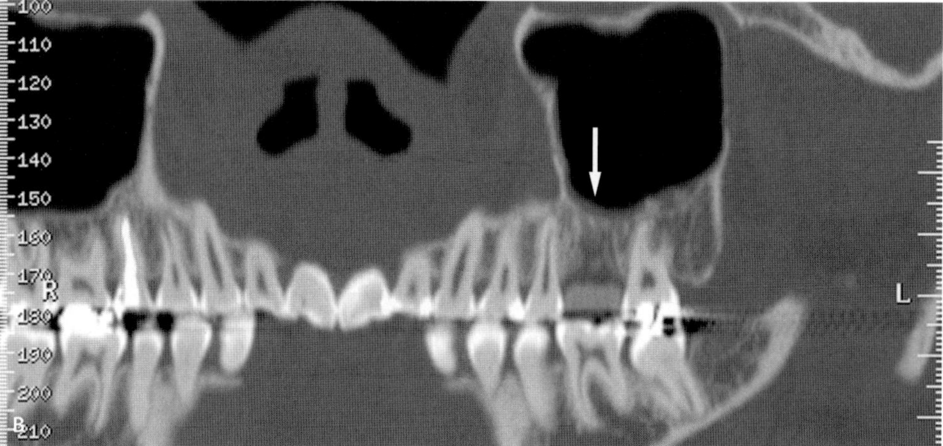

Figure 7.11

Alveolar process examination before and after dental implant surgery; one-tooth implant. **A** Axial CT image with DentaScan program, preoperative. **B** Panoramic reconstruction shows acceptable height of alveolar process, but incomplete bone regeneration after tooth extraction (*arrow*)

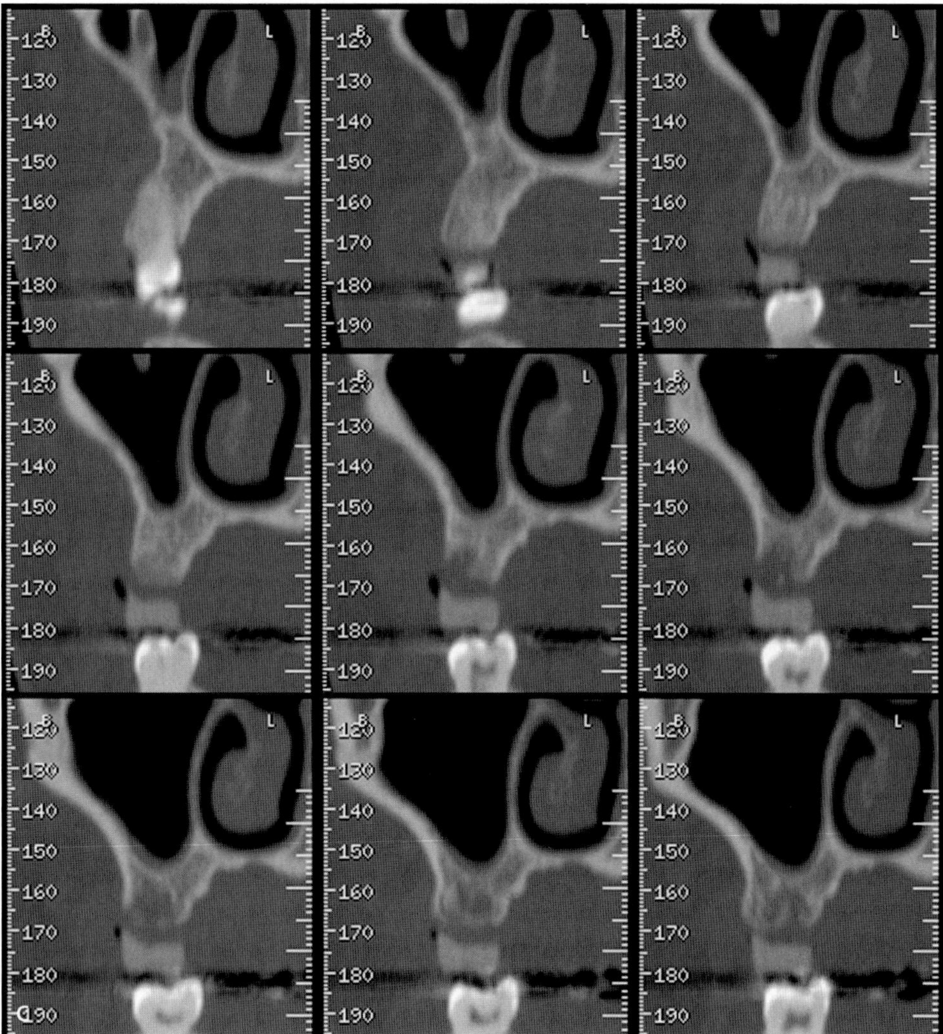

Figure 7.11 *(continued)*

C Cross-sectional images confirm that bone regeneration in edentulous site is not complete but show acceptable width of alveolar process

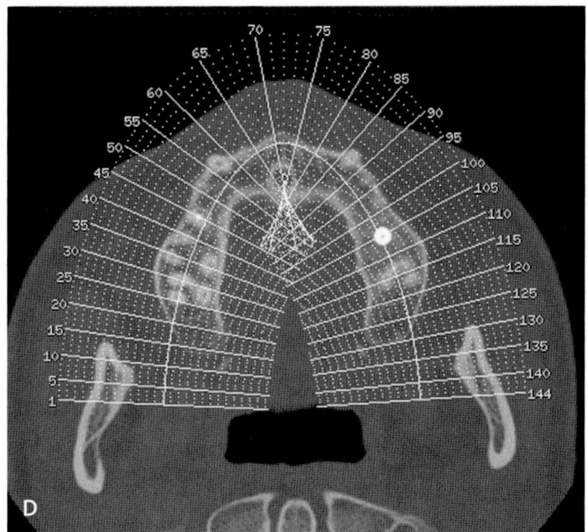

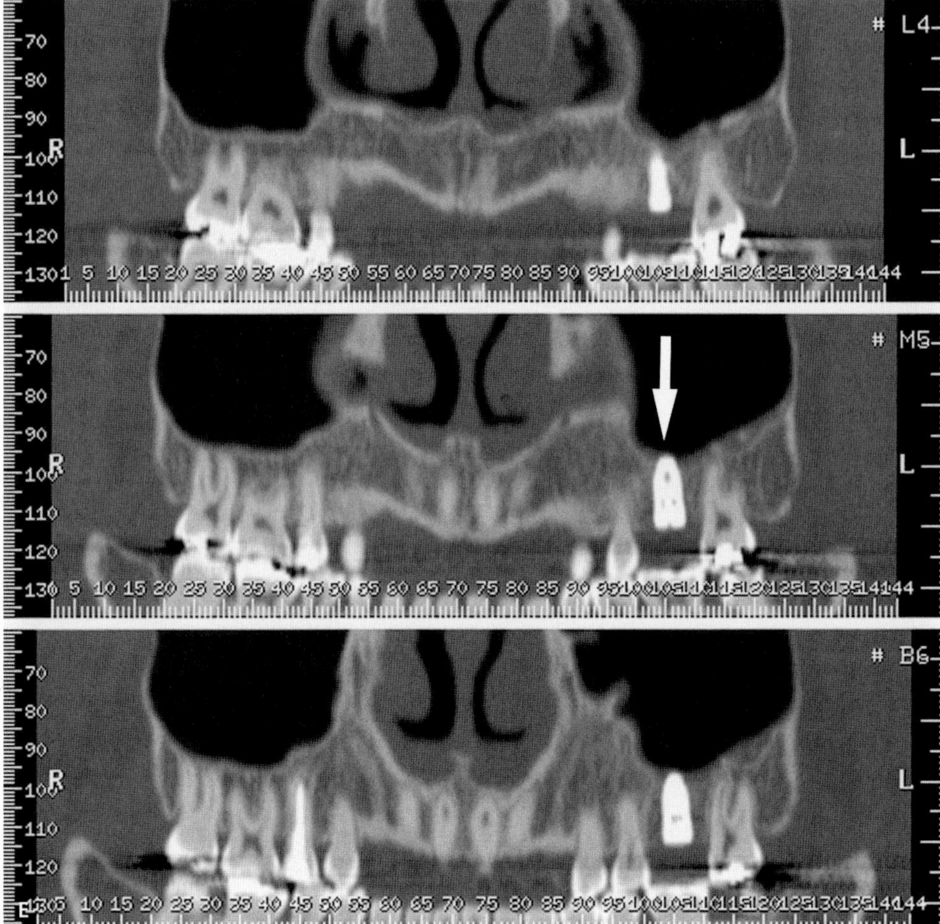

Figure 7.11 *(continued)*

D Axial CT image with DentaScan program, postoperative. E Panoramic alveolar process reconstructions shows implant correctly placed (*arrow*)

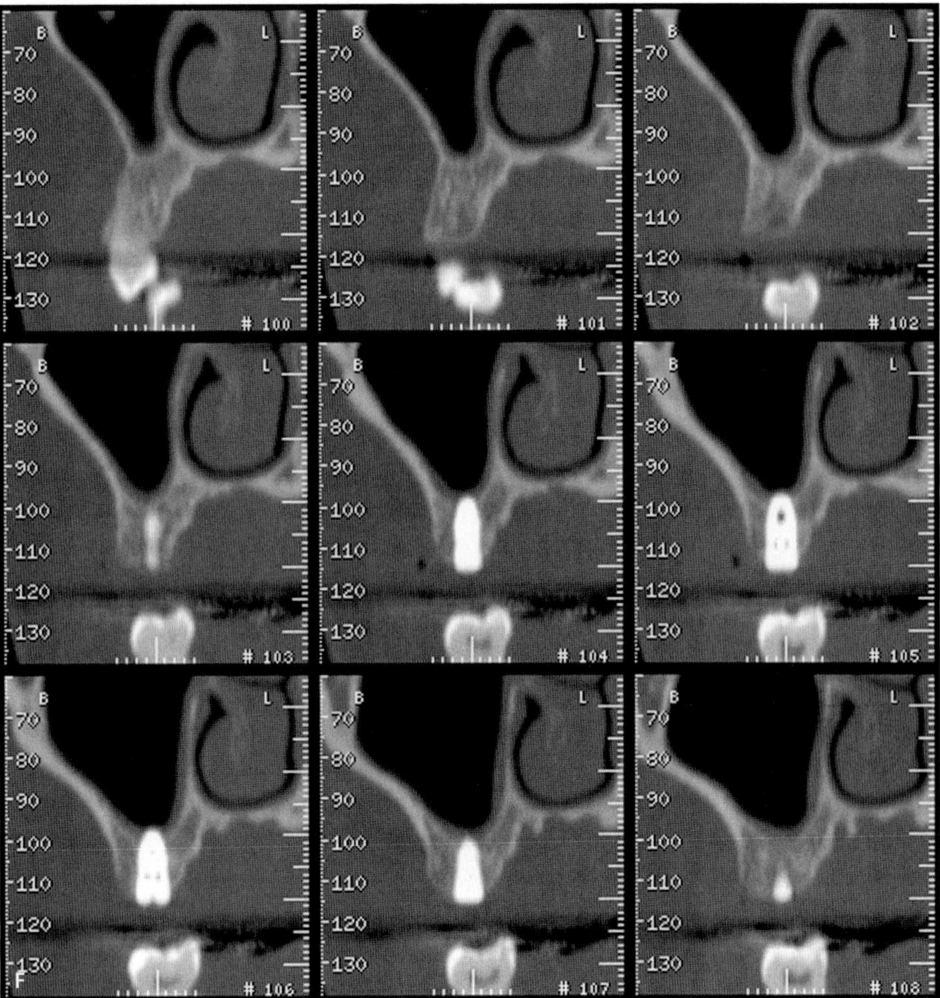

Figure 7.11 *(continued)*

F Cross-sectional images of alveolar process confirm correct placement of implant

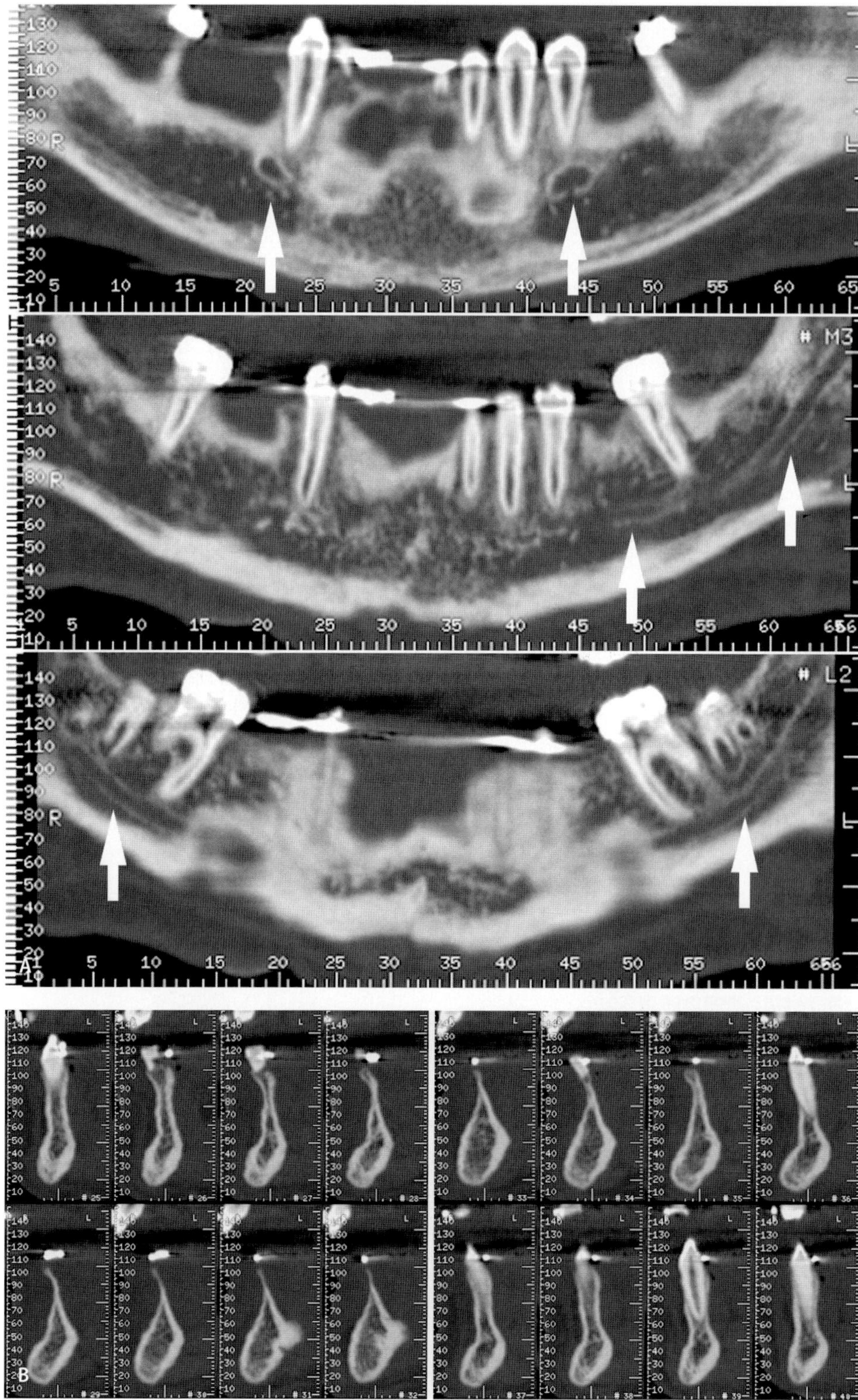

Figure 7.12

Alveolar process examination before dental implant surgery; 15-year-old male with multiple agenesia. **A** Panoramic DentaScan reconstructions of mandible showing agenesia of three incisors and two premolars; note mandibular foramina (*arrows*) and mandibular canal (*arrows*). **B** Cross-sectional images perpendicular to alveolar process of anterior mandible (altogether 16 sections) show extremely thin edentulous alveolar process

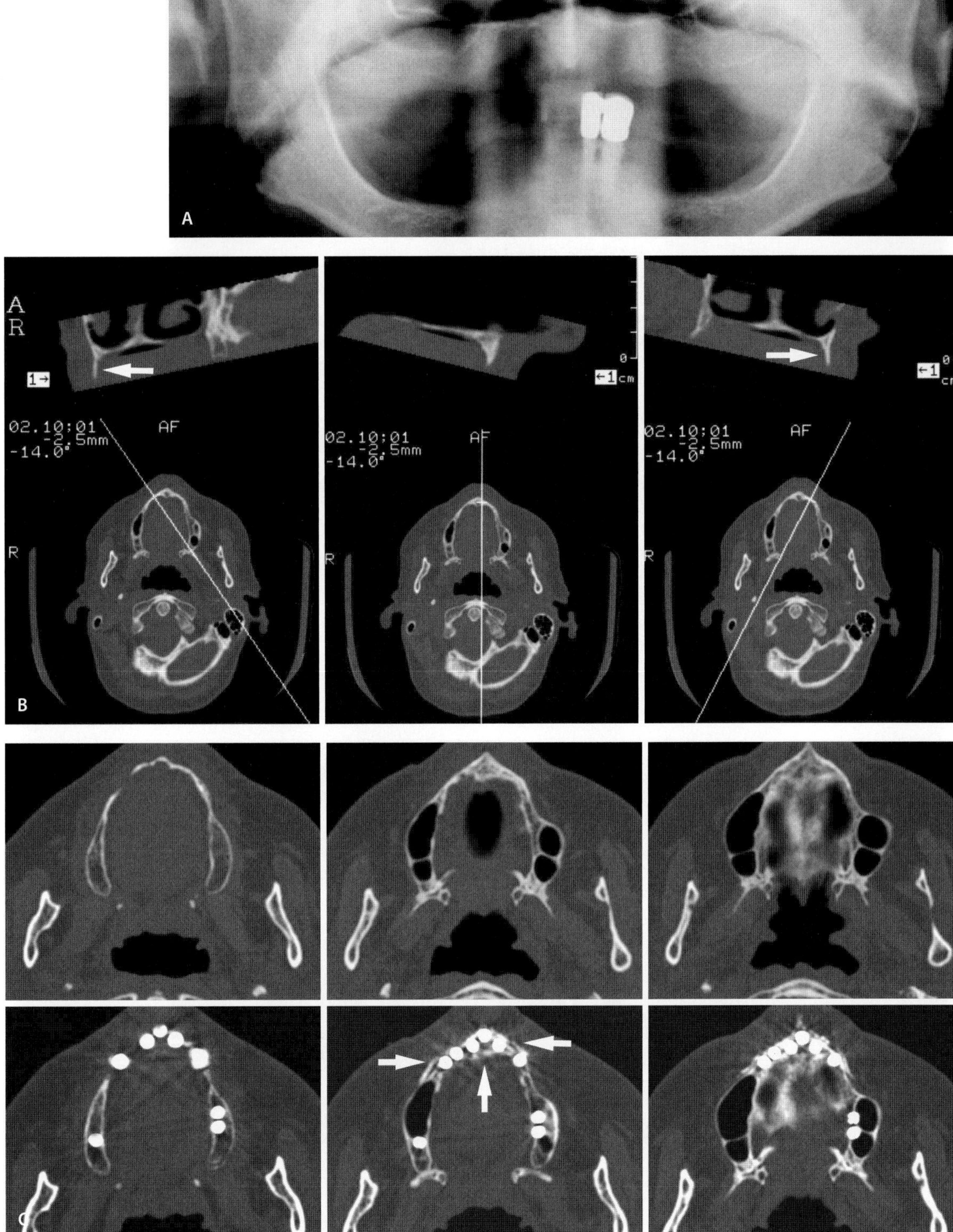

Figure 7.13

Dental implant surgery with bone graft from chin; 68-year-old female who could not accept her complete maxillary denture. **A** Panoramic view does not indicate that maxillary alveolar process is very thin. **B** Three CT sections perpendicular to anterior maxillary alveolar process corresponding to cursor lines on reference images show that alveolar process (*arrows*) is very thin (1–2 mm), but has acceptable height (about 10 mm). **C** Axial preoperative CT sections in upper row and corresponding axial CT sections in lower row after implant surgery with bone graft (*arrows*) taken from patient's chin

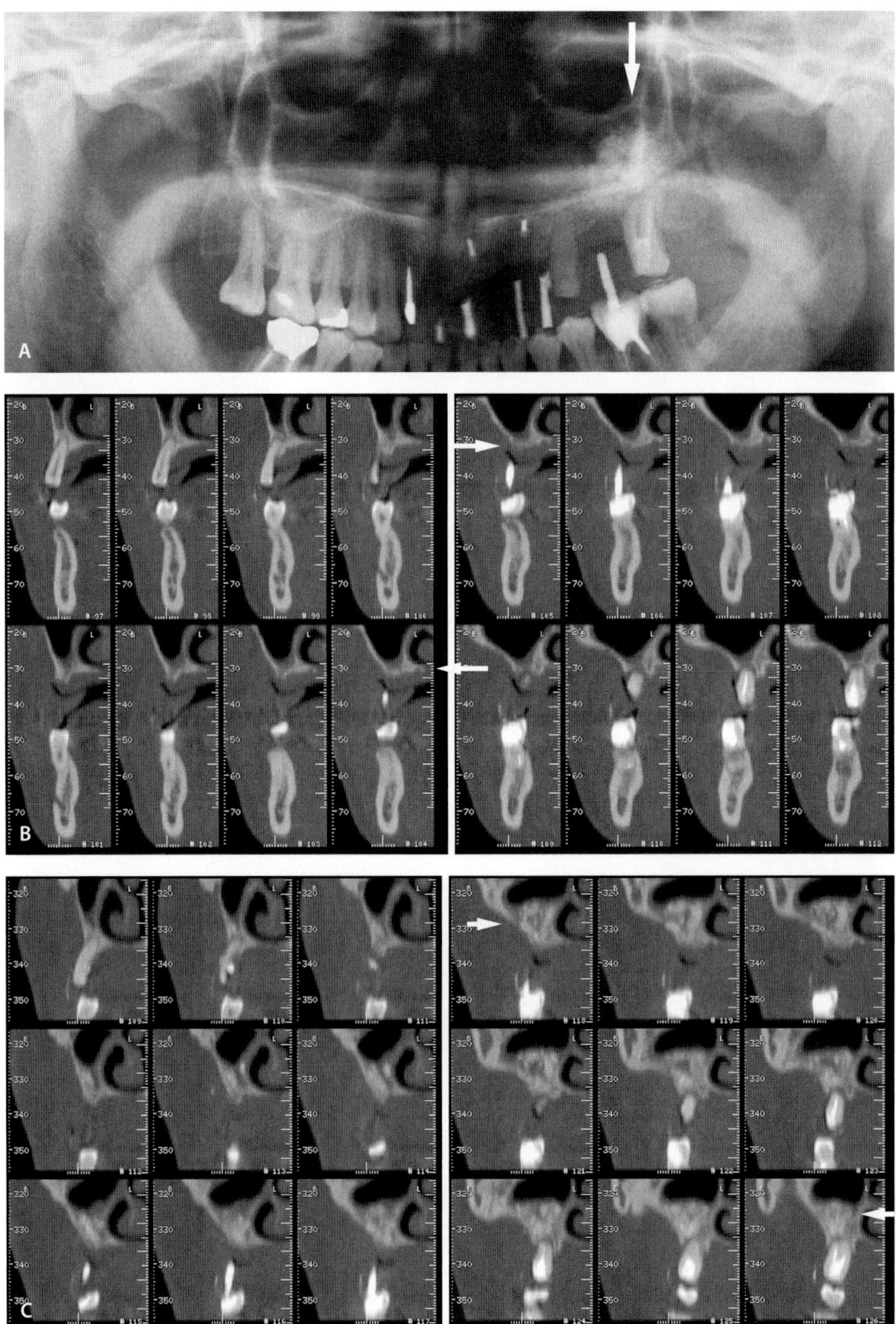

Figure 7.14

Sinus lift with bone graft from chin and artificial bone chips; 39-year-old female. **A** Panoramic view, postoperative, shows increased dimension of alveolar process in maxilla with bone from the patient's chin and artificial bone chips (*arrow*). **B** Preoperative cross-sectional DentaScan images of left maxilla show that edentulous alveolar process is too small for implant placement (*arrows*). **C** Postoperative cross-sectional DentaScan images show that new bone has increased alveolar process to an acceptable height and width (*arrows*)

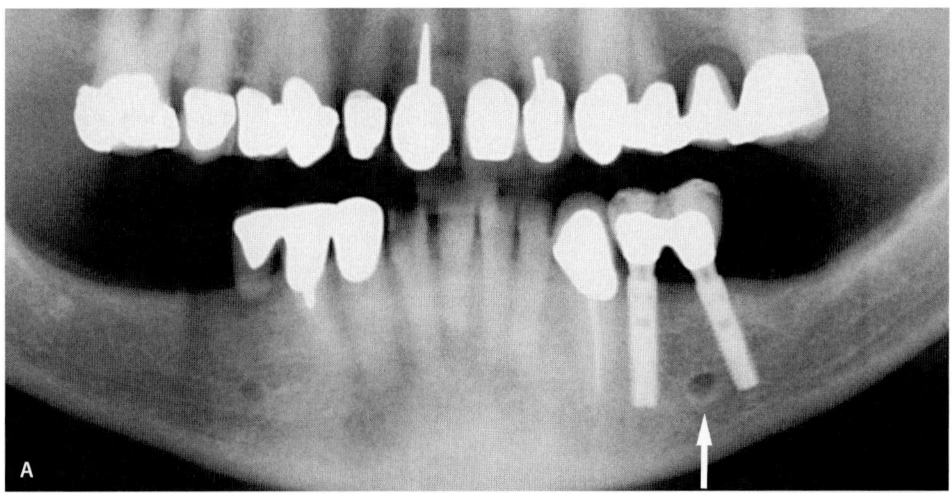

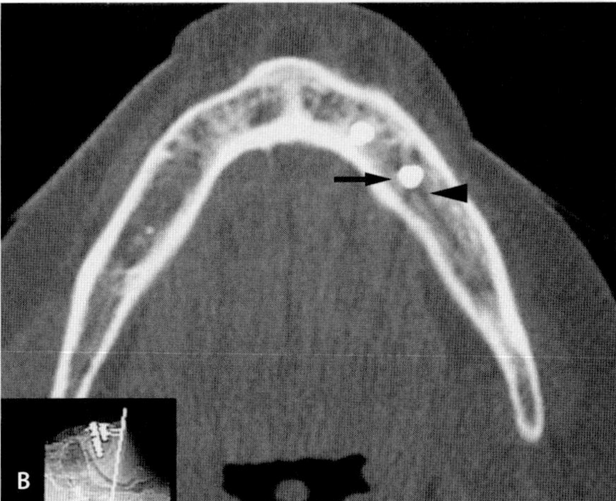

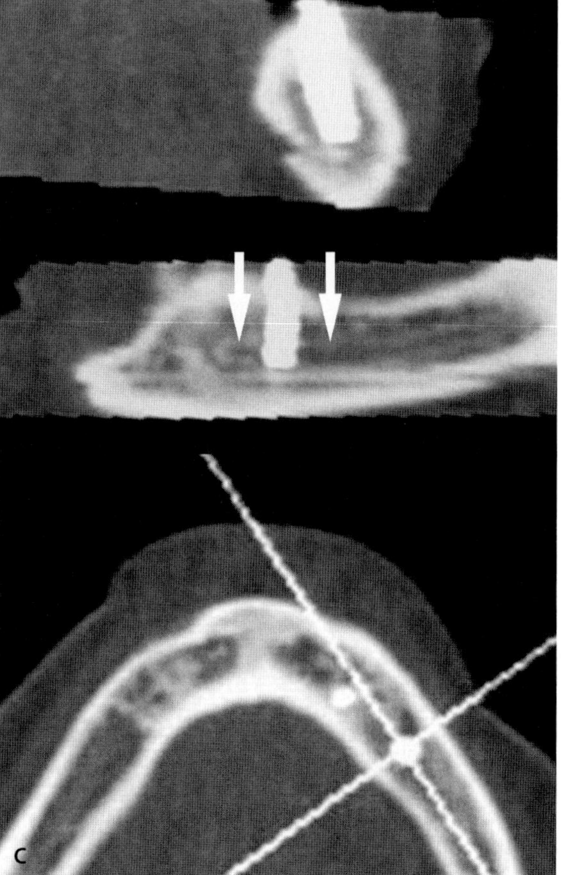

Figure 7.15

Dental implant complication; 67-year-old female with mental nerve paresthesia due to implant placement in mandibular canal. **A** Panoramic view indicates that relationship between distal implant and mandibular canal needs to be further assessed (*arrow* mental foramen). **B** Axial CT image (according to reference image) shows that implant (*arrow*) is located in middle of jaw just in area of mandibular canal (*arrowhead*). **C** CT image perpendicular and parallel to alveolar process according to reference image, shows that implant is located in mandibular canal (*arrows*); step in reformatted images due to motion artifact

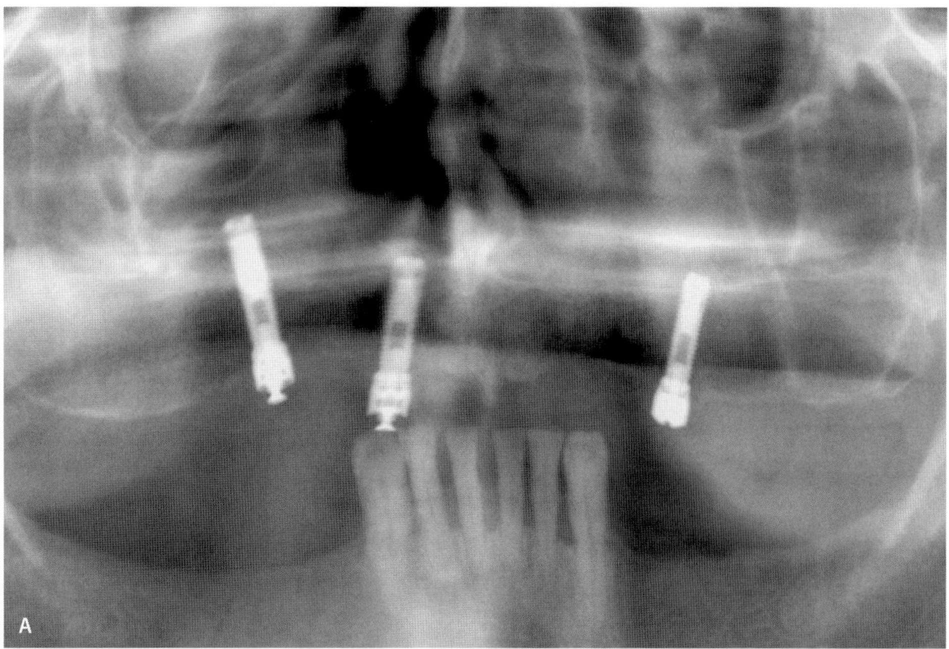

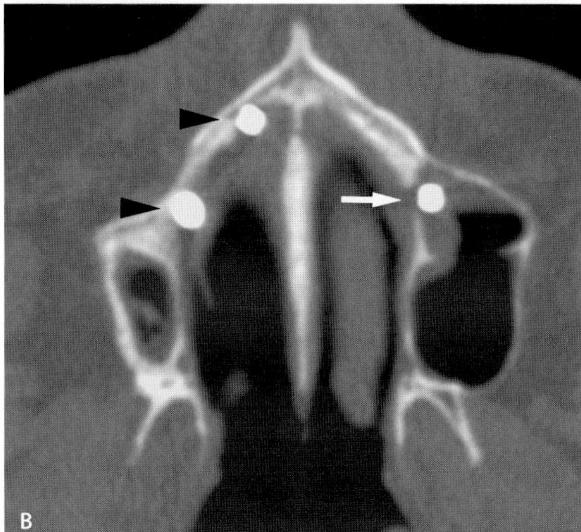

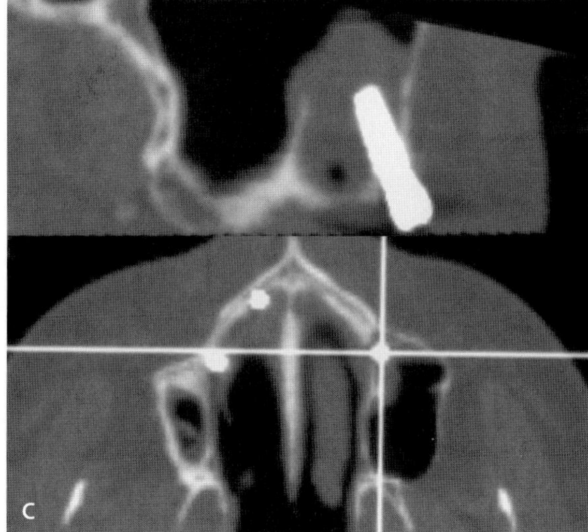

Figure 7.16

Dental implant complication; 45-year-old male with pain and implants that would not heal adequately (three already lost) because of location in nasal cavity and maxillary sinus. **A** Panoramic view shows apparently normal bone conditions around three remaining implants, but reliable evaluation impossible. **B** Axial CT image shows two implants located in nasal cavity (*arrowheads*) and one implant located in maxillary sinus (*arrow*) with resorption of medial sinus wall. Note very small maxillary sinus on right side. **C** Sagittally reformatted CT image (coronal image not shown) according to reference image, confirms implant in maxillary sinus with no bone support other than sinus wall, and some mucosal thickening around implant

Suggested Reading

Abrahams JJ, Hayt MW, Rock R (2003) Dental CT reformatting programs and dental imaging. In: Som PM, Curtin HD (eds) Head and neck imaging, 4th edn. Mosby, St. Louis, pp 907–918

Arai Y, Tammisalo E, Iwai K, Hashimoto K, Shinoda K (1999) Development of a compact tomographic apparatus for dental use. Dentomaxillofac Radiol 28:245–248

Araki K, Maki K, Seki K, Sakamaki K, Harata Y, Sakaino R, Okano T, Seo K (2004) Characteristics of a newly developed dentomaxillofacial X-ray cone beam CT scanner (CB MercuRay): system configuration and physical properties. Dentomaxillofac Radiol 33:51–59

Baba R, Ueda K, Okabe M (2004) Using a flat-panel detector in high resolution cone beam CT for dental imaging. Dentomaxillofac Radiol 33:285–290

Cohnen M, Kemper J, Mobes O, Pawelzik J, Modder U (2002) Radiation dose in dental radiology. Eur Radiol 12:634–637

Danforth RA, Peck J, Hall P (2003) Cone beam volume tomography: an imaging option for diagnosis of complex mandibular third molar anatomical relationships. J Calif Dent Assoc 31:847–852

Ericson S, Kurol J (2000) Incisor root resorptions due to ectopic maxillary canines imaged by computerized tomography: a comparative study in extracted teeth. Angle Orthod 70:276–283

Ericson S, Kurol PJ (2000) Resorption of incisors after ectopic eruption of maxillary canines: a CT study. Angle Orthod 70:415–423

Hamada Y, Kondoh T, Noguchi K, Iino M, Isono H, Ishii H, Mishima A, Kobayashi K, Seto K (2005) Application of limited cone beam computed tomography to clinical assessment of alveolar bone grafting: a preliminary report. Cleft Palate Craniofac J 42:128–137

Hashimoto K, Arai Y, Iwai K, Araki M, Kawashima S, Terakado M (2003) A comparison of a new limited cone beam computed tomography machine for dental use with multidetector row helical CT machine. Oral Surg Oral Med Oral Pathol Oral Radiol Endod 95:371–377

Heiland M, Schulze D, Adam G, Schmelzle R (2003) 3D-imaging of the facial skeleton with an isocentric mobile C-arm system (Siremobil Iso-C3D). Dentomaxillofac Radiol 32:21–25

Kobayashi K, Shimoda S, Nakagawa Y, Yamamoto A (2004) Accuracy in measurement of distance using limited cone-beam computerized tomography. Int J Oral Maxillofac Implants 19:228–231

Linsenmaier U, Rock C, Euler E, Wirth S, Brandl R, Kotsianos D, Mutschler W, Pfeifer KJ (2002) Three-dimensional CT with a modified C-arm image intensifier: feasibility. Radiology 224:286–292

Mozzo P, Procacci C, Tacconi A, Martini PT, Andreis IA (1998) A new volumetric CT machine for dental imaging based on the cone- beam technique: preliminary results. Eur Radiol 8:1558–1564

Ning R, Kruger RA (1988) Computer simulation of image intensifier-based computed tomography detector: vascular application. Med Phys 15:188– 192

Ritman EL, Kinsey JH, Robb RA, Gilbert BK, Harris LD, Wood EH (1980) Three-dimensional imaging of heart, lungs, and circulation. Science 210:273–280

Rothman SL, Chaftez N, Rhodes ML, Schwarz MS (1988) CT in the preoperative assessment of the mandible and maxilla for endosseous implant surgery. Work in progress. Radiology 168:171–175

Schulze D, Heiland M, Thurmann H, Adam G (2004) Radiation exposure during midfacial imaging using 4- and 16-slice computed tomography, cone beam computed tomography systems and conventional radiography. Dentomaxillofac Radiol 33:83–86

Vannier MW, Hildebolt CF, Conover G, Knapp RH, Yokoyama-Crothers N, Wang G (1997) Three-dimensional dental imaging by spiral CT. A progress report. Oral Surg Oral Med Oral Pathol Oral Radiol Endod 84:561–570

Facial Traumas and Fractures

Introduction

The main objective of imaging patients with traumas to the face is to detect fractures. CT is the superior imaging modality to assess bone structures and routinely the examination will include axial and coronal sections. With multidetector CT, high-quality images can be obtained in any desired plane and 3D reconstruction can be very valuable in the evaluation of the complex facial skeleton. Although some detail is lost as part of the smoothing algorithm, the 3D images will visualize the fracture segments and their relationship to one another better than different series of 2D images. In the present chapter we focus mainly on mandibular traumas and fractures.

If clinical examination indicates that only the mandible is injured in a minor trauma, a panoramic view with a supplementary posteroanterior view of the mandible and/or intraoral/occlusal views may be sufficient. However, it has been reported that coronal CT alone is more accurate than panoramic radiography alone for diagnosing mandibular condyle fractures. Thus, CT is increasingly used to assess also mandibular fractures. Tooth fractures are adequately evaluated with intraoral (digital or film) radiography but dental traumatology is beyond the scope of this chapter. In general, radiographic examination of any suspected fracture should be in at least two planes, preferably perpendicular to each other.

The diagnosis of facial fractures usually is accomplished by a combination of clinical and imaging examinations.

Non-fracture Traumas

Definition

Minor and/or blunt and/or low-velocity traumas not leading to fracture.

Clinical Features

- Pain
- Dental occlusion does not fit
- Abnormal jaw mobility, usually restricted
- Soft-tissue injury
- Hematoma, epistaxis, edema
- Mandibular luxation

Imaging Features

- Mandibular condyle displacement in fossa at closed mouth (probably due to joint effusion; frequently seen on MRI of TMJ after condyle fractures)
- Restricted condyle translation
- Articular disc displacement
- Paranasal sinus opacification or fluid-air level, or dome-shaped blood clot
- Soft-tissue swelling (subcutaneous hematoma, edema)
- Foreign body

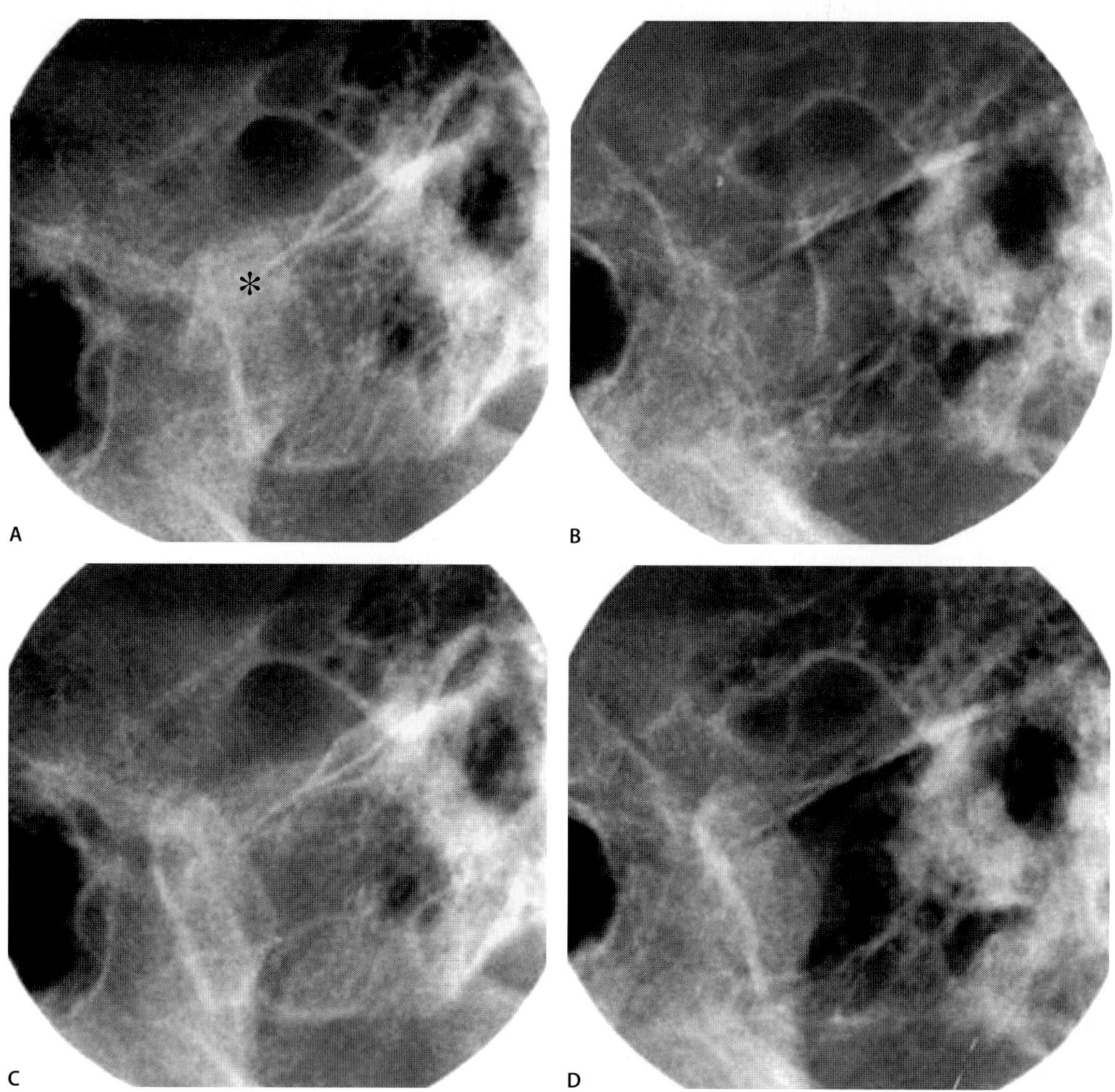

Figure 8.1

Non-fracture trauma to mandible; 14-year-old male with trauma to chin due to bicycle accident, and problems with mouth opening and dental occlusion. **A** and **B** Conventional TMJ radiography at closed mouth shows abnormal position of condyle (*asterisk*) in fossa of right joint (**A**) and wide joint space in left joint (**B**). **C** and **D** Open mouth images show restricted condylar translation of right (**C**) and left (**D**) joint (at this age condyles usually move clearly in front of eminences)

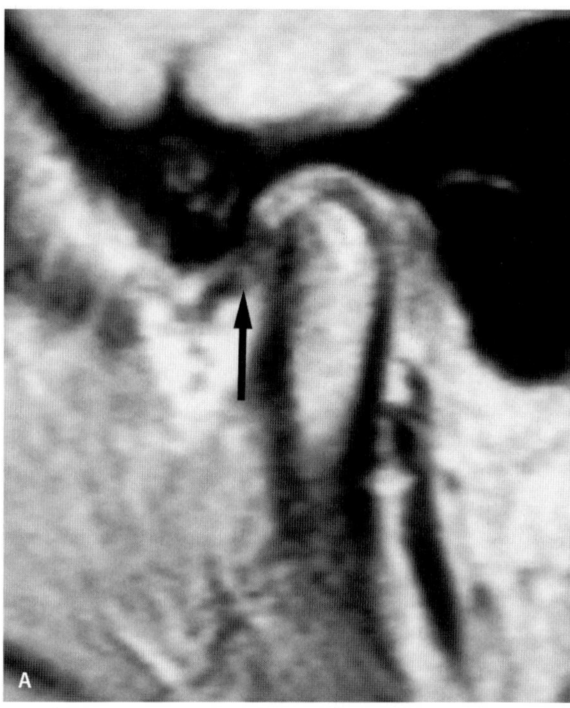

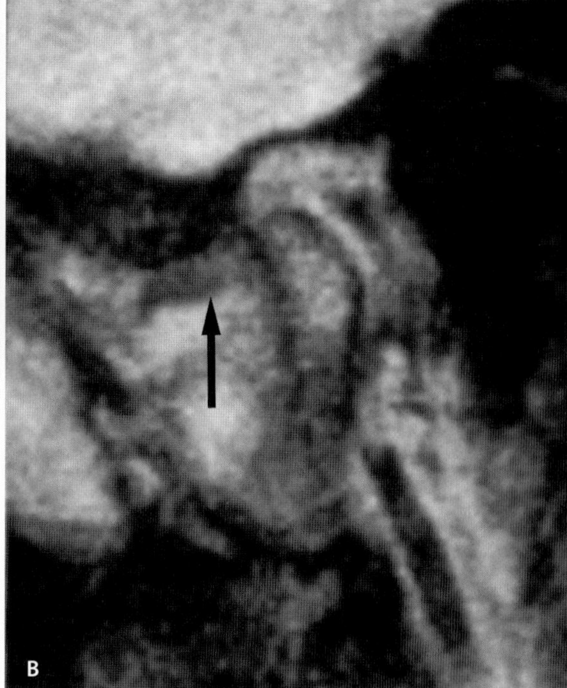

Figure 8.2

Non-fracture trauma to mandible; 20-year-old female with trauma to chin 2 months previously, still with pain and limited mouth opening capacity without joint sound; before trauma she had a clicking jaw but no pain or mouth opening problem (no fractures were found after thorough examinations). **A** and **B** Oblique sagittal TMJ MRI shows anteriorly displaced disc (*arrow*) both at closed (**A**) and at open mouth (**B**) and restricted condyle translation

Figure 8.3

Non-fracture trauma to mandible; patient with jaw luxation. 3D CT image shows condyle in front of eminence (*arrow*), also on contralateral side (not shown) (courtesy of Dr. A. Kolbenstvedt, Rikshospitalet University Hospital, Oslo, Norway)

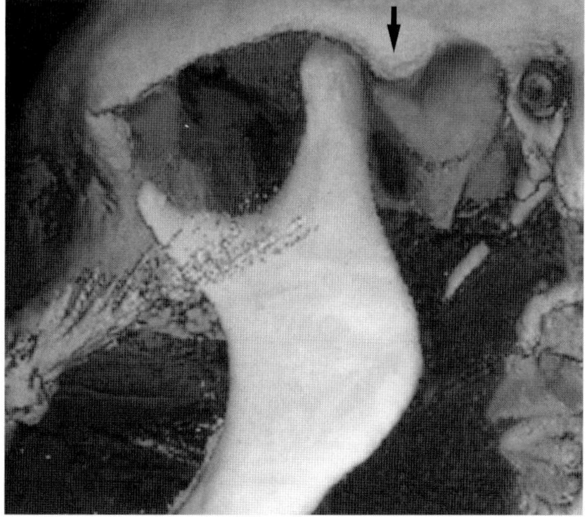

Fractures

Definition

Traumatic cortical discontinuity with or without dislocation.

Clinical Features

- See Non-fracture Traumas
- Abnormal morphology such as flattening
- Palpable step-off of bone
- Crepitation due to emphysema
- Paresthesia, anesthesia
- Hemorrhage

Imaging Features

- See Non-fracture Traumas
- Cortical discontinuity, defect
- Abnormal angulation
- Absent or displaced bone
- Abnormal linear density
- Bone overlap ("double radiopacity")
- Green-stick in young patients
- "Empty fossa" sign on axial CT images
- Localized air collection

Mandibular Fractures

Clinical Features

- See Fractures
- Most common fractures in facial skeleton after nasal fractures
- Unilateral mandibular body fracture reported as most frequent mandibular fracture in oral and maxillofacial surgery practice
- Most common site of mandibular body fracture is junction of body and ramus, followed by molar region
- Mandibular condyle fractures constitute up to about one-half of mandibular fractures and affect all age groups; reported as most frequent mandibular fracture in children
- More than one fracture of mandible common; typically, mandibular body fracture on one side and mandibular neck/condyle fracture on contralateral side; almost half of patients with condyle fractures have mandibular body fractures
- In one study of condyle fractures interpersonal violence was most frequent cause
- Symphyseal and coronoid process area uncommon sites, but in one series with interpersonal violence as a frequent cause, symphyseal fractures were second most common to mandibular angle fractures
- Assault reported to be a more frequent cause than motor vehicle accident, falls and sports, but assault also reported equally frequent to motor vehicle accident
- Males clearly more frequent than females

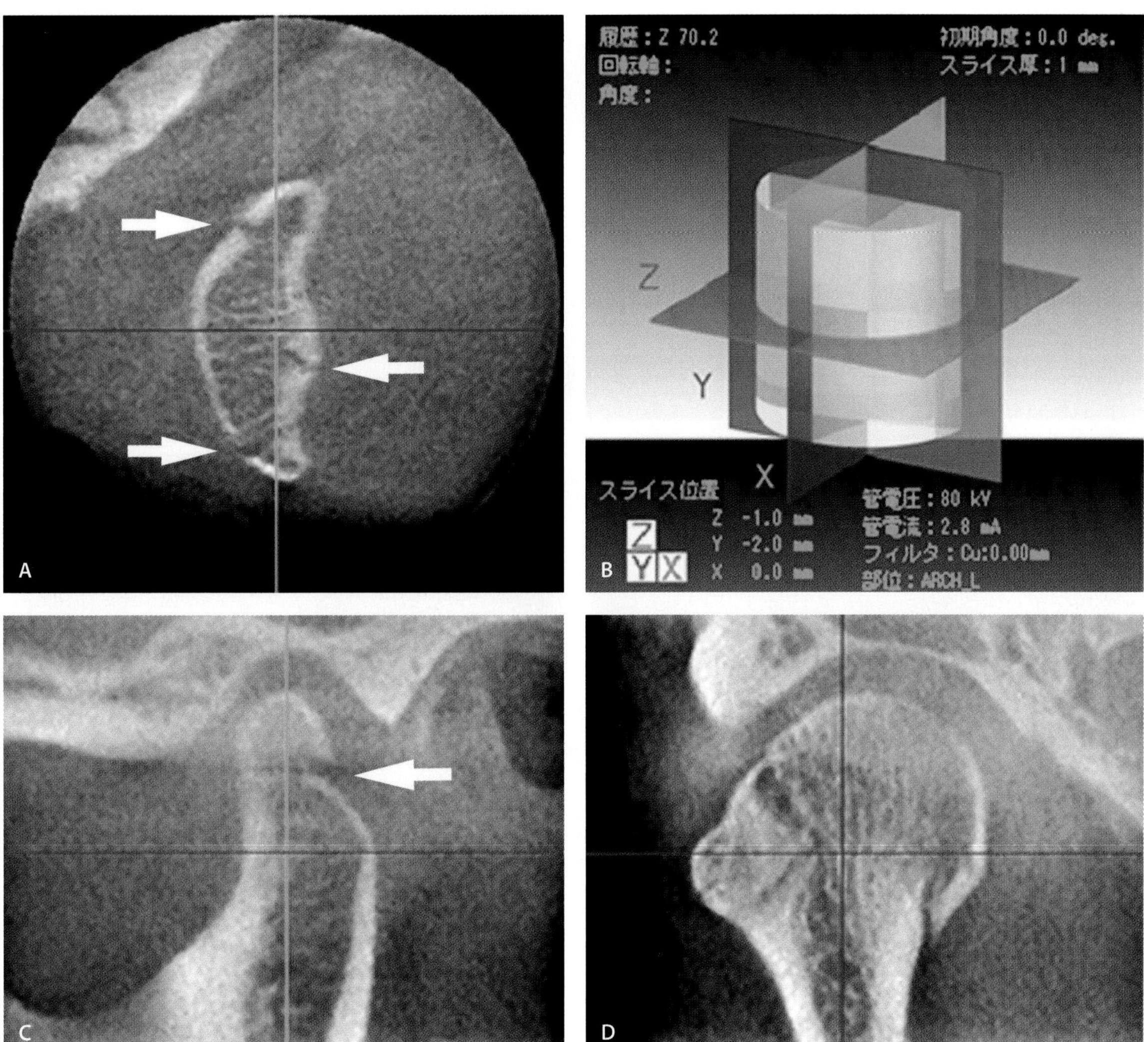

Figure 8.4

Mandibular intracapsular condyle fractures; 34-year-old male with pain after trauma to right TMJ; cone beam CT examination. **A** Axial section shows fracture lines in lateral, central and medial parts of condyle (*arrows*). **B** Three imaging planes are indicated by different colors. **C** Sagittal section shows evident fracture in posterior part of condyle (*arrow*). **D** Coronal section shows fracture lines in lateral and medial parts of condyle, with only minimal displacement (courtesy of Dr. K. Honda, Nihon University School of Dentistry, Tokyo, Japan)

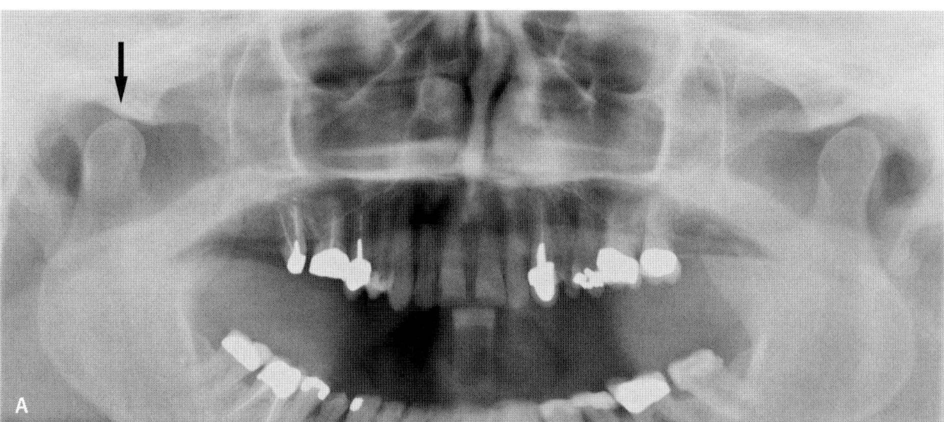

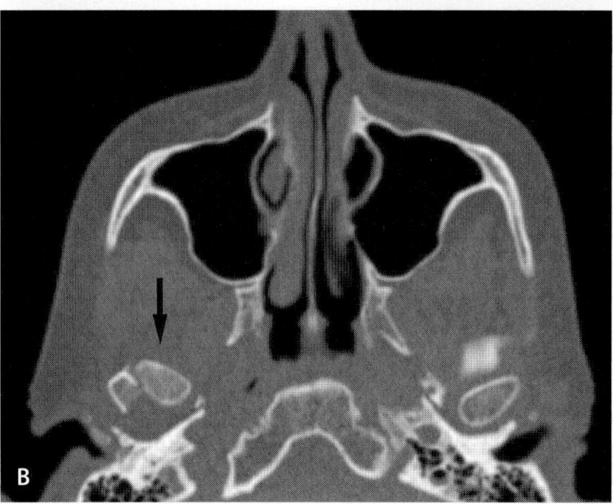

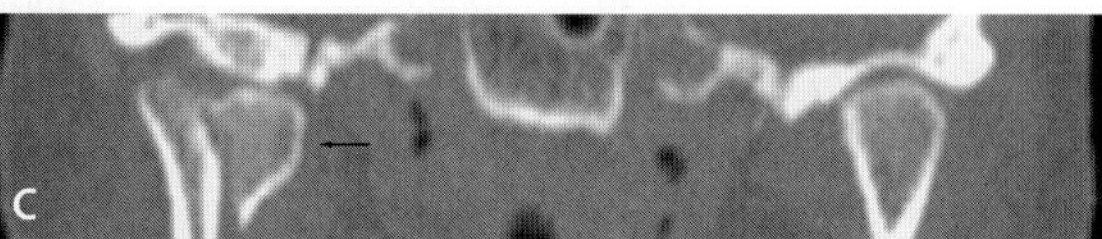

Figure 8.5

Mandibular condyle fracture, unilateral; 48-year-old female 2 weeks after trauma to mandible, now with dental occlusion problems and pain from right TMJ on mouth opening. **A** Panoramic view (open mouth) shows intracapsular fracture of right condyle, apparently without dislocation (*arrow*). **B** Axial CT image shows fragment of condyle slightly dislocated medially (*arrow*). **C** Coronal CT image shows intracapsular fracture with some dislocation of fragment (*arrow*)

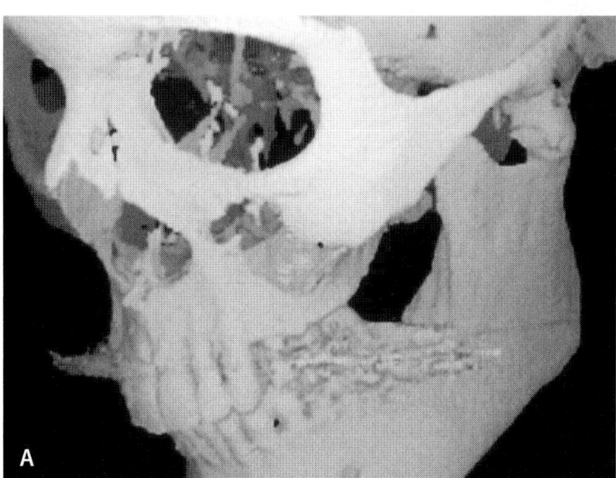

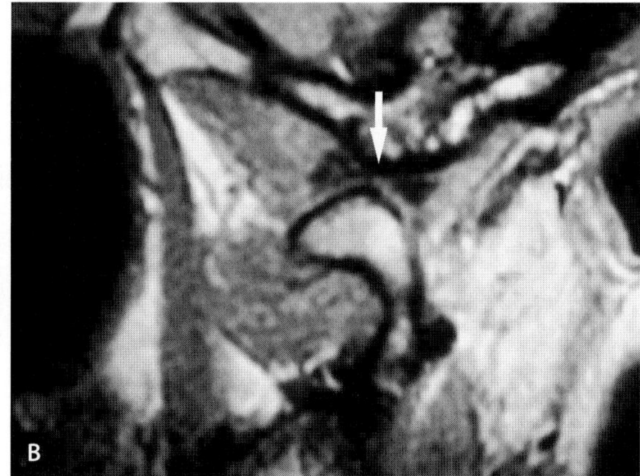

Figure 8.6

Mandibular neck fracture, unilateral, several years old and healed without symptoms or signs. **A** 3D CT image shows satisfactory dental occlusion. **B** MRI of TMJ shows mandibular condyle healed in open mouth position at closed mouth, apparently with normal disc in normal position (*arrow*)

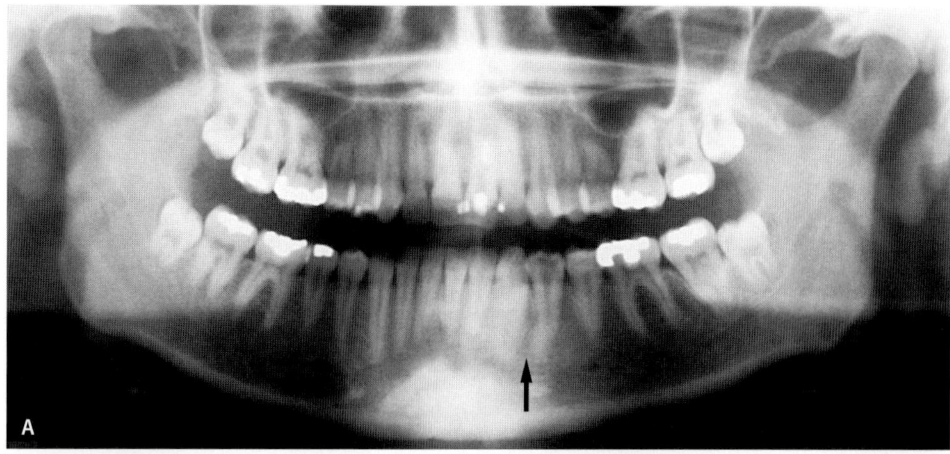

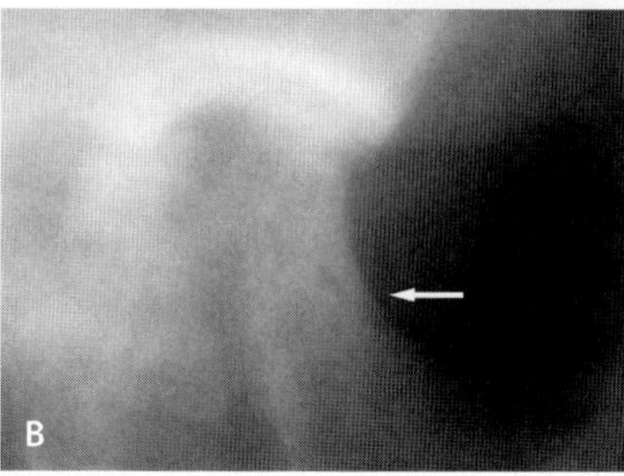

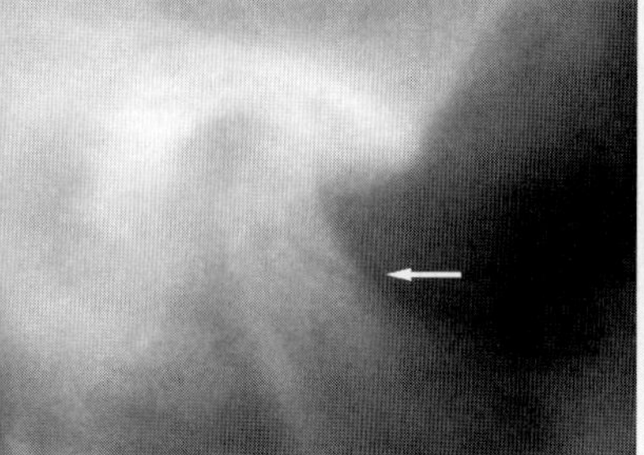

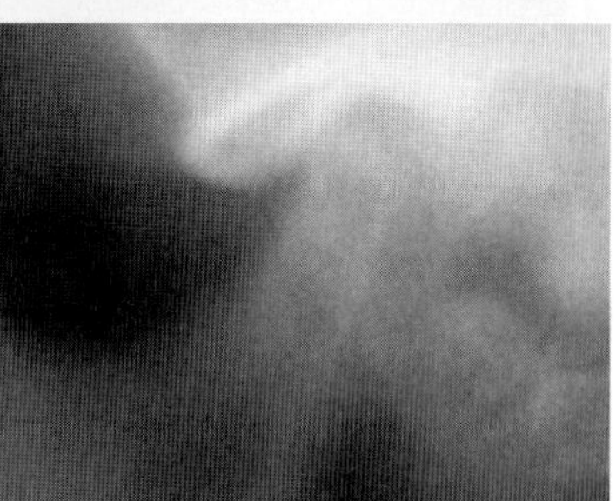

Figure 8.7

Mandibular body and contralateral neck fractures, without dislocation; 19-year-old female with tooth fracture (first premolar in left mandible) and pain with limited mouth opening due to bicycle accident. **A** Panoramic view shows fracture line in left mandibular body (*arrow*) and suggests possible fracture of right mandibular condyle/neck. **B** Conventional tomography of right TMJ at open (*left*) and closed mouth (*middle*), and of left TMJ at closed mouth (*right*) for comparison, confirms fracture line in right mandibular neck/condyle area (*arrow*), apparently without dislocation (cannot be definitely decided without coronal imaging)

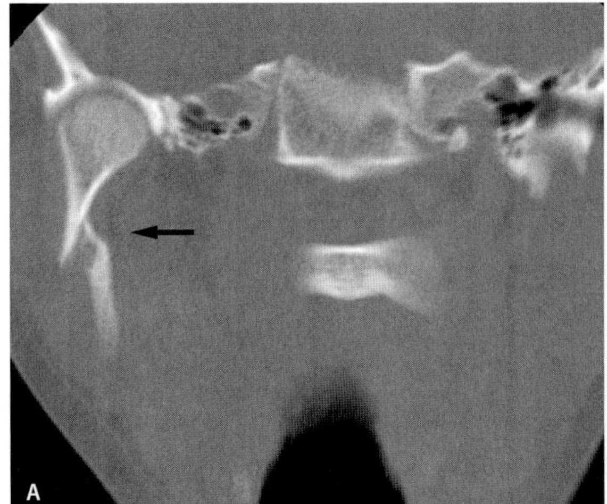

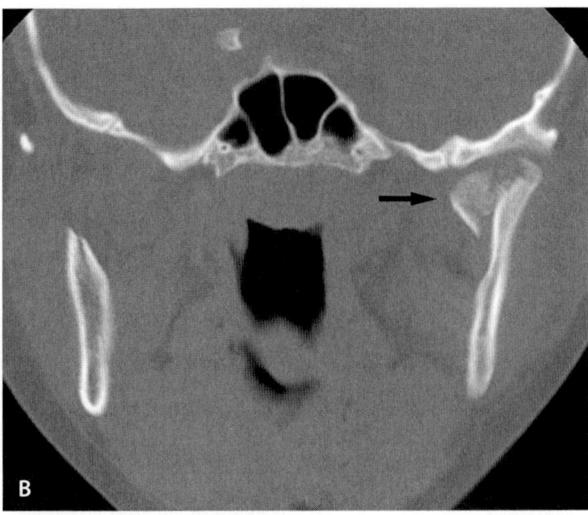

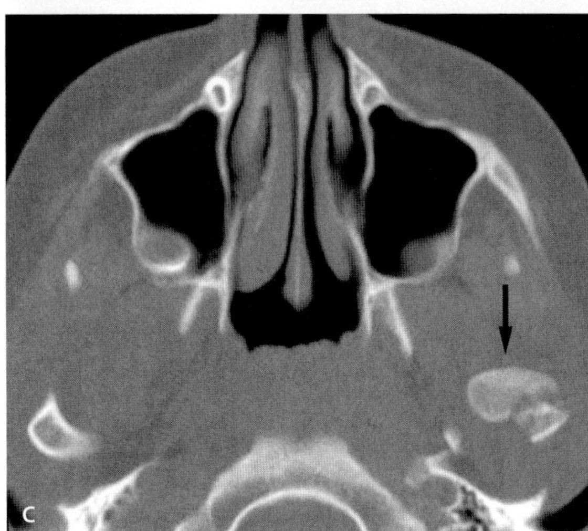

Figure 8.8

Mandibular neck and contralateral mandibular condyle fractures; 10-year-old male who fell over handlebars of his bike, landing on his chin. **A** Coronal CT shows right mandibular neck fracture (*arrow*). **B** Coronal CT shows intracapsular fracture of contralateral mandibular condyle with some medial dislocation of medial fragment (*arrow*). **C** Axial CT confirms intracapsular condyle fracture with dislocation (*arrow*)

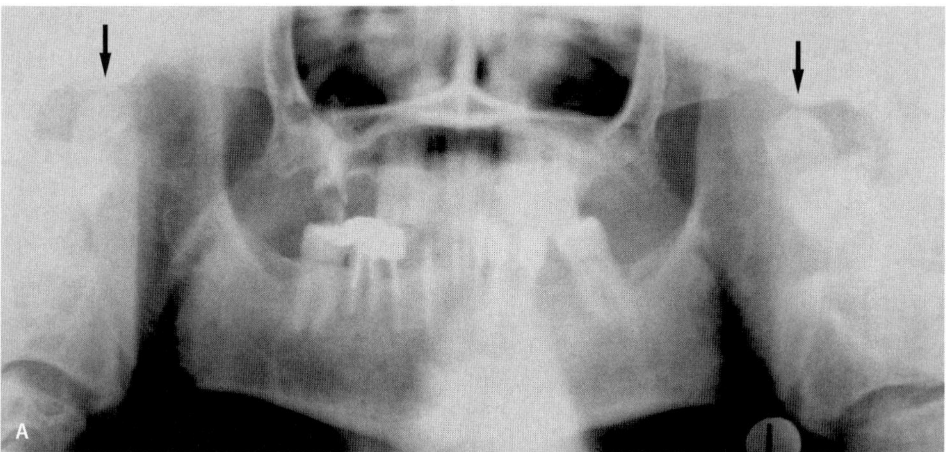

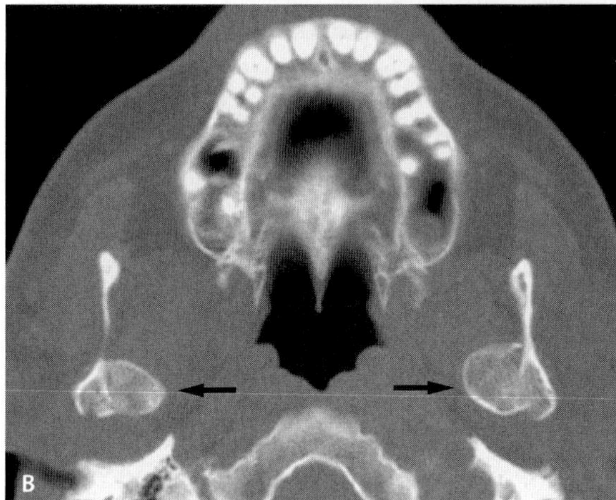

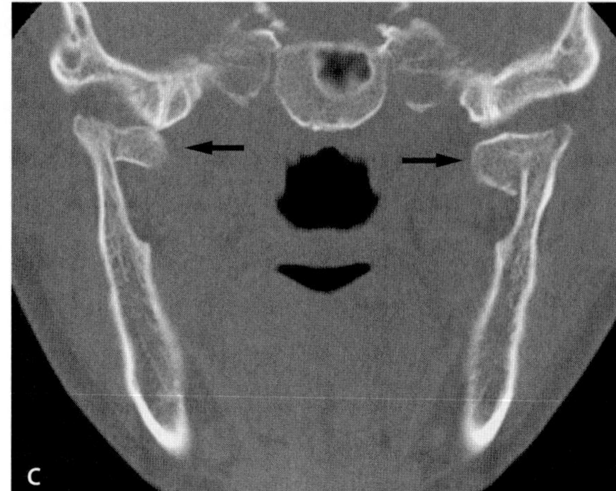

Figure 8.9

Mandibular neck fractures, bilateral; 37-year-old male with 5-year-old healed mandibular fractures without symptoms or signs and with satisfactory dental occlusion, now with new trauma to face but no new fractures. **A** Panoramic view shows deformed mandibular condyles bilaterally (*arrows*). **B** axial CT image shows bony union between fragments and remaining mandible bilaterally (*arrows*). **C** Coronal CT image shows medially displaced and healed fragments bilaterally (*arrows*)

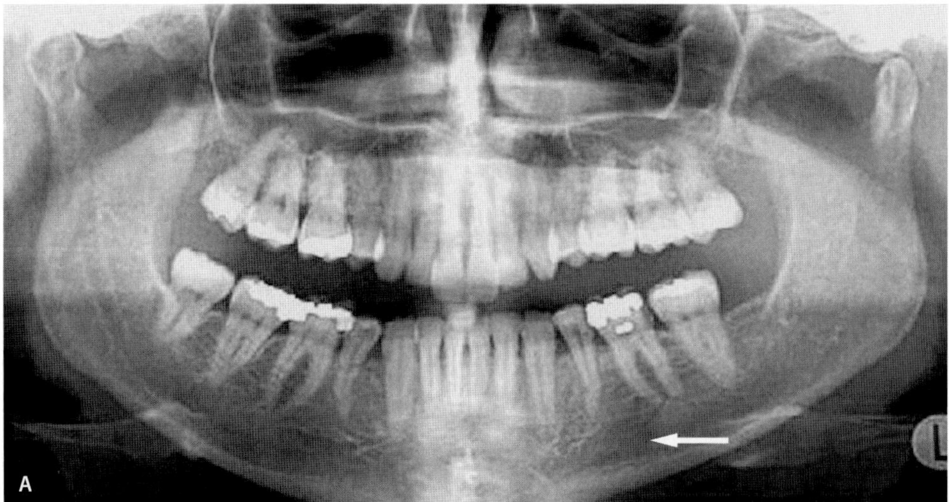

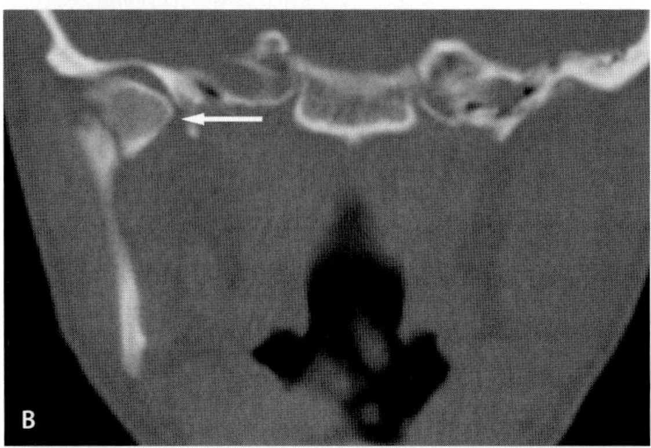

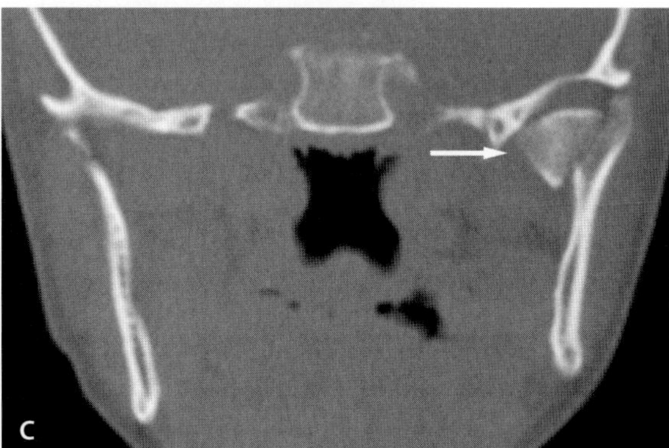

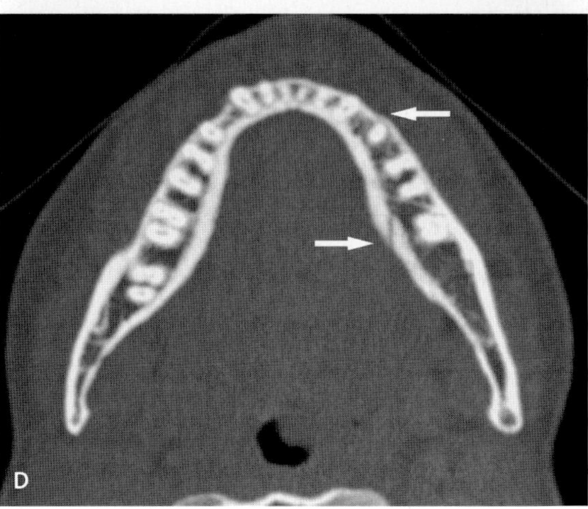

Figure 8.10

Mandibular bilateral neck and mandibular body fractures; 44-year-old female with trauma to chin 3 weeks previously, but still some problems with dental occlusion (only tooth fractures diagnosed by clinical and intraoral radiographic examinations). **A** Panoramic view shows fracture of mandibular body (*arrow*), and suggests possible fractures of condyles. **B** Coronal CT image shows intracapsular fracture of right mandibular condyle with minimal dislocation (*arrow*). **C** Coronal CT image shows intracapsular fracture of left mandibular condyle with small dislocation (*arrow*). **D** Axial CT image shows mandibular body fracture without dislocation (*arrows*).

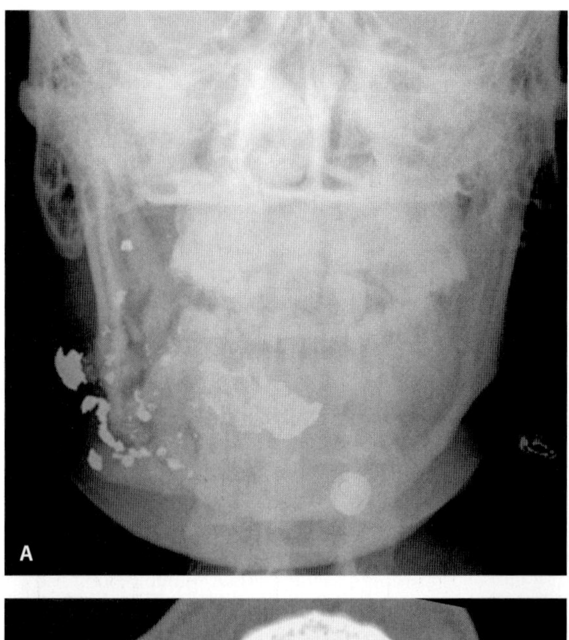

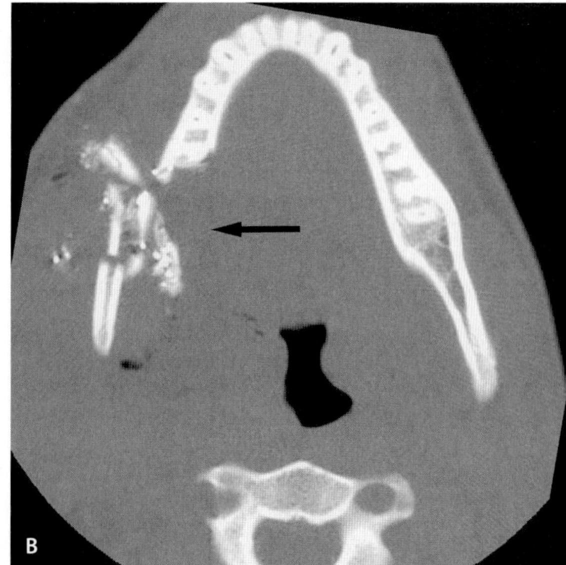

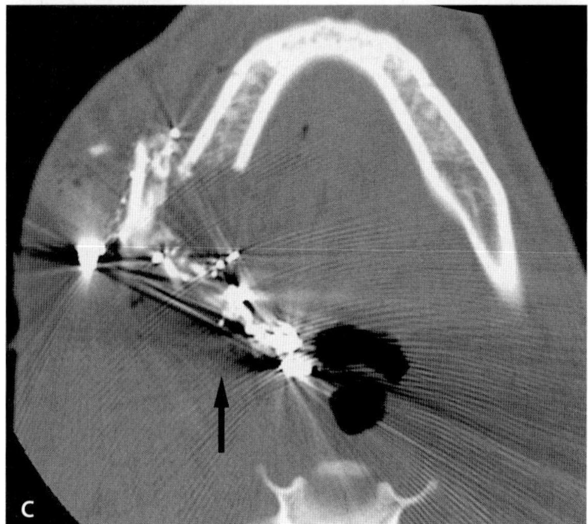

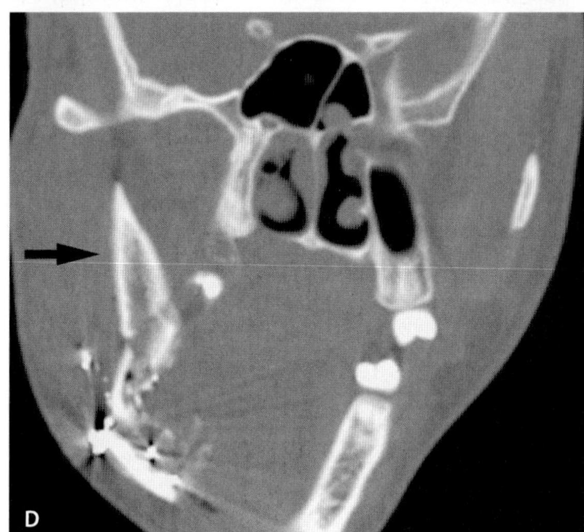

Figure 8.11

Mandibular body fracture, comminuted; 17-year-old male with gunshot to face. A En face view shows multiple bone and metallic fragments, and an intratracheal tube. B Axial CT image of tooth-bearing area shows comminuted fracture with many bone and metallic fragments (*arrow*). C Axial CT image at a more caudal level shows multiple metallic bullet fragments, from cheek area to air space with air bubbles along bullet track (*arrow*), and soft-tissue swelling. D Coronal CT image shows intact coronoid process (*arrow*). E Coronal CT image shows intact mandibular neck and condyle (*arrow*)

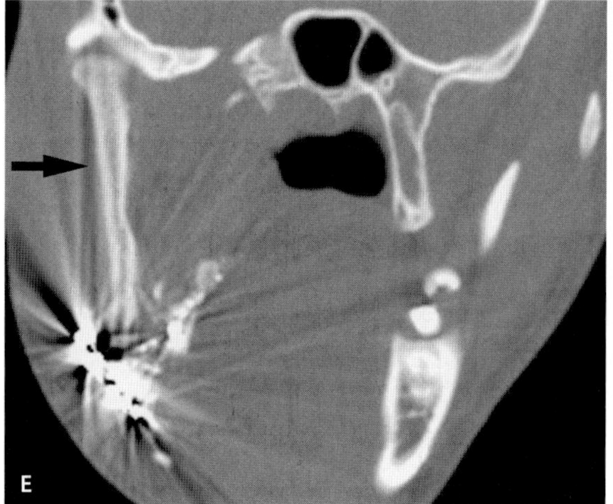

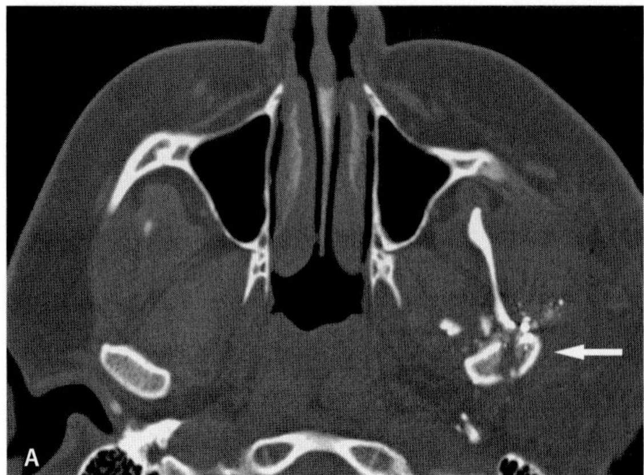

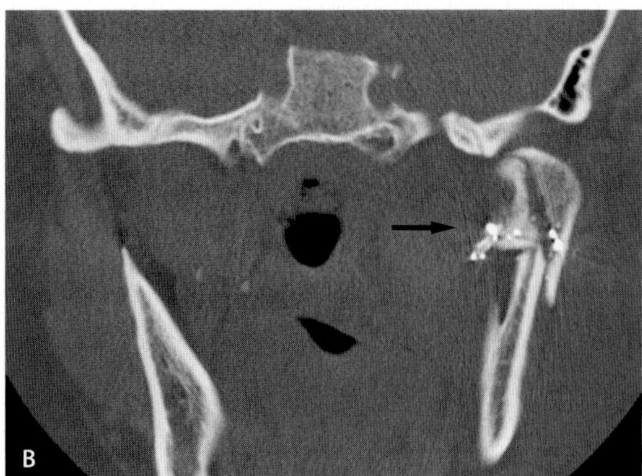

Figure 8.12

Mandibular condyle fracture, comminuted; 23-year-old female with gunshot to face. **A** Axial CT image shows multiple bone and metallic fragments and intracapsular condyle fracture (*arrow*). **B** Coronal CT image shows multiple bony and metallic fragments and condyle divided into two main pieces (*arrow*)

Mandibular Fractures Combined with Other Fractures

Clinical Features

- 15% of patients with mandibular fractures have at least one other facial bone fracture
- In patients with severe facial traumas also mandible frequently injured; in about half of LeFort fractures
- Compound fractures communicate with soft-tissue wounds

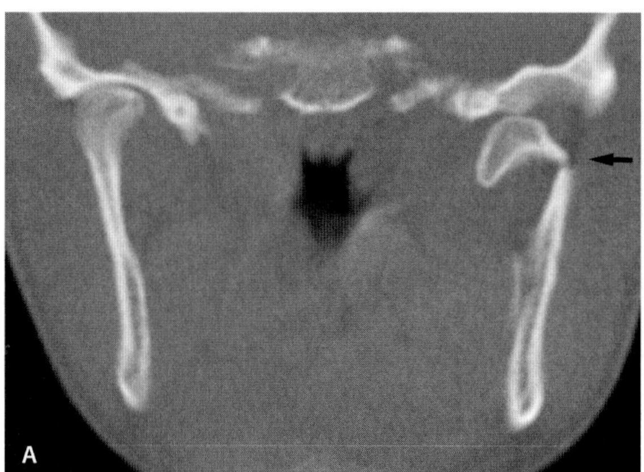

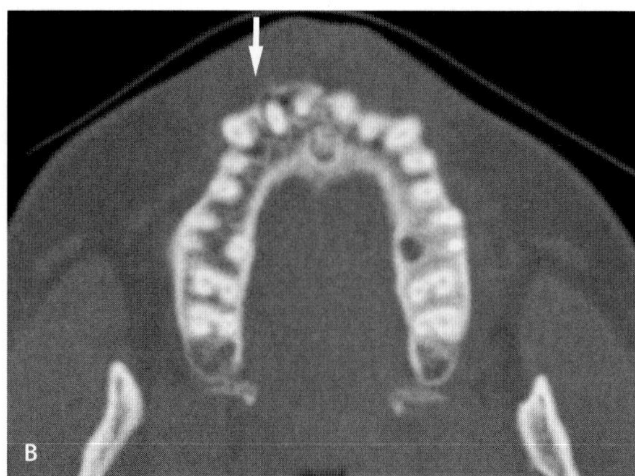

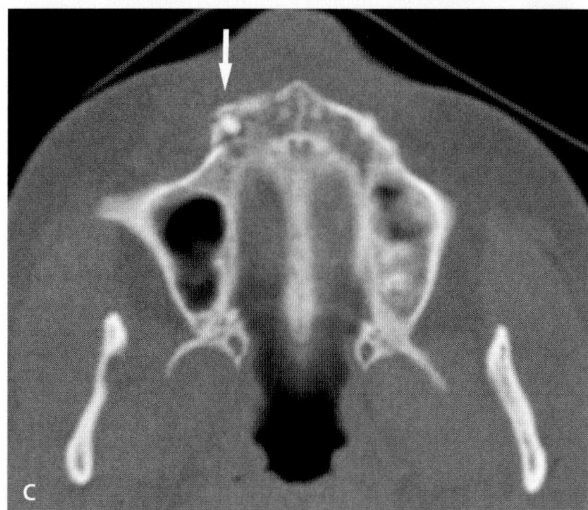

Figure 8.13

Mandibular neck and maxillary alveolar process fractures; 33-year-old female with trauma to chin and maxilla. A Coronal CT image shows fracture of left mandibular neck (*arrow*). B Axial CT image shows right maxillary alveolar process fracture with dislocated tooth (*arrow*). C Axial CT image shows comminuted fracture of maxillary alveolar process (*arrow*)

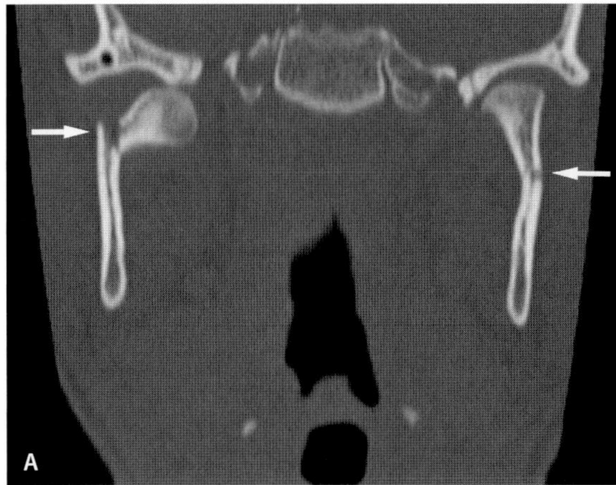

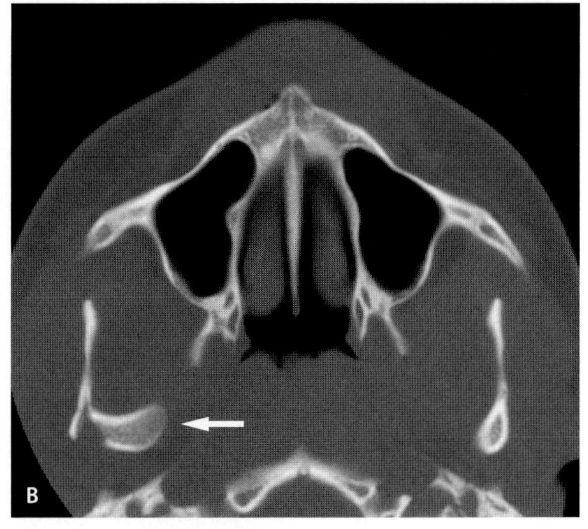

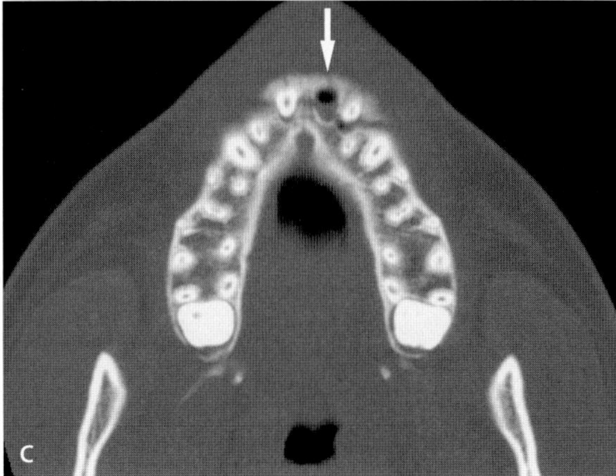

Figure 8.14

Mandibular bilateral neck (greenstick on one side) and maxillary alveolar process fractures; 14-year-old male with trauma to chin and maxilla. **A** Coronal CT image shows right mandibular neck fracture with fragment dislocated medially (*arrow*) and greenstick fracture of left mandibular neck with minimal displacement (*arrow*). **B** Axial CT image confirms displacement of right mandibular condyle (*arrow*) and no evident displacement of left side. **C** Axial CT image shows fracture of maxillary alveolar process in anterior region with loss of one incisor (*arrow*)

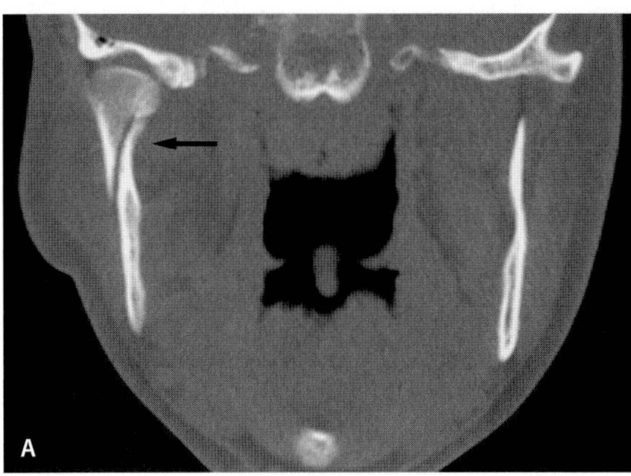

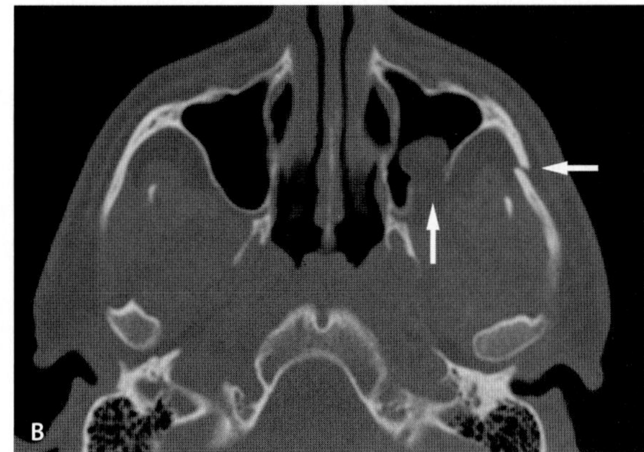

Figure 8.15

Mandibular neck, maxillary sinus wall and zygomatic arch fractures; 38-year-old male who had been assaulted 1 month previously, now with limited mouth opening, dental occlusion problem and tenderness to left zygomatic arch (1 week after trauma only sinus wall fracture was diagnosed at a hospital). **A** Coronal CT image shows mandibular neck fracture with minimal dislocation (*arrow*). **B** Axial CT image shows maxillary sinus wall fracture and zygomatic arch fracture (*arrows*)

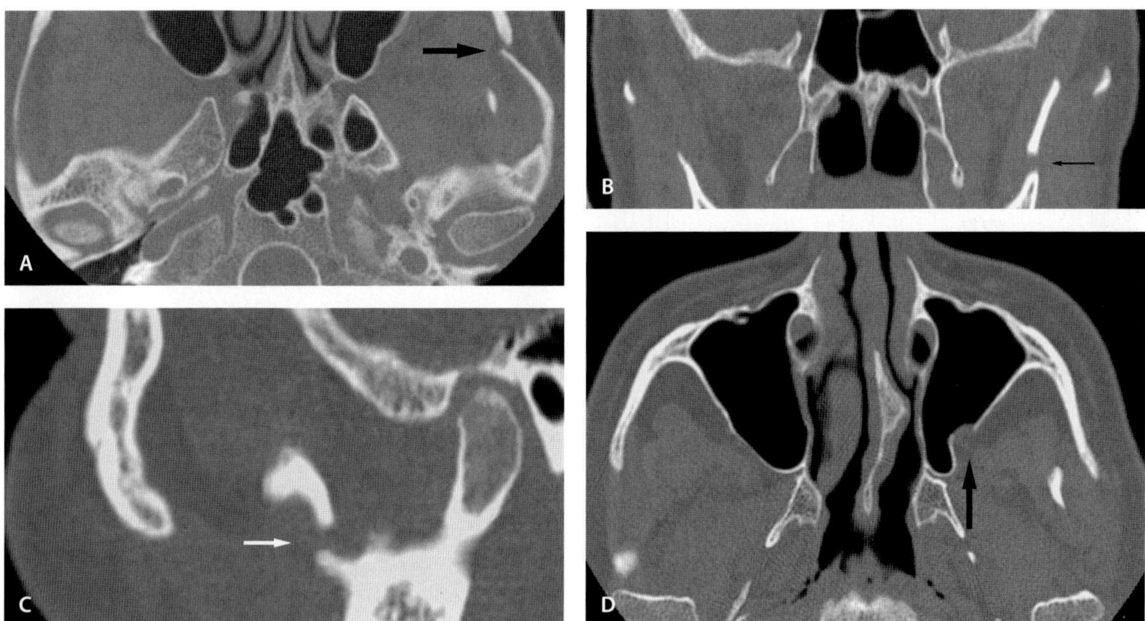

Figure 8.16

Mandibular coronoid process, maxillary sinus wall and zygomatic arch fractures; 54-year-old female with bicycle accident 3 weeks previously, but still with mouth opening problem. **A** Axial CT image shows fracture of zygomatic arch (*arrow*). **B** Coronal CT image shows fracture of mandibular coronoid process (*arrow*). **C** Sagittal CT image confirms coronoid process fracture (*arrow*), but mandibular condyle located normally in fossa. **D** Axial CT image shows maxillary sinus wall fracture (*arrow*)

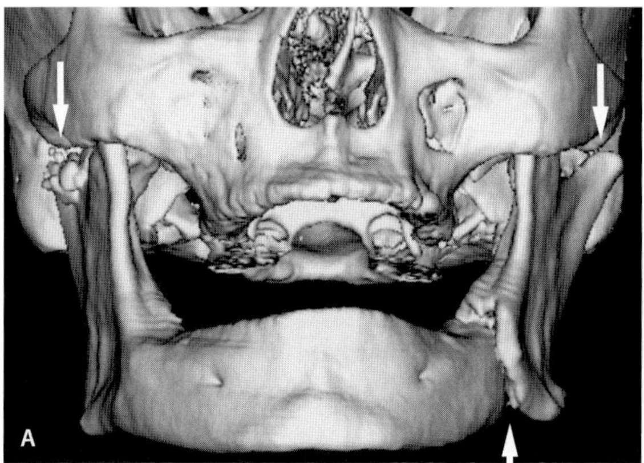

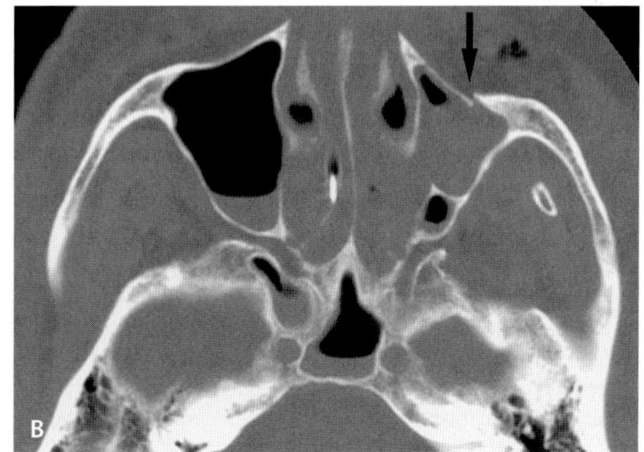

Figure 8.17

Mandibular bilateral neck, mandibular body and maxillary sinus wall fractures; 58-year-old female who was struck by a car with loss of consciousness. **A** 3D CT image shows fracture of left mandibular body (*arrow*) and bilateral mandibular neck fractures (*arrows*). **B** Axial CT image shows maxillary sinus wall fracture (*arrow*), intrasinus hemorrhage and subcutaneous air collection

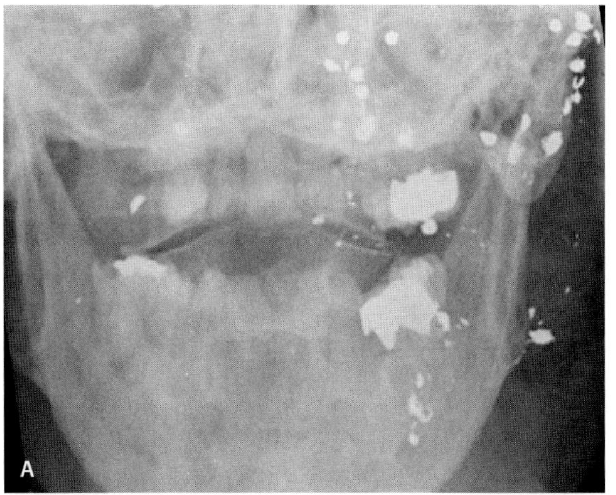

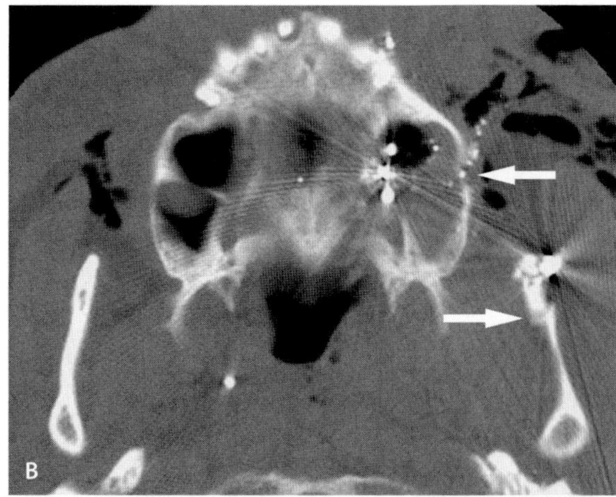

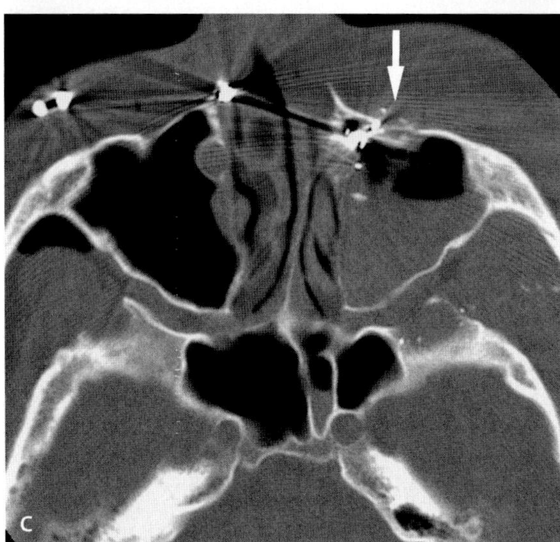

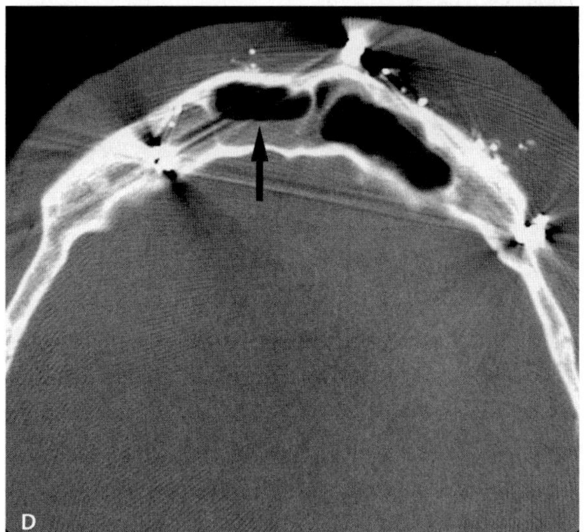

Figure 8.18

Mandibular and maxillary fractures not pronounced and without dislocations, but severe hemorrhage intracranially and in most paranasal sinuses; 60-year-old male with gunshot to face. A Posteroanterior view shows numerous bullet pellets and fragments, but no obvious fractures. B Axial CT image shows mandibular fracture (*arrow*), maxillary sinus wall fracture (*arrow*), left maxillary sinus opacification (hemorrhage), and a number of metallic fragments and air collections, in particular in the bullet track. C Axial CT image shows fracture of anterior maxillary wall (*arrow*), left maxillary sinus fluid-air level (hemorrhage) and metallic fragments. D Axial CT image shows fluid-air level (hemorrhage) of frontal sinus (*arrow*) and a number of metallic fragments. E Axial CT image shows large intraparenchymal hemorrhage in left frontotemporal lobes (*arrow*) causing some mass effect onto frontal horn of the left lateral ventricle, some widening of extra-axial space over left frontal area possibly due to subdural hematoma, pneumocephalus in the left frontal area, and bullet fragments, one in particular adjacent to occipital horn of right lateral ventricle

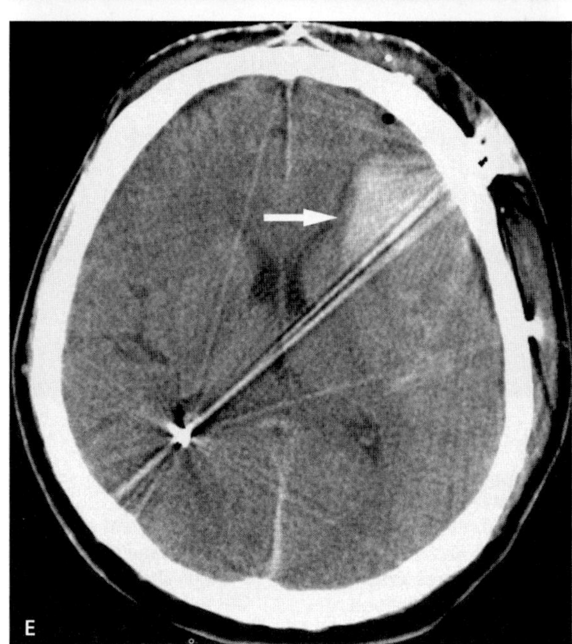

Complications of Mandibular Fractures

Clinical Features

- Mandibular fractures are easily overlooked in the diagnostic work-up of traumatized patients, particularly of those with severe head injuries
- Undetected mandibular fractures may lead to various complications, some of which could have been avoided
- Infections, osteomyelitis and nonunion seem to be the most frequent complications after surgical treatment; mandibular angle fractures have the highest overall morbidity rate
- Dental occlusion problems and marked deviation of mandible on mouth opening seem to be most frequent complications after nonsurgical treatment of condyle fractures

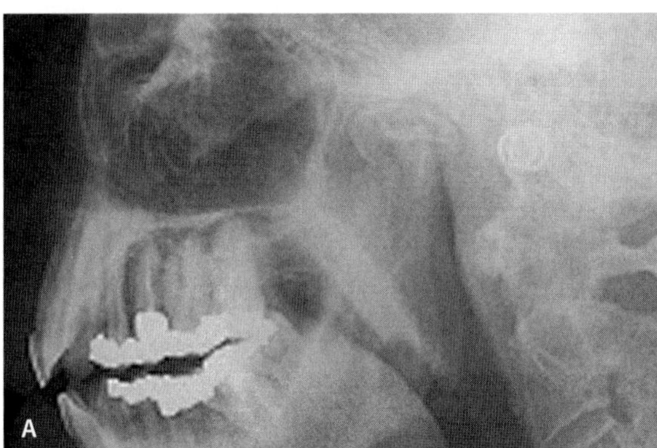
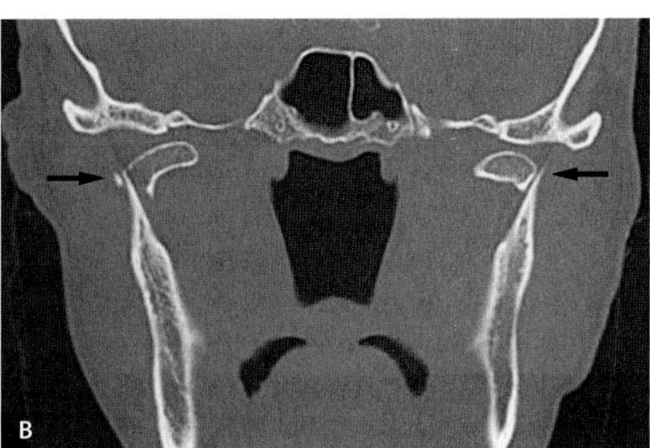

Figure 8.19

Open bite; 61-year-old male with trauma to face and head 3 weeks previously with loss of consciousness, no mandibular fractures diagnosed, now with contact only on molar teeth at closed mouth. **A** Lateral view shows anterior bite opening. **B** Coronal CT image shows bilateral mandibular neck fractures (*arrows*)

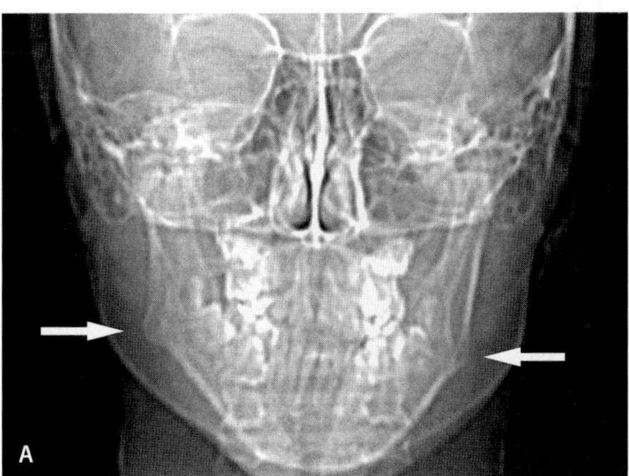
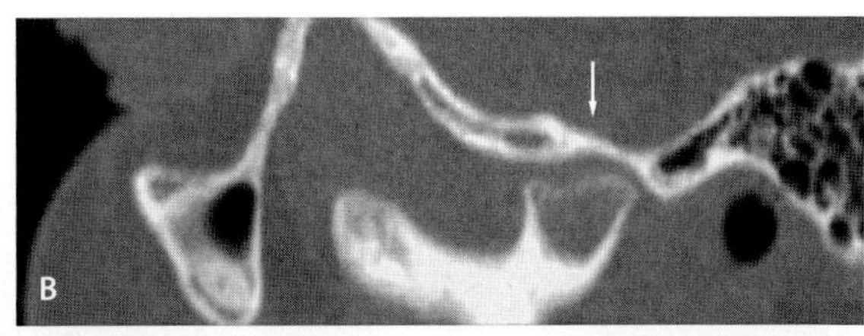
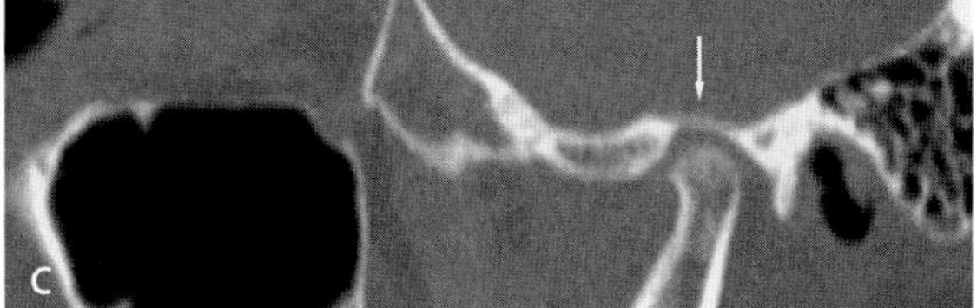

Figure 8.20

Facial asymmetry; 12-year-old female with a 4-year history of trauma to chin but no fractures diagnosed. **A** Scout view shows facial asymmetry with mandibular underdevelopment on right side (*arrows*). **B** Oblique sagittal CT image of right TMJ shows deformed mandibular condyle and flattened fossa. **C** Oblique sagittal CT image of left TMJ shows normal mandibular condyle and fossa (other images of this patient in Fig. 6.40)

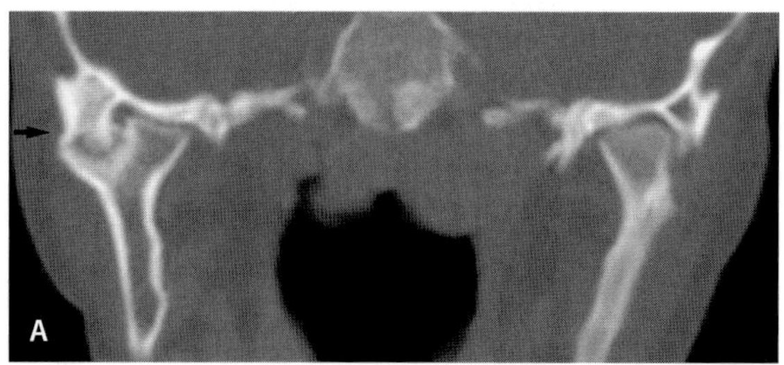

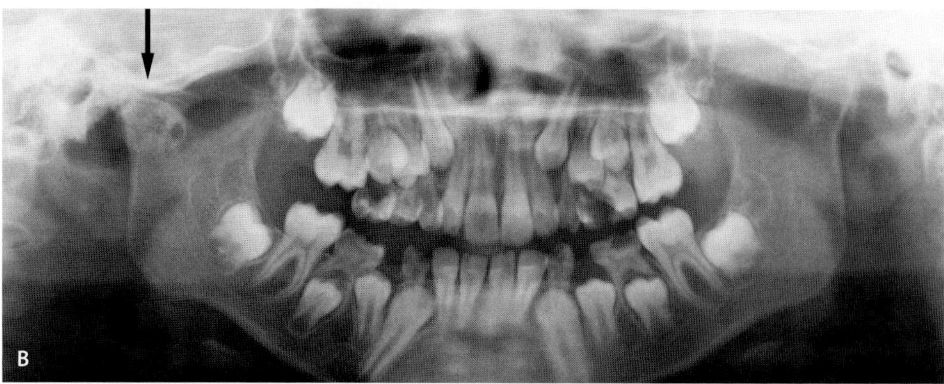

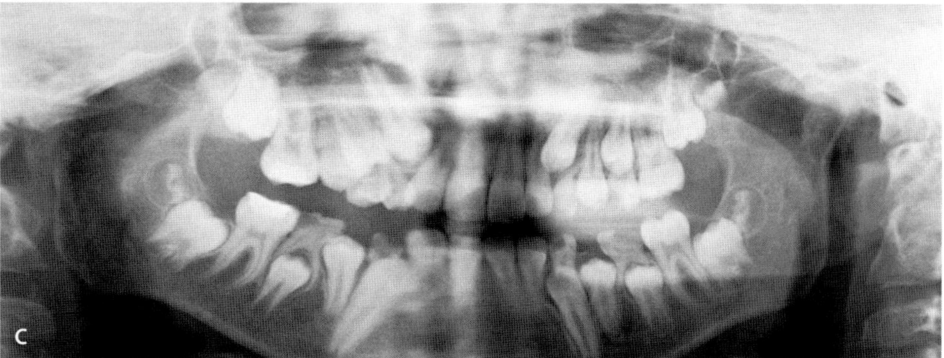

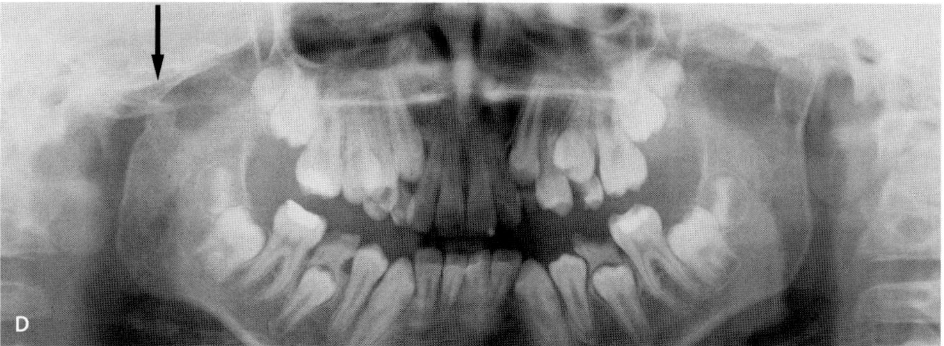

Figure 8.21

TMJ ankylosis; 10-year-old male with a 4-year history of trauma to head with loss of consciousness; no jaw fractures diagnosed, but mouth opening capacity gradually reduced to less than 10 mm; postoperatively it increased to 33 mm. **A** Coronal CT image shows fibro-osseous ankylosis of lateral part of right TMJ (*arrow*); probably also previous fracture of left joint. **B** Panoramic view shows abnormal right mandibular condyle (*arrow*). **C** Panoramic, postoperative view shows most of right mandibular condyle resected. **D** Panoramic view, 1 year postoperative, shows small, new mandibular condyle (*arrow*)

Nasal Fractures

Clinical Features

- See Fractures
- Nasal bone or nasal pyramid fractures are most frequent and constitute 40–50% of all facial bone fractures
- 66% result from a lateral force, only 13% from a frontal force
- The majority involve thinner distal third of nasal bones, with intact nasal–ethmoid margin
- More severe fractures may result in detachment of entire nasal pyramid, saddle nose, hypertelorism and telecanthus

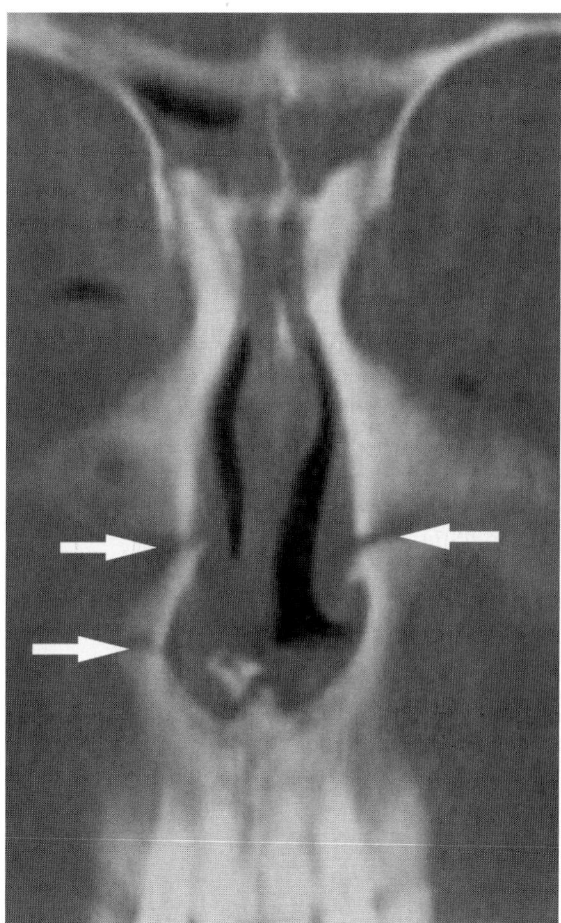

Figure 8.22

Nasal aperture fractures. Coronal CT image shows three fractures of nasal aperture (*arrows*), as well as fractures of frontal sinus with fluid-air level and nasal septum (courtesy of Dr. A. Kolbenstvedt, Rikshospitalet University Hospital, Oslo, Norway)

Midfacial Fractures

Clinical Features

- See Fractures
- Central midfacial fractures; all forms of fractures that occur between root of nose and maxillary alveolar processes, without involvement of zygomas; isolated maxillary fractures, nasal–ethmoidal–orbital fractures, LeFort fractures 1 and 2
- Lateral midfacial fractures; isolated zygomatic arch fracture, tripod fracture, blow-out fracture
- Fractures may be bilateral or unilateral
- About one-fourth as common as mandibular fractures
- Majority of severe midfacial fractures occur in road traffic accidents
- More than 80% of patients are males
- Peak age incidence third decade
- Rare in children
- Trismus is reported in about 33% of all zygomatic fractures and in about 45% of zygomatic arch fractures; a fractured arch may impinge on coronoid process or temporalis muscle
- 1% to near 15% of central–lateral midfacial fractures are reported to have accompanying fractures of anterior skull base
- Posttraumatic complications; meningitis, hypertelorism, olfactory dysfunction, mucocele

Isolated Maxillary Sinus Wall Fracture

Clinical Features

- Uncommon, but usually comminuted
- Alveolar fractures most frequent

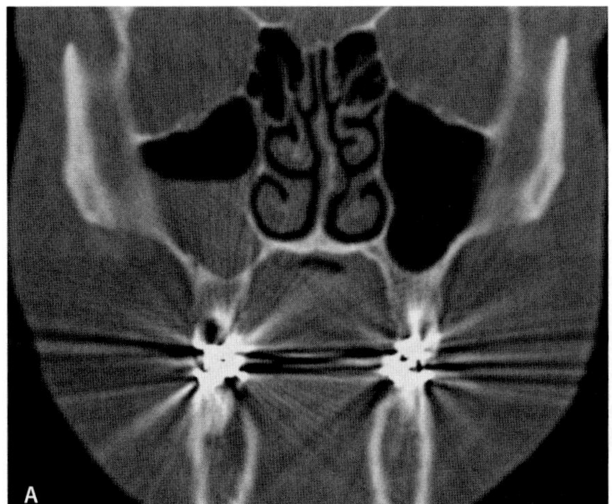

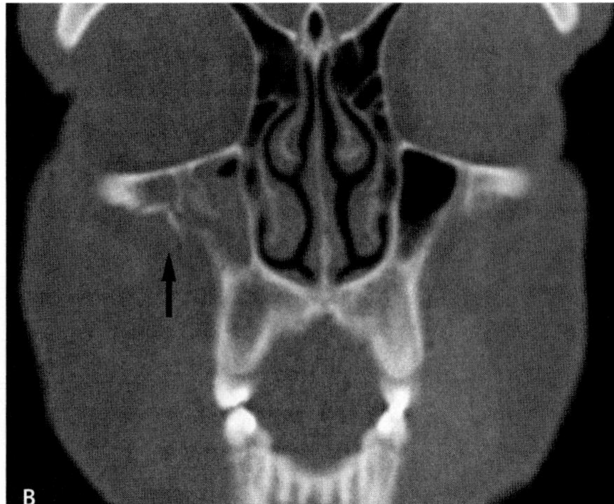

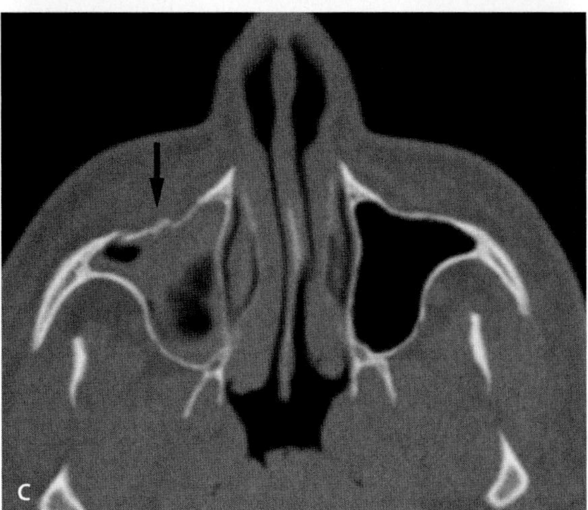

Figure 8.23

Maxillary sinus wall fracture; 32-year-old male victim of violence 3 days previously, with infra-orbital hematoma and pain. A Coronal CT image shows normal bony walls of maxillary sinuses but unilateral fluid-air level. B Coronal CT image shows comminuted fracture of lateral maxillary sinus wall (*arrow*). C Axial CT shows fracture of anterior maxillary sinus wall (*arrow*)

LeFort Fractures

Definition

LeFort 1 is characterized by fracture just above the floor of the nasal cavity with separation of the entire palate and maxillary alveolar process; fractures through the lower nasal septum, lower walls of maxillary sinuses, and lower pterygoid plates ("horizontal fracture").

LeFort 2 is characterized by fracture of the root of the nose, bilateral fractures of the lacrimal bones and medial orbital walls, the floor of the orbits near the infraorbital canals, zygomaticomaxillary sutures and anterior walls of maxilla ("pyramidal fracture") and posteriorly, infratemporal surfaces of the maxilla and lower pterygoid plates. Wassmund 1 fracture does not include the nasal bones but is otherwise identical.

LeFort 3 is characterized by separation of the entire viscerocranium from the skull base ("craniofacial dysjunction"); fracture of the root of the nose, bilateral fractures of the lacrimal bones and medial orbital walls, the floor of the orbits to the inferior orbital fissure, where one fracture line extends to the lateral orbital wall and another down across the posterior maxilla to the lower pterygoid plates and additionally, fractures of the zygomatic arches. Wassmund 3 fracture does not include the nasal bones but is otherwise identical.

Clinical Features

- Usually, different fracture types occur in combination
- Dental occlusion does not fit
- "Floating palate" (LeFort 1)
- "Dish face", hemorrhage, edema, emphysema, and in near 80% anesthesia of infraorbital nerve(s) (LeFort 2)
- "Dish face", CSF rhinorrhea, hemorrhage, edema, emphysema, damage to lacrimal apparatus, and in near 70% anesthesia of infraorbital nerve(s) (LeFort 3)

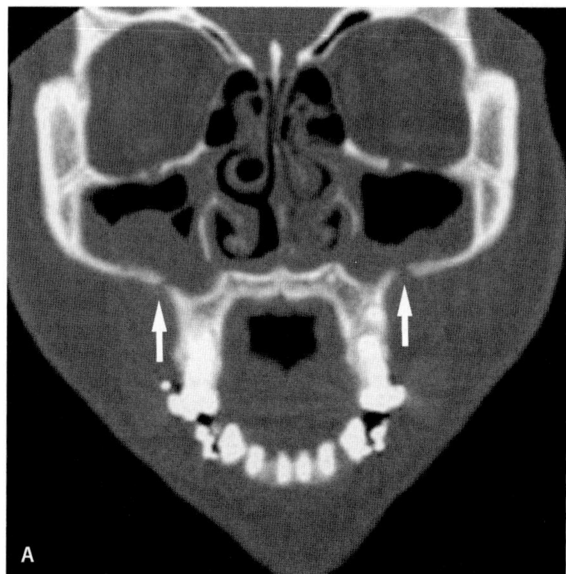

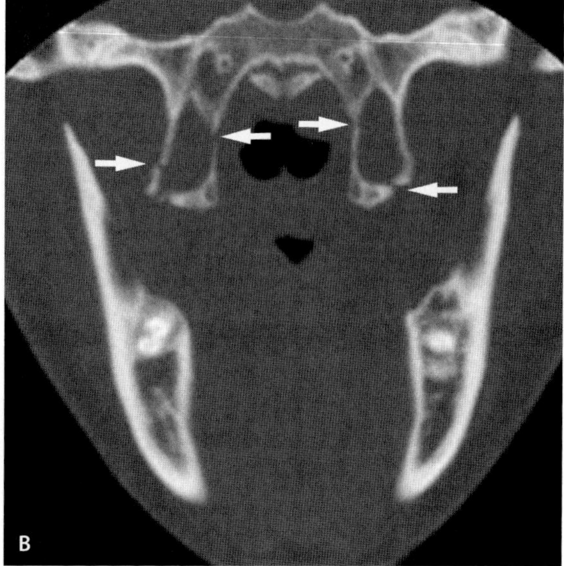

Figure 8.24

LeFort 1 osteotomies; 48-year-old female with pain and facial swelling after maxillary surgery. **A** Coronal CT image shows osteotomy defects in anterolateral maxillary walls (*arrows*) and through inferior portion of nasal cavity. Associated mucosal thickening in maxillary sinuses characteristically seen after surgery. **B** Coronal CT image shows osteotomy defects in pterygoid plates (*arrows*)

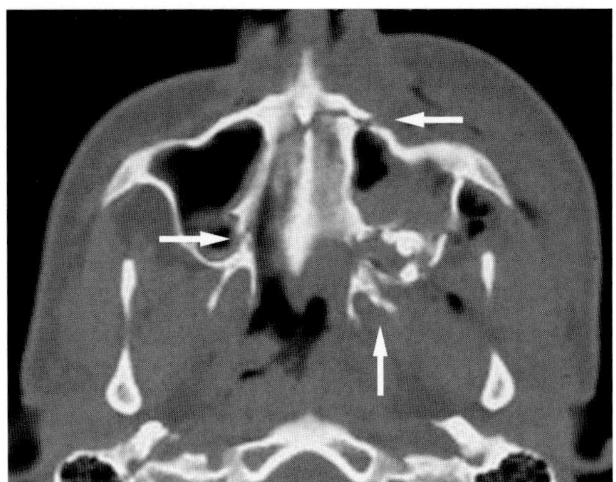

Figure 8.25

LeFort 1 fracture. Axial CT image shows fracture line in anterior, inferior part of nasal cavity (*arrow*), in posterior, inferior part of maxillary sinus, most prominent on left side and in left pterygoid plate (*arrow*). Note also fracture in right medial maxillary sinus wall (*arrow*) (courtesy of Dr. A. Kolbenstvedt, Rikshospitalet University Hospital, Oslo, Norway)

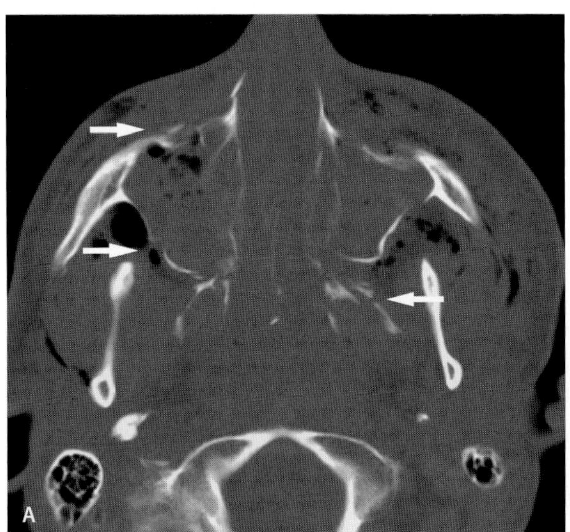

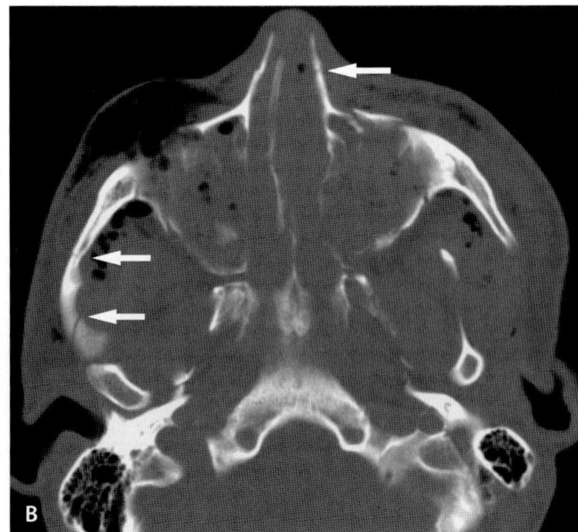

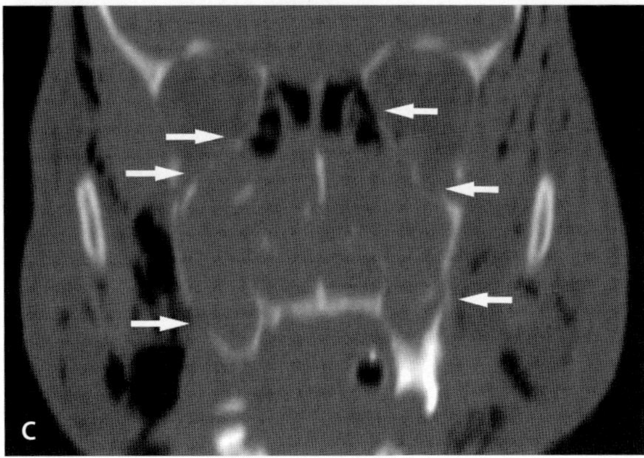

Figure 8.26

LeFort 2 fracture with a zygomatic arch nondisplaced fracture; 37-year-old male who was assaulted. **A** Axial CT image shows bilateral fractures of anterior part of maxilla (*arrow*), lateral-posterior part of maxilla (*arrow*), and pterygoid plates (*arrow*). Hemorrhage in maxillary sinuses and multiple air collections. **B** Axial CT image shows bilateral fracture of nasal bone (*arrow*) and fractures of right zygomatic arch (*arrows*). Note large emphysema in cheek. **C** Coronal, reformatted CT image shows bilateral fractures of medial orbital walls (*arrows*), superior and inferior lateral maxillary sinus walls (*arrows*), and nasal aperture. Note intratracheal tube

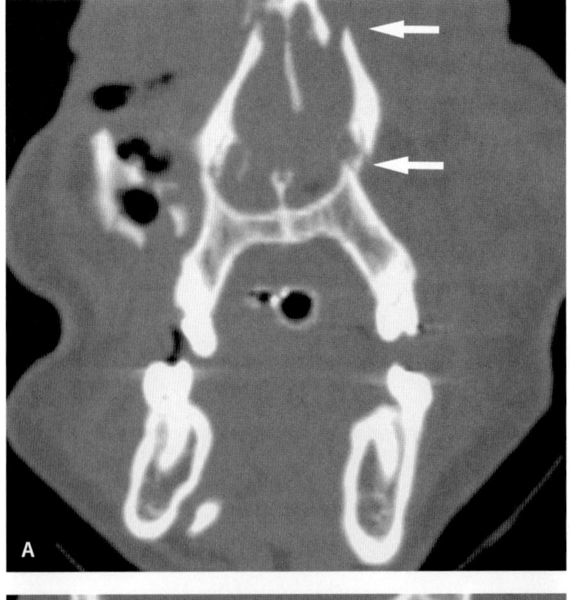

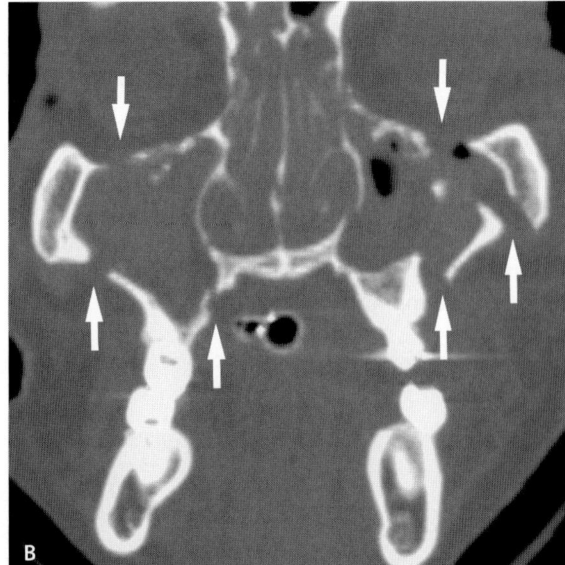

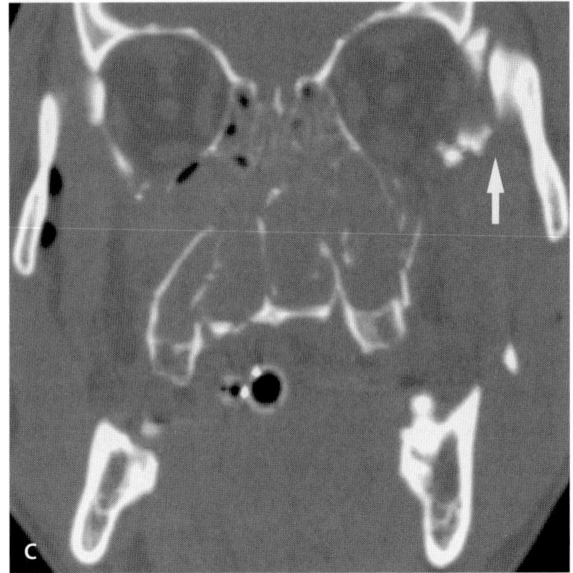

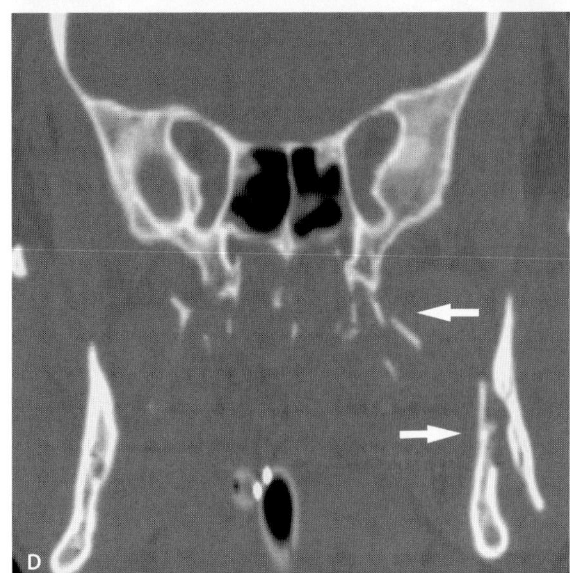

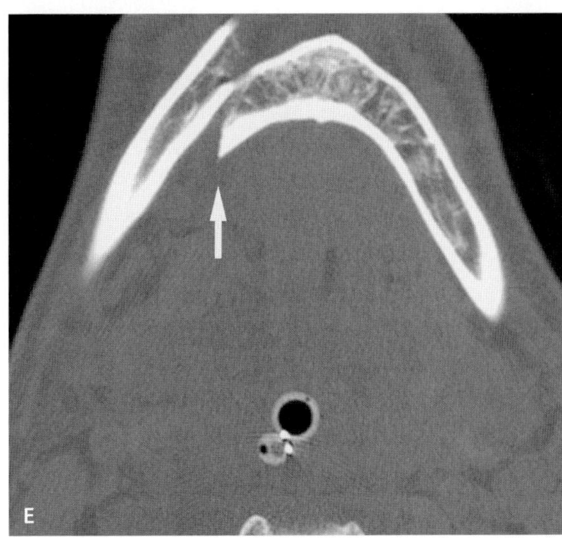

Figure 8.27

LeFort 3 and mandibular body fractures; 45-year-old male after motor vehicle crash with trauma to face and head, and loss of consciousness. **A** Coronal CT image shows bilateral fractures of superior nasal aperture near nasal bone and inferior nasal aperture above palate (*arrows*), opacification due to hemorrhage of nasal cavity, bone fragments and air collections in right cheek, and intratracheal tube. **B** Coronal CT image shows bilateral fractures of orbital floor and maxillary sinus wall (*arrows*), and opacification of nasal cavity and all sinuses except left frontal, due to hemorrhage. **C** Coronal CT image shows fracture of left lateral orbital wall (*arrow*), necessary for definition of a LeFort 3 fracture; zygomatic arch was also fractured. **D** Coronal CT image shows bilateral fractures of pterygoid plates (*arrow*) and left mandibular ramus (*arrow*). **E** Axial CT image shows fracture of right mandibular body (*arrow*)

Tripod Fracture

Synonyms: Trimalar or zygomatic fracture

Definition

Fracture through (1) lateral orbital wall with fracture site at zygomaticofrontal suture, (2) zygoma and maxilla with fracture site at zygomaticomaxillary suture, (3) zygomatic arch with fracture site at zygomaticotemporal suture.

Clinical Features

- Most common fracture of facial skeleton after nasal and mandibular fractures
- About half of all midfacial fractures (more than two-thirds in one study), either alone or in combination with other midfacial fractures
- Infraorbital nerve paresthesia or anesthesia in almost 95%

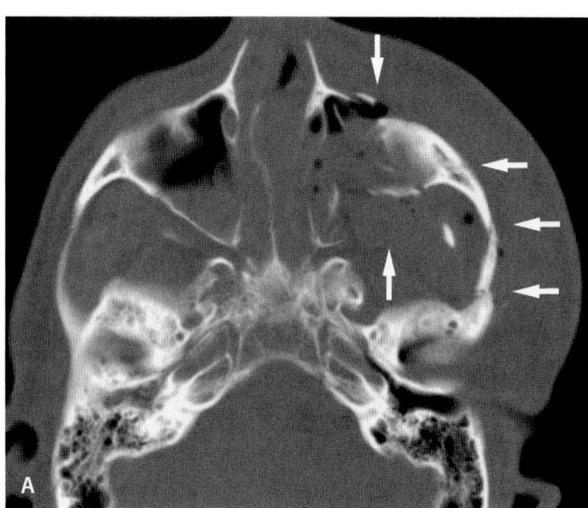

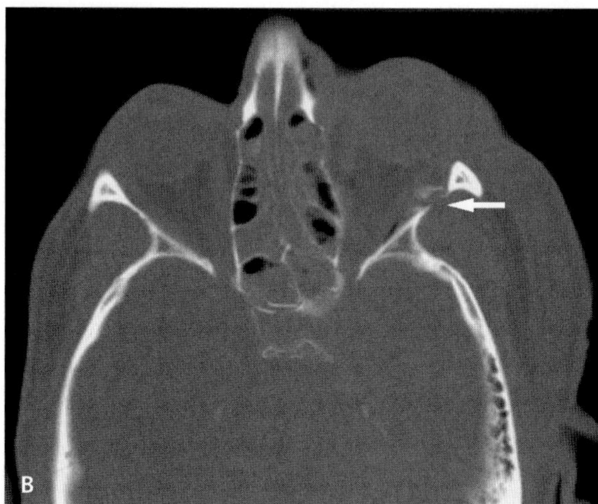

Figure 8.28

Tripod fracture, classic; 45-year-old and with facial trauma. A Axial CT image shows fractures of anterior maxillary sinus wall, lateral–posterior maxillary sinus wall and zygomatic arch (*arrows*), and intrasinus hemorrhage. B Axial CT image shows fracture of lateral orbital wall (*arrow*), hemorrhage in ethmoid cells, and swelling due to subcutaneous edema

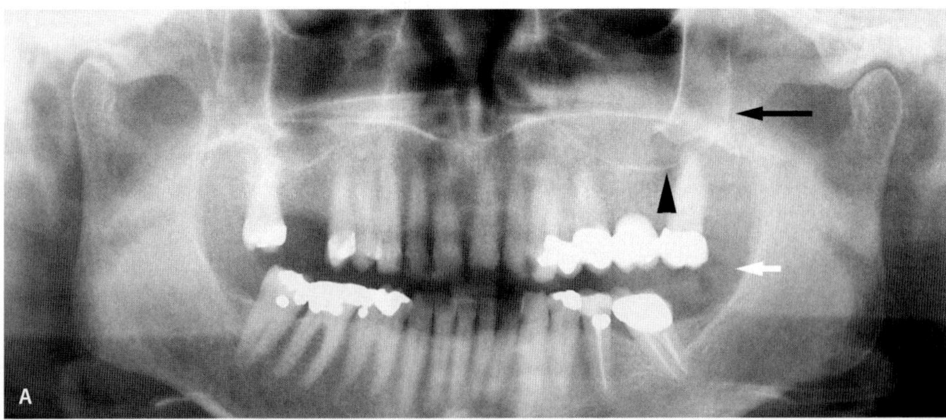

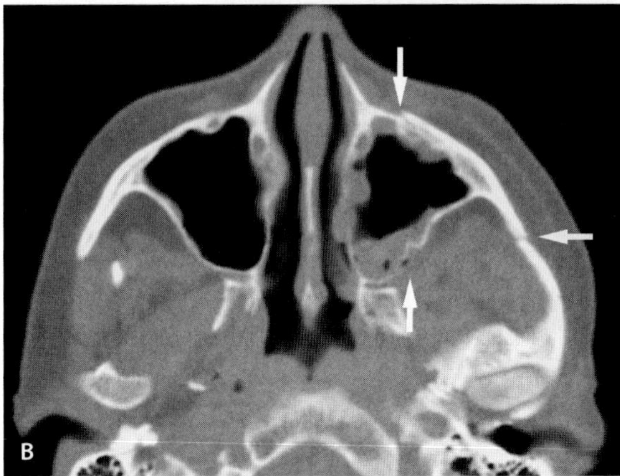

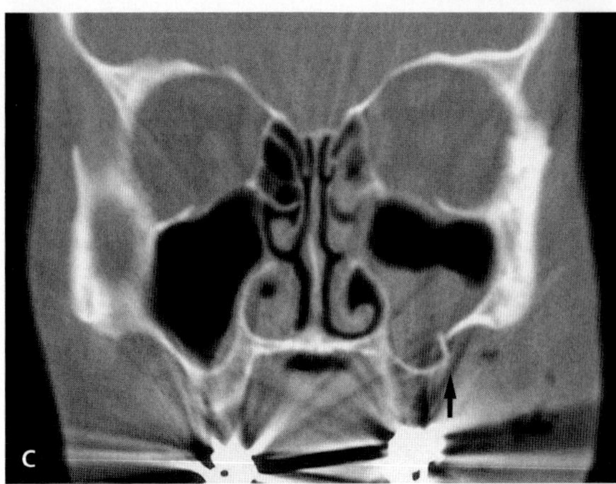

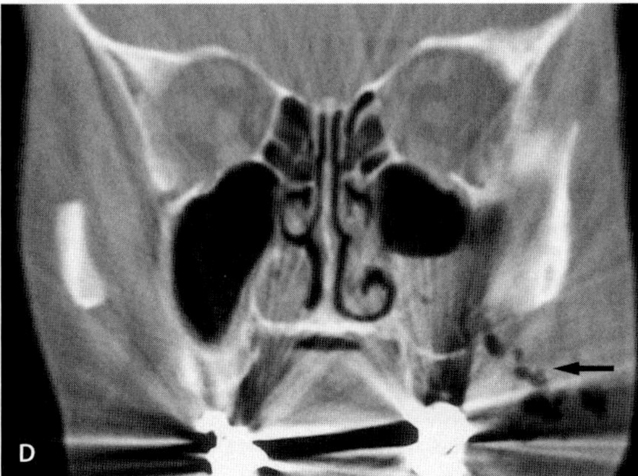

Figure 8.29

Tripod fracture, but no evident lateral orbital wall fracture; 70-year-old female with trauma to face 3 days previously. A Panoramic view shows opacification of left maxillary sinus (arrow) with abnormal structure (*arrow head*), and possibly some air collections (*white arrow*). B Axial CT image shows fractures of anterior maxillary sinus wall, lateral–posterior maxillary sinus wall and zygomatic arch (*arrows*). C Coronal CT image confirms comminuted fracture of lateral maxillary sinus wall (*arrow*) with soft-tissue swelling in sinus, probably blood clot. D Coronal CT image shows fluid-air level and collections of subcutaneous air close to destroyed maxillary sinus wall (*arrow*)

Blow-out Fracture

Definition

Fracture of orbital floor, usually not orbital rim (classic); but also of medial or other orbital walls.

Clinical Features

- Only 3–5% of all midfacial fractures
- Diplopia
- Enophthalmos, exophthalmos

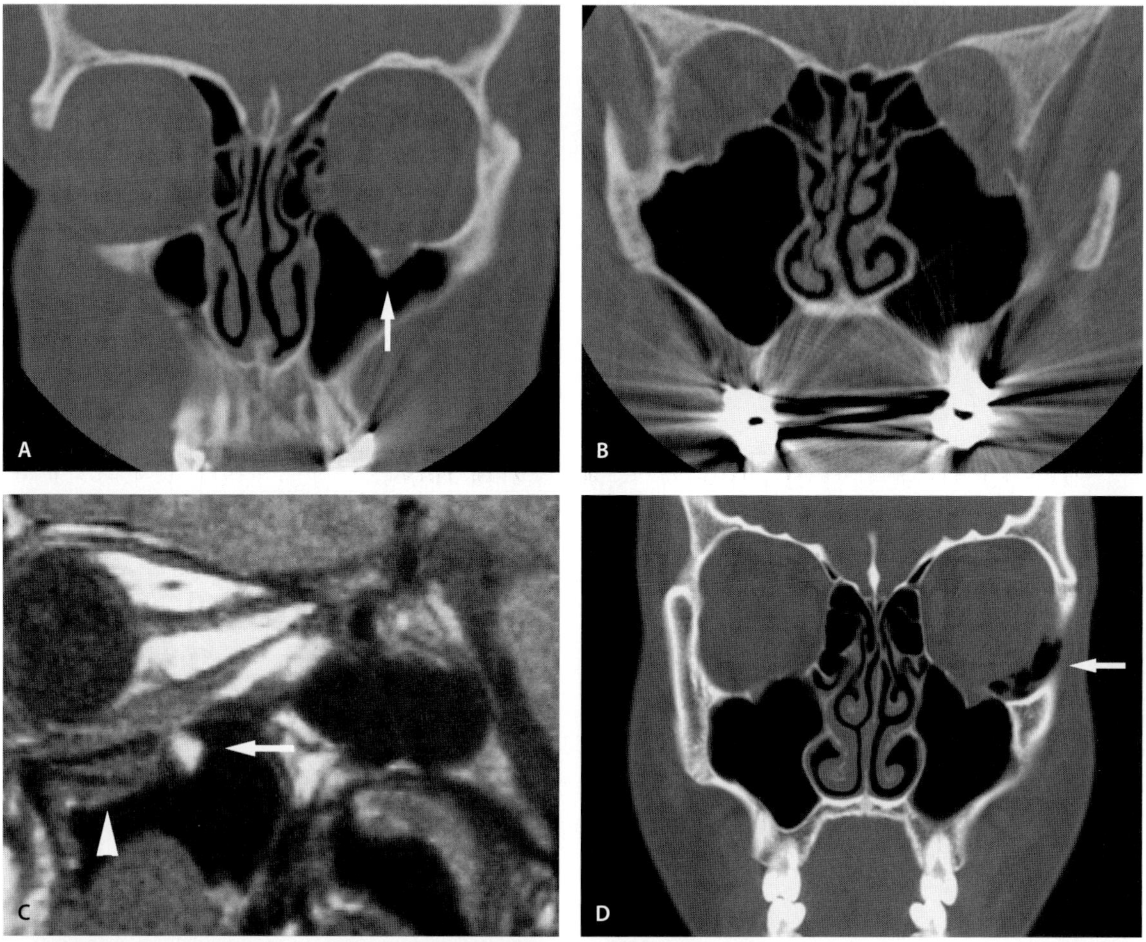

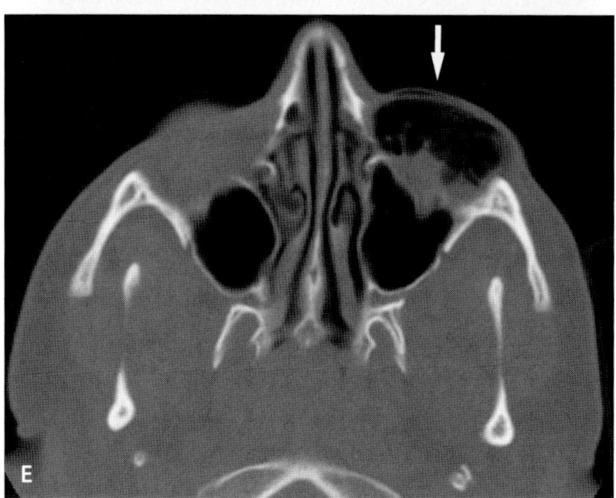

Figure 8.30

Blow-out fracture, classic; 60-year-old female with fall on face 10 days previously, with infra-orbital hematoma and some tenderness. **A** Coronal CT image shows fracture of orbital floor (*arrow*). **B** Coronal CT image, more posterior section, shows otherwise normal sinuses. **C** Sagittal MRI of another patient shows orbital fat (*arrow*), and bone fragment and mucosal swelling or muscle tissue (*arrowhead*) in maxillary sinus due to blow-out fracture; note intact orbital rim (courtesy of Dr. A. Kolbenstvedt, Rikshospitalet University Hospital, Oslo, Norway). **D** Coronal CT image of another patient shows orbital air collection (*arrow*). **E** Axial CT image of same patient as in **D** shows large subcutaneous emphysema (*arrow*)

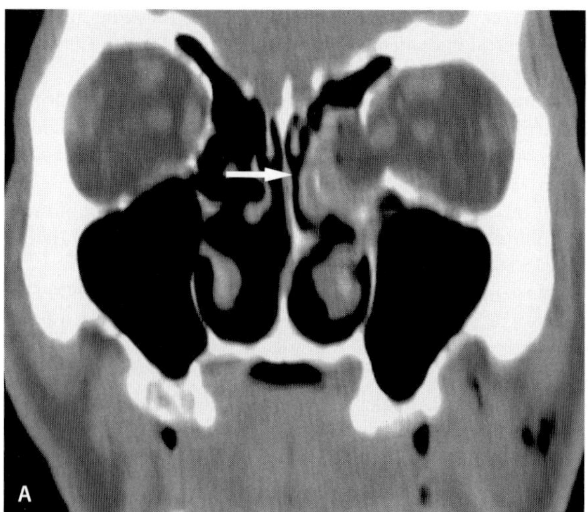

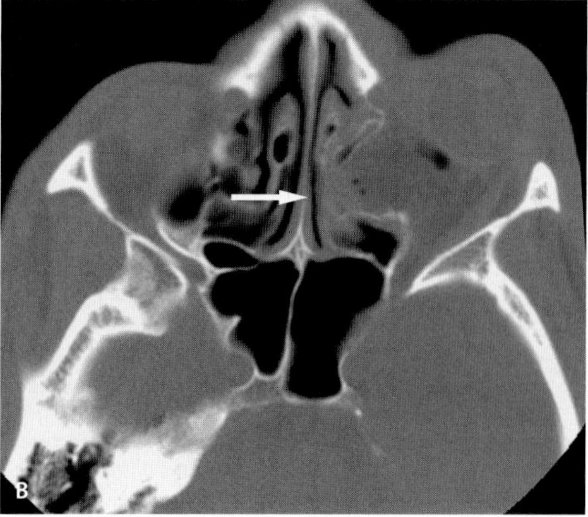

Figure 8.31

Blow-out fracture, medial; 54-year-old male who was struck by a car from behind. A Coronal CT image shows fracture of left medial orbital wall and soft tissue with periorbital fat in ethmoid cells (*arrow*). B Axial CT image shows fracture of lamina papyracea with opacification of left ethmoid cells (*arrow*), and air collection in orbit. Soft-tissue swelling over left periorbital area

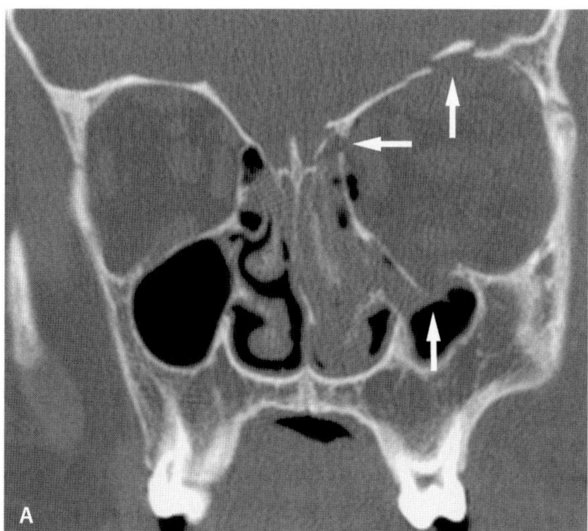

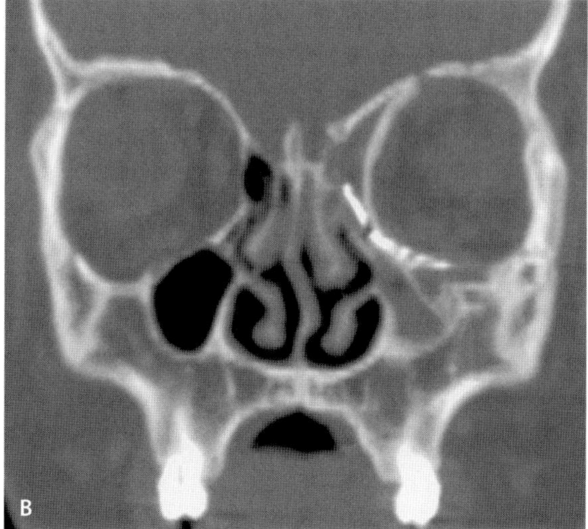

Figure 8.32

Blow-out fracture, extensive with fractures of maxillary wall and nasal bone; 15-year-old male with trauma to left face and eye; now to postoperative examination of bone graft from calvarial bone. A Coronal CT image shows fractures of left orbital floor, and medial and superior walls (*arrows*), some air collection in orbit, and soft-tissue swelling in ethmoid cells, nasal cavity and maxillary sinus. B Coronal CT image, postoperative, shows normal configuration of left orbit, with opacification of ethmoid cells and maxillary sinus

Suggested Reading

Adi M, Odgen GE, Chisholm DM (1990) An analysis of mandibular fractures in Dundee, Scotland. Br J Oral Maxillofac Surg 28:194–199

Arden RL, Crumley RL (1993) Cartilage grafts in open rhinoplasty. Facial Plast Surg 9:285–294

Chacon GE, Dawson KH, Myall RW, Beirne OR (2003) A comparative study of two imaging techniques for the diagnosis of condylar fractures in children. J Oral Maxillofac Surg 61:668–672

Cooke HE, Rowe M (1990) A retrospective study of 356 midfacial fractures occurring in 225 patients. J Oral Maxillofac Surg 48:574–578

Dolan KD, Ruprecht A (1992) Imaging of midfacial fractures. In: Westesson P-L (ed) Contemporary maxillofacial imaging. Oral and Maxillofacial Surgery Clinics of North America. Saunders, Philadelphia, pp 125–151

Farman AG, Nortje C, Wood RE (1993) Traumatic injuries. In: Oral and maxillofacial diagnostic imaging. Mosby, St. Louis, pp 158–180

Haug RH, Foss J (2000) Maxillofacial injuries in the pediatric patient – a review. Oral Surg Oral Med Oral Pathol Oral Radiol Endod 90:126–134

Heiland M, Schmelzle R, Hebecker A, Schulze D (2004) Intraoperative 3D imaging of the facial skeleton using the SIREMOBIL Iso-C3D. Dentomaxillofac Radiol 33:130–132

Henriksen LH, Trebo S (1988) Post-traumatic coronoid impingement on zygomatic arch: CT demonstration. J Comput Assist Tomogr 12:712–713

Honda K, Larheim TA, Johannessen S, Arai Y, Shinoda K, Westesson P-L (2001) Ortho cubic super-high resolution computed tomography: a new radiographic technique with application to the temporomandibular joint. Oral Surg Oral Med Oral Pathol Oral Radiol Endod 91:239–243

Kucik CJ, Clenney T, Phelan J (2004) Management of acute nasal fractures. Am Fam Physician 70:1315–1320

Lamphier J, Ziccardi V, Ruvo A, Janel M (2003) Complications of mandibular fractures in an urban teaching center. J Oral Maxillofac Surg 61:745–750

Rowe NL (1985) Maxillofacial injuries – current trends and techniques. Injury 16:513–525

Schwenzer N (1986) Corrective operations following primary surgical management of facial cleft patients (in German). Fortschr Kieferorthop 47:540–546

Schimming R, Eckelt U, Kittner T (1999) The value of coronal computer tomograms in fractures of the mandibular condyle process. Oral Surg Oral Med Oral Pathol Oral Radiol Endod 87:632–639

Schuknecht B, Graetz K (2005) Radiologic assessment of maxillofacial, mandibular, and skull base trauma. Eur J Radiol 15:560–568

Silvennoinen U, Iizuka T, Lindqvist C, Oikarinen K (1992) Different patterns of condylar fractures: an analysis of 382 patients in a 3-year period. J Oral Maxillofac Surg 50: 1032–1037

Silvennoinen U, Iizuka T, Oikarinen K, Lindqvist C (1994) Analysis of possible factors leading to problems after nonsurgical treatment of condylar fractures. J Oral Maxillofac Surg 52:793–799

Som PM, Brandwein MS (2003) Facial fractures and postoperative findings. In: Som PM, Curtin HD (eds) Head and neck imaging, 4th edn. Mosby, St. Louis, pp 374–438

Sullivan SM, Banghart PR, Anderson Q (1995) Magnetic resonance imaging assessment of acute soft tissue injuries to the temporomandibular joint. J Oral Maxillofac Surg 53:763–766

Smith PH (1967) Blow out fracture of the floor of the orbit. Aust N Z J Surg 36:319–322

Takahashi T, Ohtani M, Sano T, Ohnuki T, Kondoh T, Fukuda M (2004) Magnetic resonance evidence of joint effusion of the temporomandibular joint after fractures of the mandibular condyle: a preliminary report. Cranio 22:124–131

Tanaka H, Westesson PL, Larheim TA (1998) Juxta-articular ankylosis of the temporomandibular joint as an unusual cause of limitation of mouth opening: case report. J Oral Maxillofac Surg 56:243–246

White SW, Pharoah MJ (2004) Trauma to teeth and facial structures. In: Oral radiology. Principles and interpretation. Mosby, 5th edn. St. Louis, pp 574–587

Yanagisawa E, Smith HW (1973) Normal radiographic anatomy of the paranasal sinuses. Otolaryngol Clin North Am 6:429–457

Ziegler CM, Woertche R, Brief J, Hassfeld S (2002) Clinical indications for digital volume tomography in oral and maxillofacial surgery. Dentomaxillofac Radiol 31:126–130

Facial Growth Disturbances

In collaboration with S.I. Blaser · N. Kakimoto

Introduction

A number of growth disturbances may occur of the facial bones, of which some are rather frequent and may have an obvious impact on facial appearance and vital functions. Jaws and dentitions may be involved. Thus, such anomalies are of great interest to dental professionals.

Advanced imaging evaluation is necessary, and in particular 3D CT imaging is increasingly used to assess growth disturbances of this complicated anatomic region. The visualization of bone (and skin) morphology is superior to different series of 2D images although some detail is lost as part of the smoothing algorithm used. This chapter illustrates a number of cases, frequently with 3D CT images. A combination of 3D for overview with 2D images for bony details represents up-to-date imaging of facial growth disturbances.

Isolated Disturbances

Common Cleft Palate and/or Cleft Lip

Definition

Congenital defect involving lip only, lip and palate, or palate only.

Clinical Features

- Most common facial birth defect; cleft lip with or without cleft palate in about 1 per 1000 live births (range 0.7–1.3)
- More common in American Indians and Japanese and less common in blacks
- Almost 99% of all facial clefts
- Isolated cleft palate less frequent
- Most often unilateral
- Males more frequent than females in severe cases
- 50–70% of patients are nonsyndromic
- Part of more than 300 recognized entities
- Obvious esthetic and functional problems such as insufficient suction for feeding

Imaging Features (Bone Structures)

- Maxillary alveolar process split in lateral incisor region, either unilaterally or bilaterally
- Anterior hemimaxilla shows narrowed curvature and upward tilting of premaxillary segment on cleft side
- Palatal end of nasal septum on cleft side; anterior nasal spine on contralateral side in unilateral clefts
- Partial or complete bony defect with corticated margins of alveolar ridge and hard palate
- In newborns; premaxilla 'loosened' from remaining maxilla in bilateral cases
- Variable degrees of midfacial hypoplasia
- Teeth missing, deformed, displaced, or supernumerary

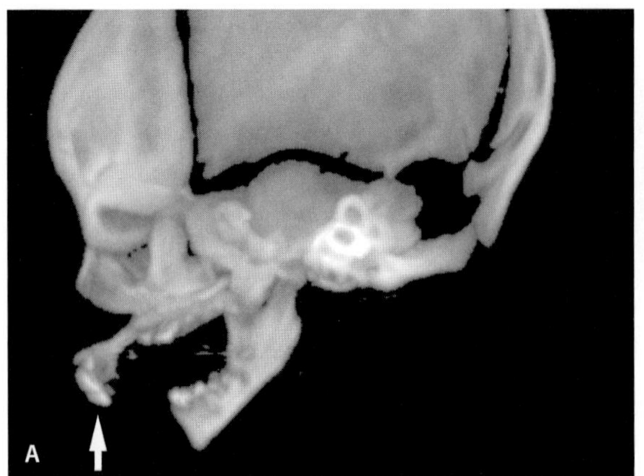

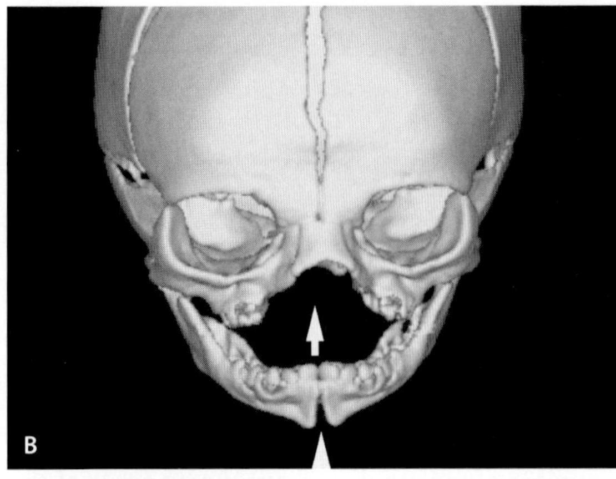

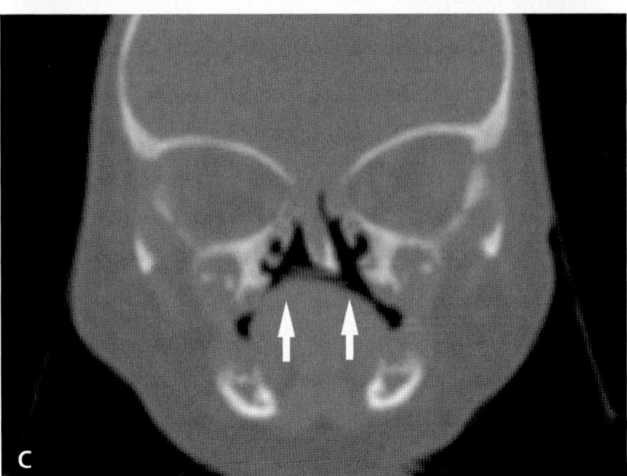

Figure 9.1

Cleft lip and palate, bilateral; 1-day-old male with multiple congenital anomalies (syndromic features). **A** Lateral CT scout image shows dislocation of premaxilla (*arrow*). **B** 3D CT image shows bilateral maxillary cleft (*arrow*) and mandibular midline cleft as well (*arrowhead*). Single nasal bone (which usually indicates intracranial abnormalities in patients with midline anomalies). **C** Coronal CT image shows bilateral maxillary cleft (*arrows*)

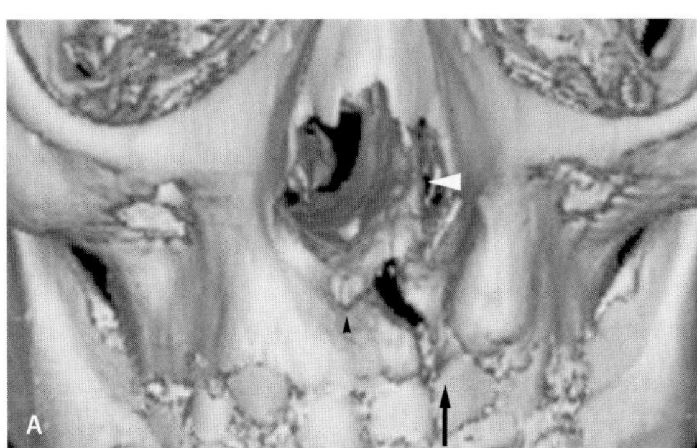

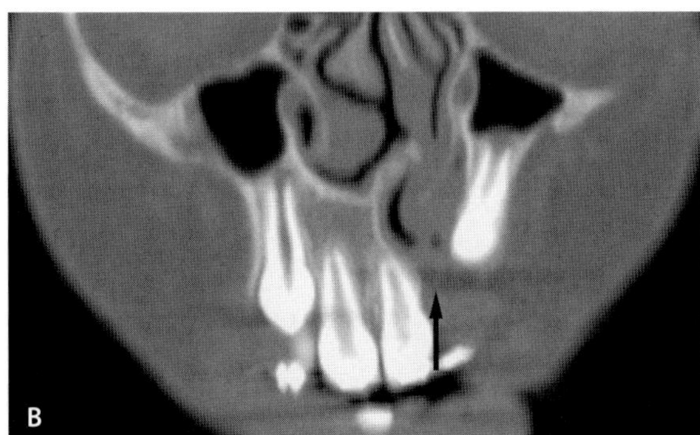

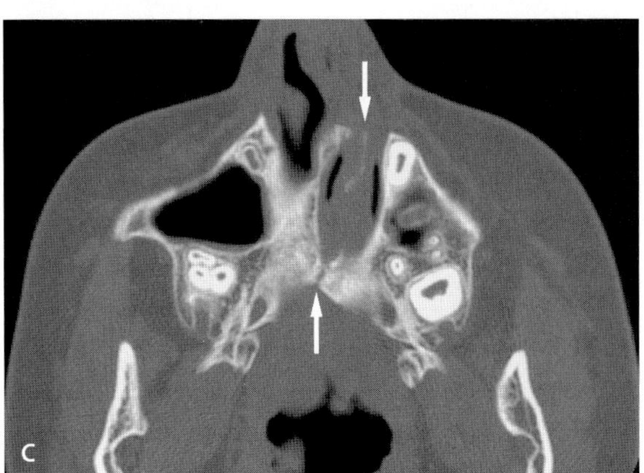

Figure 9.2

Cleft palate, unilateral; 11-year-old male with untreated deformity. **A** 3D CT image shows cleft on left side (*arrow*). Note nasal septum deviating to cleft side (*arrowhead*) and anterior nasal spina (*small arrowhead*) deviating to non-cleft side. **B** Coronal CT image shows cleft through alveolar process and nasal cavity (*arrow*). **C** Axial CT image shows that cleft is corticated and completely through palate (*arrows*)

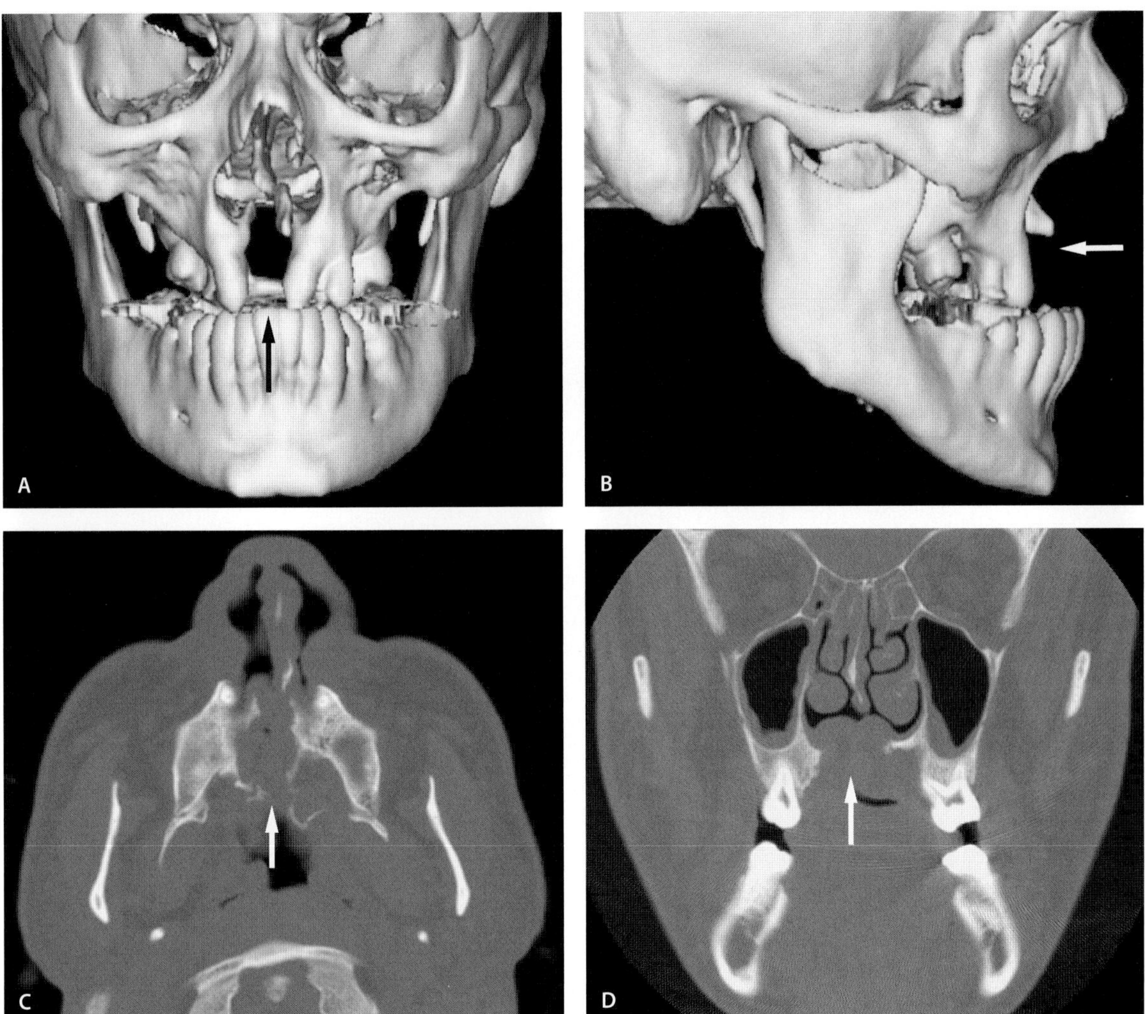

Figure 9.3

Cleft palate, midline; 31-year-old male with untreated deformity. **A** 3D CT image, en face view, shows almost symmetric cleft (*arrow*) with premaxillary segment and incisors absent. Narrow nasal bone. **B** 3D CT image, lateral view, shows hypoplastic maxilla (*arrow*). **C** Axial CT shows large, complete defect (*arrow*). **D** Coronal CT image shows soft-tissue lining to nasal cavity (*arrow*), mucosal thickening in ethmoid sinuses, and minimal mucosal thinning in maxillary sinuses

Choanal Atresia

Definition

Congenital anomaly of occluded posterior choana (either bony or membranous) with no communication between nasal cavity and nasopharynx on one or both sides.

Clinical Features

- Incidence about 1 per 5000 to 7000 births
- 20–50% of patients have other congenital anomalies such as cleft palate and a syndrome
- Males more frequent than females
- Present at birth with immediate respiratory distress, in particular if bilateral since neonates are obligate nose breathers and cannot feed because a patent nose is necessary to breathe during feeding
- Nasal stuffiness and mucoid discharge. Mucus in posterior nasal cavity can simulate a membrane

Imaging Features

- Bony plate (80–90%) or membranous web (10–20%) between vomer and lateral nasal wall
- Bony thickening of posterolateral nasal wall and posterior vomer; narrowing of posterior nasal cavity
- Two-thirds are unilateral

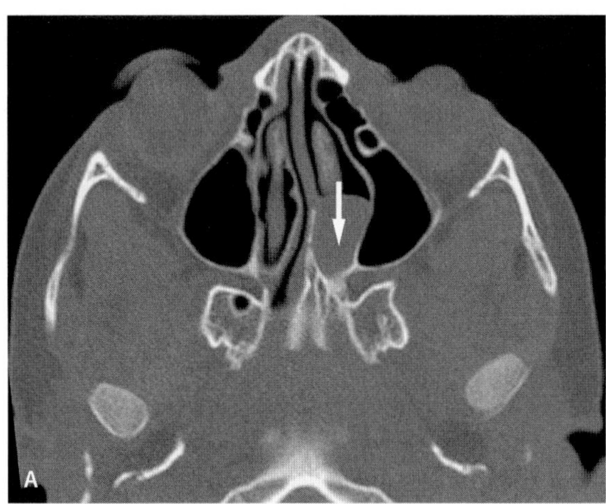

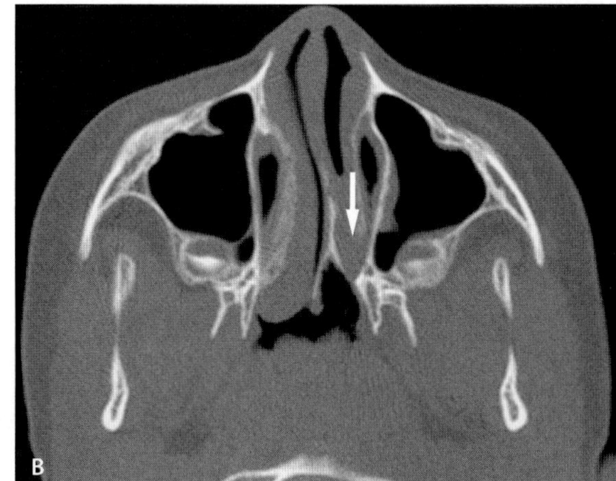

Figure 9.4

Choanal atresia; 7-year-old female presented with chronic left nasal obstruction. A Axial CT image shows bony plate between posterior vomer and posterior lateral nasal wall (*arrow*), and probable mucus plug in nasal cavity. B Axial CT image, more caudal section, shows a very thin bony plate (*arrow*)

Tori Palatinus, Maxillaris, and Mandibularis

Definition

Hyperostosis of normal cortical and medullary bone.

Clinical Features

- Torus palatinus: midline of hard palate along intermaxillary–interpalatine suture; nasal aspect of palate never affected
- Torus maxillaris: alveolar process either on buccal aspect (externus) or on palatal aspect (internus); frequently bilateral and usually in premolar area; single or multiple
- Torus mandibularis: alveolar process on lingual aspect in premolar area; frequently bilateral (80%); single or multiple

Torus palatinus:

- Found in at least 20% of a general US population
- Highly variable incidence in diverse ethnic populations; high in Amerindians and Alaskan Eskimos
- Inherited anomalies documented; 40–60% chance of occurrence with one or both affected parents compared with 5–8% chance with unaffected parents
- Only about 2% in newborns, increasing incidence with age
- Growth with individual up to 20–30 years; usually noticeable in adult age
- Females more frequent than males

See also Chapter 3.

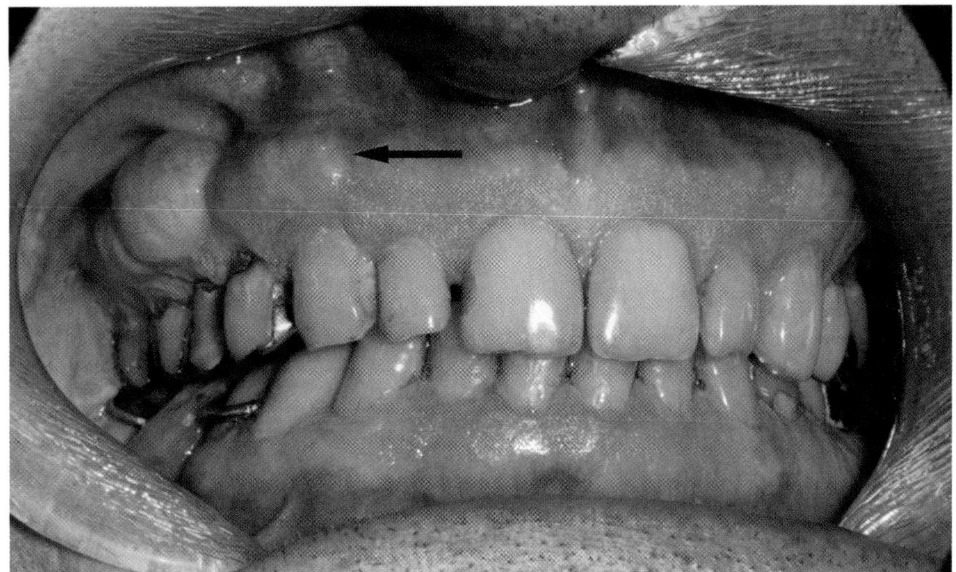

Figure 9.5

Tori maxillaris; 50-year-old male with incidental finding. Clinical photo shows multiple buccal exostoses of right maxilla (*arrow*), similar on left side (not shown)

Condylar Hyperplasia

Definition
Unilateral overgrowth of mandibular condyle.

Clinical Features
- Facial asymmetry; right or left side equally often
- Frequently noticeable in third decade
- Females more frequent than males
- Dental malocclusion

Imaging Features
- Unilaterally enlarged condyle in cranial direction
- Entire mandible on one side my also become enlarged; hemifacial hypertrophy (hyperplasia), which may be present at birth or later

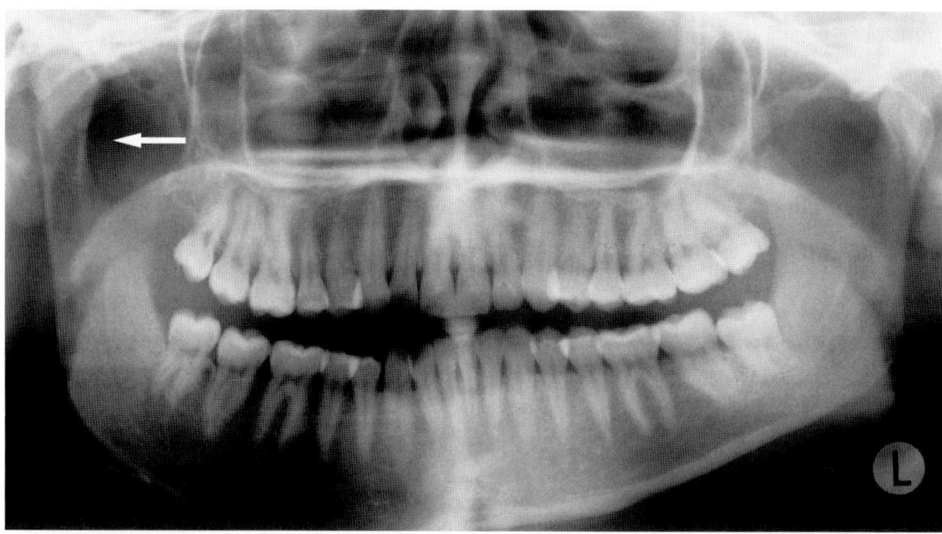

Figure 9.6

Condylar hyperplasia; 23-year-old female with facial asymmetry and dental malocclusion. Panoramic view shows enlarged right mandibular condyle and neck (*arrow*) as well as enlarged mandibular body (other images of this patient in Fig. 6.39)

Cherubism

Definition

Hereditary condition characterized by progressive bilateral swelling of mandibular angles during childhood, histopathologically similar to giant cell granuloma

Clinical Features

- Sporadic cases reported
- Usually detected during early childhood around 4 years of age
- Symmetric and painless, rarely unilateral
- Occasionally also maxilla; tuberosities
- No other parts of skeleton involved

Imaging Features

- Bilateral multilocular radiolucencies; jaw expansion may be extensive
- Displacement of mandibular canals
- Usually not condyle regions
- Displacement of teeth mesially, problematic eruption
- Premature exfoliation of primary teeth

See also Chapter 3.

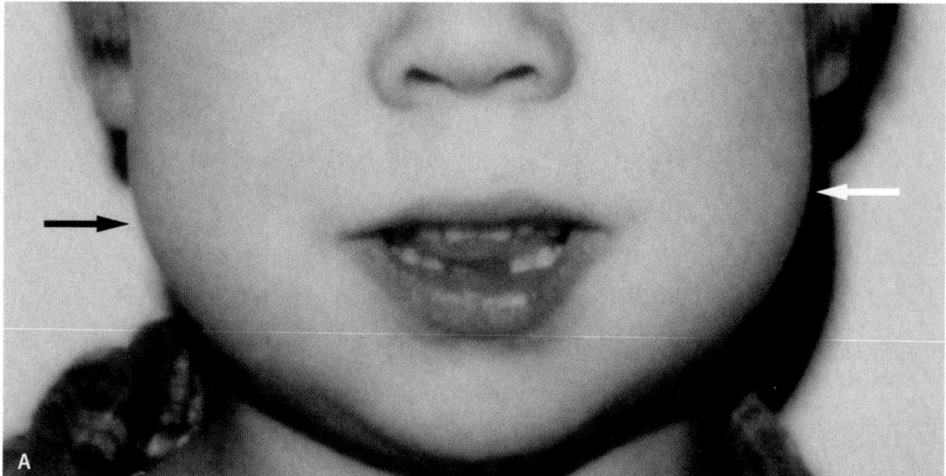

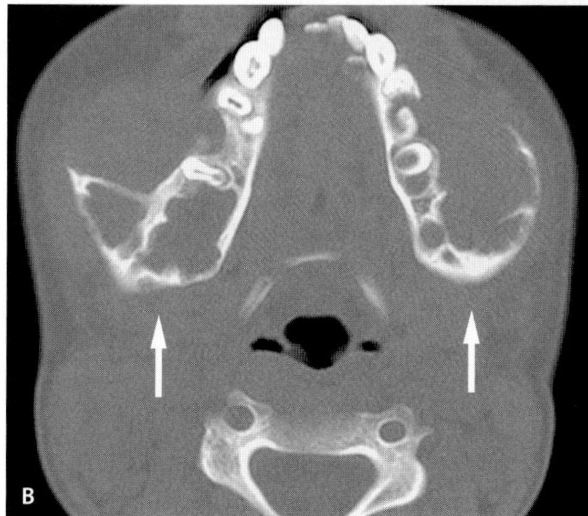

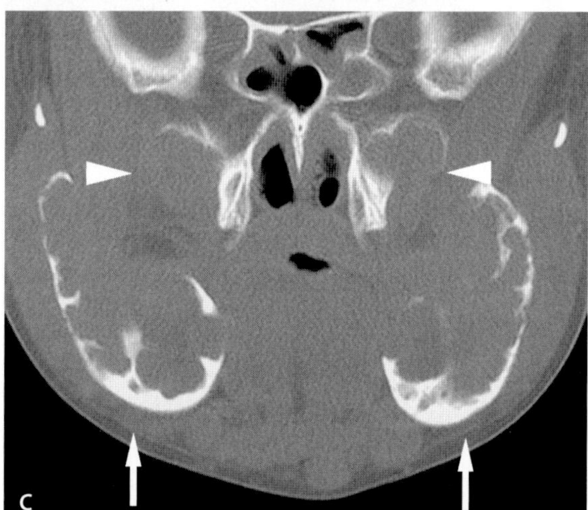

Figure 9.7

Cherubism; 6-year-old male with gradually increasing swelling of face and mandible bilaterally. **A** Clinical photograph shows bifacial swelling (*arrows*). **B** Axial CT image shows expanded jaw radiolucencies bilaterally (*arrows*). **C** Coronal CT image confirms bilateral jaw expansion (*arrows*). Note also bilateral expansion of maxilla (*arrowheads*)

Fibrous Dysplasia

Definition

Benign skeletal disorder; medullary bone replaced by metaplastic fibrous tissue.

Clinical Features

- Painless increasing bone deformity
- Most common benign skeletal disorder

Imaging Features

- Bone deformity may be extensive
- Radiolucent and/or radiopaque bone
- Ground-glass appearance characteristic; thick and sclerotic bone

See also Chapter 3.

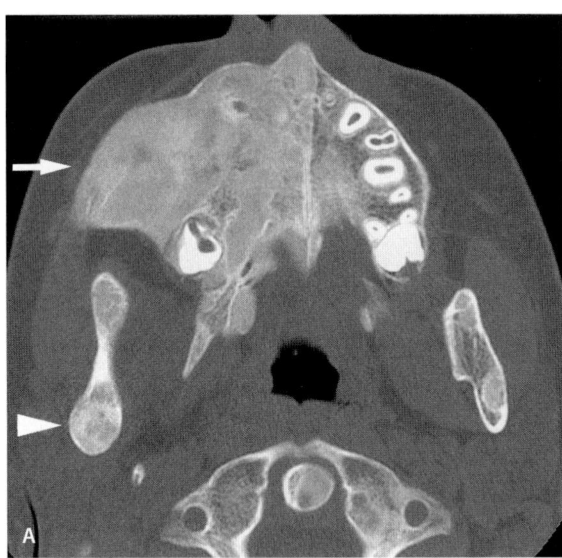

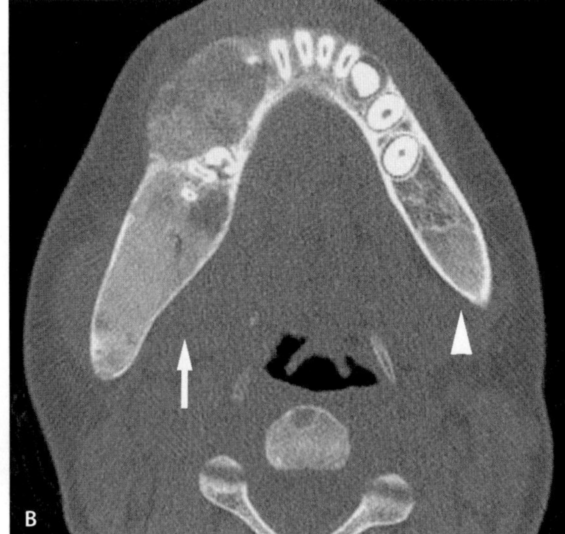

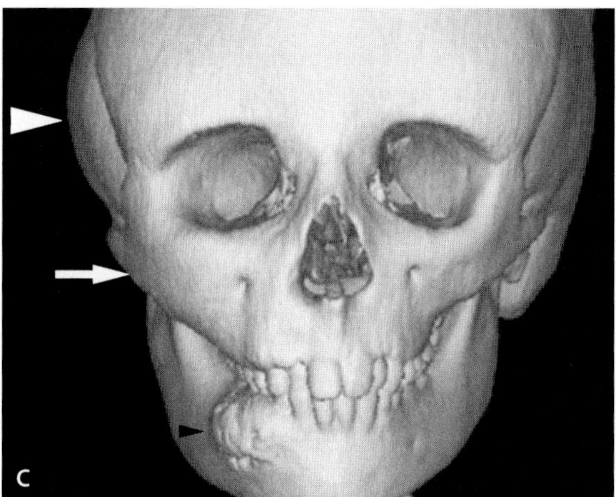

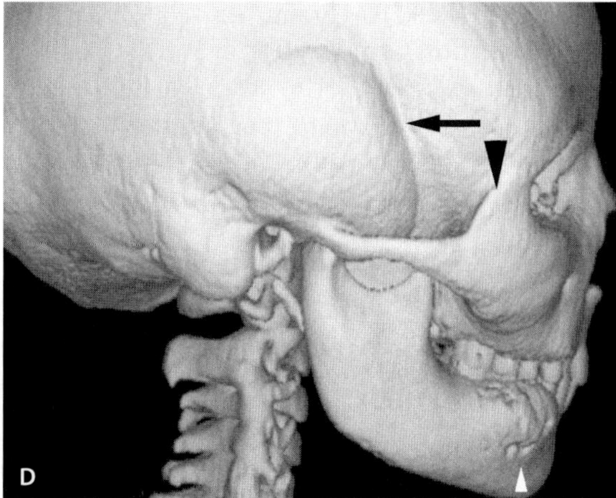

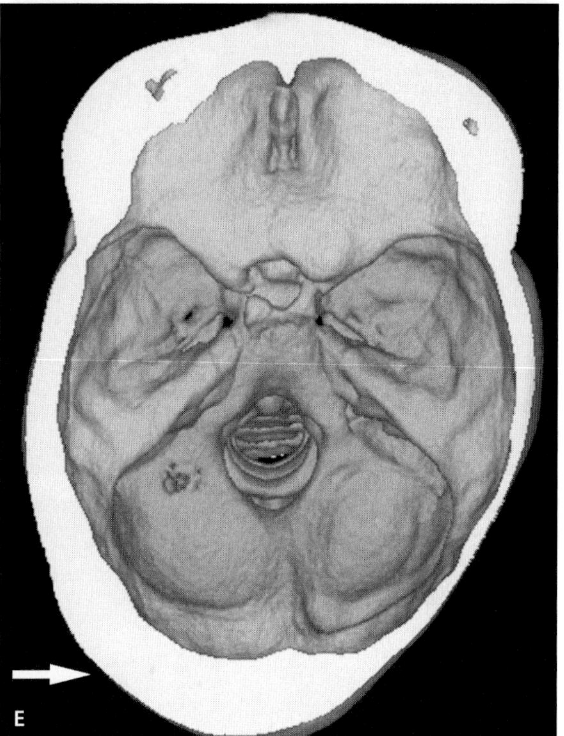

Figure 9.8

Craniofacial fibrous dysplasia; 11-year-old female with painless gradually increasing swelling of right face and mandible. **A** Axial CT image shows typical ground-glass appearance of evidently expanded right maxilla (*arrow*) and of right mandible (*arrowhead*). **B** Axial CT image shows ground-glass appearance of entire right mandibular body (*arrow*) and also in minor part of left mandible (*arrowhead*). **C** 3D CT image, en face view, shows evident growth deformity of right maxilla and zygoma (*arrow*), right temporal bone (*arrowhead*), and right mandible (*small arrowhead*). **D** 3D CT image, right side, shows growth deformity of temporal bone (*arrow*), zygoma (*arrowhead*), and mandible (*small arrowhead*). **E** 3D CT image, axial view, shows growth deformity of left occiput (*arrow*)

Mandibular Neck/TMJ Fracture or TMJ Infection Complication

Fractures or infections may lead to growth disturbances when they occur in younger patients and are not treated properly; in adults fractures may lead to dental occlusion problems such as open bite (see Fig. 8.19) or restricted mouth opening capacity due to contact between coronoid process and fractured zygomatic arch.

Clinical Features

- Micrognathic growth; bilateral complication
- Mandibular asymmetric growth; unilateral complication
- Dental malocclusion
- Variable restricted mouth opening capacity
- Deviation of mandible on opening

Imaging Features

- TMJ deformity or fibro-osseous ankylosis (see Fig. 8.21)

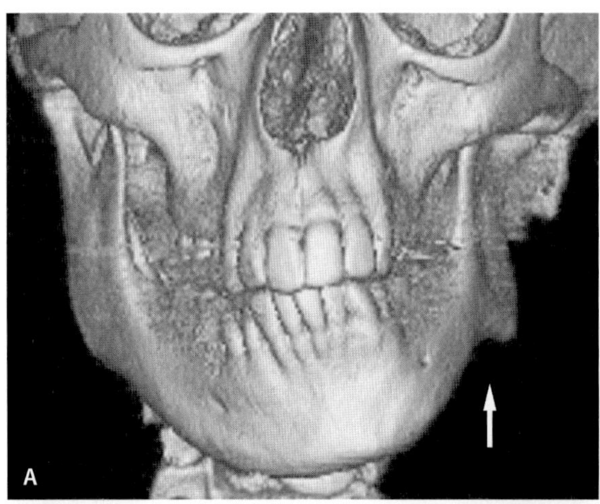

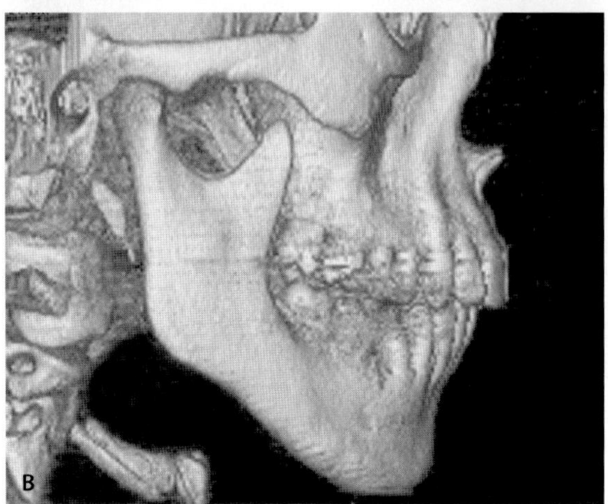

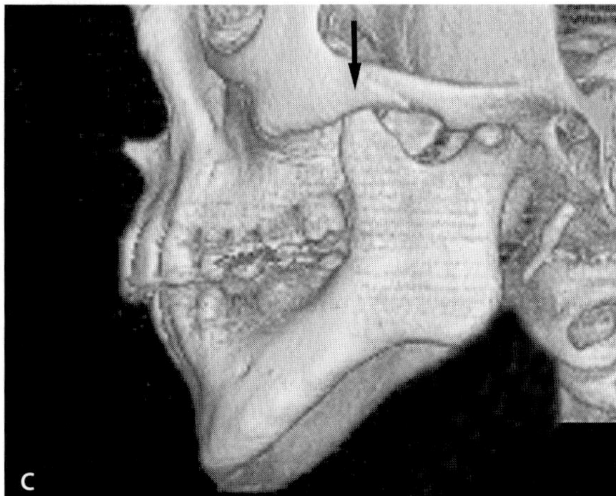

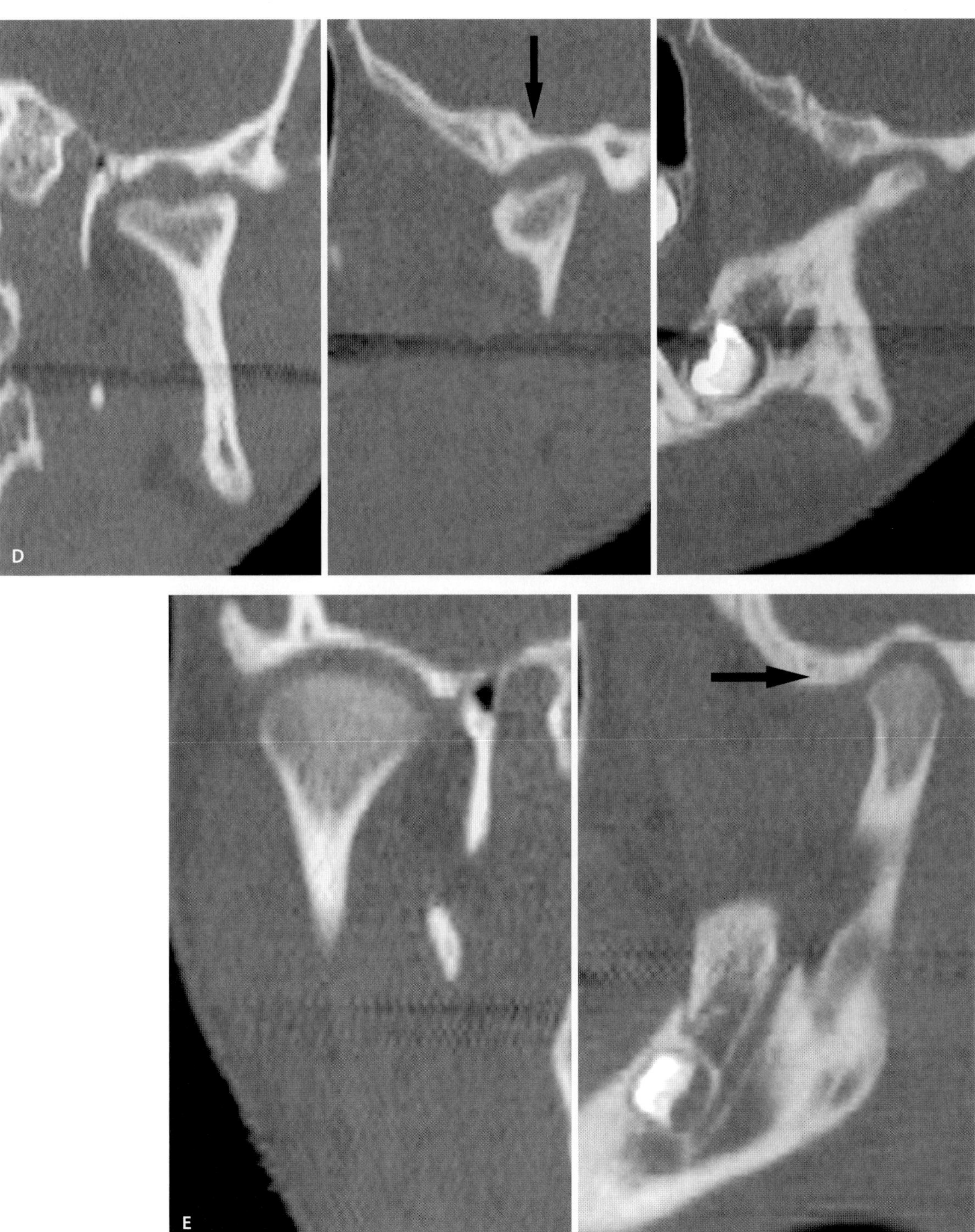

Figure 9.9

Facial asymmetry; 15-year-old male with previous trauma to mandible. **A** 3D CT image, en face view, shows evident mandibular asymmetry with antegonial notching (*arrow*) of abnormal side. **B** 3D CT image, lateral view, shows normally developed right mandible. **C** 3D CT image, lateral view, shows underdeveloped left mandible. Note large coronoid process (*arrow*) compared to contralateral normal side. **D** Oblique coronal CT image, mid-condyle section (*left*), oblique sagittal CT image, mid-condyle section (*central*), and oblique sagittal CT image, lateral section (*right*) of left TMJ shows deformed condyle and fossa; flattened with cortical irregularities (*arrow*). **E** Oblique coronal CT image, mid-condyle section (*left*) and oblique sagittal CT image, mid-condyle section (*right*) of right TMJ show normal bone and well-developed fossa (*arrow*)

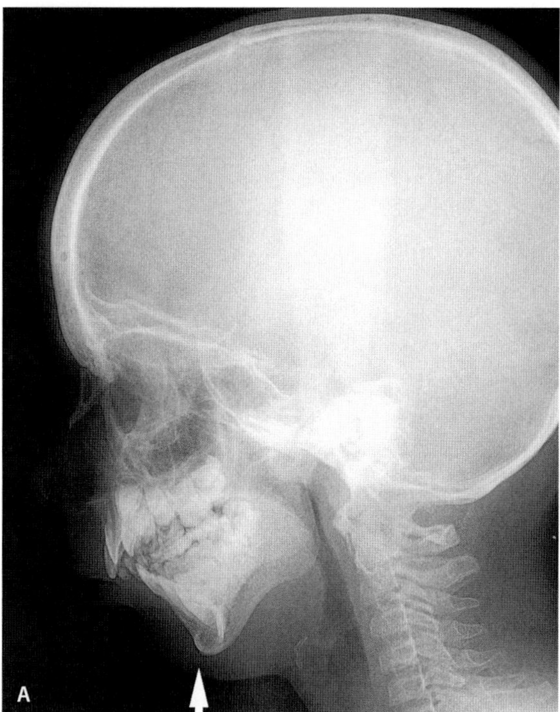

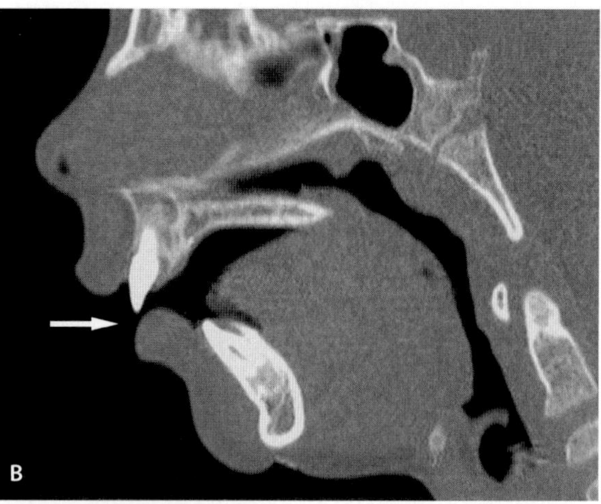

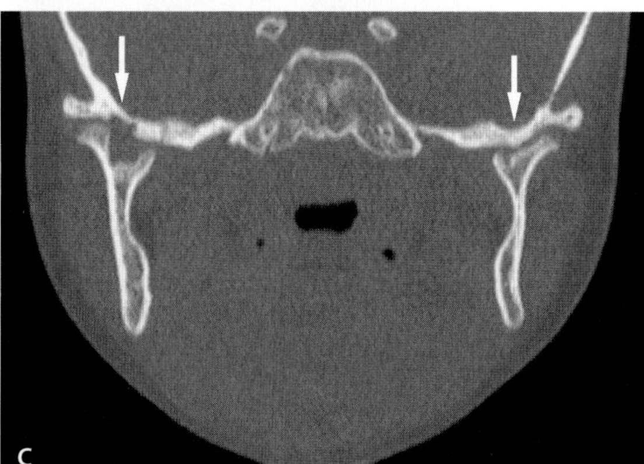

Figure 9.10

Mandibular underdevelopment; 7-year-old male with history of septic arthritis at birth with subsequent - osteomyelitis and surgery of hips, now with gradually inhibited mandibular growth and mouth opening capacity (27 mm). **A** Lateral view shows mandibular retrognathia (*arrow*) with some asymmetry. **B** Sagittal CT image shows severe dental malocclusion (*arrow*). **C** Coronal CT image shows bilaterally deformed TMJs but no ankyloses (*arrows*)

TMJ Internal Derangement Complication

There is evidence that anterior disc displacement with accompanying joint abnormalities (but without fractures) in younger age groups may have an impact on mandibular growth.

See Figs. 6.40, 6.41, and 8.20.

Systemic Disease

Juvenile Idiopathic (Rheumatoid/Chronic) Arthritis

Definition

Inflammatory synovial disease that attacks children before 16 years of age.

Clinical Features

- Micrognathia, but compensatory growth of anterior part of mandible
- Facial asymmetry
- More frequent in those with early onset and polyarticular disease; in particular with a disease course from pauciarticular (four or fewer joints) to polyarticular (five or more joints)
- Females more frequent than males

Imaging Features

- TMJ abnormalities; bilateral in micrognathia cases
- Unilateral TMJ abnormalities, or more severe on one side, in mandibular asymmetry cases
- Abnormal condyle; hypoplastic, flat
- Abnormal fossa; flat

See also Chapter 6.

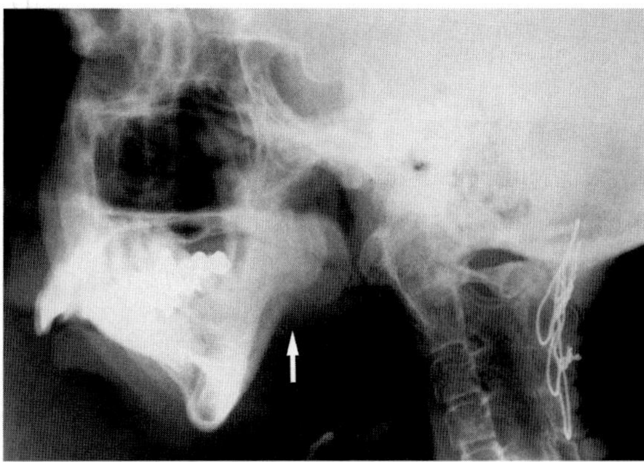

Figure 9.11

Micrognathia; 28-year-old female with juvenile idiopathic arthritis presenting before the age of 4 years and now with severe bilateral TMJ abnormalities. Lateral view shows severely underdeveloped mandible with bilateral notching (*arrow*). Note atlantoaxial dislocation and bony ankylosis of cervical spine, and surgical fixation of spine to skull

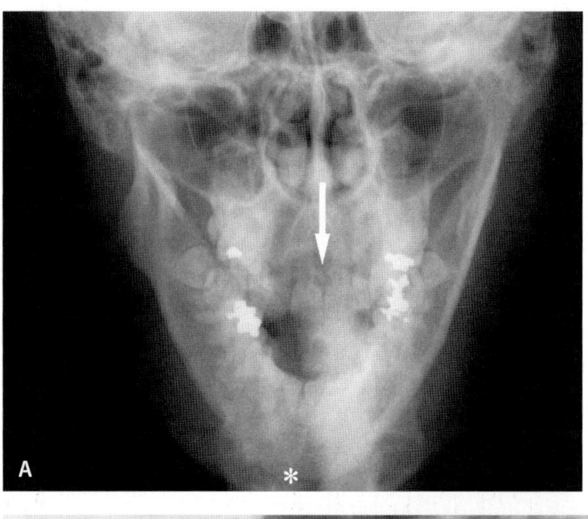

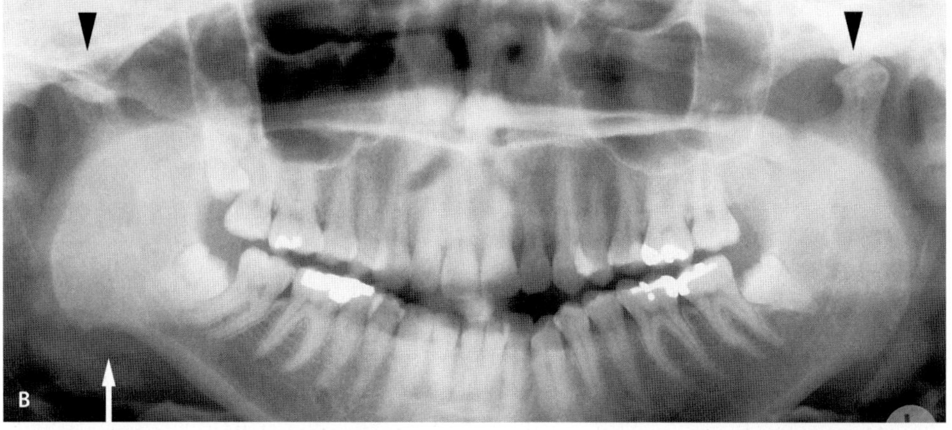

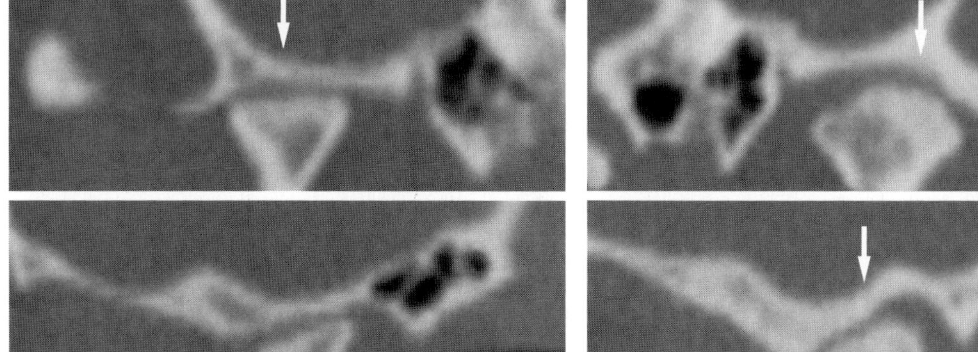

Figure 9.12

Retrognathia, slight micrognathia and facial asymmetry; 35-year-old female with juvenile idiopathic arthritis from early childhood. **A** Posteroanterior view shows asymmetric mandible (*asterisk* midpoint of chin) with deviation to right side on mouth opening (*arrow* midline of maxilla). **B** Panoramic view shows mandibular asymmetry with most underdevelopment and antegonial notching (*arrow*) on right side and bilateral condyle abnormalities (*arrowheads*) with most severe abnormalities of right joint. **C** CT images, oblique coronal (*upper*) and oblique sagittal (*lower*) views of the right TMJ show deformed, flattened condyle and fossa with cortical (irregular) outline (*arrow*). **D** CT image, oblique coronal (*upper*) and oblique sagittal (*lower*) views of the left TMJ show deformed condyle and fossa, but less pronounced than in the contralateral joint. Note also sclerosis both in condyle and fossa (*arrows*), indicating secondary osteoarthritis

Syndromes

A number of syndromes may have facial growth disturbances as part of their anomalies.

Down Syndrome

Clinical Features

- Most common genetic syndrome; incidence about 1 per 650 live births, but highly variable in different populations (1/600–1/2000)
- High association with increased maternal age
- Muscular hypotonia, large tongue
- Hyperextensibility of joints
- Short stature
- Cardiovascular anomalies
- Mental retardation
- Flattened facial profile and occiput
- Hypodontia
- Airway and hearing problems
- Average life expectancy less than half normal

Imaging Features

- Midfacial hypoplasia
- Flattened nose bridge
- Maxillary sinus hypoplasia; absent frontal and sphenoid sinuses
- Relative mandibular prognathism
- Ear abnormalities
- Atlantoaxial dislocation

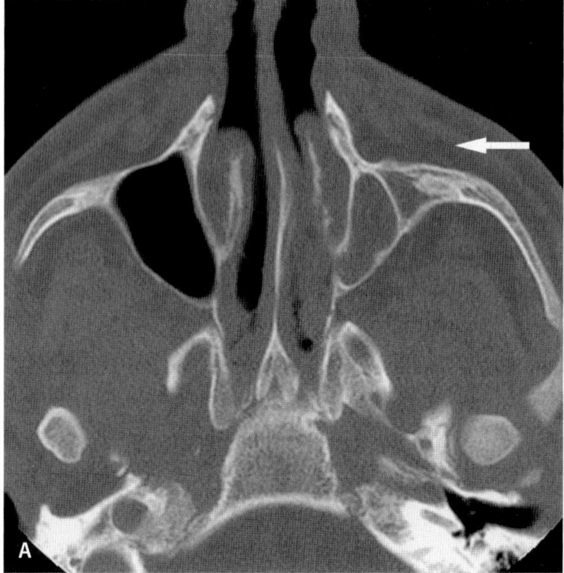

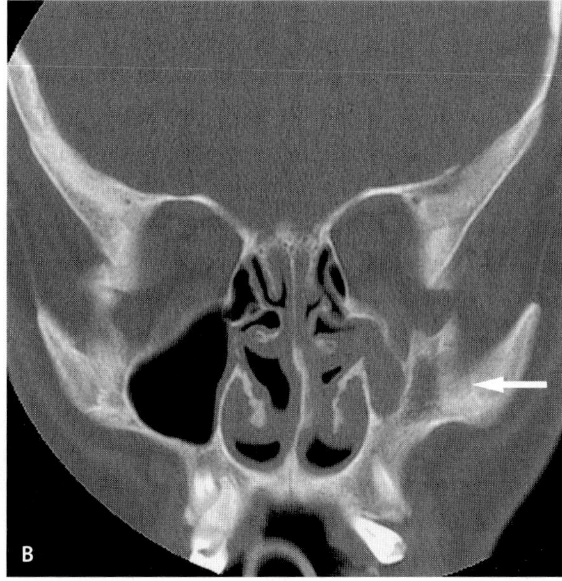

Figure 9.13

Down syndrome; 16-year-old. A Axial CT image shows hypoplastic, retruded left maxilla (*arrow*). B Coronal CT image shows hypoplastic left maxillary sinus (*arrow*)

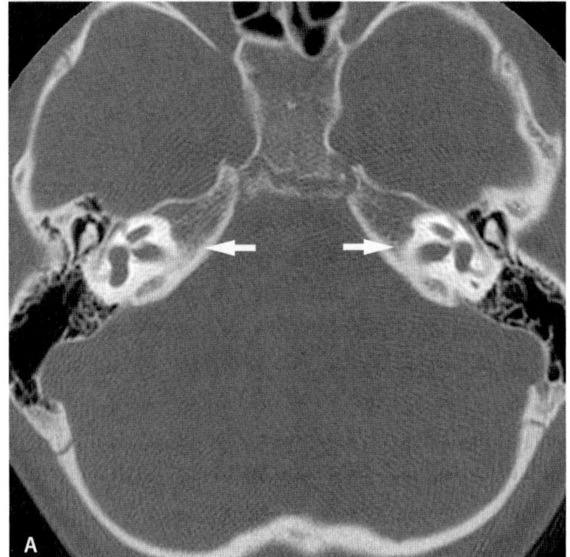

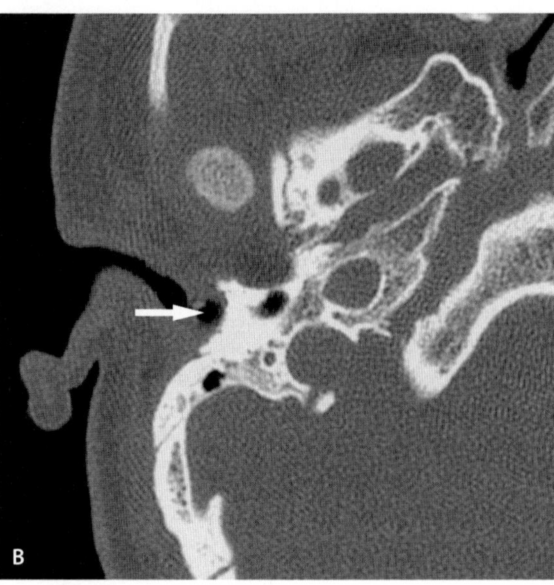

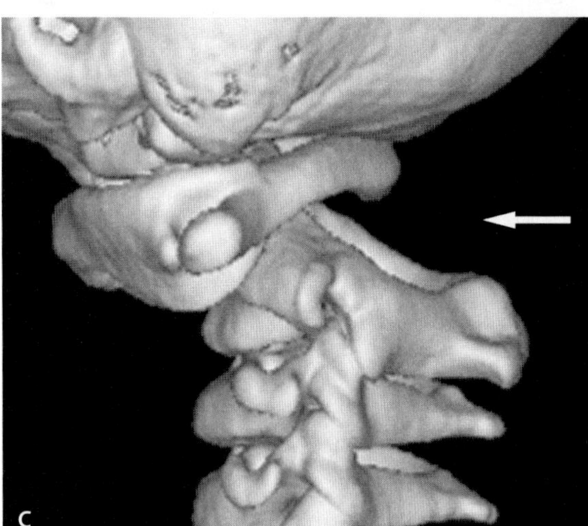

Figure 9.14

Down syndrome; 4-year-old. **A** Axial CT image shows vestibular dysplasia (*arrows*). **B** Axial CT image shows stenosis of external auditory canal (*arrow*). **C** 3D CT image shows C1–C2 dislocation (*arrow*)

Premature Cranial Synostoses

Definition

Premature fusion of one or more cranial sutures resulting in abnormal skull shape.

Clinical Features

- Estimated incidence up to 1 per 2000 live births
- Mostly isolated (85%)
- Classic types: scaphocephaly, plagiocephaly (anterior or posterior), brachycephaly, trigonocephaly, oxycephaly (turricephaly), cloverleaf skull
- Only 15% syndromic (see Syndromic Craniosynostoses)

Imaging Features

- Premature cranial suture closure; sagittal synostosis (scaphocephaly) and unilateral coronal synostosis (plagiocephaly) most frequent
- Cranial deformity of variable degree

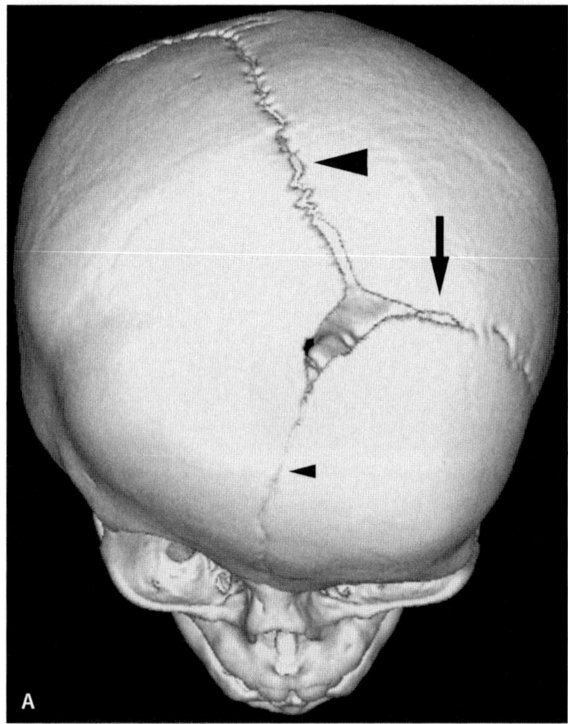

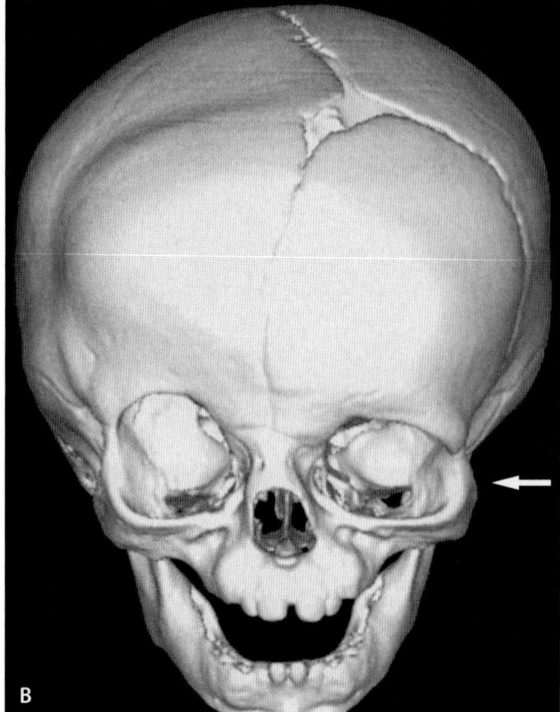

Figure 9.15

Premature unilateral synostosis, 7-month-old male. **A** 3D CT image shows closure of right side of coronal suture but left side open (*arrow*), as is sagittal suture (*large arrowhead*). Anterior fontanelle open and metopic suture closed but can be seen (*small arrowhead*). Asymmetric deformity of anterior part of head. **B** 3D CT image shows evident asymmetry of right and left orbita (*arrow*) due to the abnormal growth

Non-synostotic Occipital Plagiocephaly

Definition

Traditionally occipital plagiocephaly has been associated with lambdoid craniosynostosis, but when the American Academy of Pediatricians in 1992 suggested supine sleeping position for neonates, the incidence of "occipital plagiocephaly" increased dramatically. The majority of these cases were, however, not associated with true craniosynostosis caused by premature closure of the lambdoid, but rather were secondary to unilateral head position during sleep.

Clinical Features

- Positional molding
- Deformational plagiocephaly; flat asymmetric head
- Patent lambdoid suture
- Treatment not surgical, rather molding of head with helmets and changing sleeping position

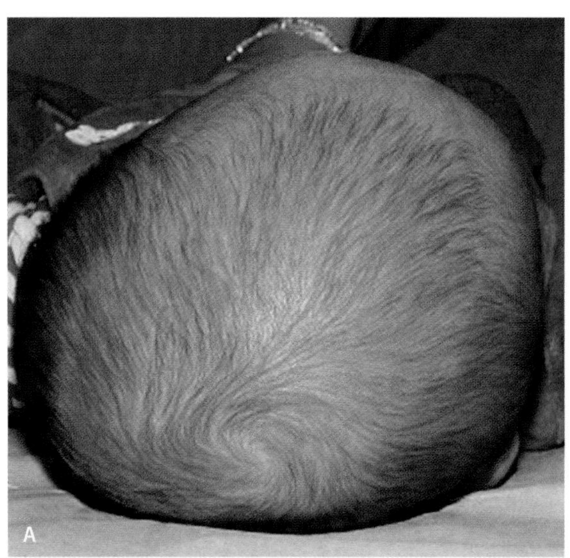

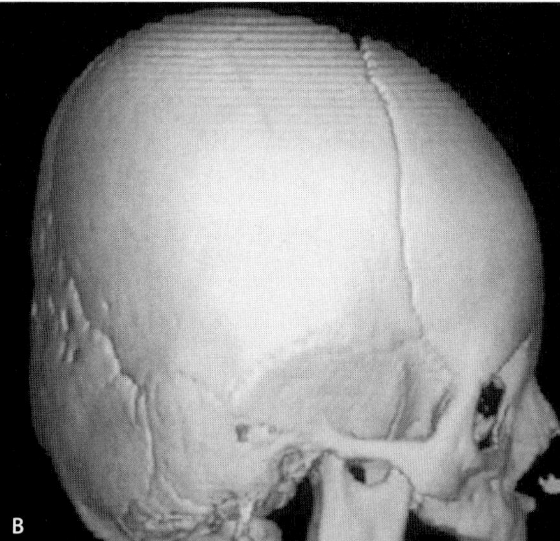

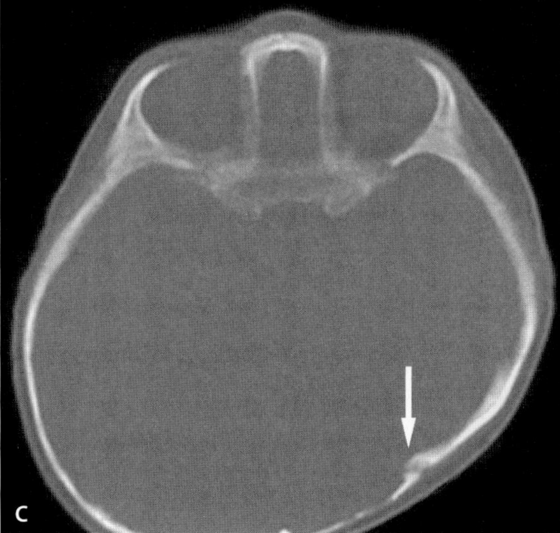

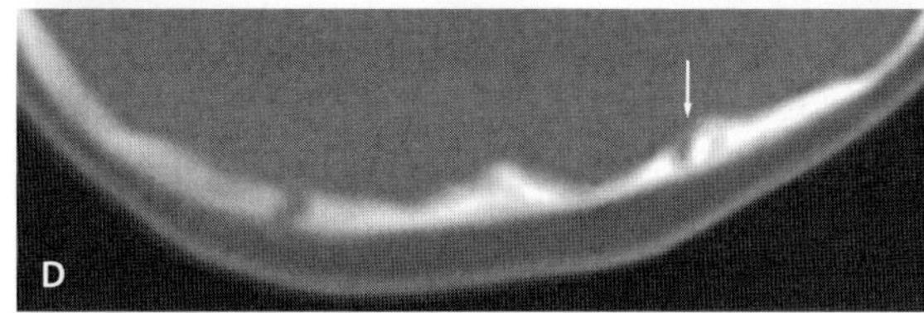

Figure 9.16

Occipital plagiocephaly unrelated to craniosynostosis; patent lambdoid suture. **A** Baby sleeping supine on one side. **B** 3D CT image shows flat head. **C** Axial CT image shows patent suture (*arrow*) but left occipital plagiocephaly. **D** Axial CT image shows complete closure of lambdoid suture (*arrow*) representing true lambdoid craniosynostosis from different patient for comparison

Turner Syndrome

Clinical Features

- Incidence about 1 per 2500 live female births
- Sex chromosome anomaly; only females
- Short stature
- Webbed neck
- Absent secondary sex characteristics
- Heart defects
- Mental deficiency; not consistently
- High palate
- Hypertelorism

Imaging Features

- Facial retrognathism
- Small mandible
- Delayed fusion of epiphyses
- Hypoplasia of odontoid process of C2
- Short metacarpals

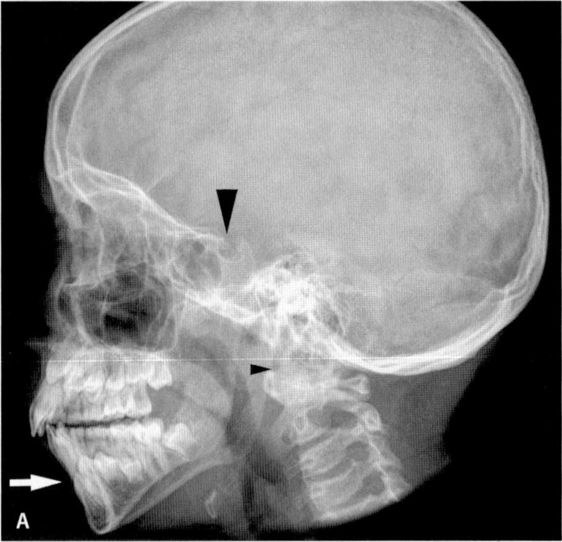

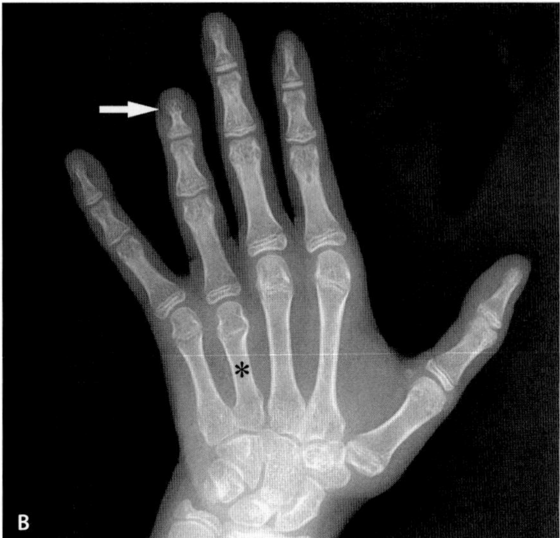

Figure 9.17

Turner syndrome; 10-year-old. **A** Lateral view shows facial retrognathism (*arrow*), bridged sella (*large arrowhead*) and odontoid hypoplasia (*small arrowhead*). **B** Hand view shows shortening of the fourth finger due to short fourth metacarpal bone (*asterisk*), drumstick distal phalanges; slender shaft and large distal heads (*arrow*), phalangeal predominance (proximal phalanges dominate over metacarpals in length)

Goldenhar Oculoauriculovertebral (OAV) Spectrum

Definition

Heterogeneous and complex group of overlapping conditions with ocular, auricular, vertebral and facial anomalies from first and second branchial arches; Goldenhar first described the triad of ocular, auricular, and mandibulofacial dysostosis in 1952, today known as Goldenhar syndrome. Later, cases with vertebral anomalies, as well as unilateral facial hypoplasia, previously named hemifacial microsomia, have been included in the expanded OAV complex. Up to about 80% of OAV complex cases are sporadic. Extreme variability of expression is characteristic.

Goldenhar Syndrome

Clinical Features

- Unilateral facial hypoplasia
- Ear anomalies; external and middle ear frequent, inner ear at least 6%
- Seven nerve palsy frequent
- Eye anomalies; dermoid of eyeball, coloboma (vertical fissure of eyelid)
- Variable vertebral anomalies may occur

Hemifacial Microsomia

Clinical Features

- Second most common facial birth defect after cleft palate/lip; about 1 per 5000 live births, but variable frequencies reported
- Males more frequent than females
- Most frequent syndrome from first and second branchial arches
- May not be appreciable in infancy; usually evident by the age of about 4 years
- Facial asymmetry and ear anomalies are characteristic
- Right side facial underdevelopment more frequent than left side
- Skin tags between ear and corner of mouth
- Seven nerve palsy frequent
- Dental malocclusion, hypodontia
- Plagiocephaly in 10%
- Bifacial microsomia has been reported

Imaging Features

- Underdeveloped mandible without mandibular condyle
- Flat zygomatic arch without glenoid fossa; may be absent
- Auricular malformations

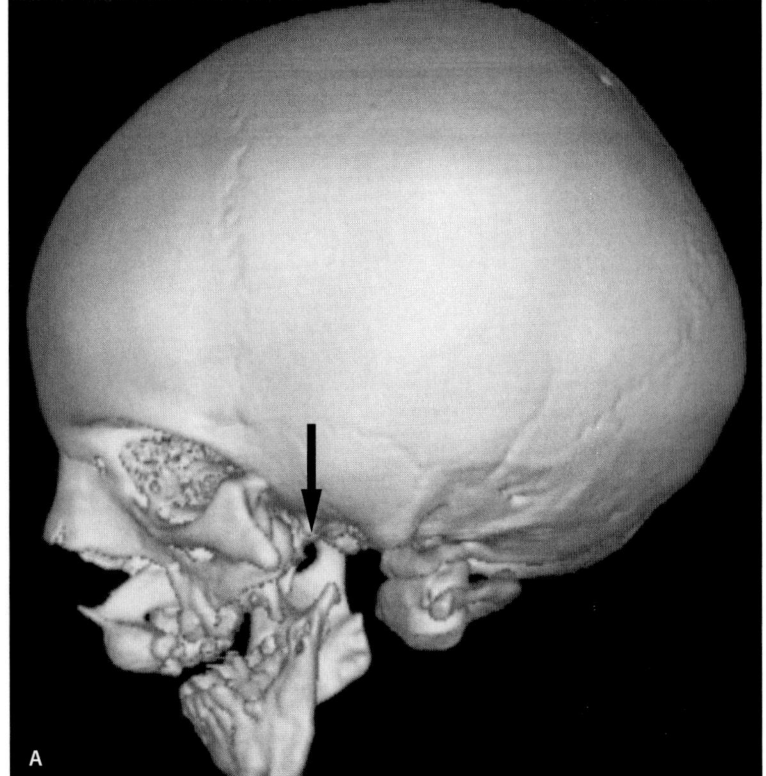

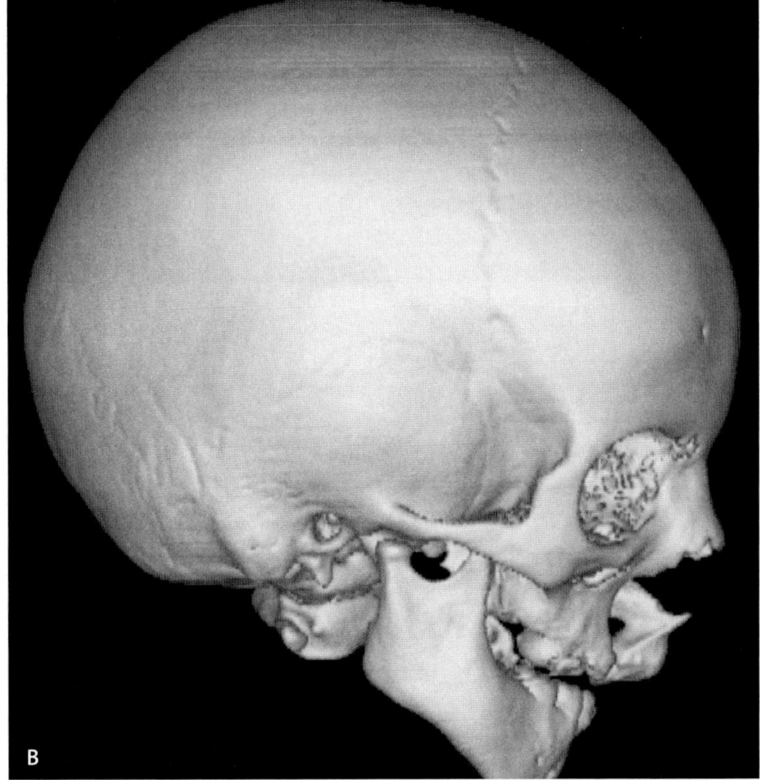

Figure 9.18

Hemifacial microsomia; 4-year-old male with multiple anomalies including cleft palate and lip. **A** 3D CT image, lateral view, shows left-sided severely hypoplastic mandible and absent zygomatic arch (*arrow*). **B** 3D CT image, lateral view, shows normal right side for comparison

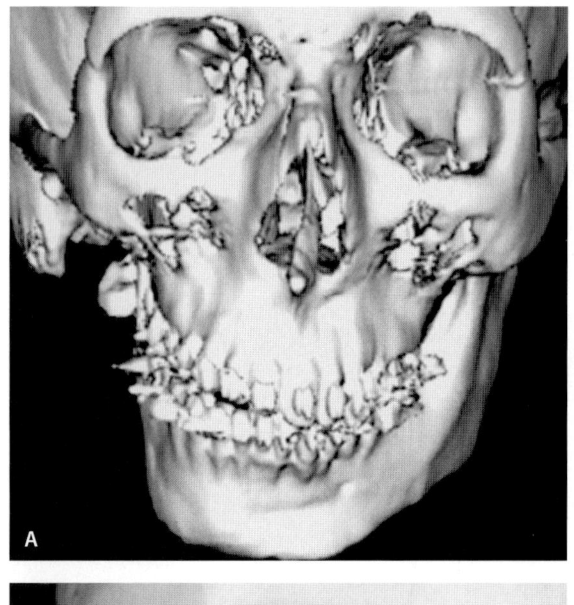
A

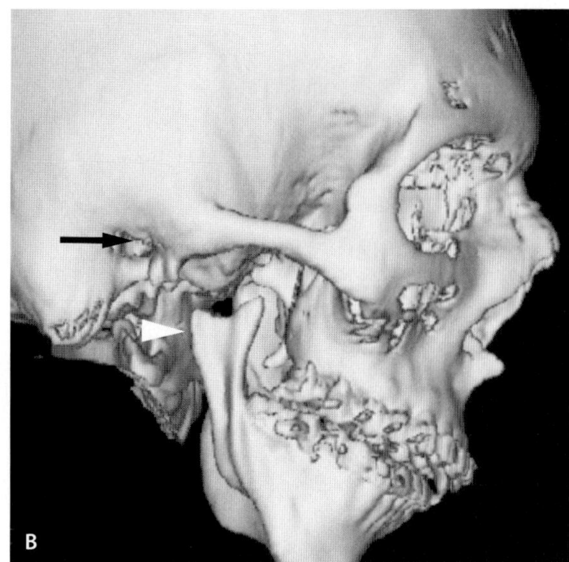
B

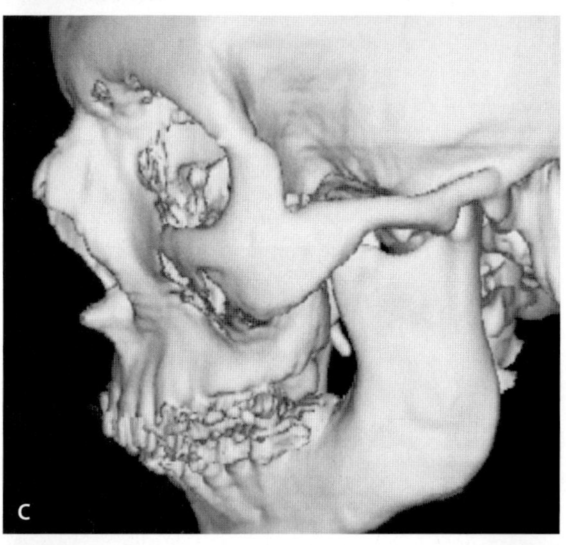
C

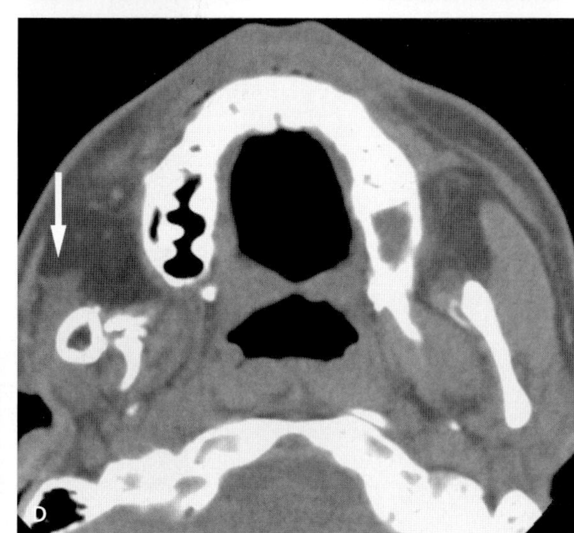
D

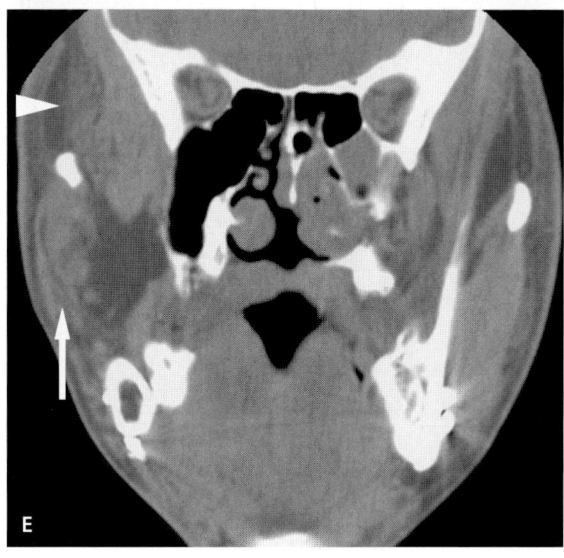
E

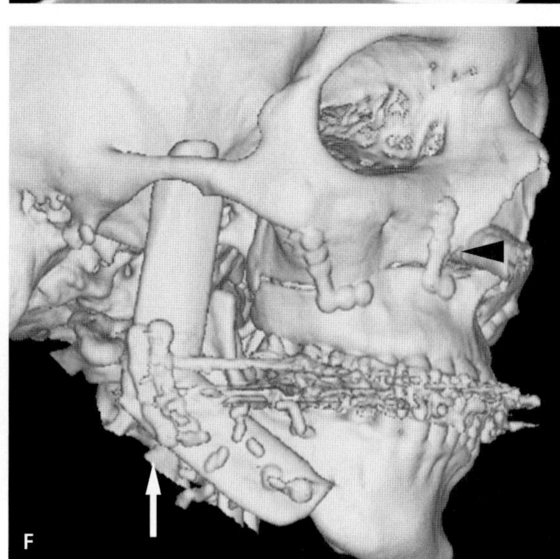
F

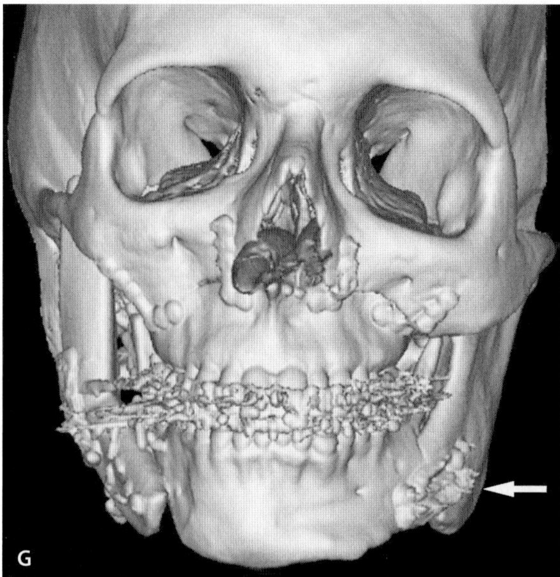

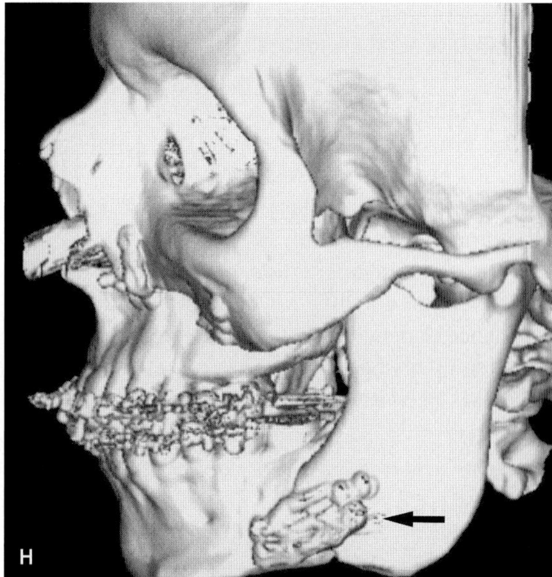

Figure 9.19

Hemifacial microsomia; 17-year-old male; pre- and postoperatively. A 3D CT image, en face view, shows facial asymmetry due to right-sided mandibular hypoplasia. B 3D CT image, lateral view, shows right-sided zygomatic arch without glenoid fossa (*arrow*), and hypoplastic mandible without mandibular condyle (*arrowhead*). Note orthodontic braces on teeth. C 3D CT image, lateral view, shows normal left side for comparison. D Axial CT image, soft tissue, shows severe atrophy of right masseter muscle (*arrow*) compared to normal left side. E Coronal CT image, soft tissue, shows severe atrophy of masseter muscle (*arrow*) and temporalis muscle (*arrowhead*) compared to normal left side. F 3D CT image, postoperative lateral view, shows right-sided fibula graft with miniplates and screws to reinforce the created mandibular angle of the graft (*arrow*). Note also miniplates and screws after LeFort 1 osteotomy (*arrowhead*). G 3D CT image, postoperative en face view, shows osteotomy of left mandible with miniplate fixation (*arrow*) to obtain symmetric facial skeleton. H 3D CT image, postoperative lateral view, shows osteotomy correction of normal left side with miniplates (*arrow*). I Coronal CT image, postoperative view, shows fibula graft "articulating" against infratemporal fossa (*arrow*)

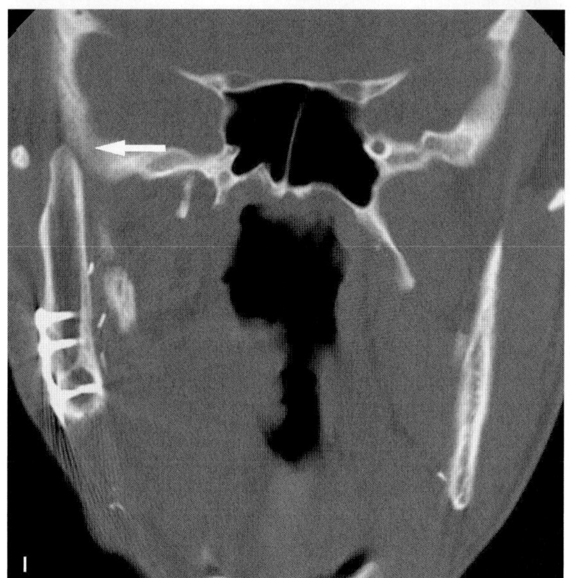

Treacher Collins Syndrome (Mandibulofacial Dysostosis)

Clinical Features

- Syndrome from first and second branchial arches; about 1 per 50,000 live births
- Micrognathia ("bird face"); symmetric underdevelopment of mandible
- Antimongoloid angulation of palpebral fissures with vertical notching or coloboma of outer parts
- Absence or deficiency of medial eyelashes
- Flattening of cheeks
- Ear tags between tragus and angle of mouth may occur

Imaging Features

- Mandibular hypoplasia; very short rami, bilateral antegonial notching, compensatory growth of anterior part
- Dental malocclusion
- Bilateral hypoplasia or agenesia of malar bone
- Malformation of external and middle ear
- Disproportionately small facial bones
- Paranasal sinuses often small, may be absent
- Lacrimal duct atresia
- Narrow palate
- Cleft palate in about one-third

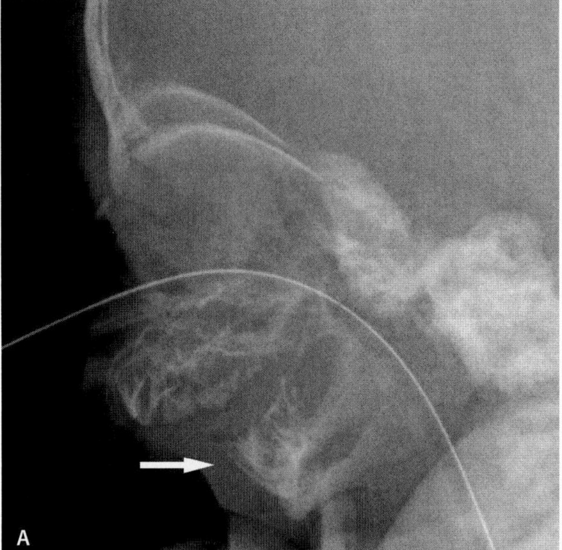

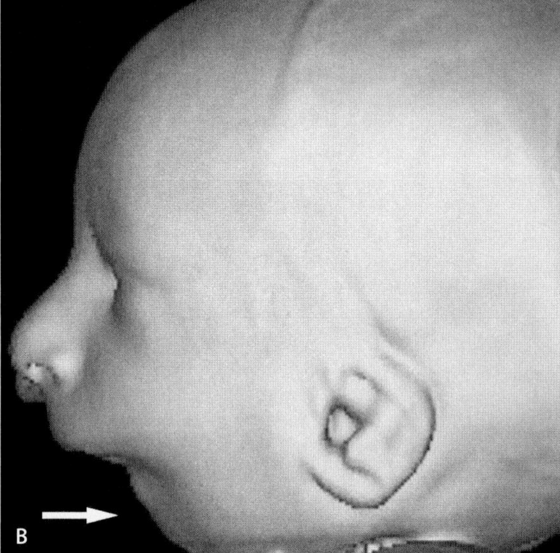

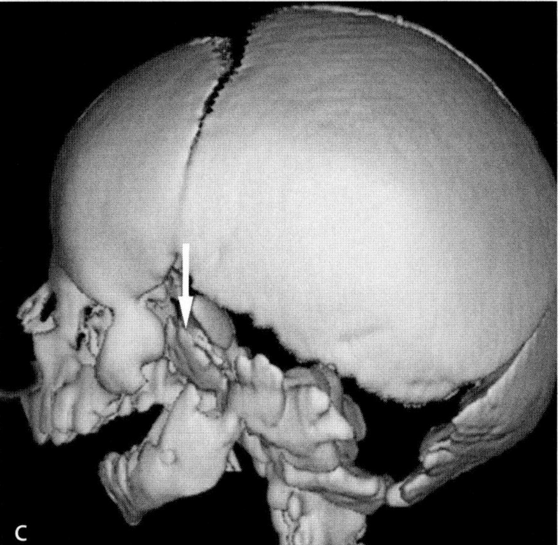

Figure 9.20

Treacher Collins syndrome; newborn with respiratory distress. **A** Lateral view shows very small and retruded mandible (*arrow*), and air-way tube. **B** 3D CT image of skin, lateral view, shows severe micrognathia (*arrow*). **C** 3D CT image, lateral view, shows absent zygoma (*arrow*)

Figure 9.21

Treacher Collins syndrome; 4-year-old male. A 3D CT image of left side shows underdeveloped mandible with antegonial notching and part of zygoma with zygomatic arch absent (*arrow*); micrognathia with open bite, and small facial skeleton compared to skull. B 3D CT image of right side; similar absence of zygoma (*arrow*) and appearance of mandible as contralateral side, except less developed condylar process

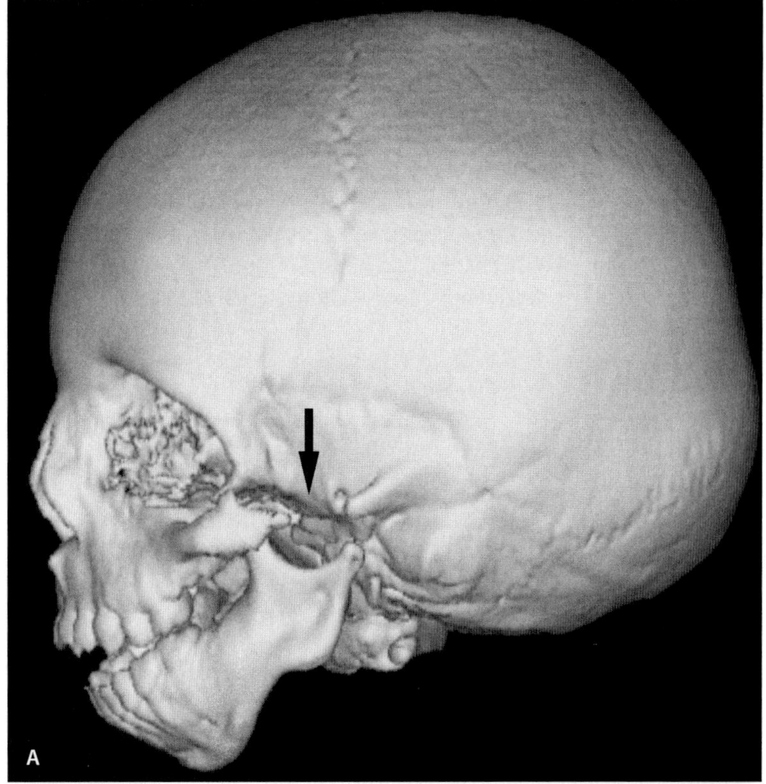

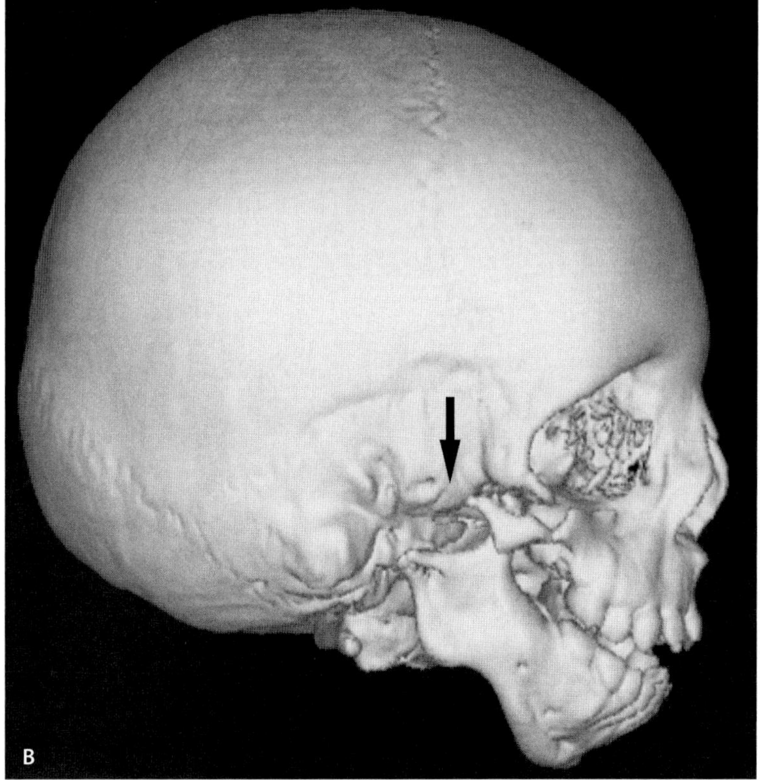

Syndromic Craniosynostoses (Craniofacial Dysostoses)

Definition

Group of syndromes showing both premature synostoses as a prominent feature and facial growth disturbances; about 15% of all craniosynostoses.

More than 100 such syndromes are recognized, but Crouzon is probably best known because craniofacial dysostosis is frequently used synonymously with this syndrome.

Crouzon Syndrome

Clinical Features

- Most frequent craniofacial dysostosis; about 1 per 25,000 births
- About one-half are familial and one-half are sporadic
- Absence of major limb abnormalities
- Oxycephaly
- Hypertelorism, exorbitism
- Shallow orbits
- Midfacial hypoplasia; relatively prominent mandible

Imaging Features

- Oxycephaly
- Bilateral coronal synostosis with brachycephaly but also sagittal synostosis with narrowing in transverse dimension
- Hypertelorism, exorbitism
- Shallow orbits
- Maxillary hypoplasia
- Partial obstruction of nasal passages, narrow palate
- Relative mandibular prognathism
- Cervical spine abnormalities; C2–C5 fusion 40%
- Calcification of stylohyoid ligament, 50%
- Intracranial anomalies common, including venous drainage and hydrocephalus

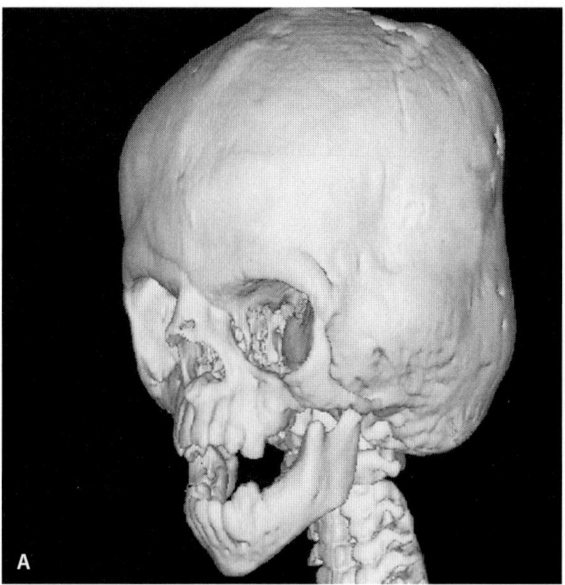

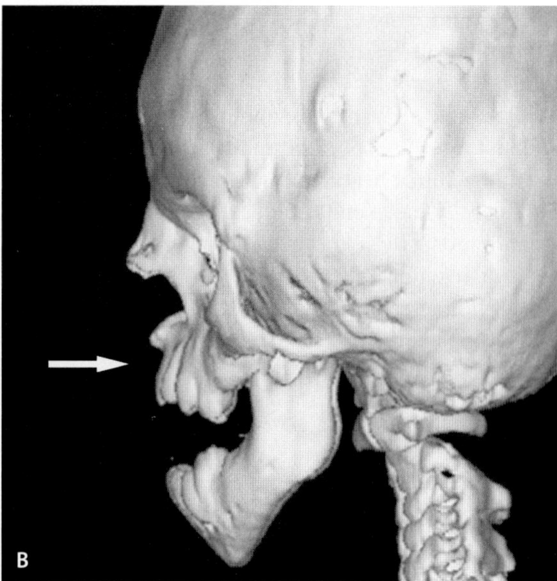

Figure 9.22

Crouzon syndrome; 2-year-old. A 3D CT image, oblique view, shows superior elongation of skull and typically "opened mouth". The maxilla and zygomas are hypoplastic. B 3D CT image, lateral view, shows maxillary hypoplasia (*arrow*)

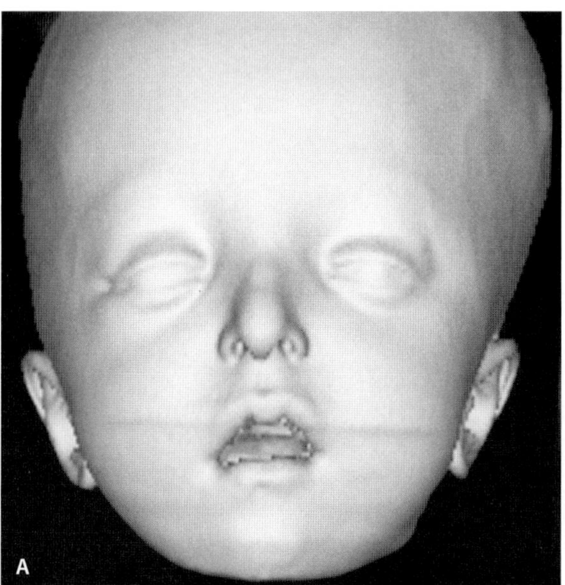

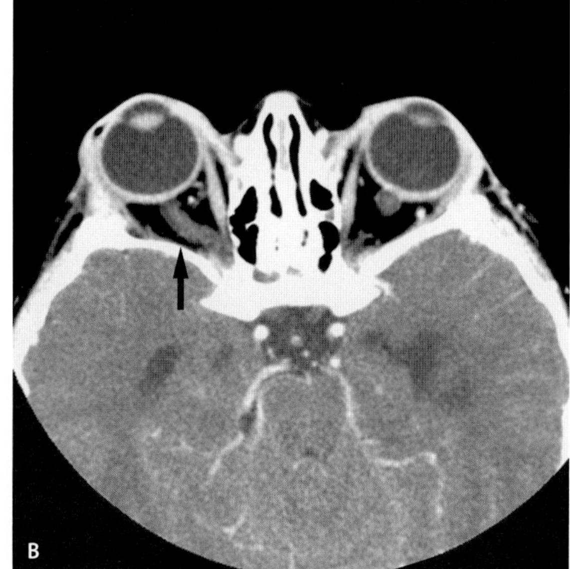

Figure 9.23

Crouzon syndrome; 3-year-old. A 3D CT image of skin, en face view, shows hypertelorism, exorbitism, and open down-turned mouth. B Axial CT image, soft-tissue, shows shallow orbits with exorbitism, and apparently enlarged optic nerve (*arrow*); MRI would probably have shown prominent perineural subarachnoid spaces and normal nerves bilaterally

Apert Syndrome

Clinical Features

- Craniofacial dysostosis; about 1 per 100,000 births
- Most cases are sporadic
- Many similar features to Crouzon syndrome, but generally more enhanced, except varying degrees of syndactyly or brachydactyly; various acrocephalosyndactyly types
- Hearing loss common
- Cleft palate in 30–42%

Imaging Features

- Similar skull type to Crouzon syndrome but more severe abnormalities; midfacial hypoplasia present at birth
- Choanal stenosis common
- Cervical spine abnormalities; fusion of C5–C6 70%
- Calcification of stylohyoid ligament 38–88%
- Intracranial anomalies

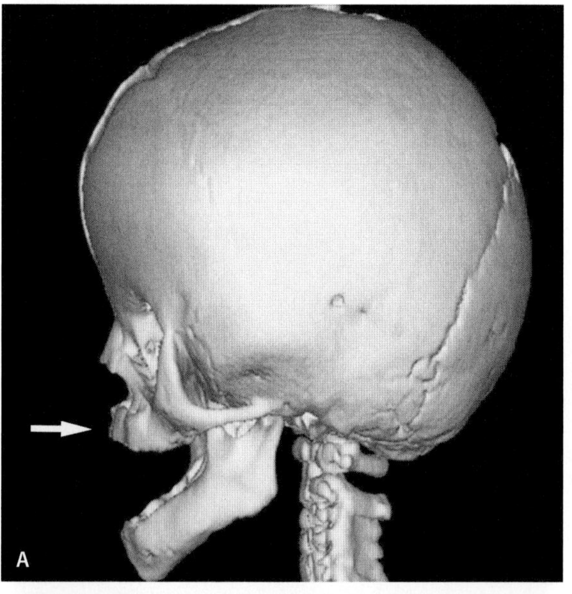

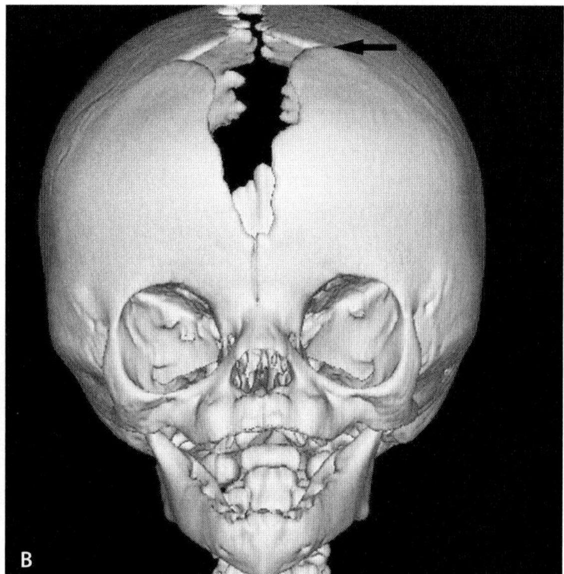

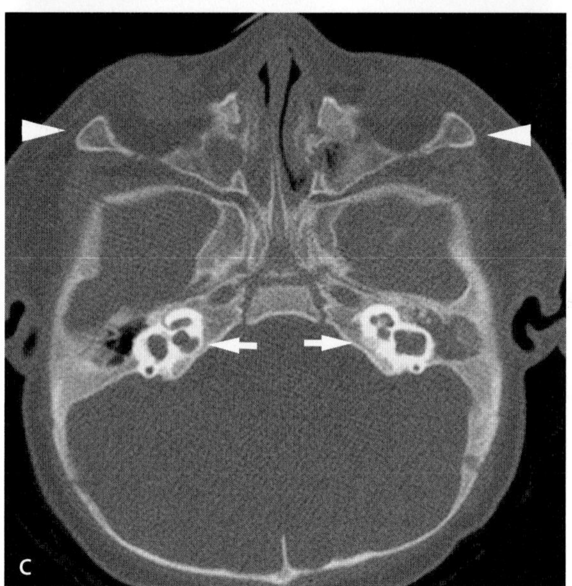

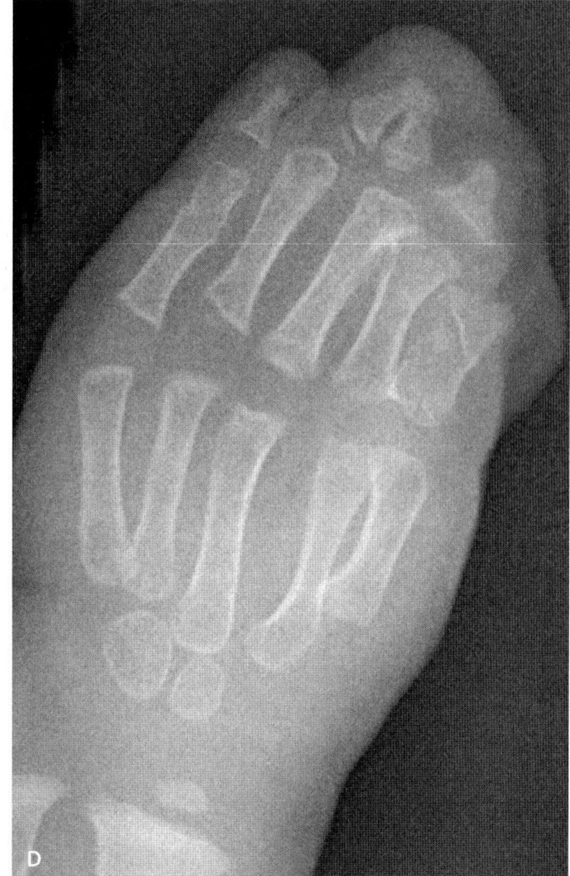

Figure 9.24

Apert syndrome; 6-month old. **A** 3D CT image, lateral view, shows oxycephaly and midfacial hypoplasia (*arrow*), and typically "opened mouth". **B** 3D CT image, en face view, shows large, open anterior fontanelle, brachycephaly with fused coronal sutures bilaterally. **C** Axial CT image shows vestibular dysplasia (*arrows*) and shallow orbits (*arrowheads*). **D** Hand view shows syndactyly (fusion of fingers)

Achondroplasia

Clinical Features

- Familial or sporadic
- Most common form of dwarfism
- Defect of generalized endochondral osteogenesis
- Disproportionately short limbs
- Lumbar lordosis
- Large, brachycephalic head with a prominent forehead
- Midfacial underdevelopment
- Nasal bone deformed (saddle nose)
- Normal lower third of face; relative mandibular prognathism
- Occurs in several dominant disorders often associated with neurologic complications such as hydrocephalus, brain stem compression, and small foramina magnum, which can result in sleep apnea, sudden infant death, and spinal cord compression

Imaging Features

- Disproportionately enlarged calvaria
- Maxillary retrognathia
- Saddle nose
- Normal mandible due to periosteal chondrogenesis

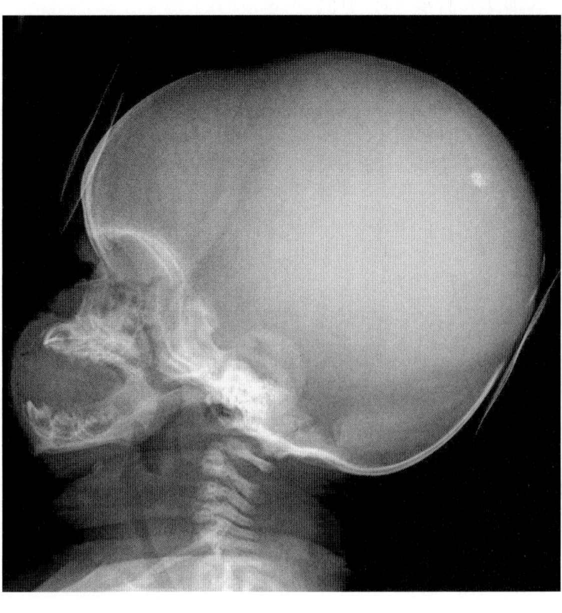

Figure 9.25
Achondroplasia; newborn. Lateral view shows midfacial hypoplasia, relative mandibular prognathism, and large tongue

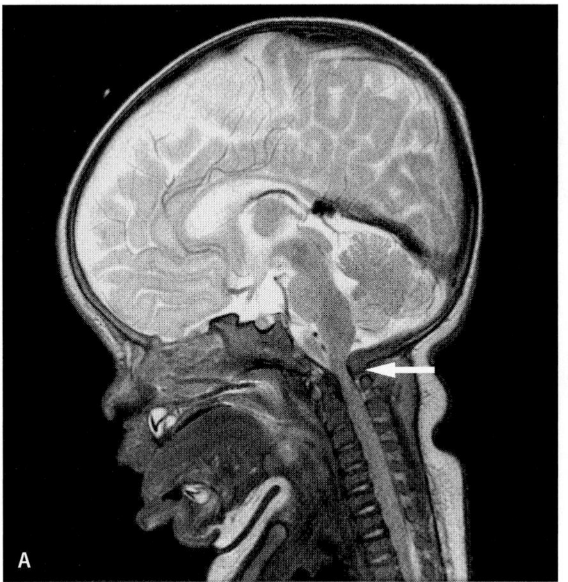

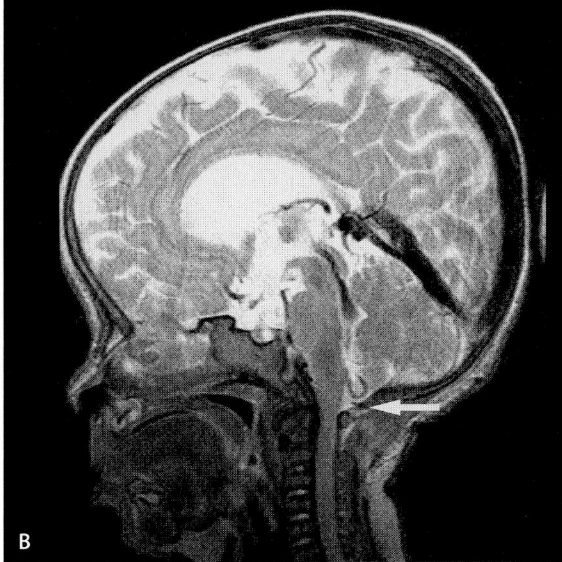

Figure 9.26
Achondroplasia; 3-month-old female. **A** Sagittal T2-weighted MRI shows spinal cord narrowing; at foramen magnum (*arrow*). **B** Sagittal T2-weighted MRI after surgery shows removal of posterior margin of foramen magnum (*arrow*) with decreased compression of brain stem/medulla/upper cervical spinal cord

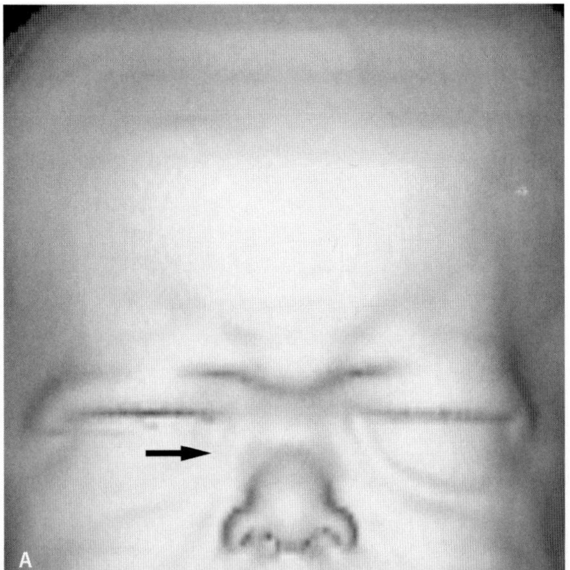

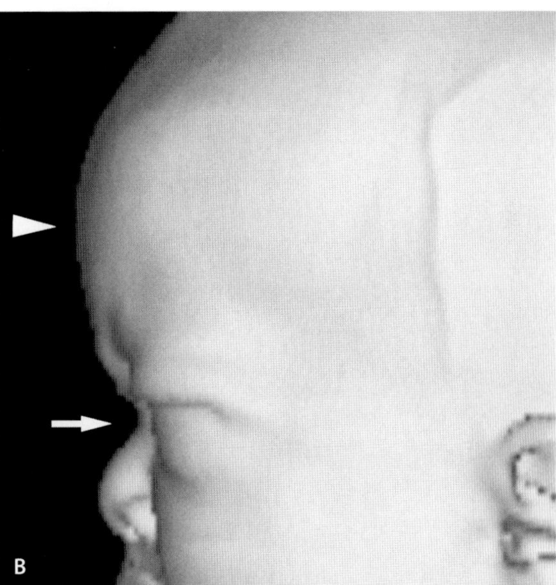

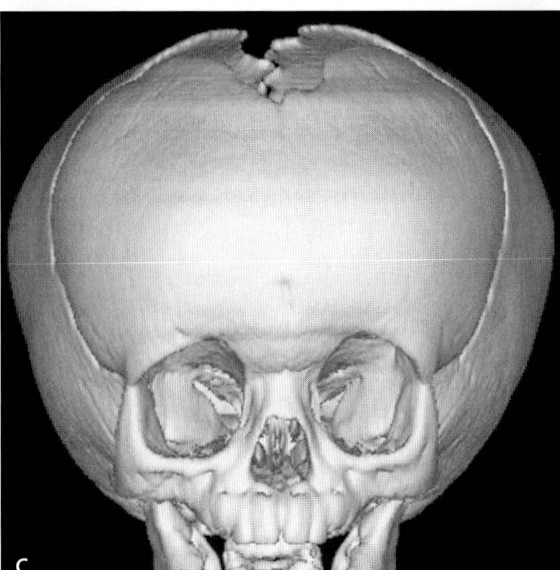

Figure 9.27

Achondroplasia; 7-month old. **A** 3D CT image, en face view of skin shows saddle nose (*arrow*). **B** 3D CT image, lateral view of skin shows saddle nose (*arrow*) and prominent forehead (*arrowhead*). **C** 3D CT image, en face view, shows macrocephaly with parietal prominence and open anterior fontanelle

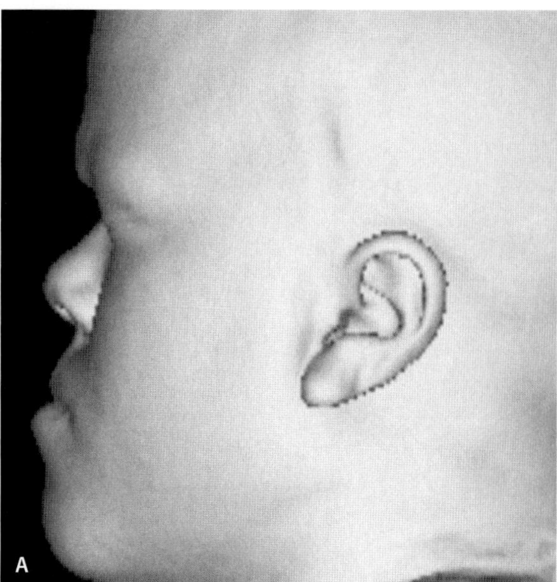

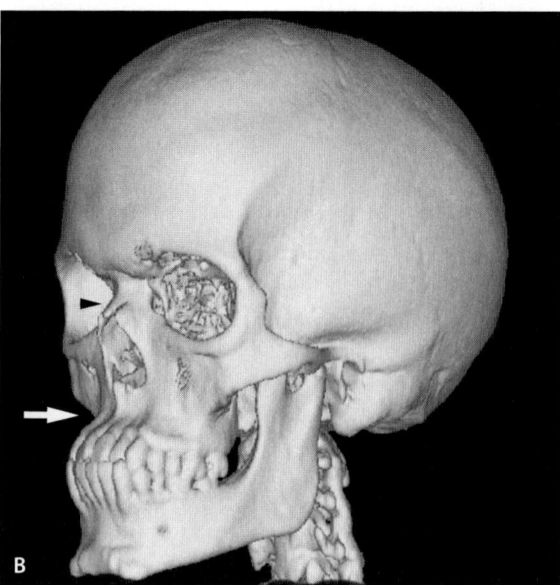

Figure 9.28

Achondroplasia; teenage. **A** 3D CT lateral of skin shows midfacial hypoplasia and saddle nose. **B** 3D CT image, oblique view, shows maxillary hypoplasia (*arrow*) and short, deformed, depressed nasal bone (*arrowhead*)

Pyknodysostosis

Clinical Features

- Rare, inherited form of dwarfism
- Short stature
- Dense, fragile bones
- Predisposed to osteomyelitis

Imaging Features

- Open fontanelles, cranial sutures
- Partial agenesia of terminal phalanges of hands and feet
- Hypoplasia of maxilla, mandible, paranasal sinuses
- Dense, fractured bones
- Abnormal dental eruption, crowding of teeth

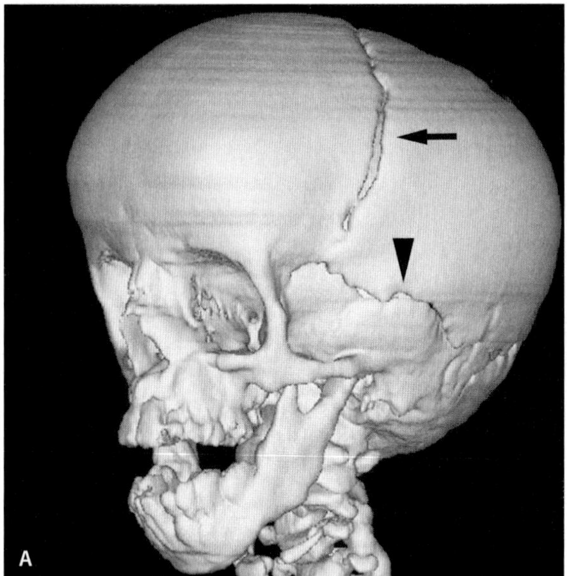

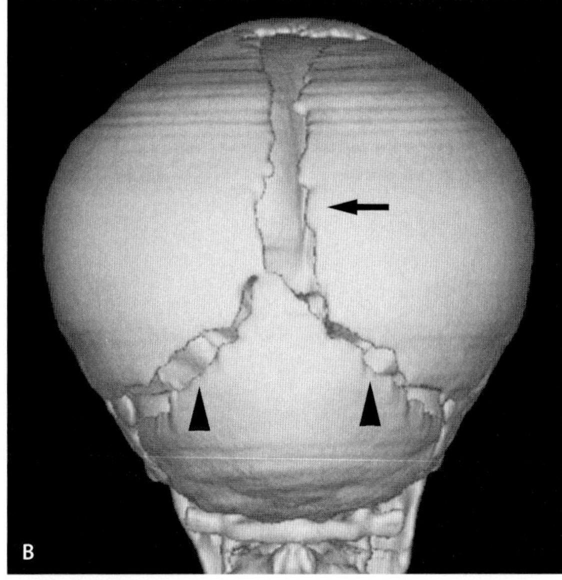

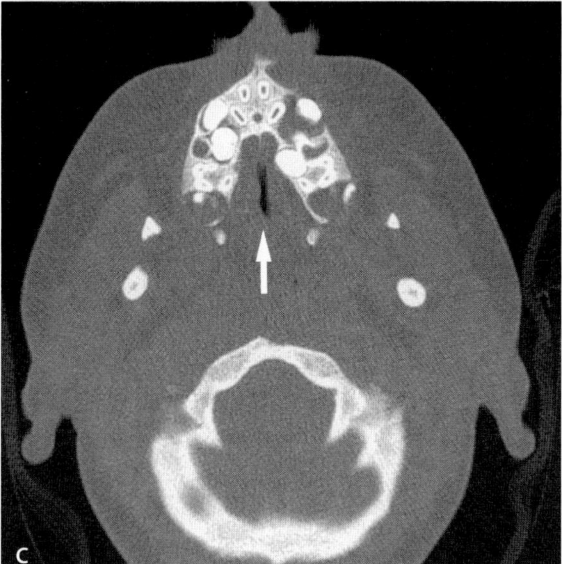

Figure 9.29

Pyknodysostosis; 9-year-old. A 3D CT image, oblique view, shows hypoplasia of maxilla and mandible and open coronal suture (*arrow*) and squamosal suture (*arrowhead*). B 3D CT image, axial view, shows wide open sagittal suture (*arrow*), open anterior fontanelle, and open lambdoid sutures (*arrowheads*). C Axial CT image shows narrow, dense maxilla and crowded teeth (some with widened follicles); incisors almost in sagittal line (*arrow*)

Ectodermal Dysplasia

Clinical Features

- Developmental abnormalities of ectodermal tissues
- Many types with various inheritance patterns
- Abnormal hearing
- Abnormal or missing sweat glands
- Multiple agenesia of teeth
- Poorly developed alveolar processes
- Sebaceous glands, hair follicles, and salivary glands (xerostomia) may also be defective

Imaging Features

- Lack of tooth germs both in permanent and primary dentition
- Disproportionately small facial skeleton compared with calvaria
- Mandible anteriorly rotated

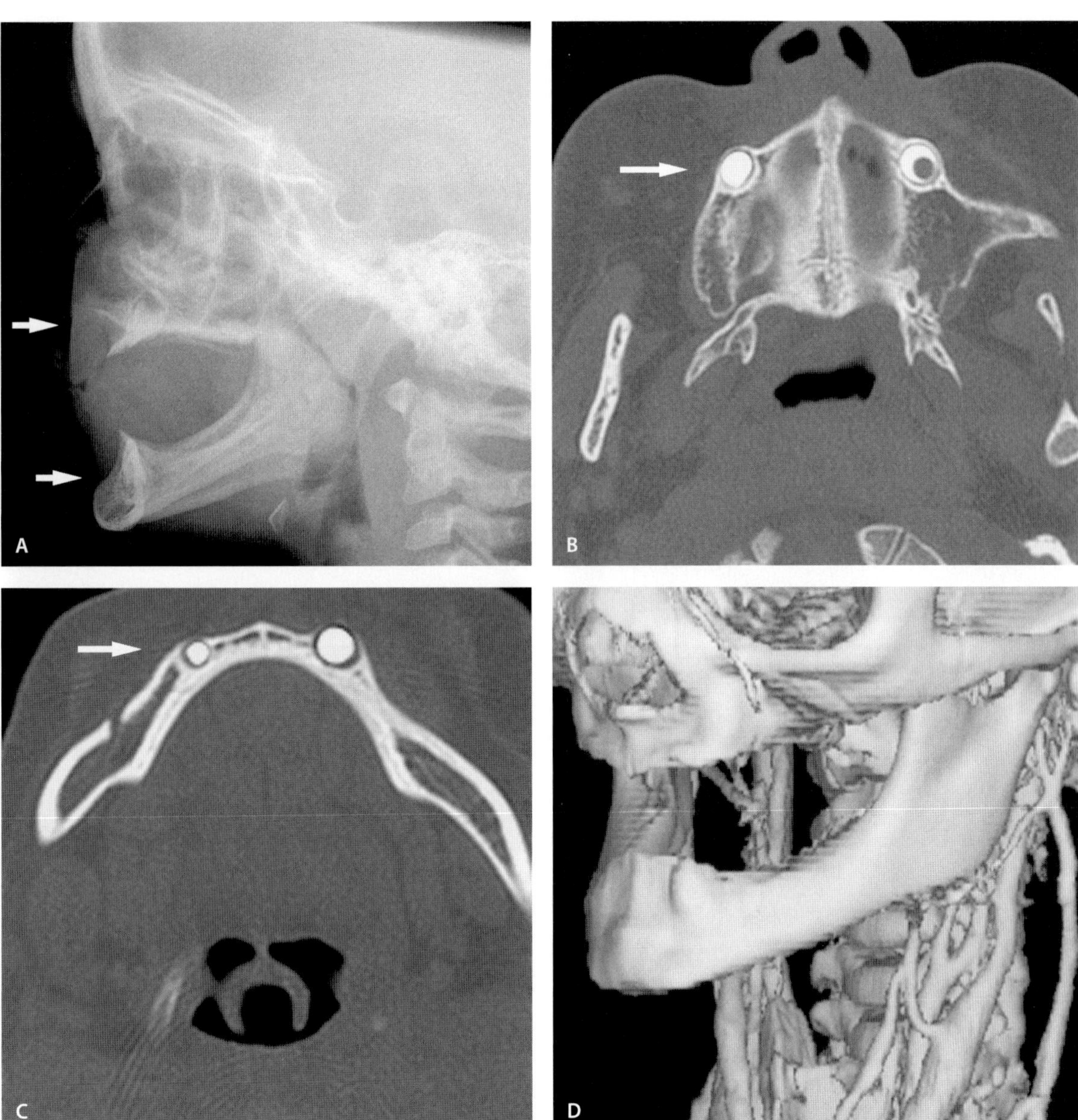

Figure 9.30

Ectodermal dysplasia; 3-year old female. **A** Lateral view shows only a couple of tooth germs (*arrows*) in anterior maxilla and mandible, and poorly developed alveolar processes (as if they were old and atrophic). **B** Axial CT image shows two teeth, possibly canines, in upper jaw (*arrow*). **C** Axial CT image shows two teeth, possibly canines, in lower jaw (*arrow*). **D** 3D CT image, oblique view, shows underdeveloped jaws without other teeth

Miscellaneous Conditions

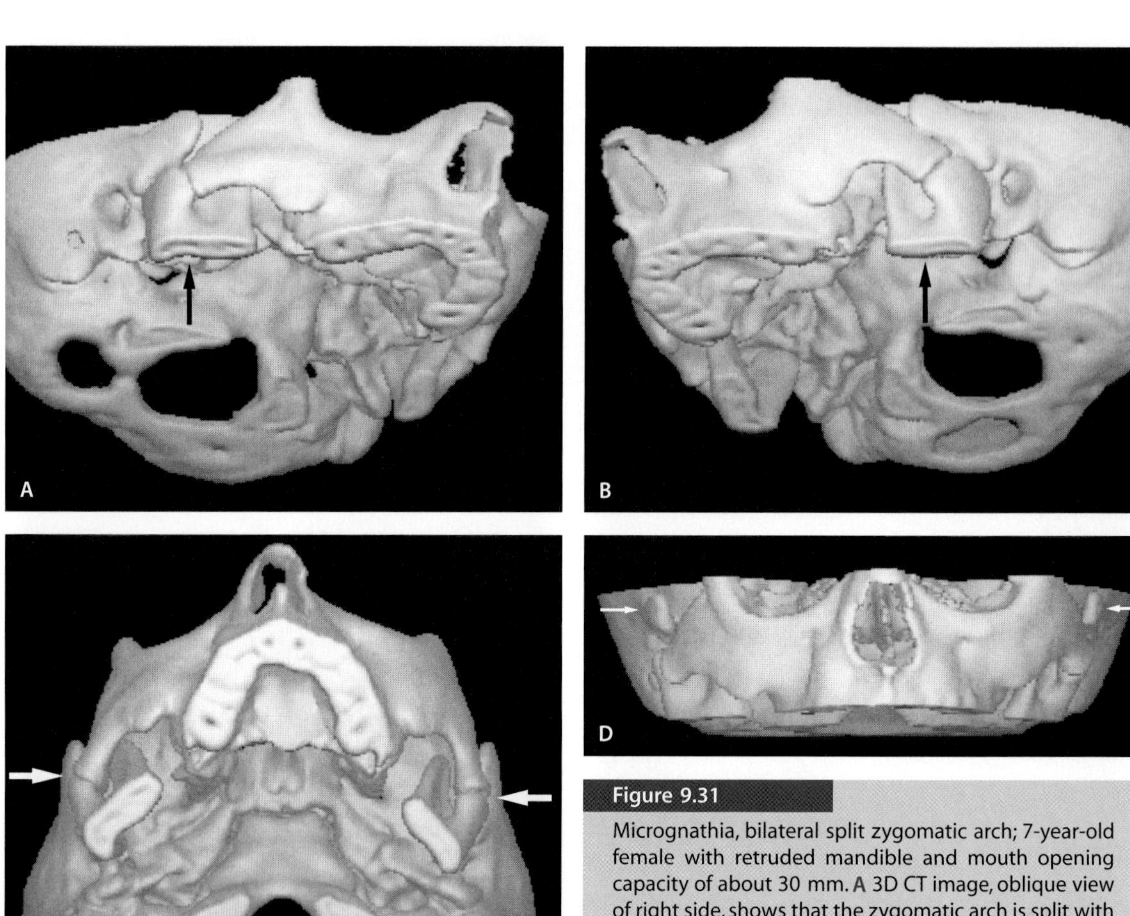

Figure 9.31

Micrognathia, bilateral split zygomatic arch; 7-year-old female with retruded mandible and mouth opening capacity of about 30 mm. **A** 3D CT image, oblique view of right side, shows that the zygomatic arch is split with the anterior part articulating with the mandible (*arrow*). **B** 3D CT image, oblique view of contralateral side, shows similar deformities (*arrow*). **C** 3D CT image, axial view, shows the symmetric deformity (*arrows*). **D** 3D CT image, en face view, shows the posterior "free" part of the split zygomatic arch bilaterally (*arrows*)

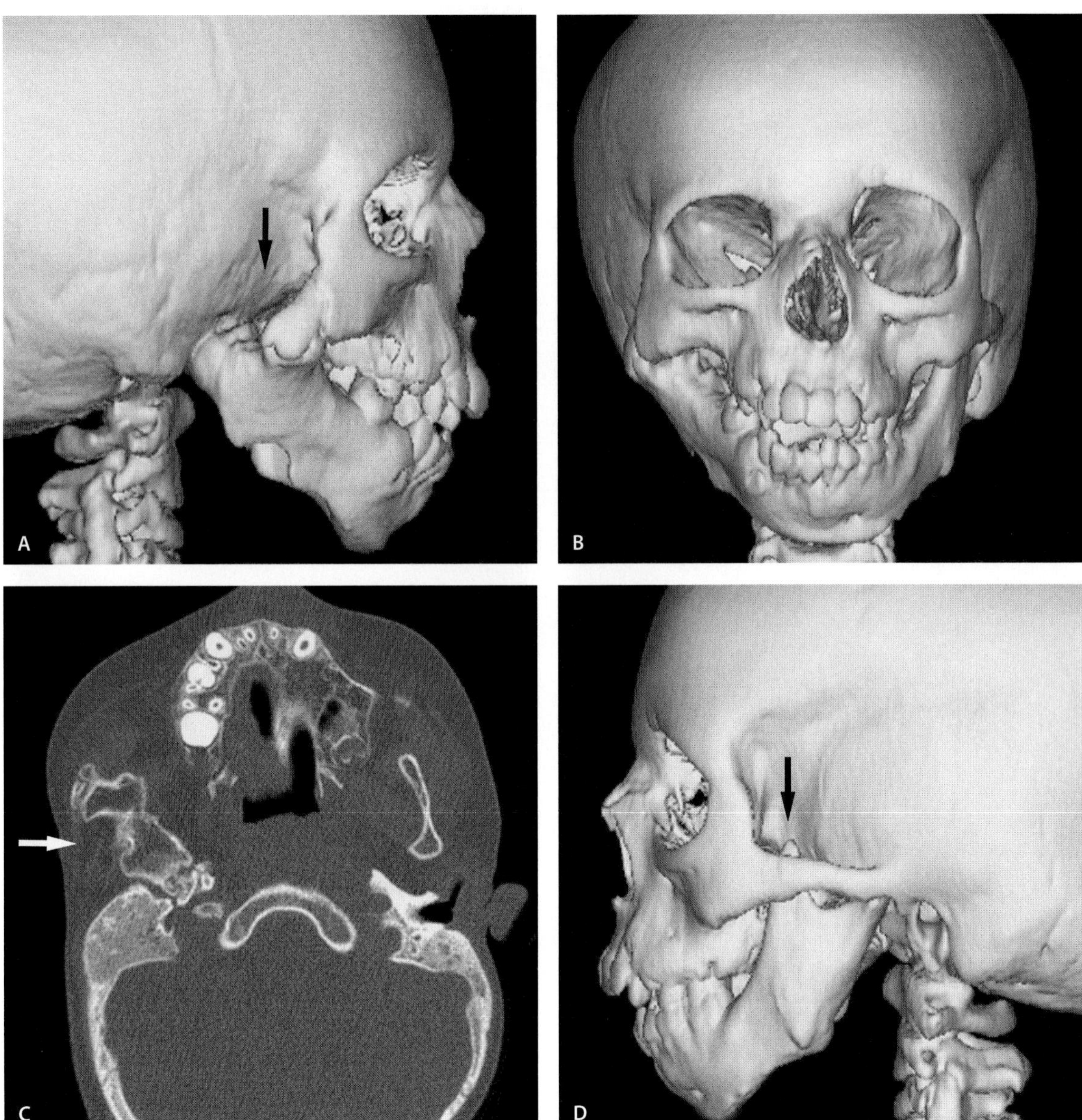

Figure 9.32

Facial asymmetry, unilateral ankylosis and absent zygomatic arch; 8-year-old. **A** 3D CT image, lateral view of right side, shows absent zygomatic arch (*arrow*) and thus no glenoid fossa; ankylosis between mandible and remaining abnormal zygomatic bone. **B** 3D CT image, en face view, shows mandibular asymmetry and open anterior bite, and some maxillary asymmetry as well. **C** Axial CT image shows bony union between mandible and zygomatic bone (*arrow*). **D** 3D CT image, lateral view of left side, shows normal zygomatic arch but coronoid hyperplasia (*arrow*), probably of a compensatory nature

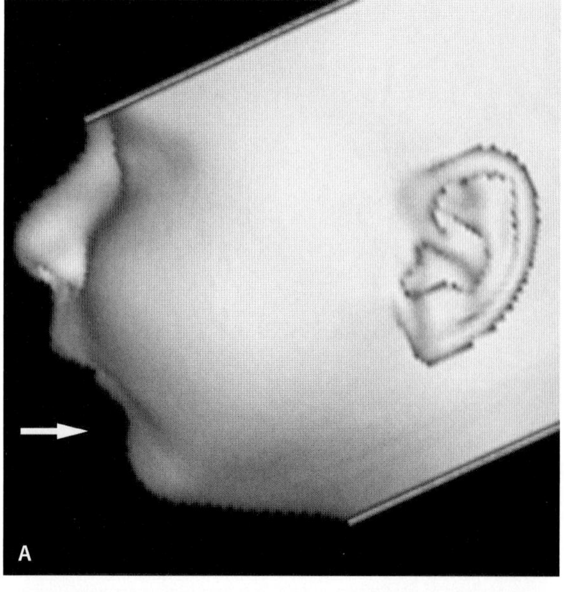

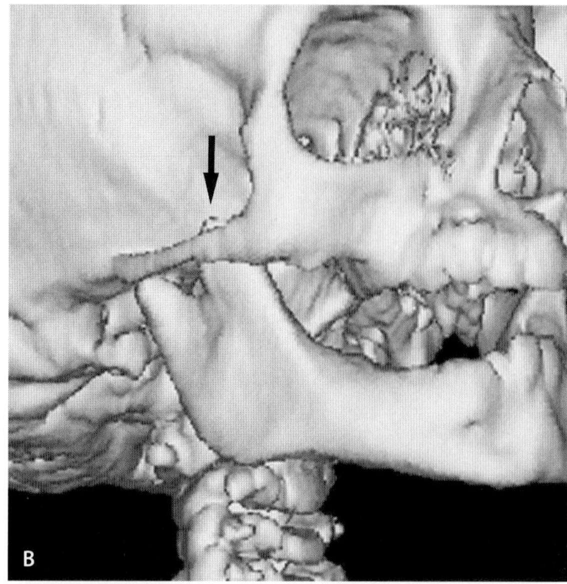

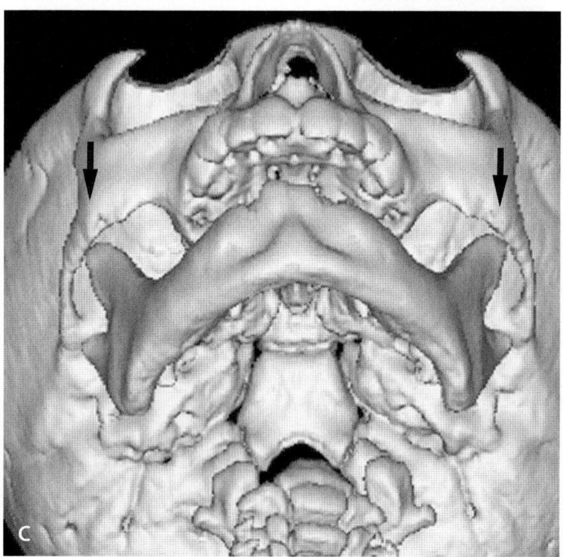

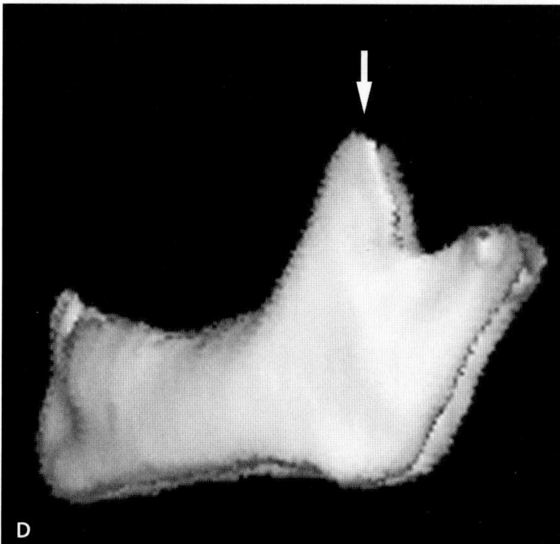

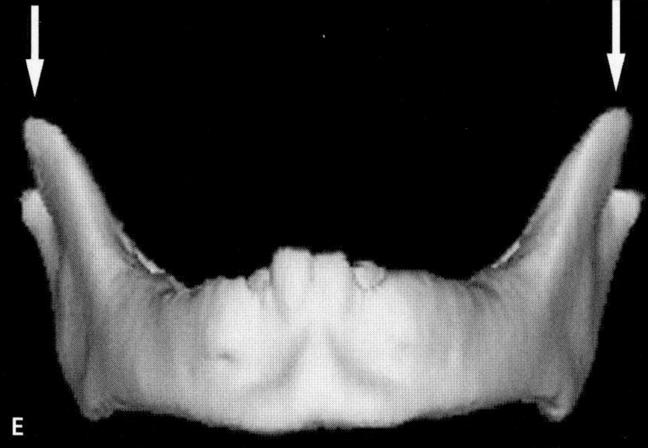

Figure 9.33

Micrognathia, coronoid hyperplasia with blocking on mouth opening; 10-month old. **A** 3D CT image of skin surface shows micrognathia ("bird face"). **B** 3D CT image shows coronoid hyperplasia (*arrow*). **C** 3D CT image, oblique axial view, shows that both coronoid processes are blocking against zygomatic arch (*arrows*). **D** Segmented 3D CT image, lateral view of mandible, shows bilateral coronoid hyperplasia (*arrow*). **E** Segmented 3D CT image, en face view of mandible, shows bilateral coronoid hyperplasia (*arrows*)

Suggested Reading

Carinci F, Pezzetti F, Scapoli L, Martinelli M, Carinci P, Tognom M (2000) Genetics of nonsyndromic cleft lip and palate: a review of international studies and data regarding the Italian population. Cleft Palate Craniofac J 37:33–40

David DJ, Mahatumarat C, Cooter RD (1987) Hemifacial microsomia: a multisystem classification. Plast Reconstr Surg 80:525–535

Farman AG, Nortje C, Wood RE (1993) Developmental anomalies of the skull and jaws. In: Oral and maxillofacial diagnostic imaging. Mosby, St. Louis, pp 105–157

Goldenhar M (1952) Associations malformatives de l'oeil et de l'oreille, en particulier le syndrome dermöide epibulbaire-appendices auriculaires-fistula auris congenita et ses relations avec la dysostose mandibulo-faciale. J Genet Hum 1:243–282

Fogh-Andersen P (1965) Rare clefts of the face. Acta Chir Scand 129:275–281

Gorlin RJ, Cohen MM Jr, Levin LS (1990) Syndromes of the head and neck. 3rd edn. Oxford University Press, New York, pp 33–35, 54, 521, 524, 641, 649, 695

Naidich TP, Blaser SI, Bauer BS, Armstrong DK, McLone DG, Zimmerman RA (2003) Embryology and congenital lesions of the midface. In: Som PM, Curtin HD (eds) Head and neck imaging, 4th edn. Mosby, St. Louis, pp 3–86

Naidich TP, Smith MS, Castillo M, Thompson JE, Sloan GM, Jayakar P, Mukherji SK (1996) Facies to remember. Number 7. Hemifacial microsomia. Goldenhar syndrome. OAV complex. Int J Neuroradiol 2:437–449

Murray JC (1995) Invited editorial. Face facts: genes, environment, and clefts. Am J Hum Genet 52:227–232

Stabrun AE, Larheim TA, Hoyeraal HM, Rosler M (1988) Reduced mandibular dimensions and asymmetry in juvenile rheumatoid arthritis. Pathogenetic factors. Arthritis Rheum 31:602–611

Van der Meulen J, Mazzola R, Stricker M, Raphael B (1990) Classification of craniofacial malformations. In: Stricker M, Van der Meulen J, Raphael B, Mazzola R (eds) Craniofacial malformations. Churchill Livingstone, Edinburgh, pp 149–309

Paranasal Sinuses

Introduction

Diseases of the paranasal sinuses are common and may cause symptoms simulating dental disease. Due to the close relationship between the dental structures and the sinuses it may also be the opposite: dental disease causing sinusitis. Thus, diseases of the paranasal sinuses are important both in medicine and dentistry. Tumors of the paranasal sinuses are rare, but may present with oral mucosa or dental symptoms.

Advanced imaging modalities are routinely used for diagnostic assessment of paranasal sinus problems and in general they have replaced conventional radiography. CT is the primary method to evaluate diseases of the paranasal sinuses. MRI is used as a supplement primarily to determine the extent of soft-tissue abnormalities extending outside the confinement of the sinus cavities. In this chapter we present a number of cases illustrated with these imaging modalities so professionals in the dental field may become more familiar with the different conditions and their imaging appearances.

Inflammatory Diseases

Acute Rhinosinusitis

Definition

Acute inflammation in nose and paranasal sinuses.

Clinical Features

- One of most common medical afflictions.
- Viral rhinosinusitis most common (common cold, influenza).
- Bacterial rhinosinusitis may develop secondarily (*Haemophilus influenzae*, *Streptococcus pneumoniae*).
- Pain over sinuses; cheek, frontal, between eyes, or suboccipital.
- Toothache, teeth tenderness to percussion; more than one tooth of maxillary lateral segment(s).
- Headache seldom.
- Dental etiology in 10–20%; larger frequencies have been reported depending on patient materials.

Imaging Features

- Nodular or smooth mucosal thickening or complete sinus opacification
- Contrast-enhanced inflamed mucosa lining; variable amounts of submucosal edema and surface secretions
- Air-fluid level, most frequent in maxillary sinus, due to bacterial sinusitis with obstruction of ostium, but only in 25–50% of patients with this disease
- T1-weighted MRI: low to intermediate
- T2-weighted MRI: high signal of inflamed mucosa and fluid
- T1-weighted post-Gd MRI: intense enhancement of inflamed mucosa; no enhancement of fluid

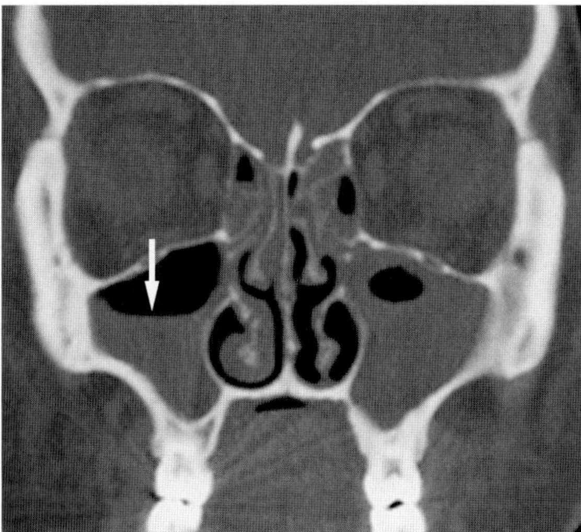

Figure 10.1

Acute rhinosinusitis secondary to common cold. Coronal CT shows fluid-level in right maxillary sinus (*arrow*), probably also in left sinus, and mucosal thickening of ethmoid cells bilaterally. Normal bone structures

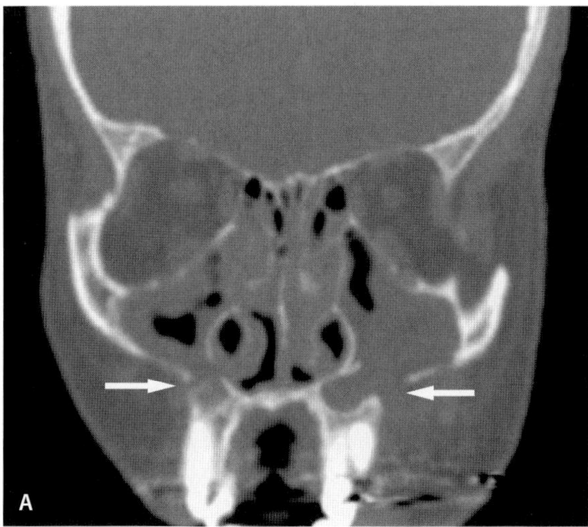

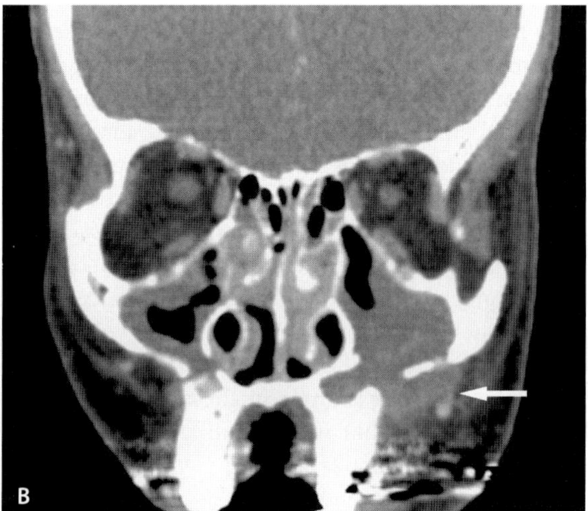

Figure 10.2

Acute sinusitis; 37-year-old female with a history of LeFort I osteotomy now with facial pain and swelling. **A** Coronal CT image shows bilateral osteotomies through maxilla and nasal cavity (*arrows*) and mucosal thickening of ethmoid and maxillary sinuses, and nasal cavity. **B** Coronal CT image, soft-tissue window, shows inflammatory tissue penetrating left maxillary osteotomy being responsible for facial swelling (*arrow*). Sinusitis does normally not cause facial swelling but since there was a passage from the maxillary sinus to the facial soft tissue via the osteotomy defect in this patient facial swelling resulted

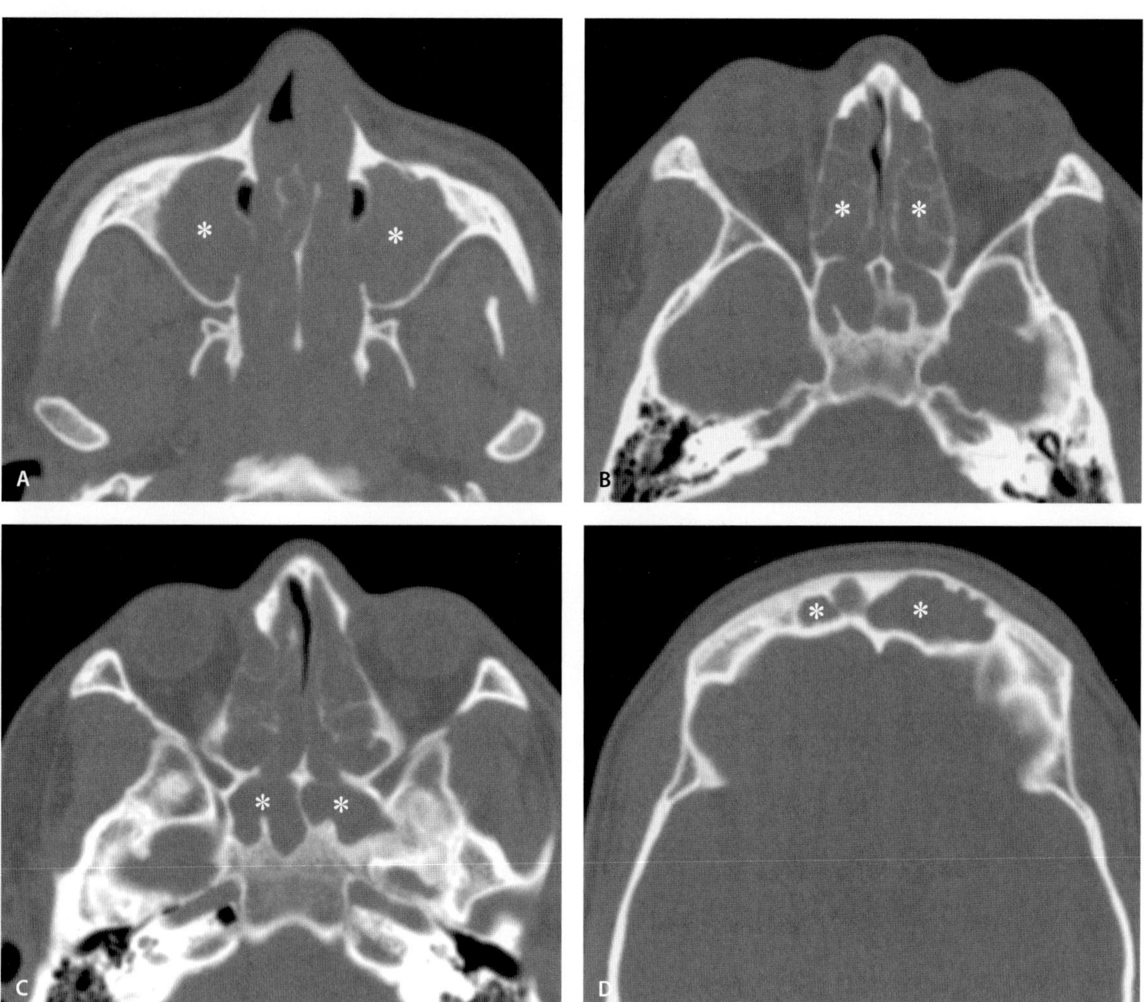

Figure 10.3

Pansinusitis; 19-year-old male with history of sinusitis and cough, now with headache, eye and cheek pain. **A** Axial CT image shows complete opacification of the maxillary sinuses (*asterisks*). **B** Axial CT image shows complete opacification of ethmoid sinuses (*asterisks*). **C** Axial CT image shows complete opacification of sphenoid sinuses (*asterisks*). **D** Axial CT image shows complete opacification of frontal sinuses (*asterisks*)

Chronic Sinusitis

Definition

Develops from either persistent acute inflammation or repeated episodes of acute or subacute sinusitis.

- Allergic sinusitis
- Vasomotor rhinitis
- Fungal sinusitis (90% *Aspergillus fumigatus*; may be fulminant and invasive in immunosuppressed patients)

Clinical Features

- Anaerobic microorganisms frequently isolated

Imaging Features

- Varying mucosal swelling, smooth or irregular swelling due to edema and secretion.
- Thickened, sclerotic, fibrotic sinus walls, particularly of maxillary sinuses.
- Dystrophic calcification.
- T1-weighted MRI: low to intermediate.
- T2-weighted MRI: usually high signal of inflamed mucosa, low signal of sclerosis and fibrosis. Inspissated mucus can be dark on all sequences resulting in false-negative MR diagnosis of chronic sinusitis.

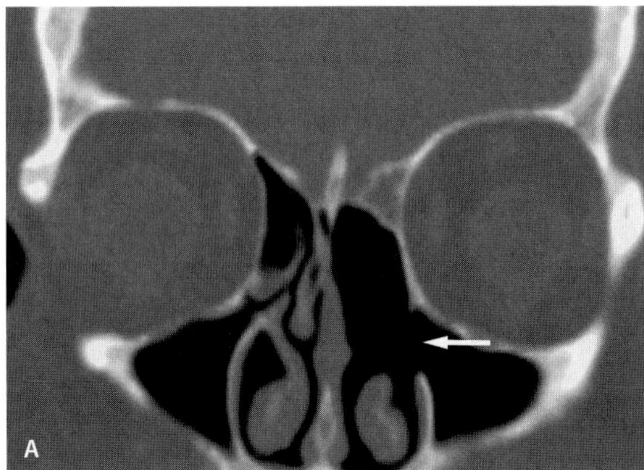

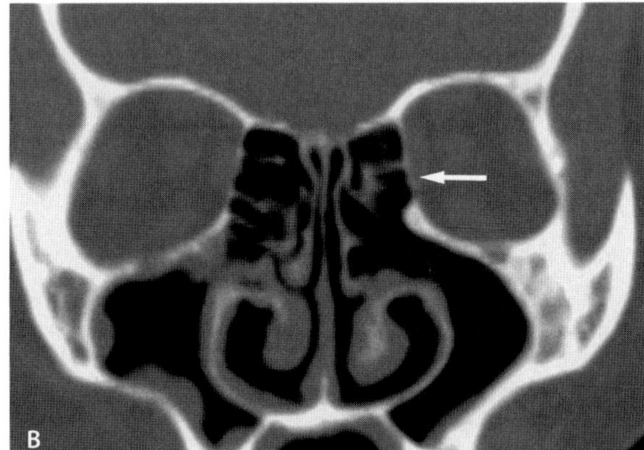

Figure 10.4

Post endoscopic surgery; 41-year-old female 9 years after septoplasty with left concha bullosa and partial ethmoid sinus resection, now with „nose problem". **A** Coronal CT image shows that left medial maxillary sinus wall is removed (*arrow*), together with left middle turbinate and ethmoid cells; otherwise normal bone and air. **B** Coronal CT image, more posterior section, shows that ethmoid cells are partially intact (*arrow*). Only minimal mucosal thickening of right maxillary sinus

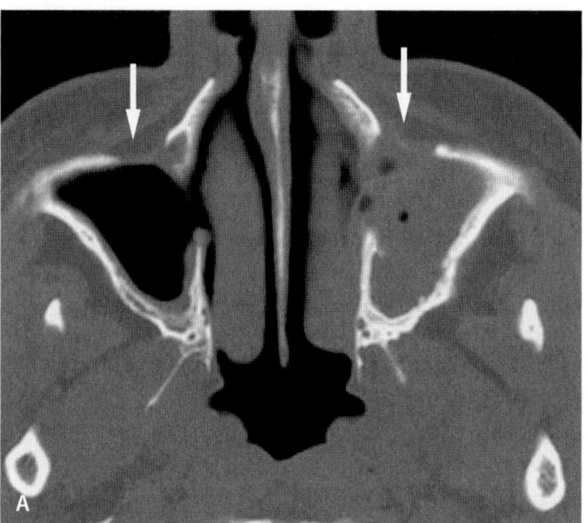

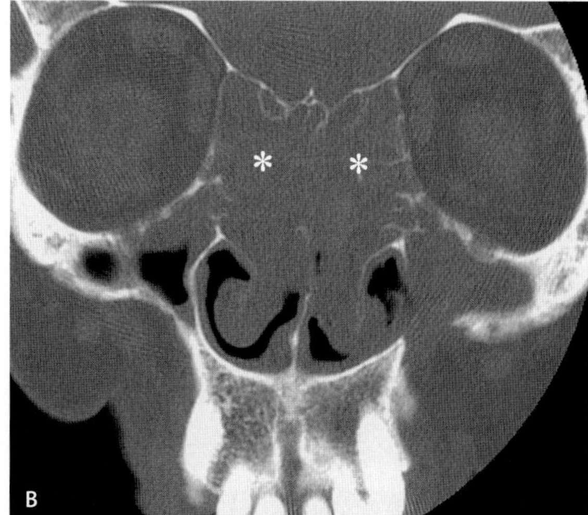

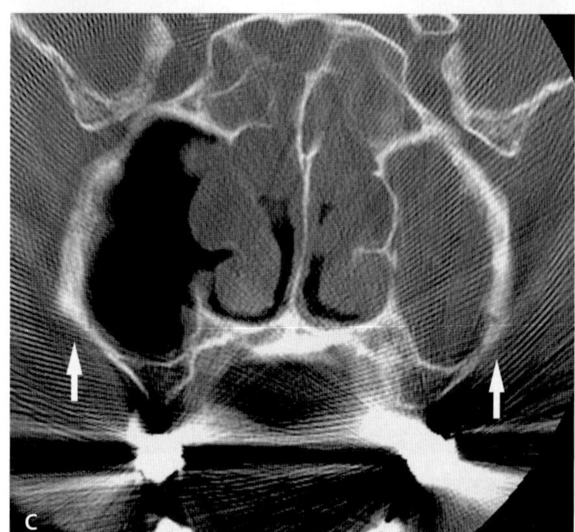

Figure 10.5

Chronic sinusitis; 61-year-old female with history of previous surgery for sinusitis. **A** Axial CT image shows surgical maxillary defects bilaterally (*arrows*), opacification of left sinus, and thickening with sclerosis of sinus walls bilaterally. **B** Coronal CT image shows opacification of ethmoid sinuses bilaterally (*asterisks*). **C** Coronal CT image shows evenly thickened maxillary sinus wall in entire sinus bilaterally (*arrows*)

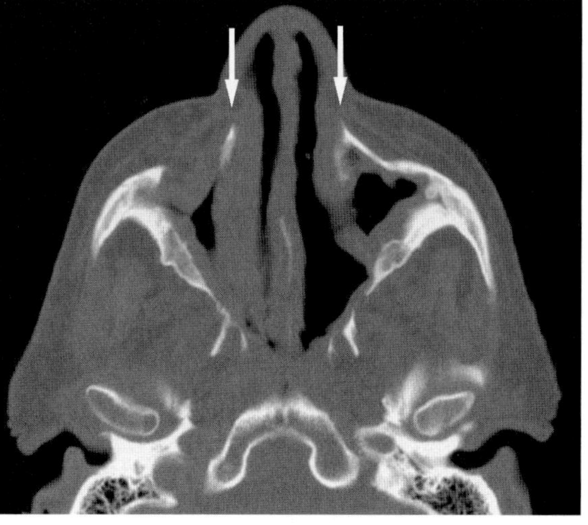

Figure 10.6

Chronic sinusitis; 69-year-old male with history of previous sinus surgery, now with history of motor vehicle accident and trauma to head. Axial CT image shows that medial maxillary sinus walls are removed surgically (*arrows*), as also part of right anterior maxillary sinus wall dot some bilateral mucosal thickening and uneven sinus wall sclerosis

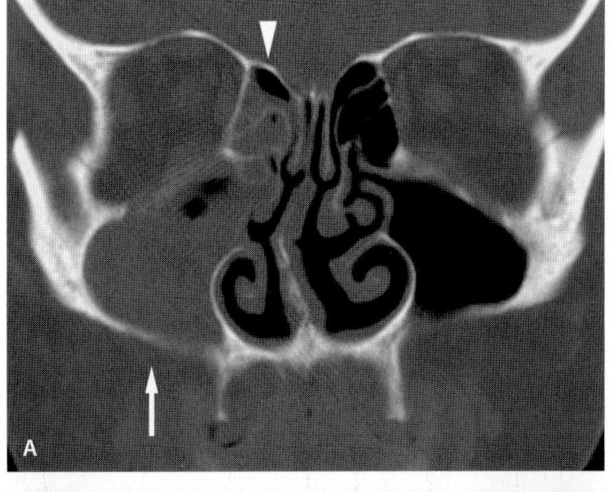

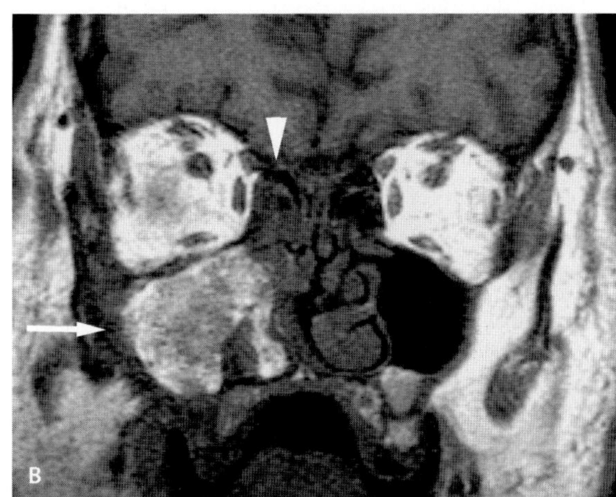

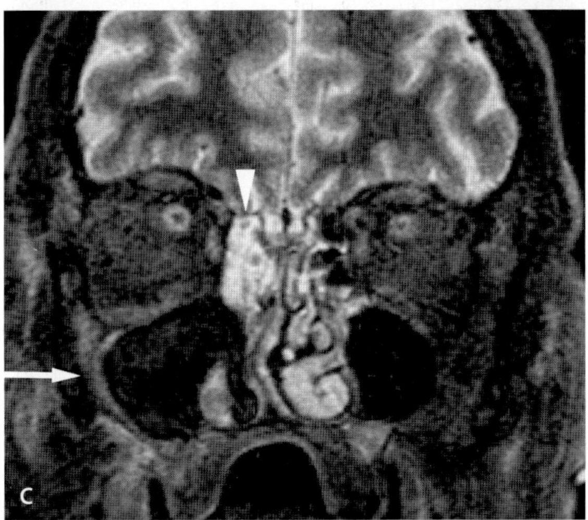

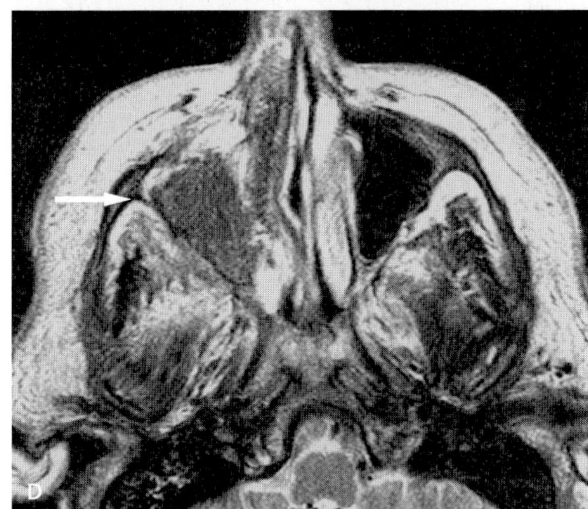

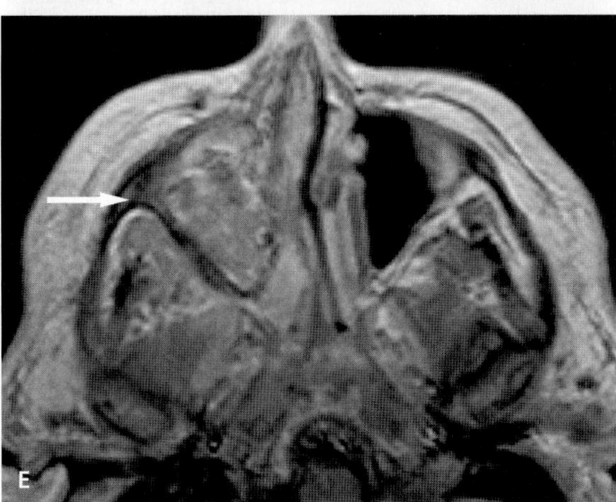

Figure 10.7

Chronic aspergillus sinusitis; 57-year-old female with history of acute lymphatic leukemia, neutropenic status post chemotherapy, now with eye and cheek pain. **A** Coronal CT image shows opacification of right maxillary sinus (*arrow*) and ethmoid sinus (*arrowhead*). **B** Coronal T1-weighted MRI shows intermediate to high signal in maxillary sinus (*arrow*) and low signal in ethmoid sinus (*arrowhead*). **C** coronal T2-weighted MRI shows low „normal" signal in right maxillary sinus (*arrow*) and high signal in ethmoid sinus (*arrowhead*). **D** Axial T1-weighted MRI shows intermediate to low signal in right maxillary sinus (*arrow*). **E** Axial T1-weighted post-Gd MRI shows heterogeneous contrast enhancement (*arrow*)

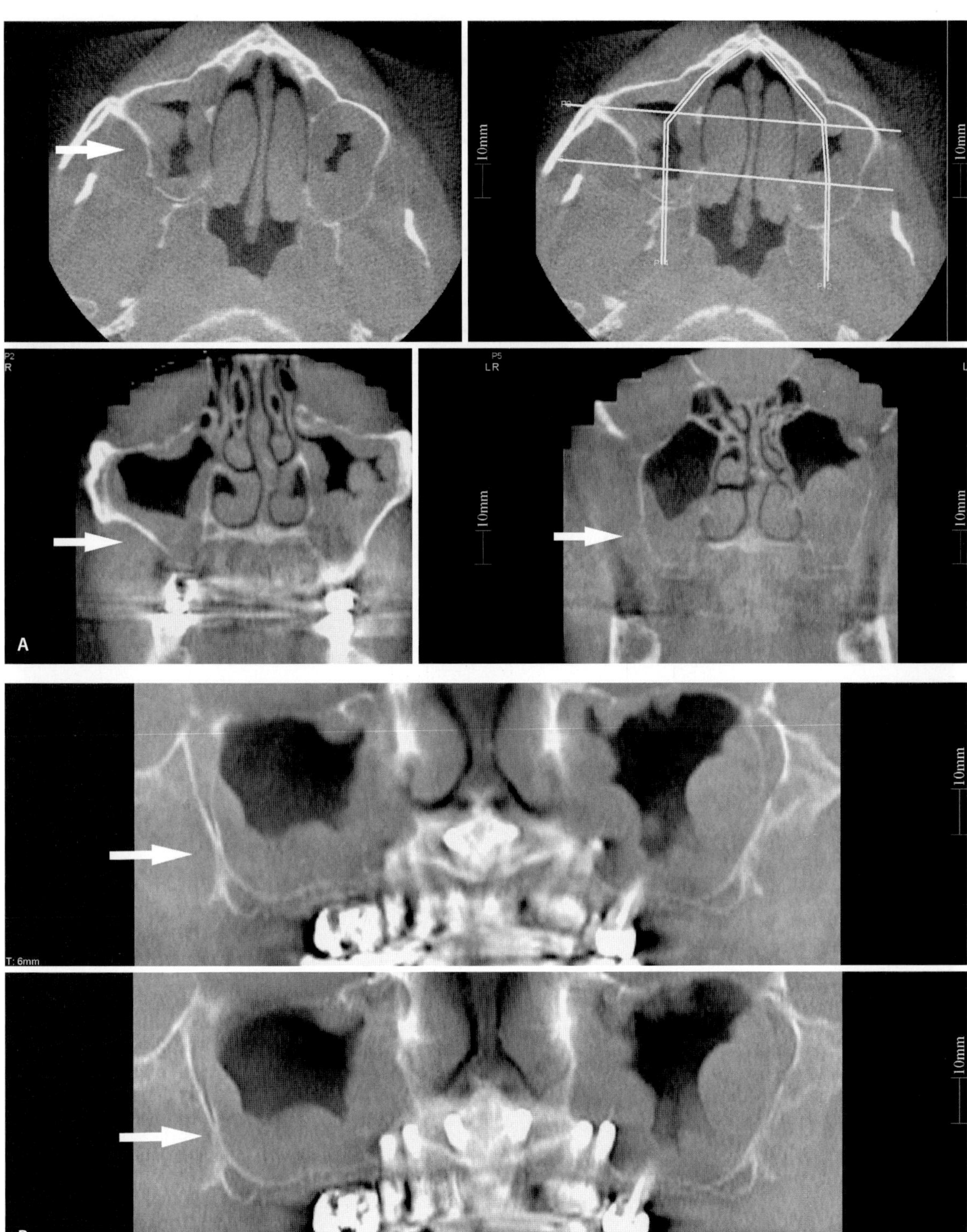

Figure 10.8

Mucosal maxillary thickening; incidental finding in 43-year-old male under treatment for dental implants and examined with cone beam CT. **A** Axial sections (*upper*) and coronal sections (*lower*) with reference lines (*upper right*) show maxillary mucosal thickening bilaterally (*arrows*). **B** Panoramic images (reference lines in **A** upper right) show maxillary mucosal thickening bilaterally (*arrows*) (courtesy of Drs. S. C. White and S. Tetradis, UCLA School of Dentistry)

Mucosal Imaging Findings in Asymptomatic Individuals

MRI findings of paranasal sinuses in patients with brain imaging.

- Mucosal thickening up to 3 mm may be present in clinically normal individuals.
- Clinically silent focal areas of mucosal thickening occur from about one-fourth and up to two-thirds of asymptomatic individuals.

Retention Cysts, Mucous and Serous

Definition

Mucous retention cyst: obstruction of submucosal mucinous gland, thus cyst wall of duct epithelium and gland capsule.

Serous retention cyst: accumulation of serous fluid in submucosal layer of sinus mucosa, thus cyst lining of elevated mucosa.

Clinical Features

- Incidental finding

Imaging Features

- Smooth, spherical soft tissue mass.
- Retention cysts found incidentally in 10–35% of patients, most commonly in maxillary sinus, but can occur in any sinus.
- Frequently small, may become large but always some air.
- Almost in every case normal bone.
- T1-weighted MRI: usually low to intermediate signal, but may show high signal if cyst has high protein content.
- T2-weighted MRI: high signal.

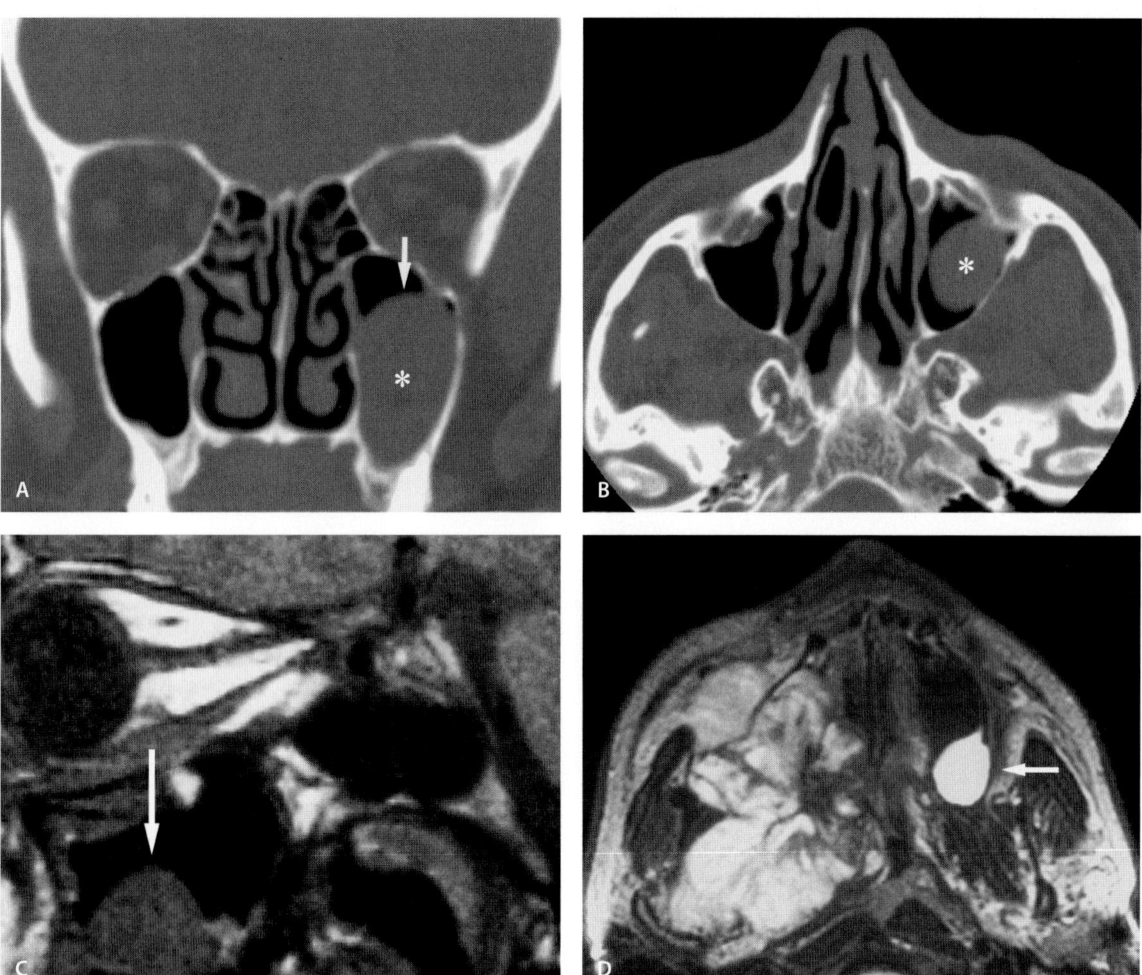

Figure 10.9

Retention cyst in maxillary sinus; incidental finding. A Coronal CT image shows retention cyst in maxillary sinus (*asterisk*) with soft-tissue lining (*arrow*), without expansion of sinus walls, but with remaining air. B Axial CT image of same patient shows soft-tissue lined retention cyst (*asterisk*). C Sagittal T1-weighted MRI shows retention cyst with intermediate signal (*arrow*) in patient with blow-out fracture. D Axial T2-weighted MRI shows retention cyst with high signal (*arrow*) in patient with osteosarcoma of right maxilla

Polyps

Definition

Expansion of fluids in deeper lamina propria of Schneiderian mucosa in nasal fossa and paranasal sinuses.

Clinical Features

- Most common expansile condition in nasal cavity; about 4% in general population.
- Nasal polyps most often associated with allergy, and frequently multiple and symmetric, but may result from infectious rhinosinusitis, vasomotor rhinitis, cystic fibrosis, diabetes mellitus, aspirin intolerance, and nickel exposure.
- In patients with polyps up to about 70% with asthma.
- Nasal stuffiness.
- When seen in children, cystic fibrosis should be ruled out.

Imaging Features

- Smooth, spherical soft tissue mass
- If multiple, complete opacification of nasal cavity and sinuses
- T1-weighted MRI: low to intermediate signal
- T2-weighted MRI: high signal
- Heterogeneous MR signal characteristic in chronic polyps; can also enhance

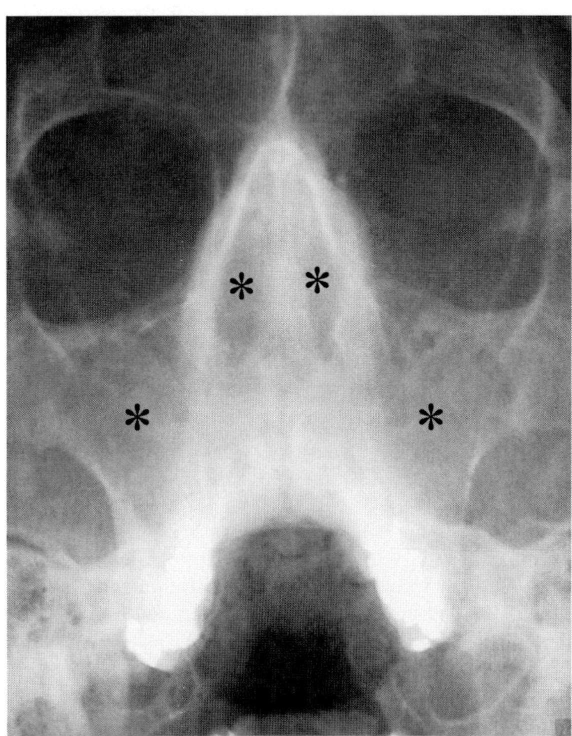

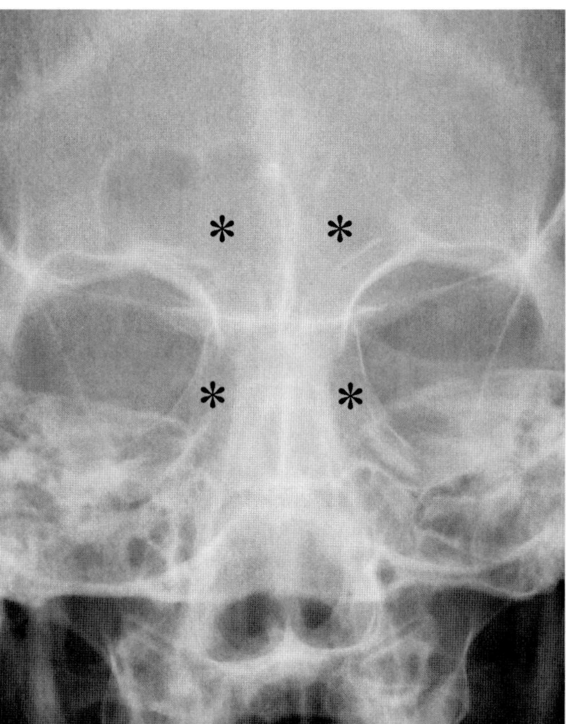

Figure 10.10

Nasal polyposis; 38-year-old male with nasal obstruction. Conventional films show complete opacification of nasal cavity and all paranasal sinuses (*asterisks*), except some air in right frontal sinus (courtesy of Dr. A. Kolbenstvedt, Rikshospitalet University Hospital, Oslo, Norway)

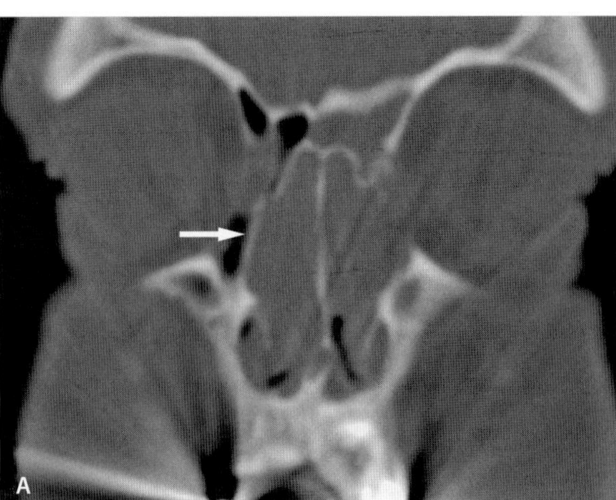

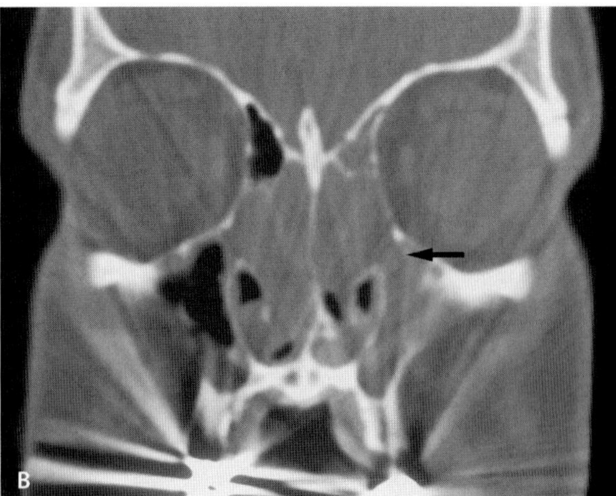

Figure 10.11

Nasal polyposis; patient with history of chronic nasal obstruction and sinusitis. **A** Coronal CT image shows opacification of nasal cavity (*arrow*). **B** Coronal CT image shows opacification of nasal cavity with soft tissue bulging through widened ostiomeatal complex particularly on left side (*arrow*) but to a lesser extent also on right, with secondary sinusitis

Figure 10.12

Nasal polyposis; 43-year-old male with previous surgery for nasal polyposis, now with recurrence. Coronal CT image shows polyps in nose bulging through ostiomeatal complex (*arrow*), but also mucosal thickening in ethmoid and maxillary sinuses (courtesy of Dr. A. Kolbenstvedt, Rikshospitalet University Hospital, Oslo, Norway)

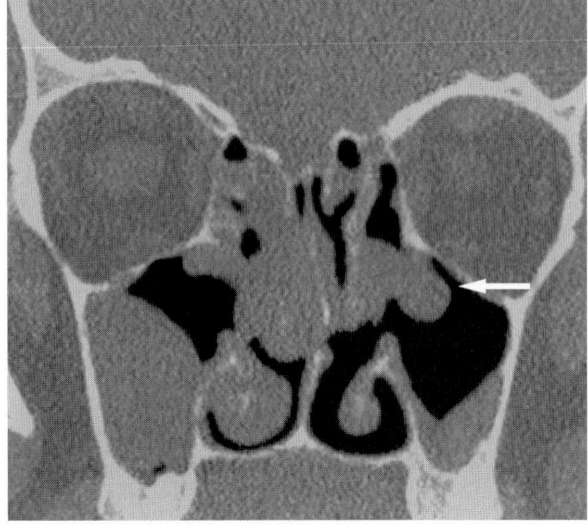

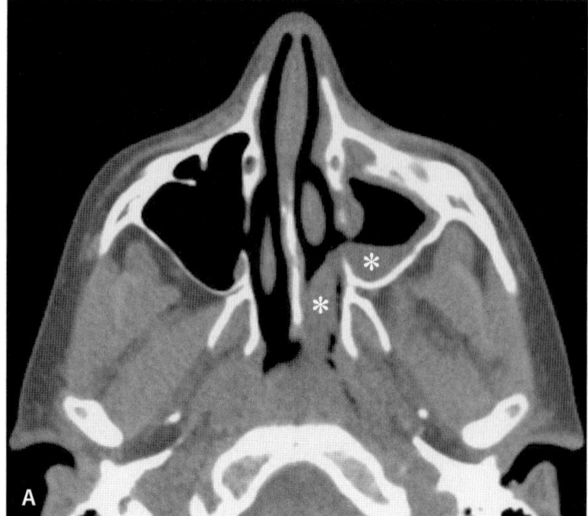

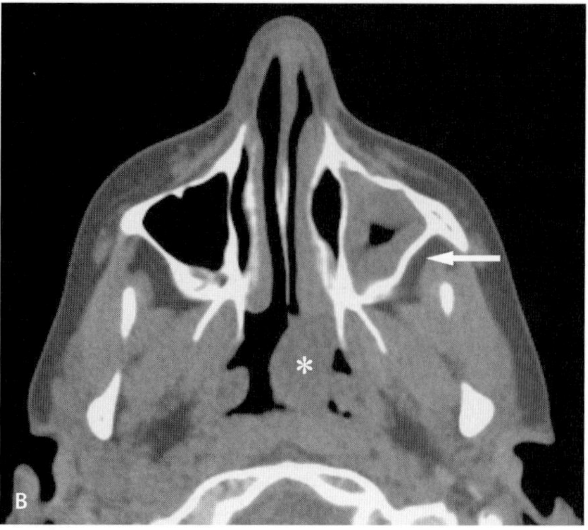

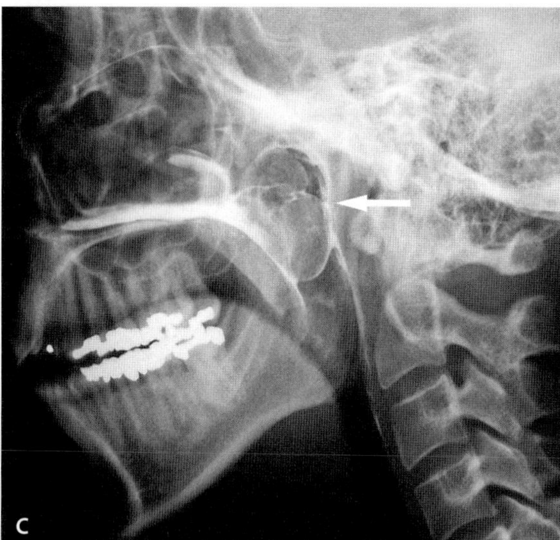

Figure 10.13

Antrochoanal polyp; 12-year-old male with history of sinusitis and nasopharyngeal mass. **A** Axial CT image shows left maxillary sinus thickening (*asterisk*) with extension of soft tissue mass into posterior nasal cavity down to nasopharynx (*asterisk*), via ethmoidal infundibulum. No bone destruction. **B** Axial CT image shows polyp in nasopharynx (*asterisk*) and soft tissue thickening in maxillary sinus (*arrow*). **C** Lateral view with contrast in nose of another patient shows how polyp blocks nasopharynx (*arrow*) (C: courtesy of Dr. A. Kolbenstvedt, Rikshospitalet University Hospital, Oslo, Norway)

Mucoceles

Definition

Collection of mucoid secretions surrounded by mucus-secreting respiratory epithelium.

Both retention and mucocele cysts consist of mucous secretions surrounded by epithelial lining, but are distinguished by their clinical and imaging features. Mucocele develops due to obstruction of sinus ostium or a compartment of a sinus with the sinus mucosa as the mucocele wall and always with expanded sinus walls.

Clinical Features

- Most common expansile condition in paranasal sinuses.
- Most frequent in frontal sinuses (60–65 %); only 5–10 % in sphenoid as well as in maxillary sinuses.
- Both sexes, wide range of age: 20 to 60 years.
- Classic mucocele is sterile with signs and symptoms from mass effect.
- Pain uncommon.
- If infected, pain; mucopyocele or pyocele.
- Ostial obstruction may be caused by inflammatory scar, trauma, or tumor.

Imaging Features

- Initially, intact but remodeled, expanded surrounding bone.
- With progressive growth sinus wall will be destroyed.
- Completely airless sinus.
- T1-weighted and T2-weighted MRI: variable MR signals depending on protein content, state of dehydration, and viscosity of content; most frequently observed patterns are moderate-to-marked high signal on T1 and T2, or moderate-to-marked low signal on T1 and T2, usually low to intermediate T1 and high T2.
- T1-weighted post-Gd MRI: no enhancement except of thin peripheral rim.

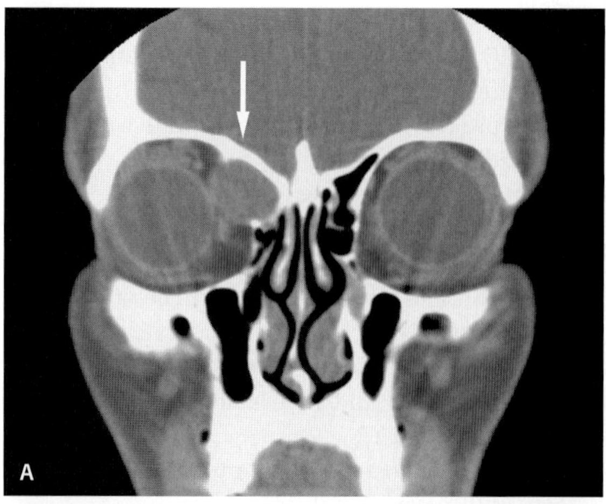

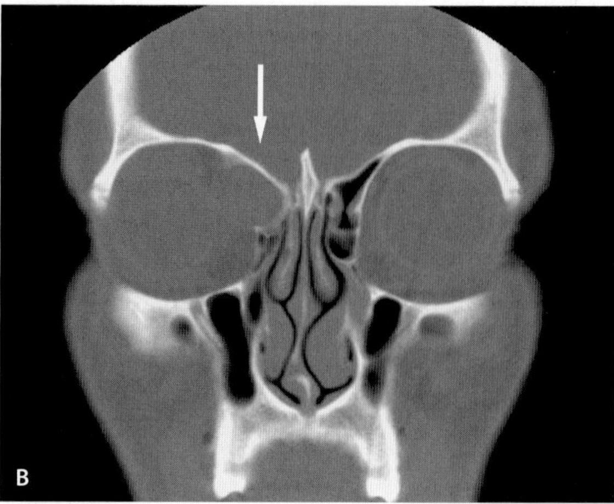

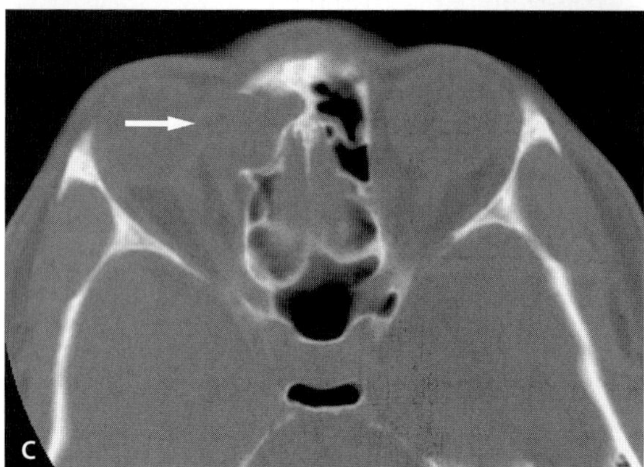

Figure 10.14

Frontal sinus mucocele; 50-year-old male with diplopia and right eye down and laterally deviated. **A** Coronal CT image, soft-tissue window, shows ovoid well-defined soft tissue mass in right orbit (*arrow*) with displacement of globe laterally down. **B** Coronal CT image, bone window, shows bone expansion and absent frontal sinus wall against orbit (*arrow*), but otherwise normal bone structures. **C** Axial CT image shows well-defined delineation of bone expansion (*arrow*)

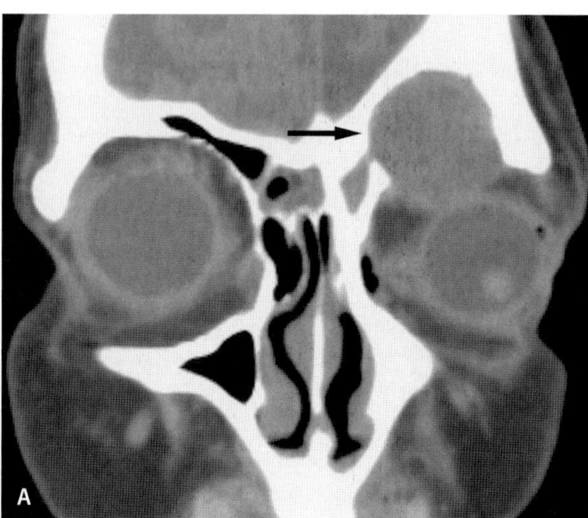

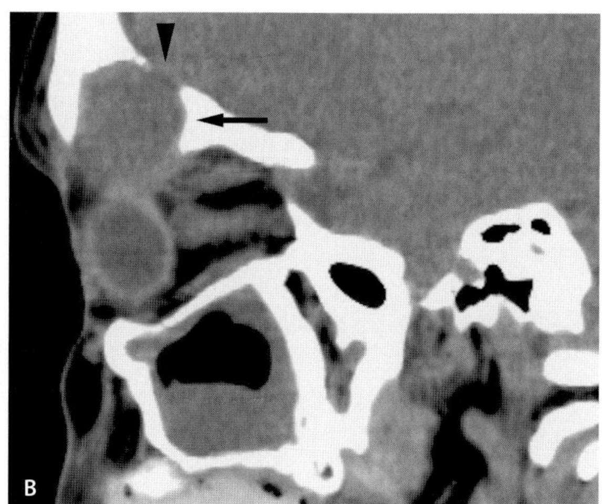

Figure 10.15

Frontal sinus mucocele; 52-year-old female with headache and diplopia. **A** Coronal CT image shows well-defined soft-tissue mass with no air in left frontal sinus with bone expansion (*arrow*), displacing globe down and laterally. **B** Sagittal CT image shows mucocele with bone expansion (*arrow*) and destroyed bone delineation to anterior cranial fossa (*arrowhead*). Note mucosal thickening in maxillary sinus

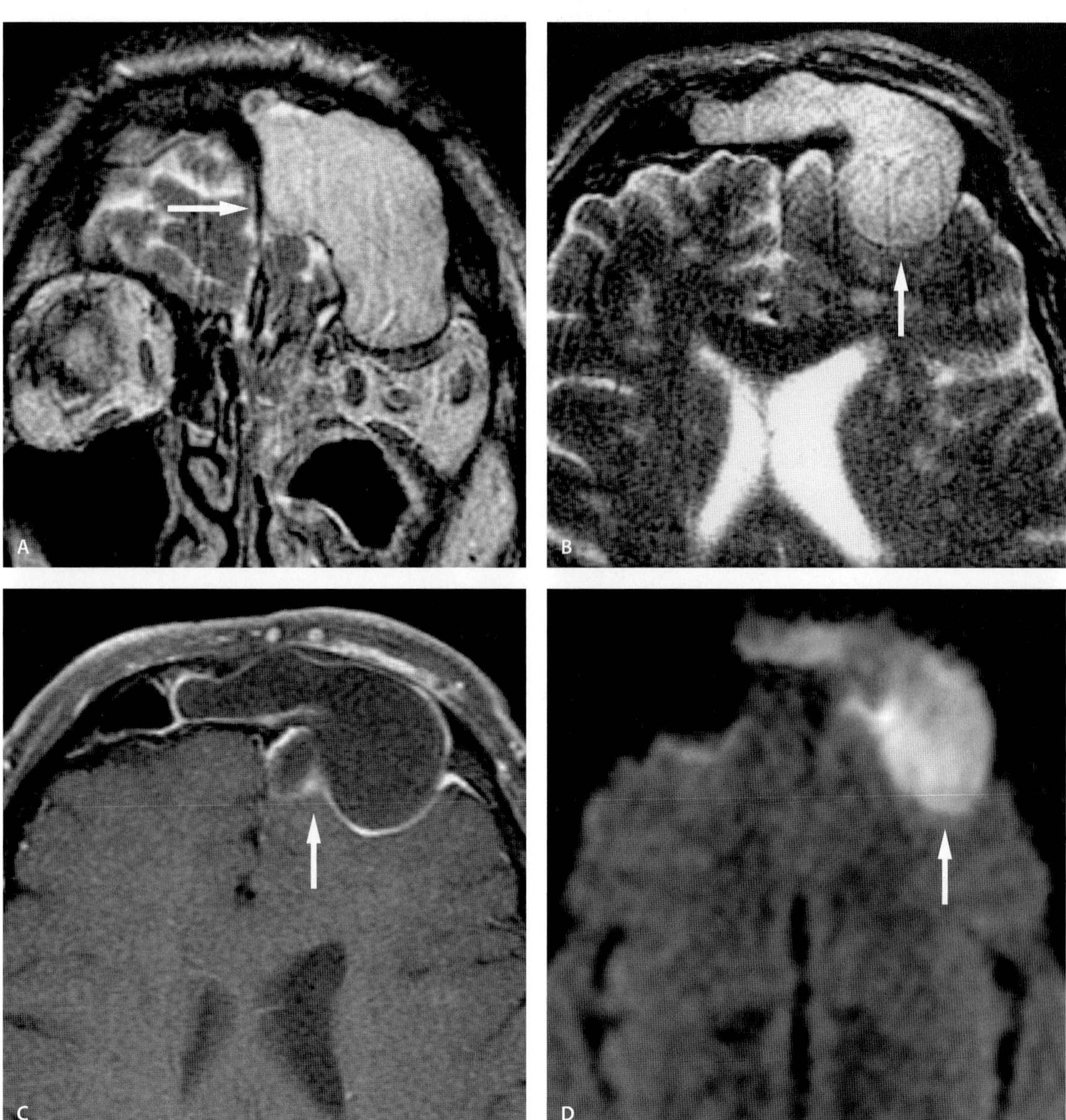

Figure 10.16

Frontal sinus mucocele; 60-year-old male presented with headache and diplopia. **A** Coronal T2-weighted MRI shows intermediate signal large expansive mucocele (*arrow*). **B** Axial T2-weighted MRI shows expansion into cranial fossa with displacement of left frontal lobe (*arrow*). **C** Axial T1-weighted post-Gd MRI shows no enhancement except in thin peripheral rim (*arrow*). **D** Axial diffusion-weighted MRI shows high signal (*arrow*)

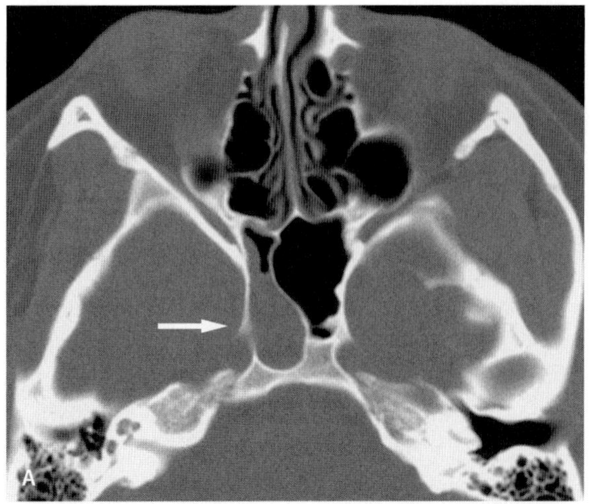

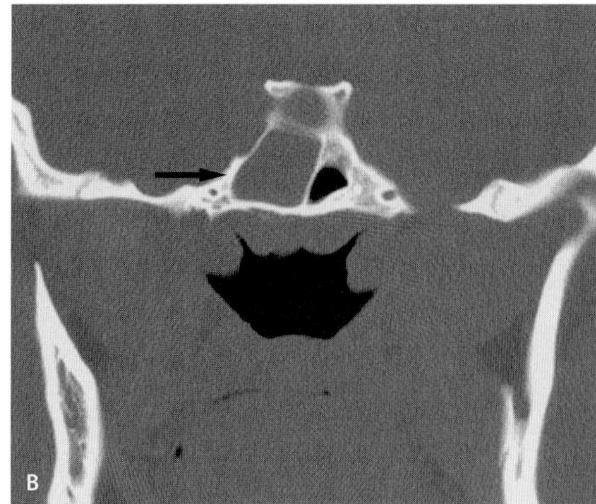

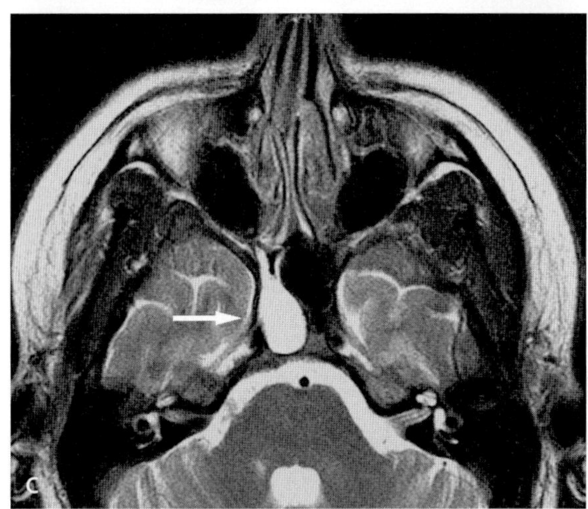

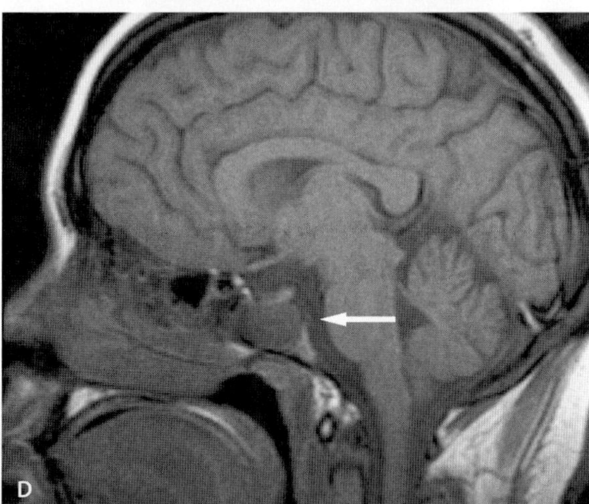

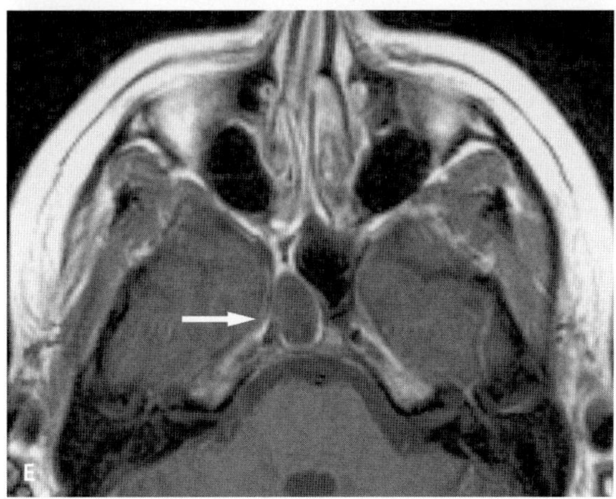

Figure 10.17

Sphenoid sinus mucocele; 19-year-old female with past medical history significant for morbid obesity who presented with history of head ache for 6 weeks, as well as occasional nausea and vomiting; initially evaluated for suspicion of brain tumor, pseudotumor cerebri, and venous thrombosis. **A** Axial CT image shows expansive mass in right compartment of sphenoid sinus with intact cortical outline (*arrow*). **B** Coronal CT image shows mucocele in right compartment of sphenoid sinus (*arrow*). **C** Axial T2-weighted MRI shows high signal of mucocele (*arrow*). **D** Sagittal T1-weighted MRI shows intermediate to low signal (*arrow*). **E** Axial T1-weighted post-Gd MRI shows no enhancement except in thin peripheral rim (*arrow*)

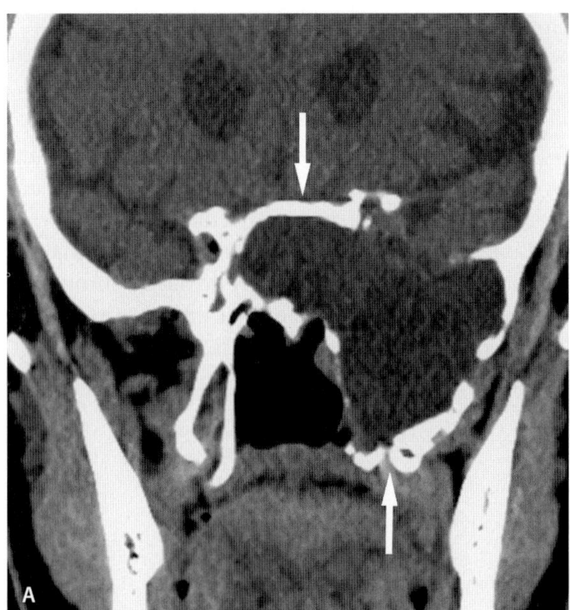

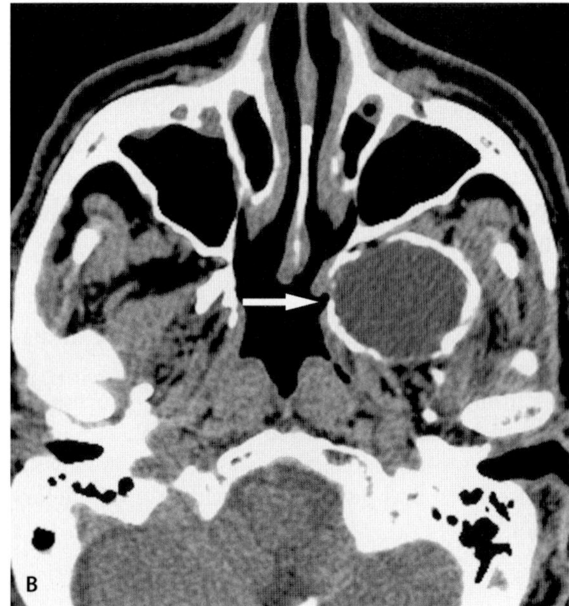

Figure 10.18

Sphenoid sinus mucocele; 85-year-old male with known chronic sinusitis, now with headache. **A** Coronal CT image, soft tissue, shows large expansive mass (*arrows*) with homogeneous hypodense content extending into clivus and pterygoid process of sphenoid bone. **B** Axial CT image, soft tissue, shows mucocele extending into parapharyngeal space (*arrow*)

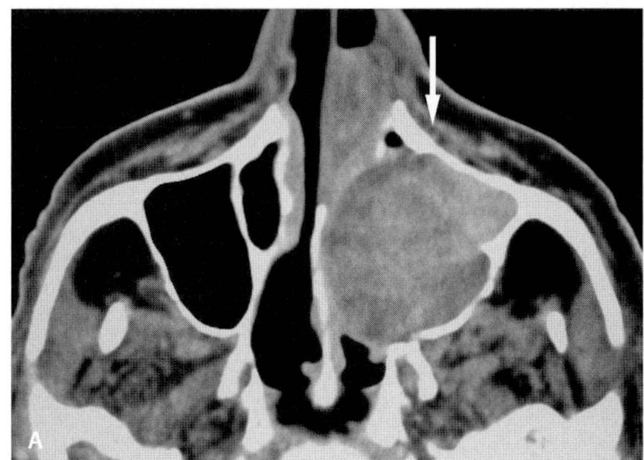

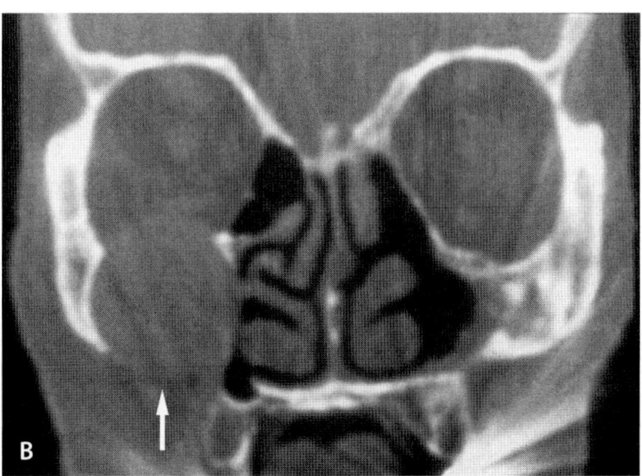

Figure 10.19

Maxillary sinus mucocele; two patients with long history of chronic sinusitis and sinus surgery. **A** Axial CT image shows expansive process in entire left maxillary sinus (*arrow*) extending to midline of nasal cavity. **B** Coronal CT image shows expansive mass in entire right maxillary sinus extending into orbit (*arrow*)

Noninfectious Destructive Sinonasal Disease (Wegener's Granulomatosis)

Definition

Necrotizing granulomatous vasculitis that usually affects upper and lower respiratory tracts and causes renal glomerulonephritis, with a limited form only in sinonasal tract with a more benign course.

Clinical Features

- Rare; diagnosis difficult to establish early in disease course.
- Chronic, nonspecific inflammatory process of nose and sinuses for more than a year.
- Nasal septum affected in more than 90%, with ulceration and perforation („saddle nose“ deformity).

Imaging Features

- Nasal involvement precedes sinus disease; secretions, soft-tissue mass of nasal septum, septal erosion.
- Sinuses affected in more than 90%; nonspecific inflammation with mucosal thickening of maxillary and ethmoid sinuses in particular.
- Bones of nasal vault and affected sinuses may be thickened and severely sclerotic due to chronic inflammation, but also bone destruction reflecting either osteomyelitis or necrosis.

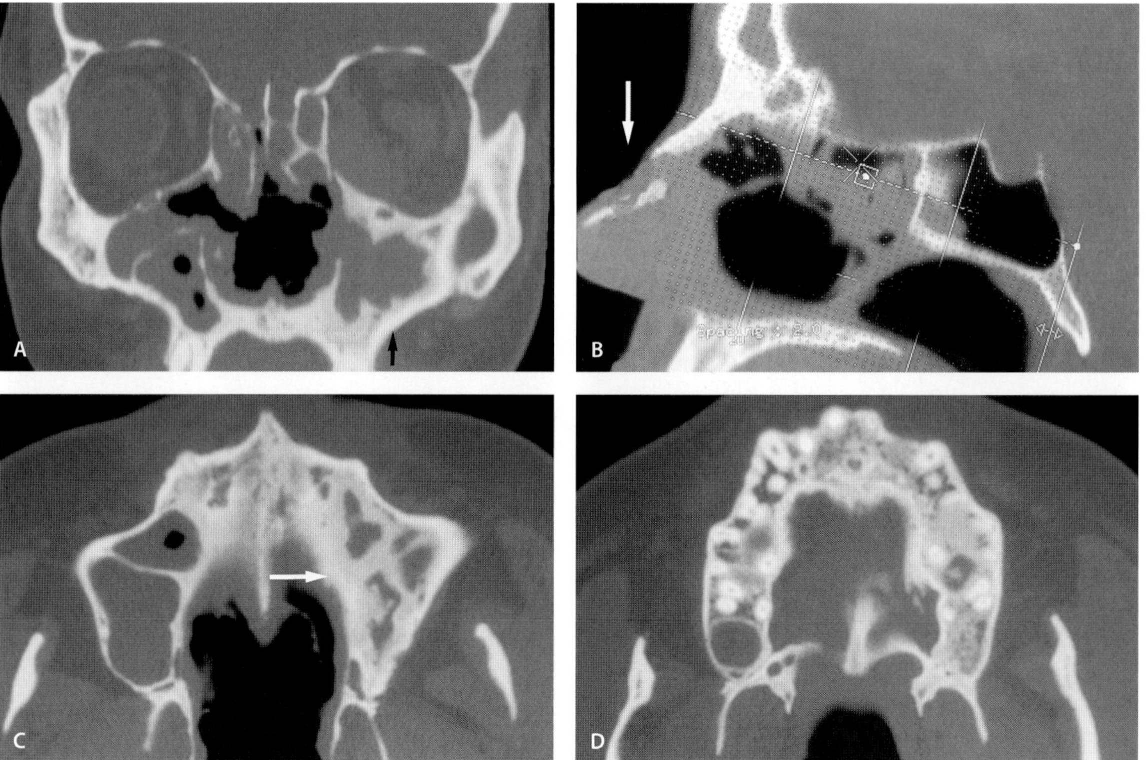

Figure 10.20

Wegener's granulomatosis; 46-year-old male with long history of nonspecific sinus problems Mucosal biopsy consistent with Wegener's granulomatosis. **A** Coronal CT image shows destruction of nasal cavity structures, and chronic sinusitis; opacification, mucosal thickening of ethmoid cells and maxillary sinuses, with severe sclerosis of maxillary sinus walls (*arrow*). **B** Sagittal CT image shows destruction of nasal bone, saddle nose (*arrow*). **C** Axial CT image shows severe sclerosis of sinus walls (*arrow*) and palate, crossing midline. **D** Axial CT image shows sclerotic bone in maxillary alveolar process

Inflammatory Dental Conditions

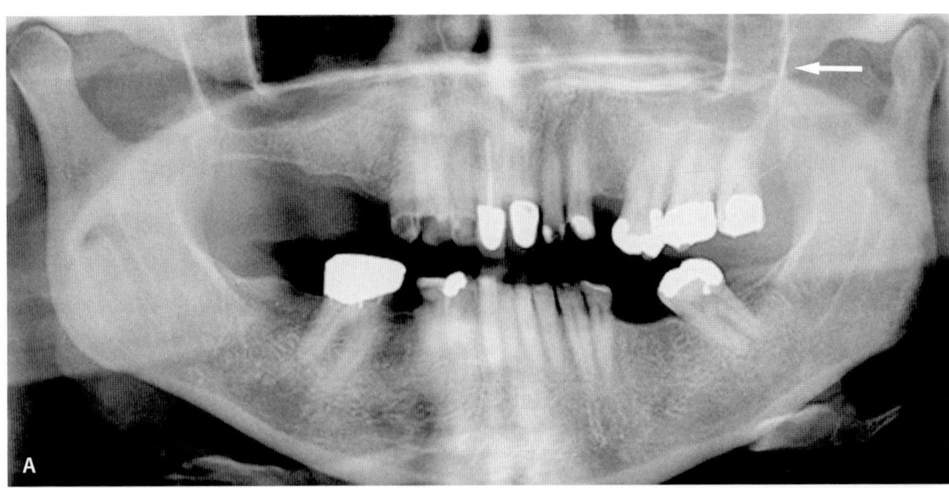

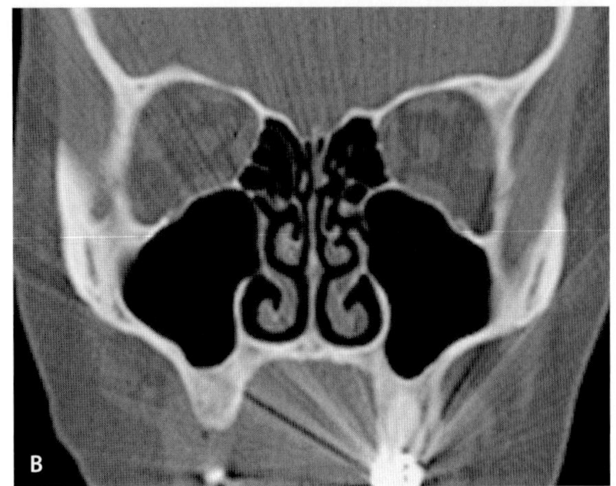

Figure 10.21

Normal paranasal sinuses; false-positive panoramic view opacification of maxillary sinus. **A** Panoramic view indicates opacification of left maxillary sinus (*arrow*). **B** Coronal CT image shows normal air and bony walls of maxillary and ethmoid sinuses

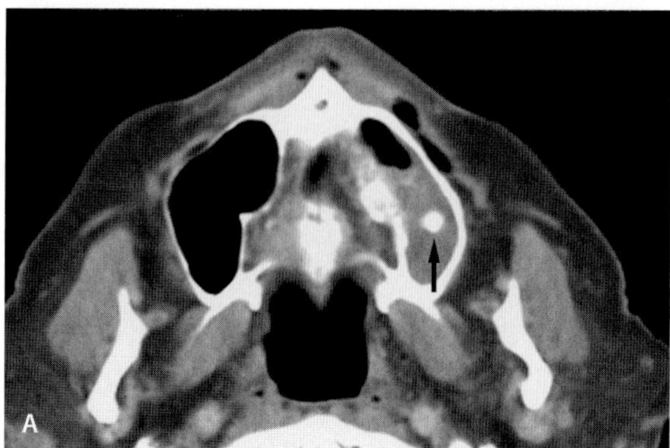

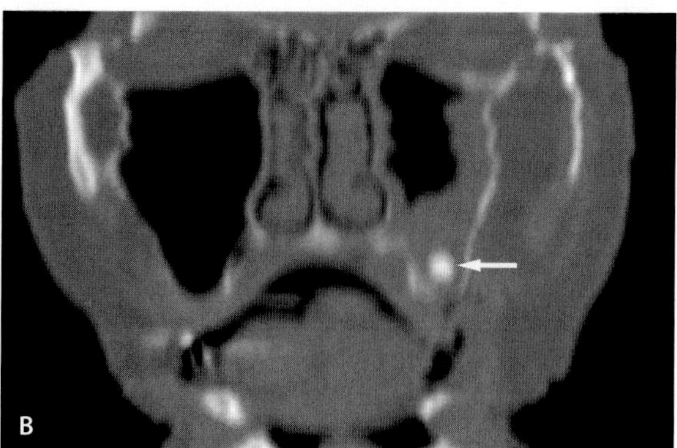

Figure 10.22

Maxillary sinusitis due to displaced root; patient with history of problematic tooth extraction. **A** Axial CT image shows root in maxillary sinus with mucosal thickening (*arrow*). **B** Coronally reformatted CT image shows root in alveolar part of sinus (*arrow*)

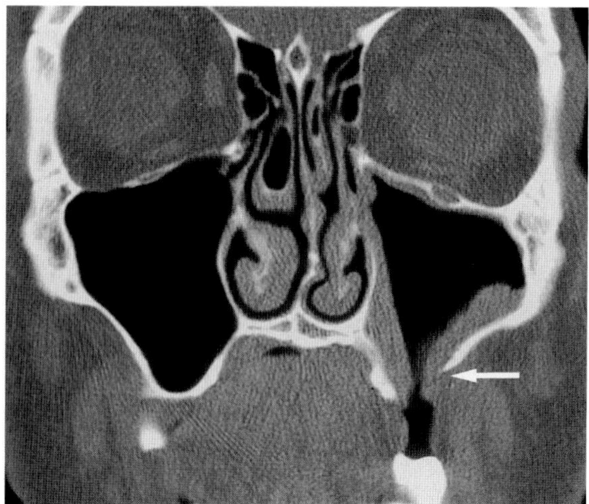

Figure 10.23

Oroantral fistula; patient with history of previous problematic tooth extraction. Coronal CT shows opening between oral cavity and maxillary sinus (*arrow*) and minimal mucosal thickening

Tumors and Tumor-like Conditions

Clinical Features

- Tumors and tumor-like expansile masses are generally rare.
- Benign more frequent than malignant.
- Vague symptoms; masses frequently extensive when detected.

Imaging Features

- Soft-tissue mass.
- Benign: expansion, remodeling of bone, bone or dental hard-tissue production, may resorb teeth.
- Malignant: destruction of bone, occasionally bone production, „floating" teeth.
- T1-weighted MRI: intermediate.
- T2-weighted MRI: intermediateto high.
- T1-weighted post-Gd MRI: contrast enhancement.
- May be difficult to decide whether mass originated in sinus or not.

Papilloma

Definition

Benign tumor of nasal cavity composed of vascular connective tissue covered by well-differentiated stratified squamous epithelium that tends to grow under and elevate mucosa (inverted).

Clinical Features

- Less common than allergic polyps; less than 3% in general population.
- Most common in males aged 40–70 years.
- Unilateral from lateral sinus wall near ethmoids.
- Nasal stuffiness or obstruction.
- Secondary bacterial sinusitis.
- Postoperative recurrence 35–40%.
- May be associated with malignancy (about 10%).

Imaging Features

- Small to extensive mass
- Bone remodeling that may deviate, not cross nasal septum
- Mass may extend into ethmoid or maxillary sinuses
- T1-weighted MRI: low or intermediate
- T2-weighted MRI: infermediate to high, usually high
- T1-weighted post-Gd MRI: some contrast enhancement

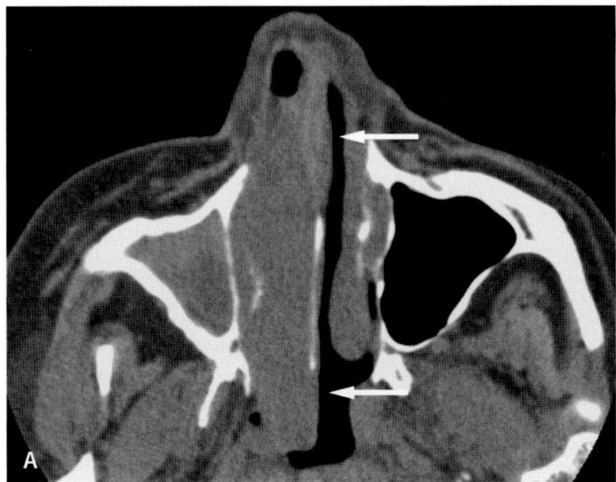

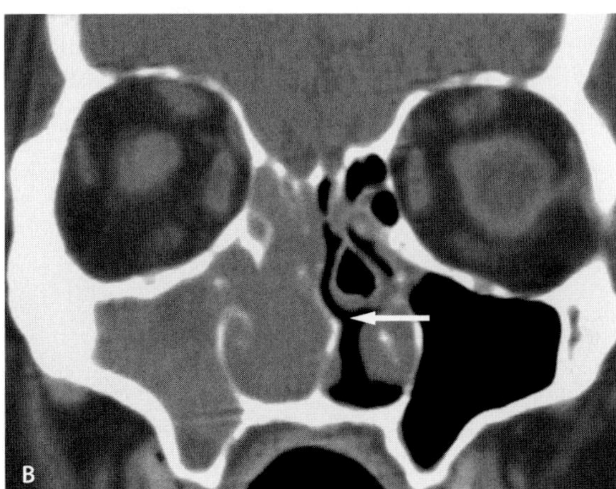

Figure 10.24

Inverted papilloma; 71-year-old male with history of nasal papilloma that developed malignancy. **A** Axial CT image shows soft-tissue mass in right nasal cavity with some deviation of nasal septum extending into nasopharynx (*arrows*). **B** Coronal CT image shows complete opacification of right nasal cavity, maxillary sinus (*arrow*), and right ethmoid sinus, and some widening of the ostiomeatal complex

Osteoma

Definition

Benign tumor of normal mature bone.

Clinical Features

- Usually an incidental finding

Imaging Features

- Most common in frontal sinuses, followed by ethmoid and maxillary sinuses
- May occlude sinus ostia causing sinusitis or mucocele formation

See also Chapter 3.

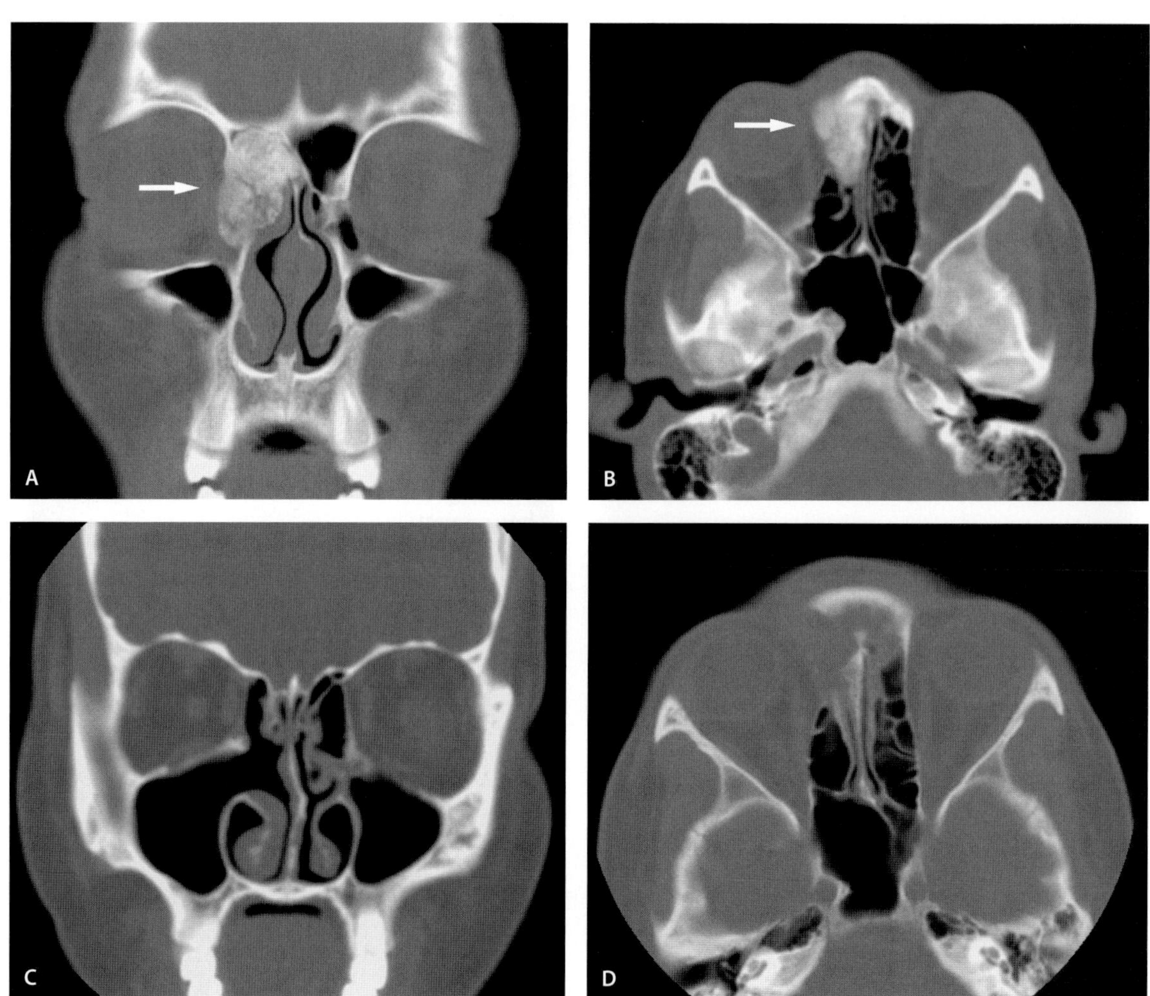

Figure 10.25

Frontal/ethmoid osteoma; 19-year-old female. **A** Coronal CT image shows well-defined bone mass in right frontal and ethmoid sinuses crossing midline (*arrow*), with left ethmoid and maxillary sinuses normal. **B** Axial CT image shows osteoma extending to frontal recess of maxilla anteriorly (*arrow*), with otherwise normal ethmoid and sphenoid sinuses. **C** Coronal CT image, post-surgery, shows resection of right middle turbinate and part of ethmoid sinus but otherwise normal bone structures and sinus air. **D** Axial CT image, post-surgery, shows partial resection of ethmoid sinus, but otherwise normal bone structures and sinus air

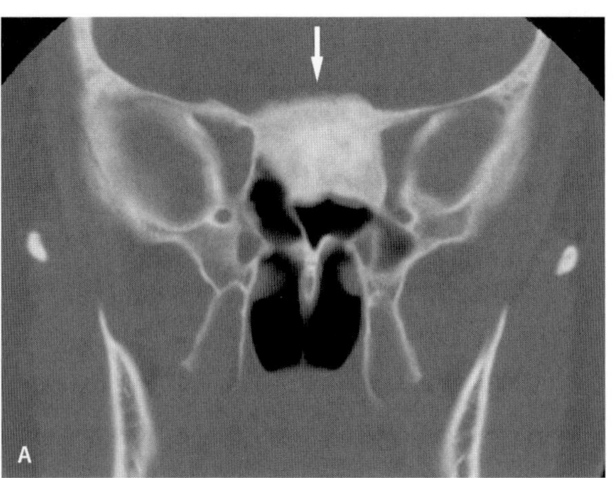

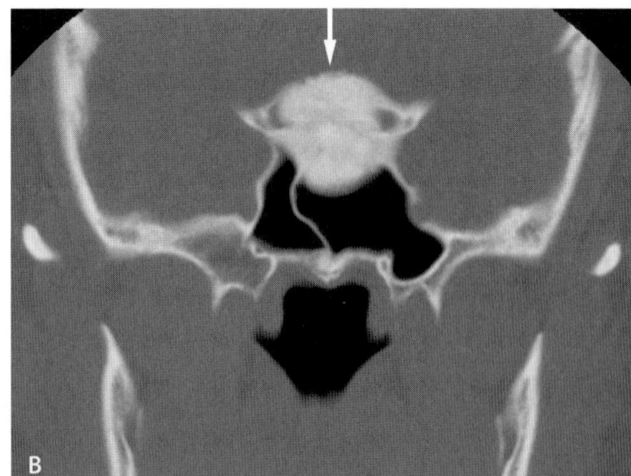

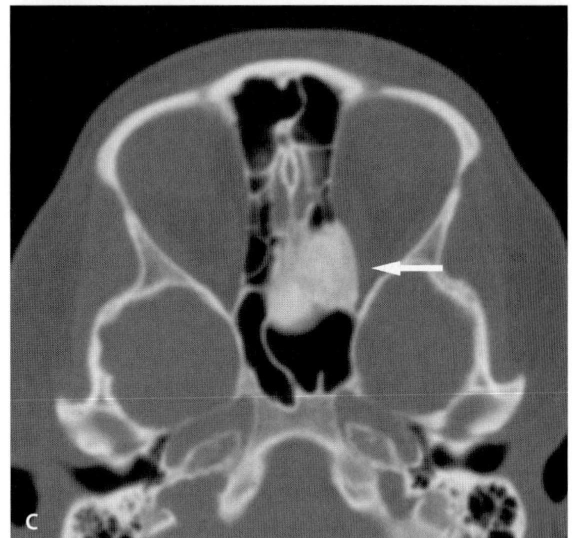

Figure 10.26

Sphenoid/ethmoid osteoma surgically confirmed, 24-year-old female with headache. A Coronal CT image shows well-defined dense mass in sphenoid bone extending into sinus (*arrow*). B Coronal CT image shows mass involving sella turcica (*arrow*). C Axial CT image shows mass extending into ethmoid and sphenoid sinuses (*arrow*)

Fibrous Dysplasia

Definition

Benign bone disease; metaplastic fibrous tissue.

Clinical Features

- Painless swelling, deformity

Imaging Features

- Radiolucent and/or radiopaque areas, depending on amount of fibrous tissue
- Ground-glass appearance typical

See also Chapter 3.

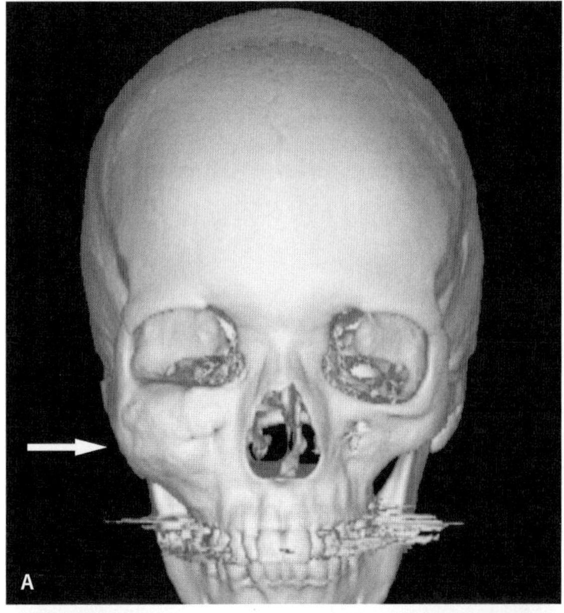

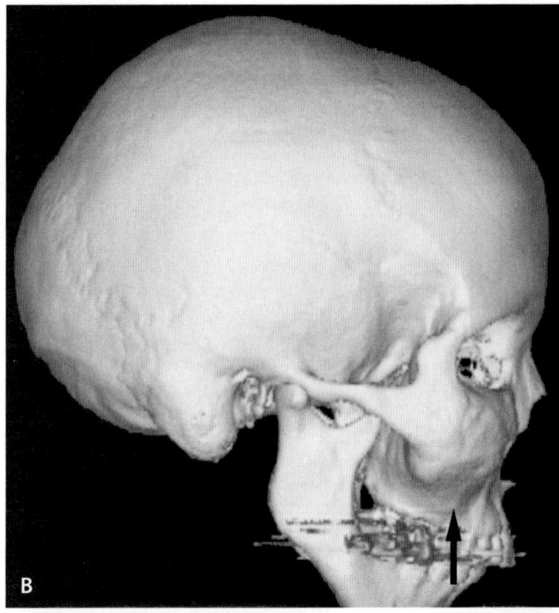

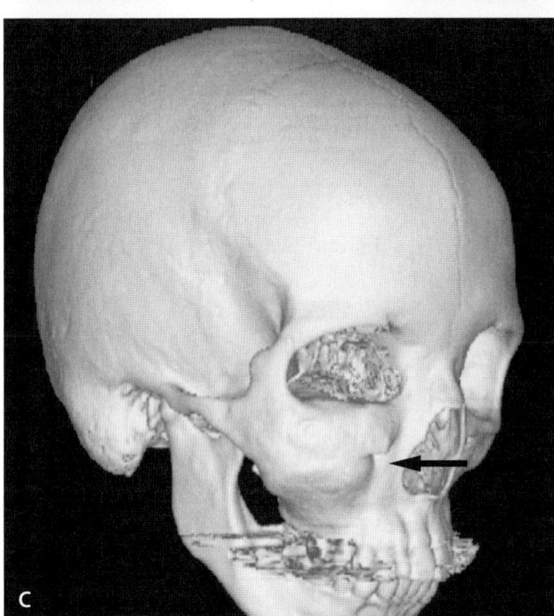

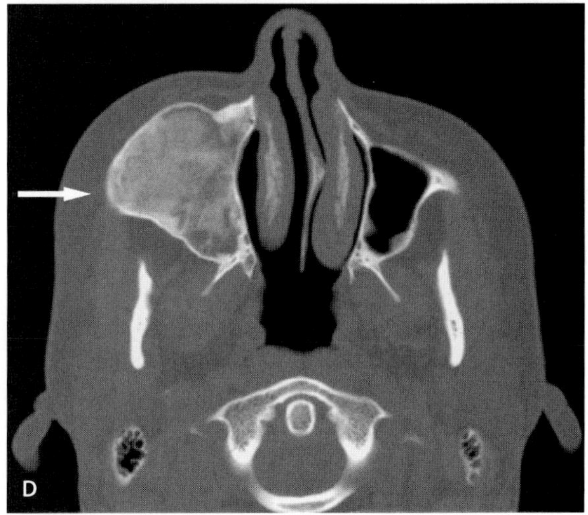

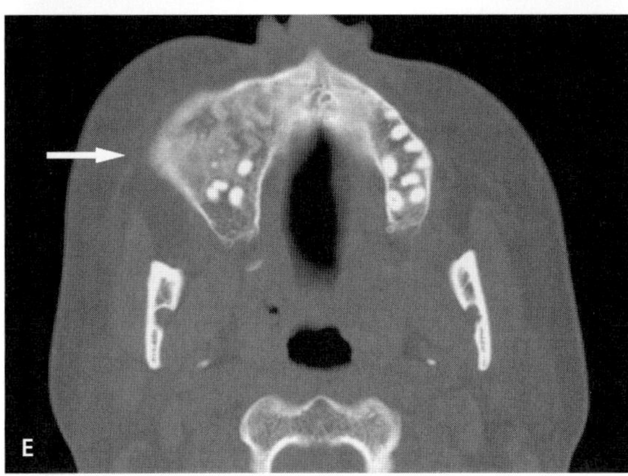

Figure 10.27

Fibrous dysplasia; 23-year-old female with painless swelling of cheek. **A** 3D CT image, en face, shows expanded right maxilla and zygoma (*arrow*) with elevated orbital floor. **B** 3D CT image, lateral, shows expanded frontal process and anterior wall of maxilla (*arrow*). **C** 3D CT image, oblique view, shows elevated orbital floor and expansion around infraorbital foramen (*arrow*). **D** Axial CT image shows ground-glass appearance (*arrow*). **E** Axial CT image of alveolar process shows no evident displacement or resorption of teeth (*arrow*)

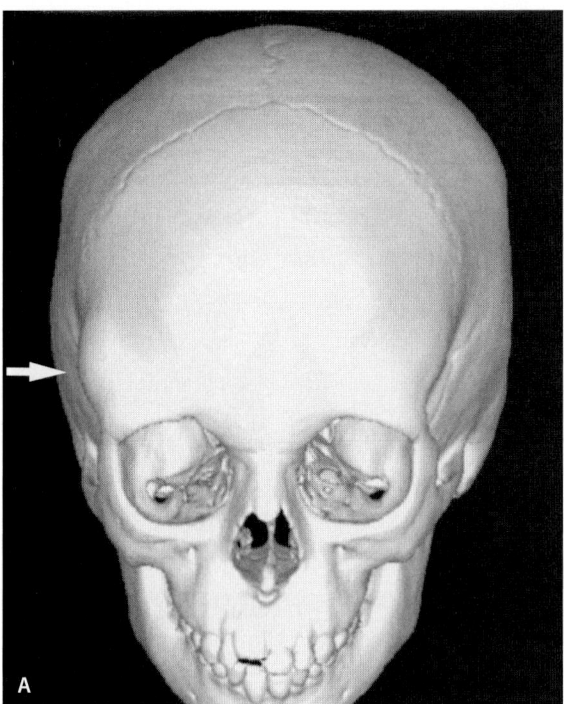

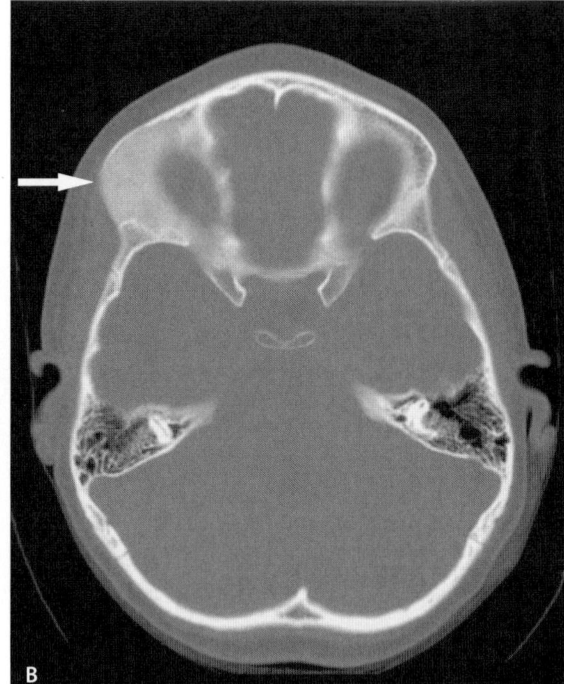

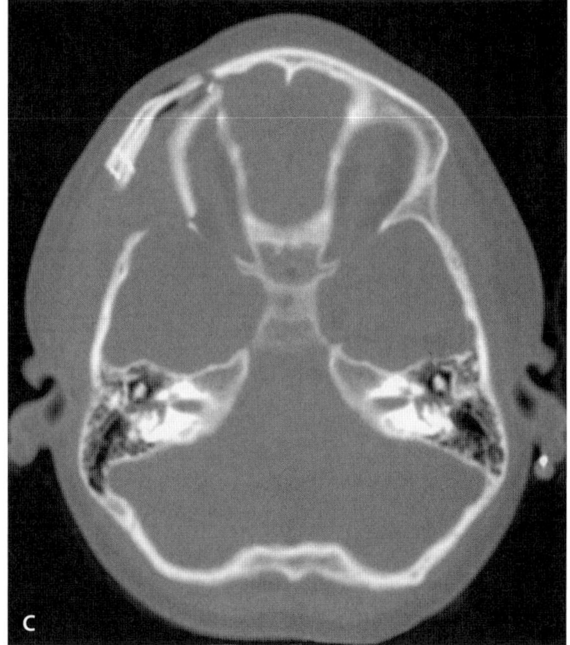

Figure 10.28

Frontal fibrous dysplasia; 6-year-old female with painless swelling of right frontal bone. A 3D CT image, en face, shows well-defined and smooth swelling (*arrow*). B Axial CT image shows ground-glass appearance (*arrow*). C Axial CT image, postoperative, shows normal morphology in the area

Nasolabial Cyst

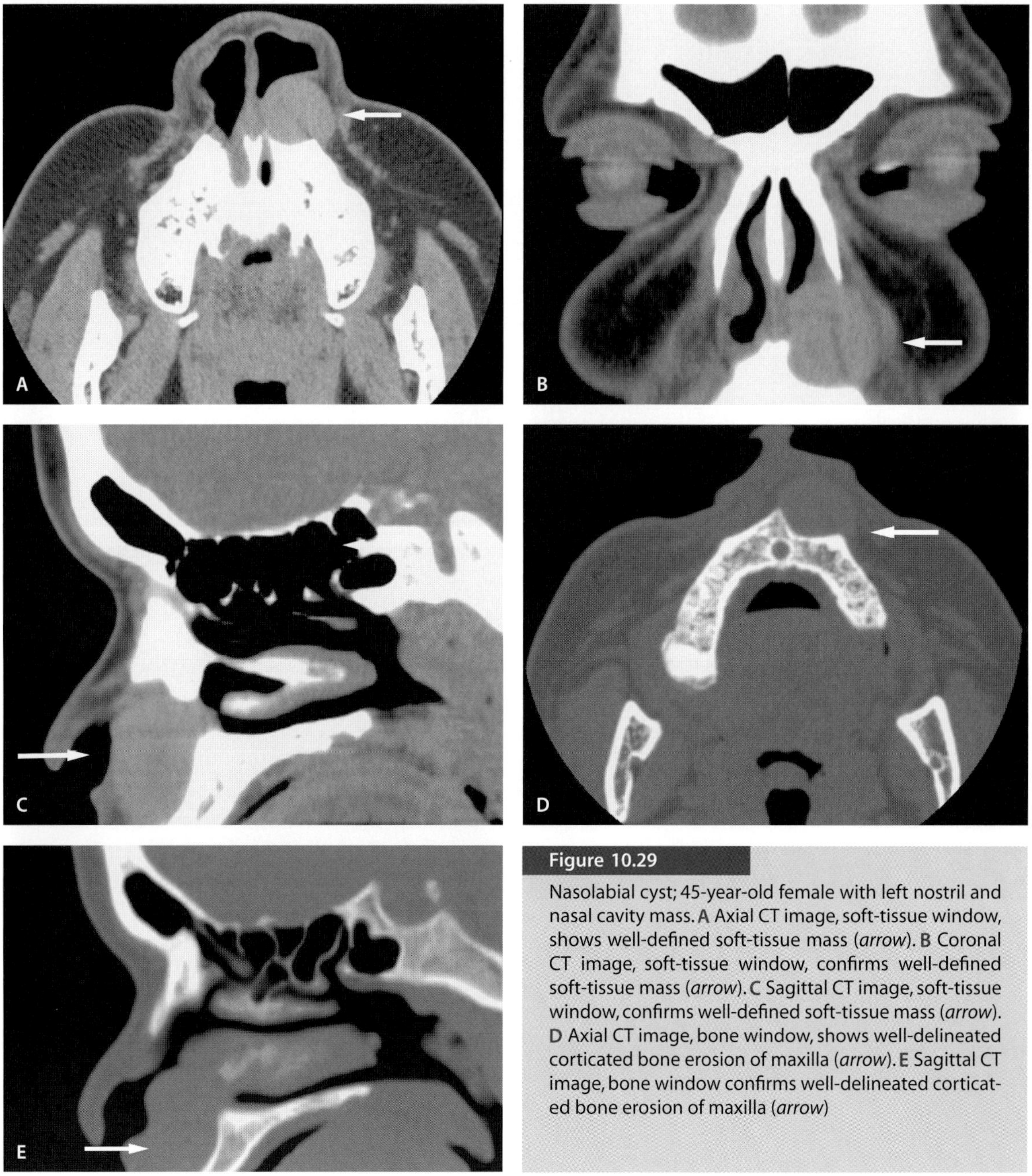

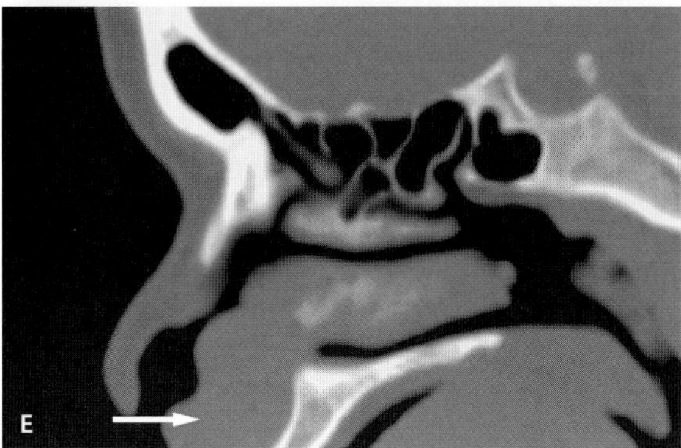

Figure 10.29

Nasolabial cyst; 45-year-old female with left nostril and nasal cavity mass. A Axial CT image, soft-tissue window, shows well-defined soft-tissue mass (*arrow*). B Coronal CT image, soft-tissue window, confirms well-defined soft-tissue mass (*arrow*). C Sagittal CT image, soft-tissue window, confirms well-defined soft-tissue mass (*arrow*). D Axial CT image, bone window, shows well-delineated corticated bone erosion of maxilla (*arrow*). E Sagittal CT image, bone window confirms well-delineated corticated bone erosion of maxilla (*arrow*)

Malignant Tumors

See also Chapter 4.

Squamous Cell Carcinoma

Definition
Malignant epithelial tumor.

Clinical Features
- 50–80% of all malignant sinus masses.
- More than 60% originate in maxillary sinuses, followed by nasal cavity, and ethmoid sinuses.
- Oral symptoms and signs may be initial; occasionally considered an intraoral cancer clinically.

Imaging Features
- Usually advanced when detected; bone destruction in 80%.
- Alveolar bone destruction reported in half of patients with maxillary sinus carcinoma.

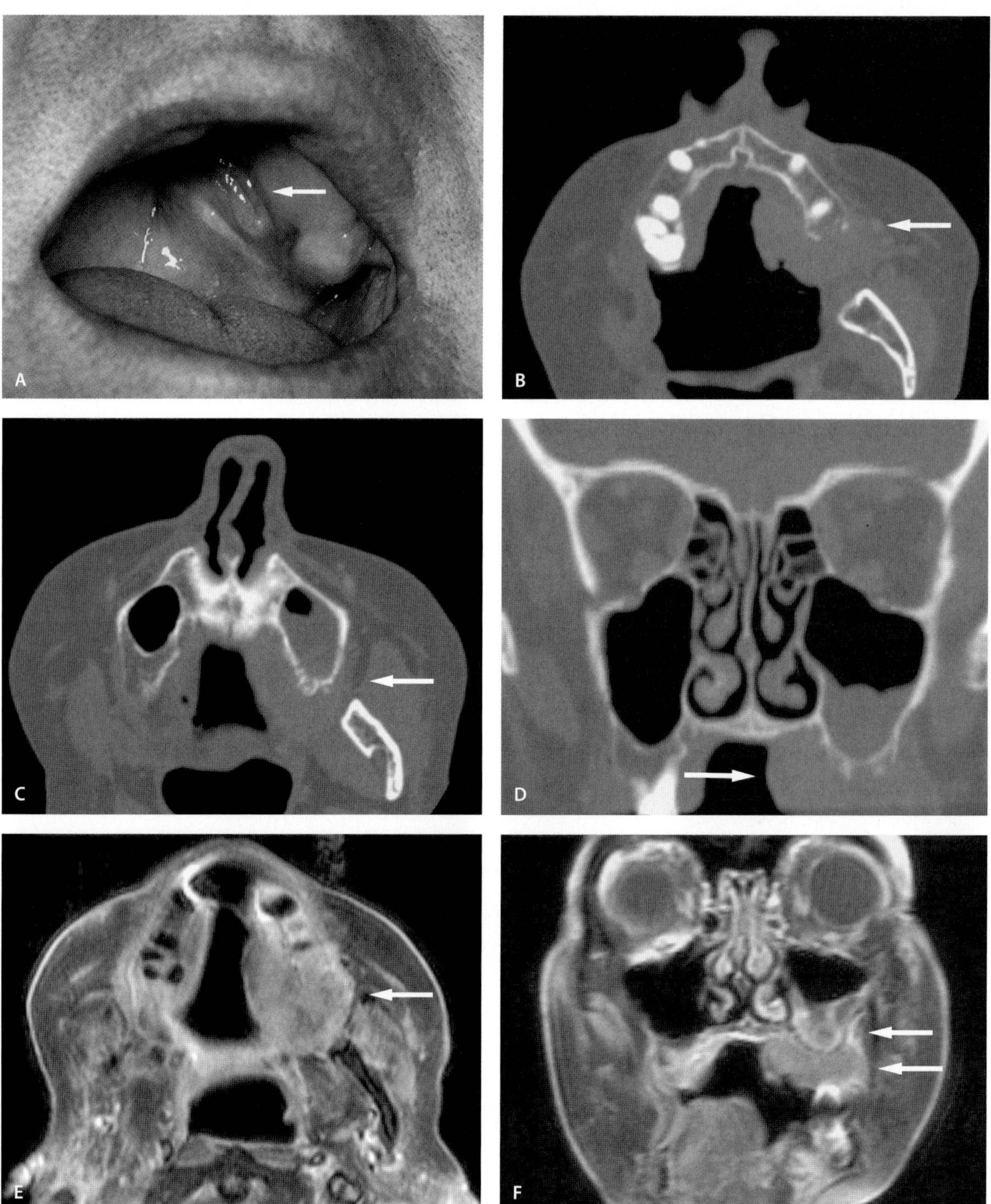

Figure 10.30

Squamous cell carcinoma of left maxillary sinus; 80-year-old female with 13-year history of successfully treated tongue cancer, now with mass in oral cavity. **A** Clinical photograph of another patient with left maxillary sinus squamous cell carcinoma shows palatal swelling (*arrow*) posterior to complete denture (removed) as initial tumor sign. **B** Axial CT image shows destruction of left maxilla and soft-tissue swelling (*arrow*). **C** Axial CT image shows intrasinus mass and irregular destruction of maxillary sinus wall (*arrow*). **D** Coronal CT image confirms intraoral and intrasinus mass with irregular destruction of maxillary sinus wall, alveolar ridge (*arrow*). **E** Axial T1-weighted post-Gd MRI shows contrast enhancement of mass (*arrow*). **F** Coronal T1-weighted post-Gd MRI confirms contrast enhancement of intrasinus and intraoral mass (*arrows*)

Adenocarcinoma

See also Chapter 12.

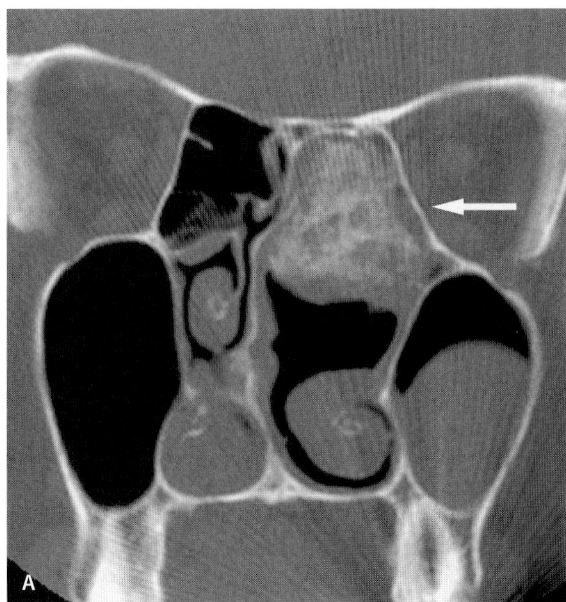

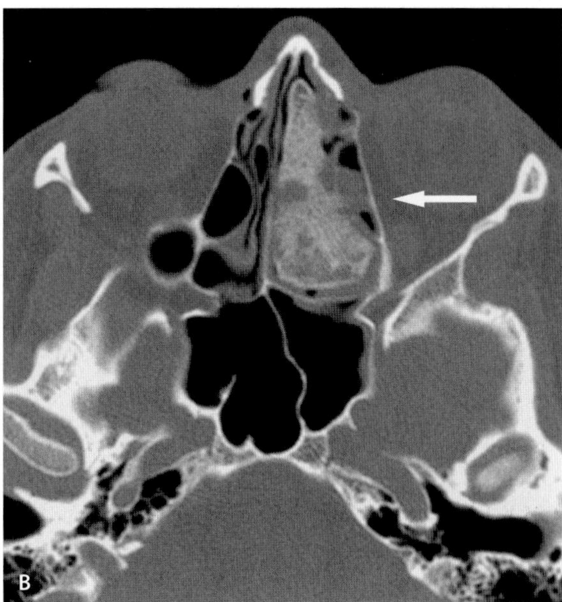

Figure 10.31

Ethmoid adenocarcinoma (low-grade); 18-year-old female, complaining of headache, following biopsy of ethmoid sinus mass. **A** Coronal CT image shows rather well-defined, dense mass in left ethmoid sinus (*arrow*) with some displacement of nasal septum to right and expanding into nasal cavity. Left middle turbinate not seen (removed during biopsy and/or incorporated in tumor). Incidental finding of a retention cyst in left maxillary sinus. **B** Axial CT image shows tumor occupying entire ethmoid sinus with some expansion of medial orbit wall and nasal septum, without penetration (*arrow*)

Lymphoma

Lymphoma is one of the most common malignancies in human immunodeficiency virus (HIV) patients and occurs much more commonly than in the general population, and may be highly aggressive but paranasal sinus involvement is rare in HIV patients.

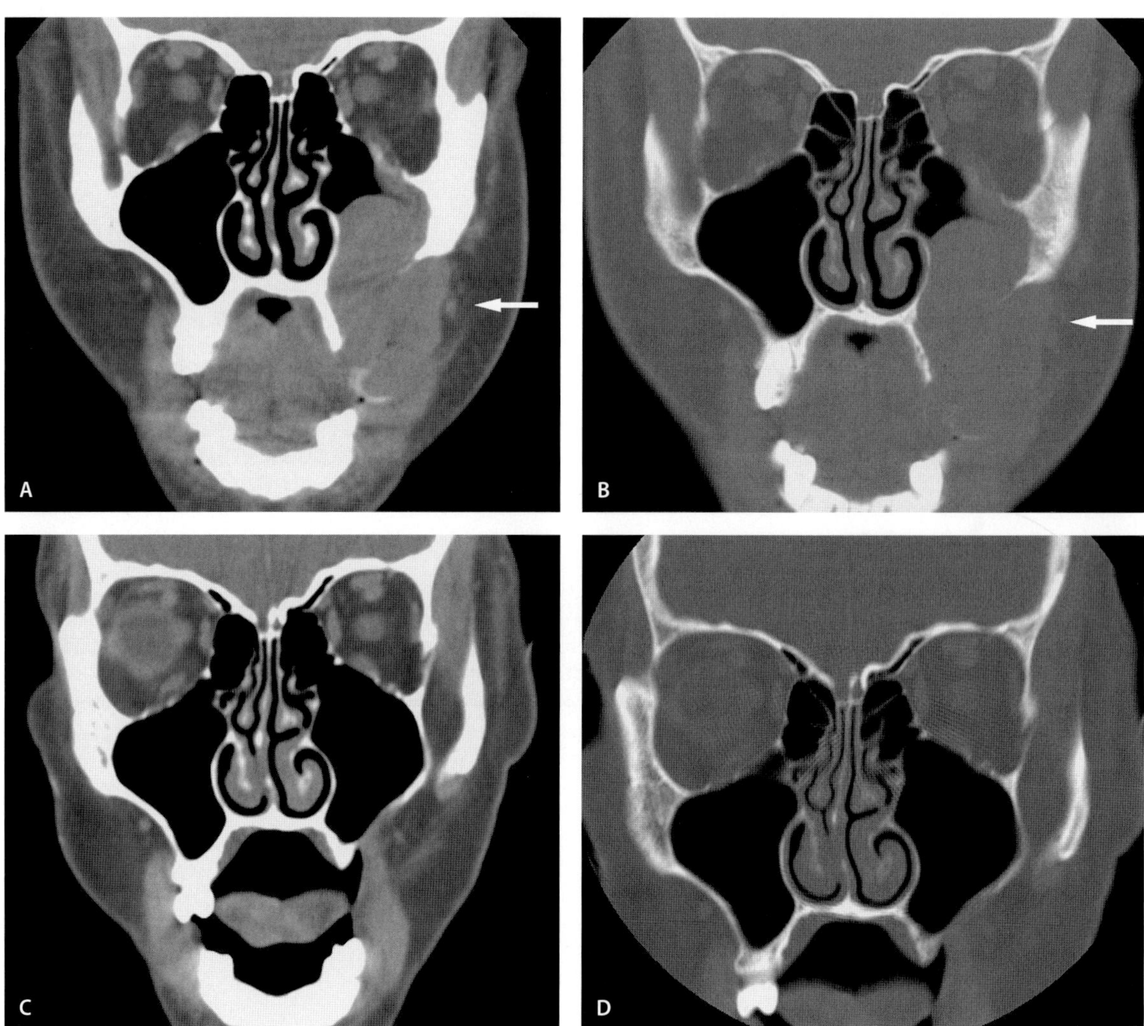

Figure 10.32

Maxillary plasmablastic lymphoma; 39-year-old male, HIV-positive status, presented with left facial pain and swelling. **A** Coronal CT image, soft tissue window, shows soft-tissue mass in infratemporal fossa that invades left maxillary sinus with bone destruction (*arrow*). **B** Coronal CT image shows severe destruction of maxillary sinus wall, alveolar ridge (*arrow*). **C** Coronal CT image, soft tissue window, posttreatment shows normal structures. **D** Coronal CT, posttreatment, shows almost normal maxillary sinus wall

Osteosarcoma

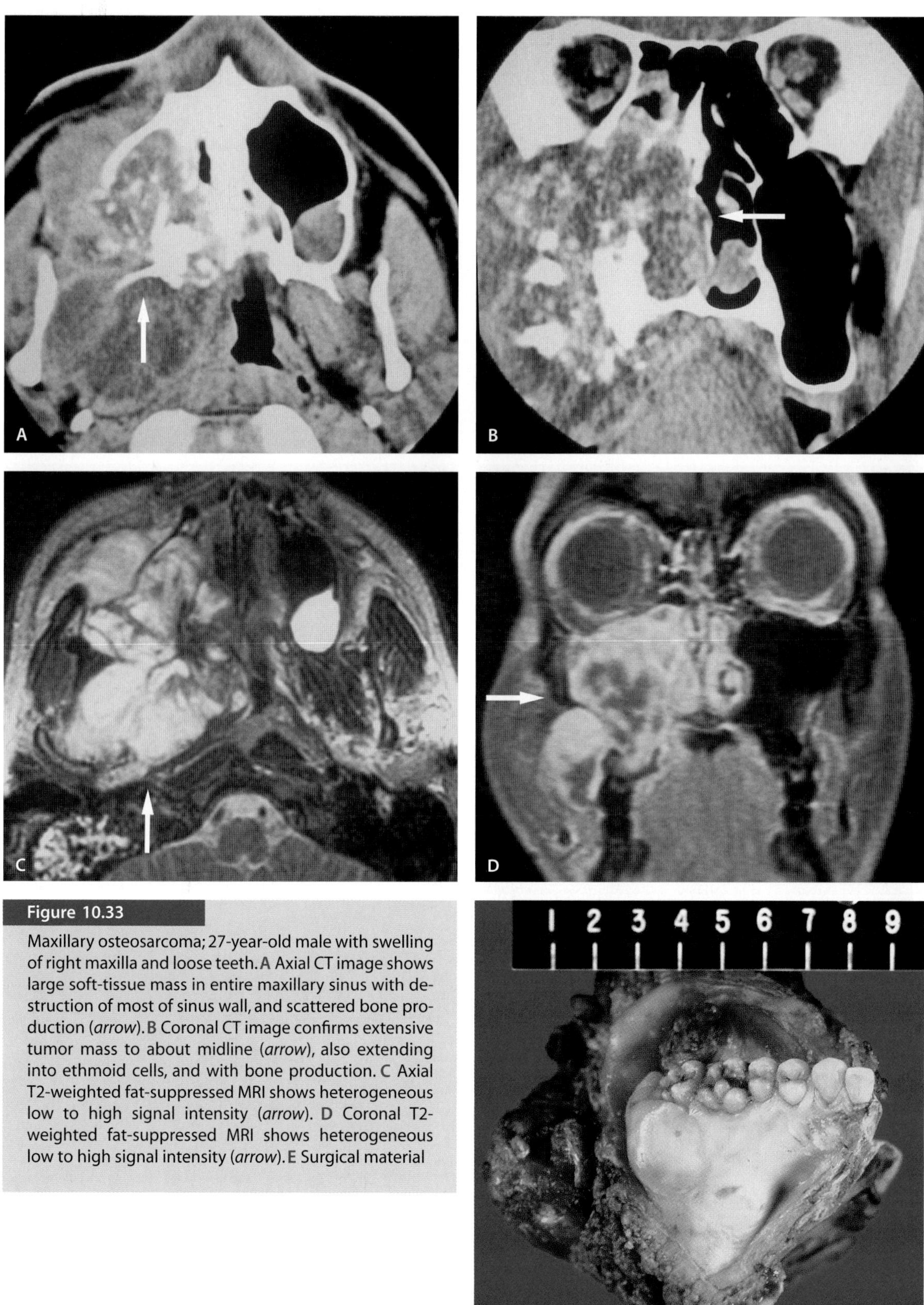

Figure 10.33

Maxillary osteosarcoma; 27-year-old male with swelling of right maxilla and loose teeth. **A** Axial CT image shows large soft-tissue mass in entire maxillary sinus with destruction of most of sinus wall, and scattered bone production (*arrow*). **B** Coronal CT image confirms extensive tumor mass to about midline (*arrow*), also extending into ethmoid cells, and with bone production. **C** Axial T2-weighted fat-suppressed MRI shows heterogeneous low to high signal intensity (*arrow*). **D** Coronal T2-weighted fat-suppressed MRI shows heterogeneous low to high signal intensity (*arrow*). **E** Surgical material

Ewing sarcoma

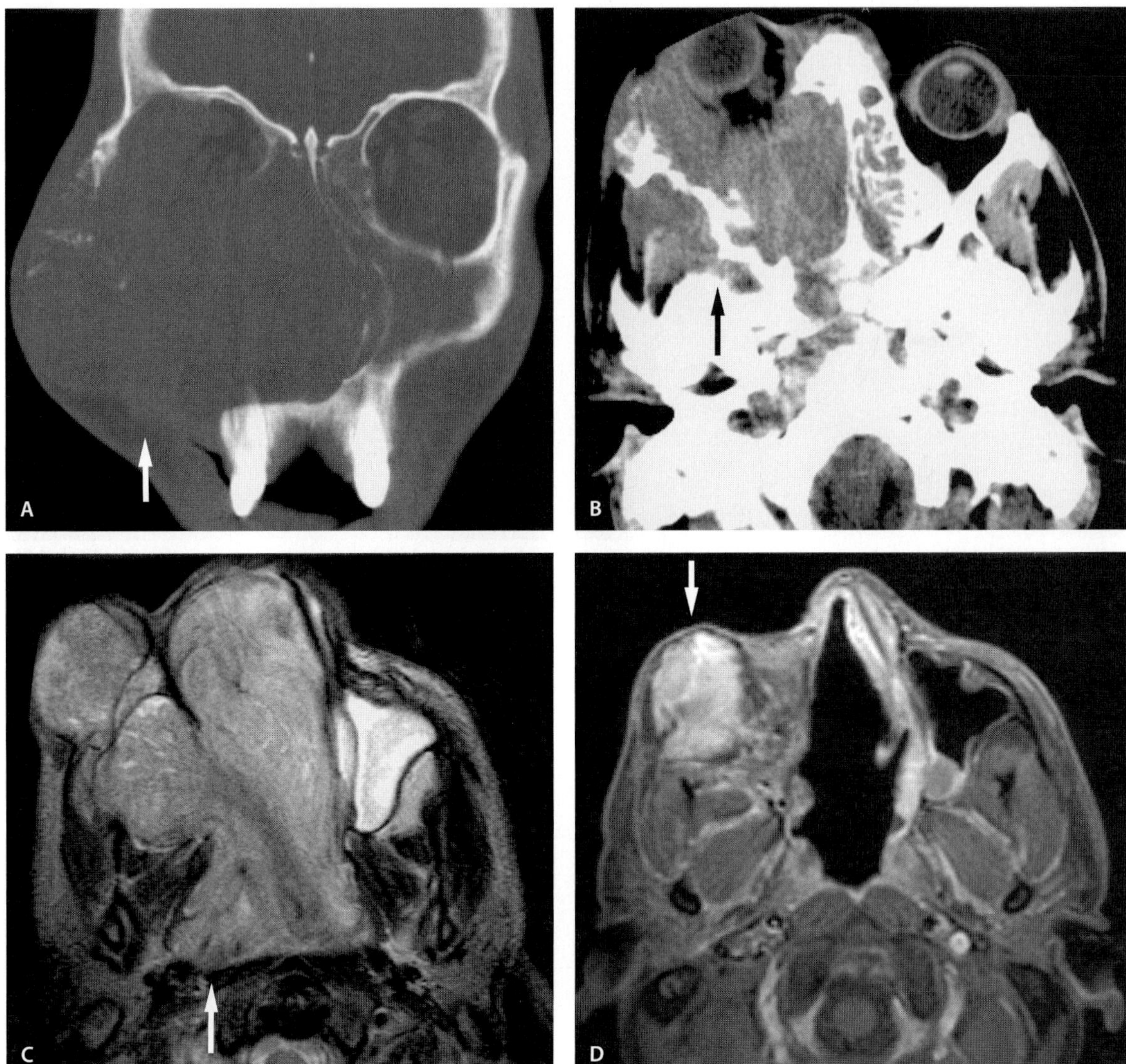

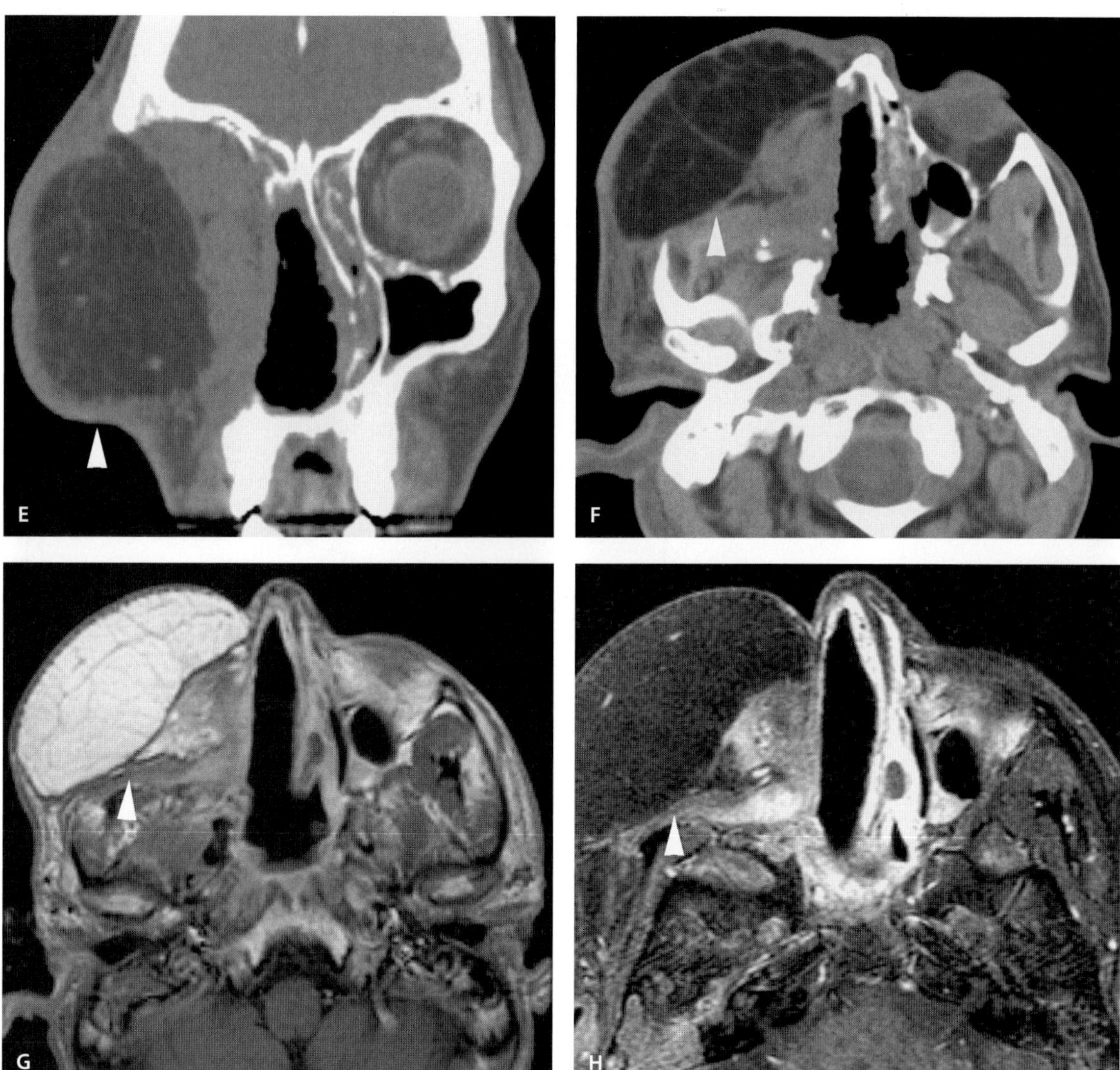

Figure 10.34

Maxillary Ewing sarcoma; 30-year-old male with huge facial mass, proptosis, shortness of breath and dysphasia. **A** Coronal CT image shows enormous tumor (*arrow*) with destruction of maxilla, zygoma, orbital floor, and nasal cavity, crossing midline with expanding medial wall of left maxillary sinus. **B** Axial CT image shows the huge destruction and displacement of right globe (*arrow*). **C** Axial T1-weighted fat suppressed MRI shows the huge exophytic tumor (*arrow*) sparing only left maxillary sinus. **D** Axial T1-weighted post-Gd MRI after first surgery, showing contrast enhancement of tumor recurrence (*arrow*). **E** Coronal CT image, after second surgery with facial flap (*arrowhead*). **F** Axial CT image shows facial flap (*arrowhead*). **G** Axial T1-weighted MRI shows facial flap (*arrowhead*). **H** Axial T1-weighted fat-suppressed MRI shows facial flat (*arrowhead*)

Expansile Odontogenic Conditions

See also Chapters 2 and 3.

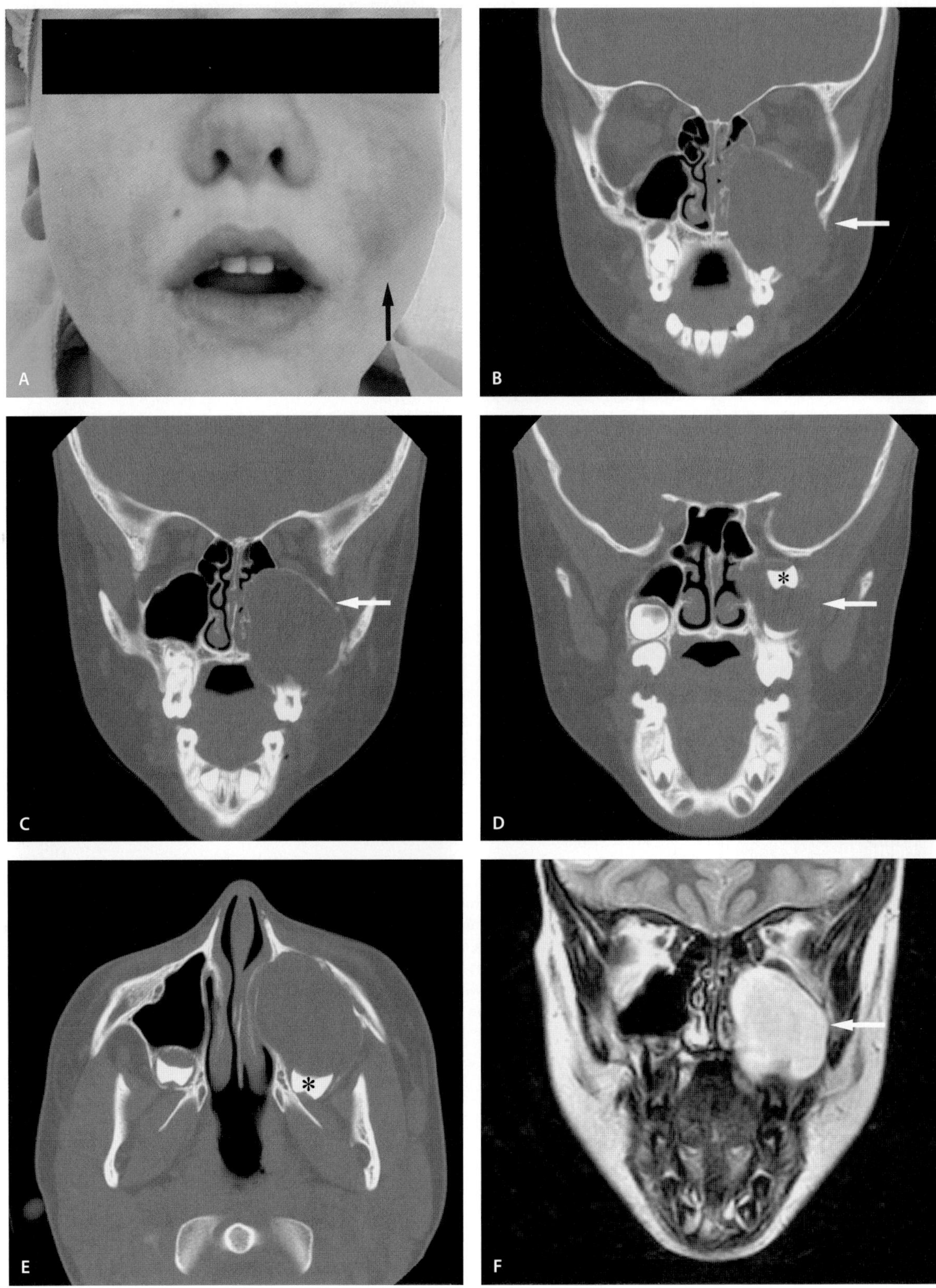

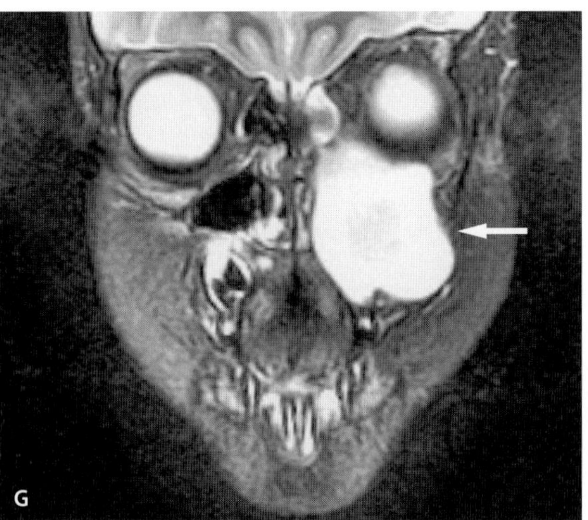

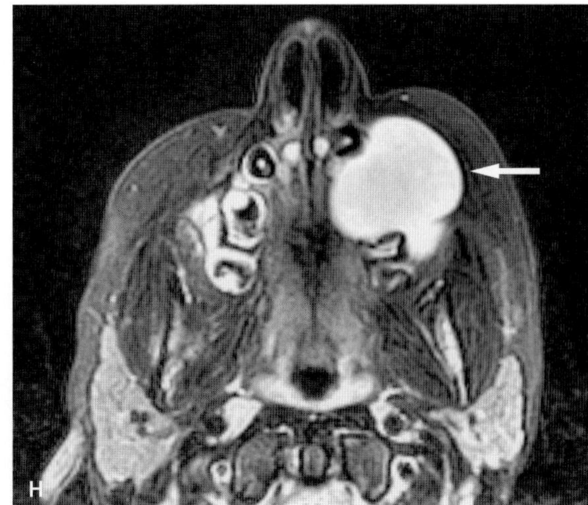

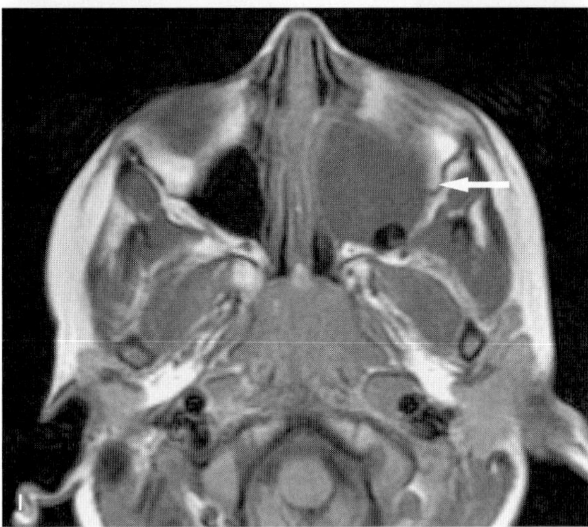

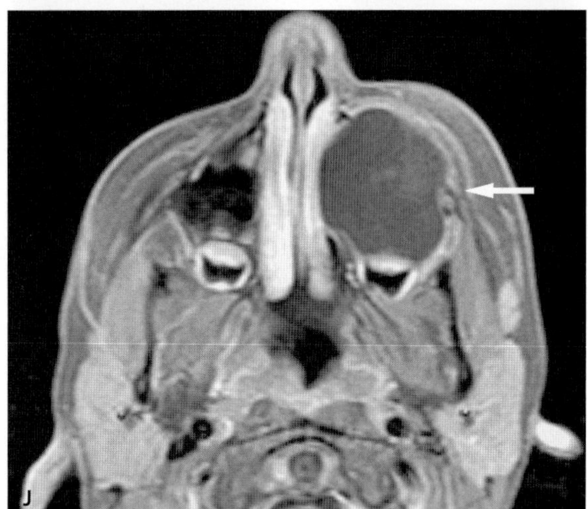

Figure 10.35

Maxillary follicular (dentigerous) cyst; 7-year-old male with painless facial swelling. **A** Clinical photograph before surgery shows facial swelling (*arrow*). **B** Coronal CT image shows cyst (*arrow*) filling entire left maxillary sinus, most of left nasal cavity, and extending into ethmoid cells, hard palate, and facial soft tissues. **C** Coronal CT shows corticated outline (*arrow*) and root resorption. **D** Coronal CT image shows cyst (*arrow*) with impacted tooth (*asterisk*) displaced to cranial part of maxillary sinus. **E** Axial CT image shows impacted tooth (*asterisk*) with follicular cyst appearance. **F** Coronal T2-weighted MRI shows homogeneous high signal content (*arrow*). **G** Coronal T2-weighted fat-suppressed MRI shows homogeneous high signal content (*arrow*). **H** Axial T2-weighted fat-suppressed MRI shows homogeneous high signal content (*arrow*). **I** Axial T1-weighted MRI without fat suppression shows intermediate signal content (*arrow*). **J** Axial T1-weighted post-Gd fat-suppressed MRI shows no enhancement of cyst (*arrow*). **K** Surgically removed cyst containing impacted tooth

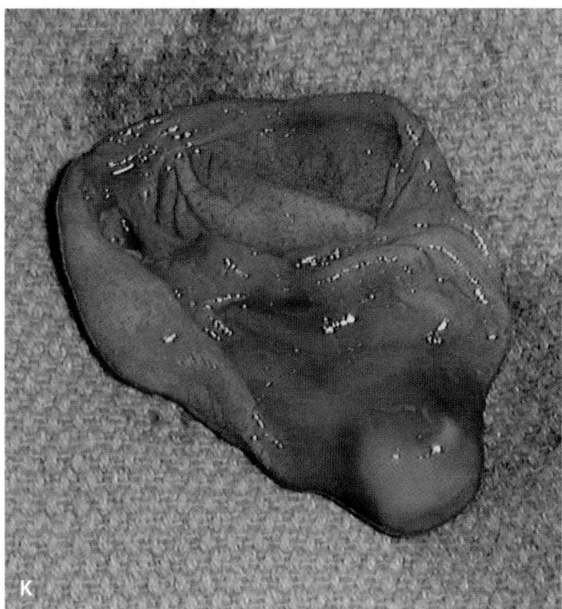

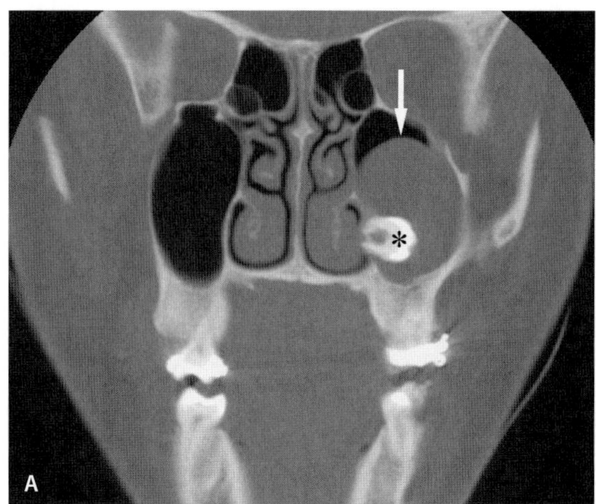

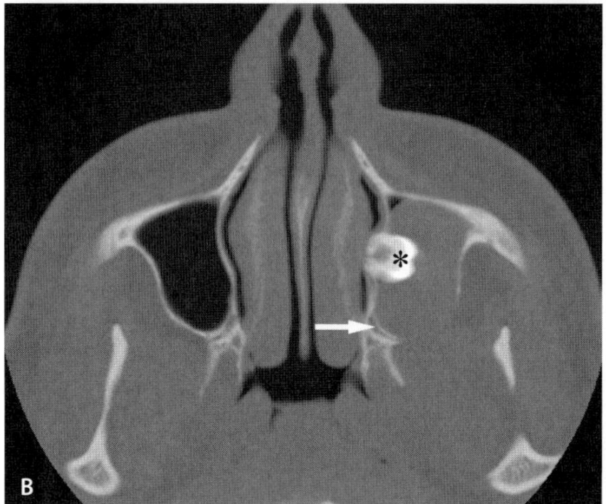

Figure 10.36

Maxillary follicular (dentigerous) cyst; 16-year-old female with impacted tooth. **A** Coronal CT image shows impacted tooth (*asterisk*) with corticated follicular cyst around tooth crown (*arrow*). **B** Axial CT image shows evident corticated outline (*arrow*)

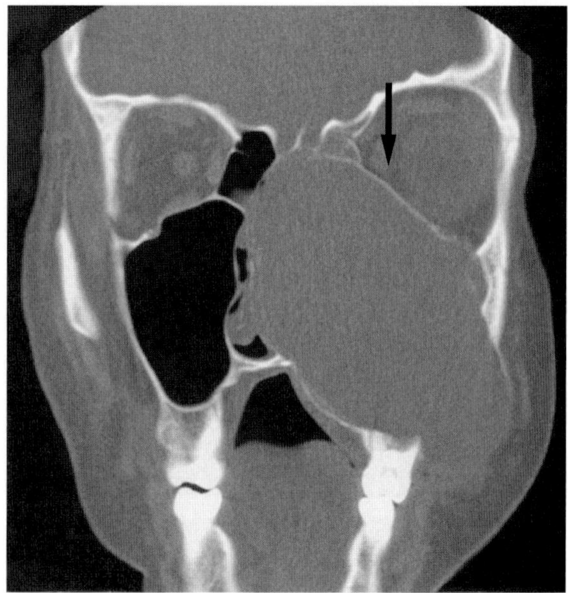

Figure 10.37

Keratocystic odontogenic tumor; 28-year-old female with some pressure in nose. Coronal CT image shows expansive mass with thin, corticated outline (*arrow*), occupying entire maxillary sinus, almost entire nasal cavity, much of ethmoid sinuses, and displacing orbital floor and hard palate. Root resorption (courtesy of Dr. A. Kolbenstvedt, Rikshospitalet University Hospital, Oslo, Norway)

Miscellaneous Conditions

Figure 10.38

Foreign body in ethmoid sinus; 37-year-old female with left ethmoid sinus mass. Axial CT image shows piece of calcified mass in ethmoid sinus (*arrow*); all other sinuses clear. This was surgically removed and turned out to be a piece of wood with local mucosal swelling and some calcification

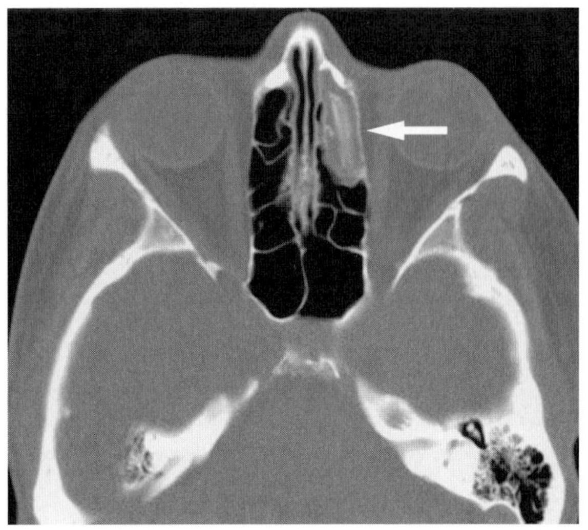

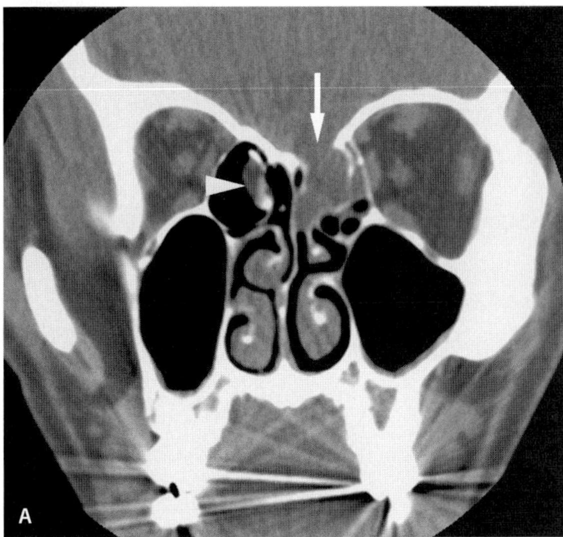

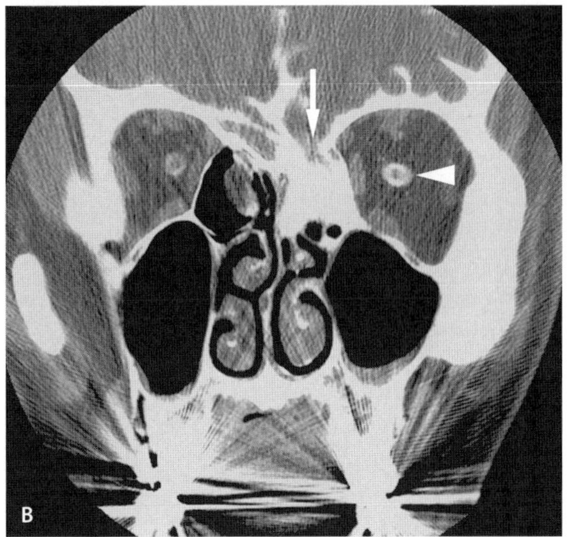

Figure 10.39

Leakage of CSF; 28-year-old male with history of gun shot wound to vertex a few years ago with multiple fractures including left maxilla, orbital floor, lamina papyracea, and left cribriform plate, the latter surgically repaired on right aspect. Clinical course complicated by bacterial meningitis; now referred for CT cisternography to locate continued rhinorrhea. **A** Coronal CT image shows defect of left cribriform plate and lamina papyracea with opacification of left ethmoid sinus (*arrow*). Surgical plate of right aspect of cribriform plate (*arrowhead*). **B** Coronal CT image after lumbar puncture with contrast injection shows CSF leakage through bony defect in the left cribriform plate and into ethmoid sinus (*arrow*). There is also contrast around optical nerve (*arrowhead*) which is normal in cisternography. Small air-fluid level in left maxillary sinus that may represent CSF

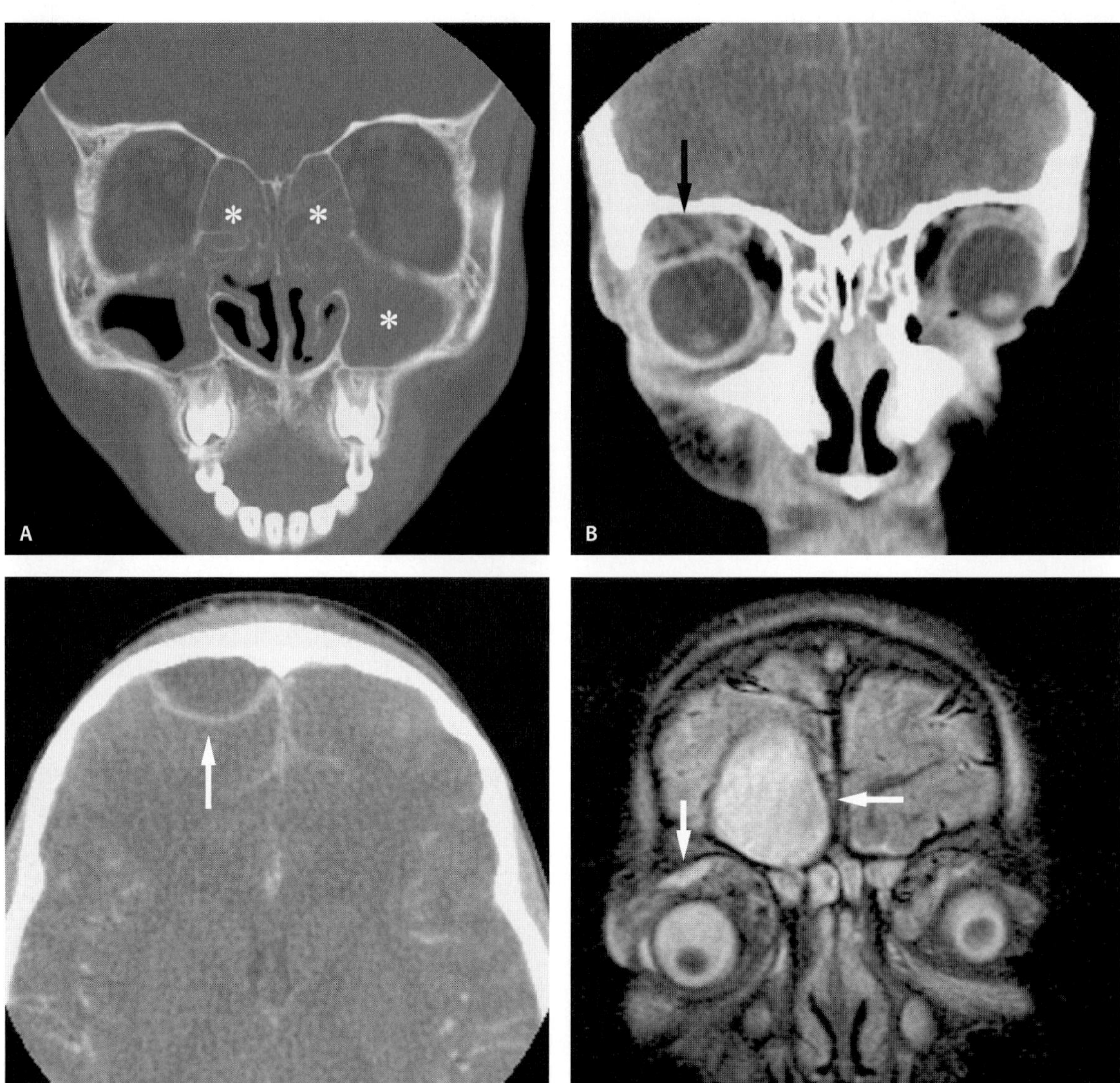
A
B
C
D

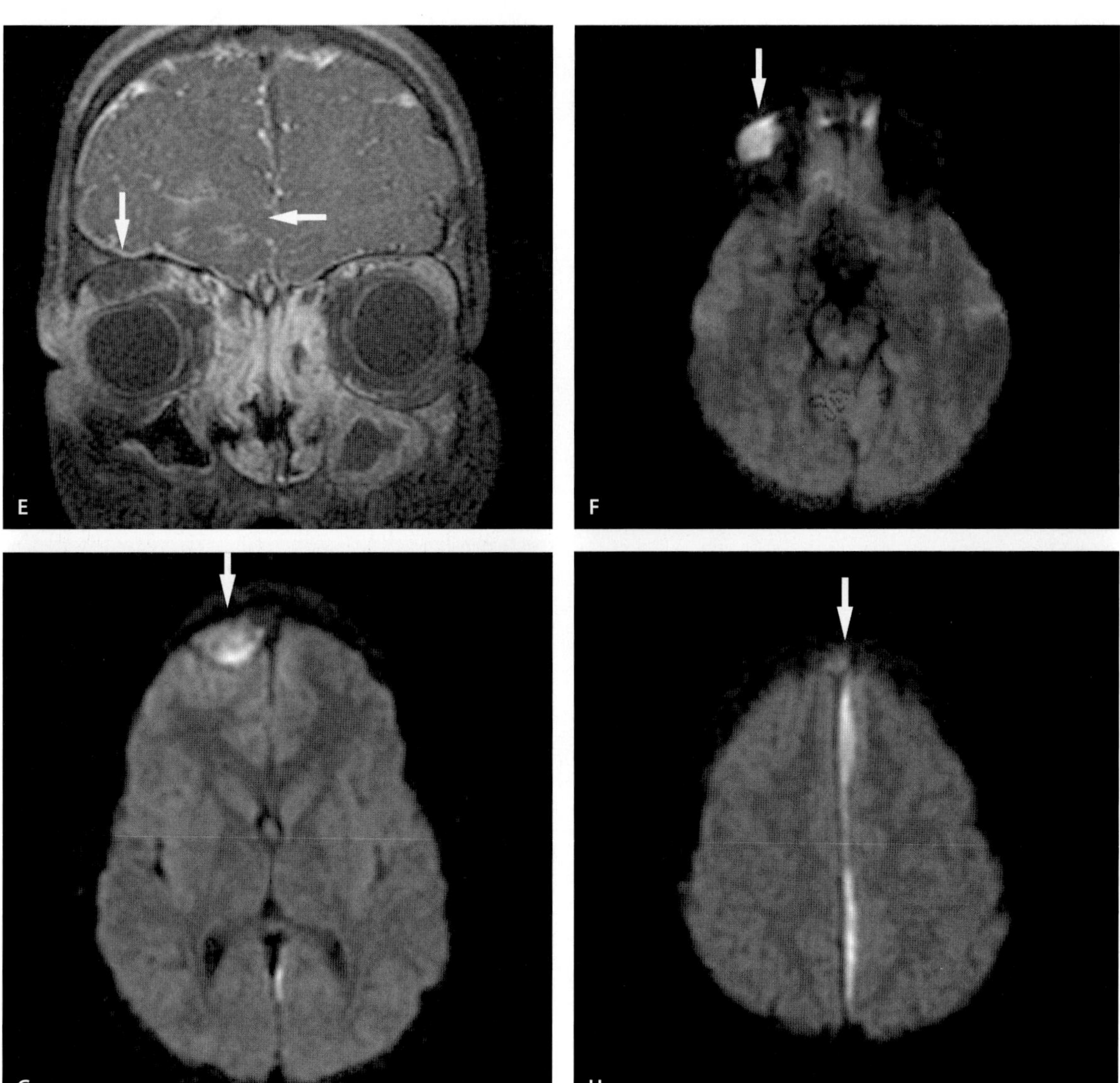

Figure 10.40

Intracranial empyema from sinusitis; 9-year-old female presenting to emergency department with headache, fever, right eye edema, and ecchymosis. **A** Coronal CT image shows complete opacification of both ethmoid and left maxillary sinuses (*asterisk*), and mucosal thickening of right maxillary sinus; also sphenoid and frontal sinuses showed opacification (not shown). **B** Coronal CT image, soft tissue window, shows hypodense central area with hyperdense periphery consistent with abscess in superior right orbit with displaced globe (*arrow*). **C** Axial CT image, soft tissue window, shows abscess in right frontal region (*arrow*). **D** Coronal FLAIR MRI shows high signal in orbit superiorly and anterior to right frontal lobe consistent with abscesses (*arrows*). There is also high signal sinusitis in ethmoid cells. **E** Coronal T1-weighted post-Gd fat-suppressed MRI shows dural and subarachnoid enhancement in right frontal region (*arrows*). There is granulation tissue and fluid in ethmoid cells. **F** Axial diffusion-weighted MRI shows high signal (= restricted diffusion) in superior aspect of right orbital cavity consistent with abscess (*arrow*). **G** Diffusion-weighted MRI shows high signal in right frontal lobe area consistent with an intracranial empyema/abscess (*arrow*). **H** diffusion weighted MRI shows high signal along falx consistent with spread of pus in subdural space along falx (*arrow*).

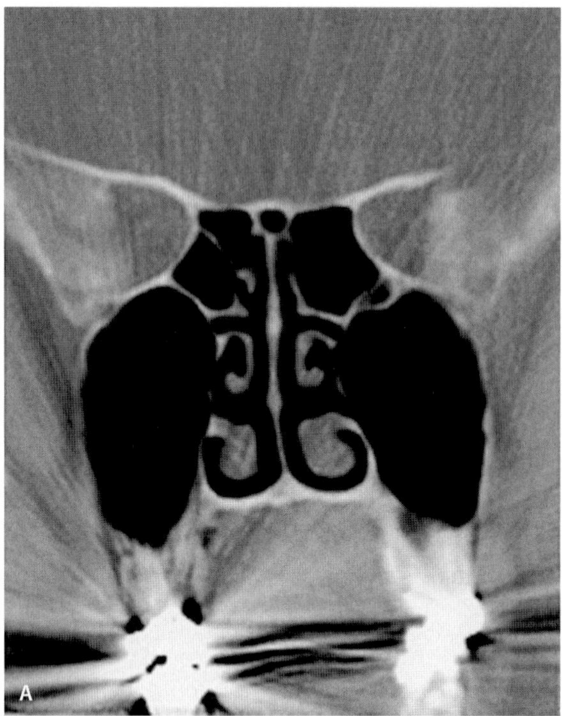

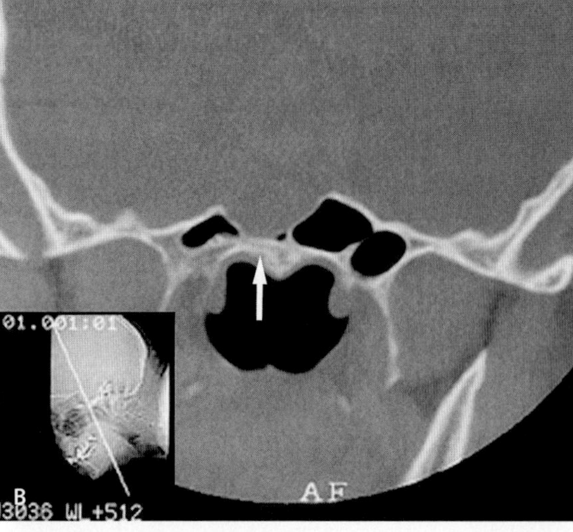

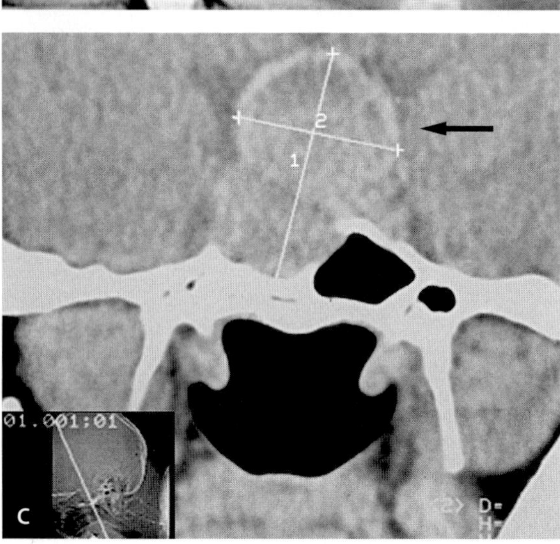

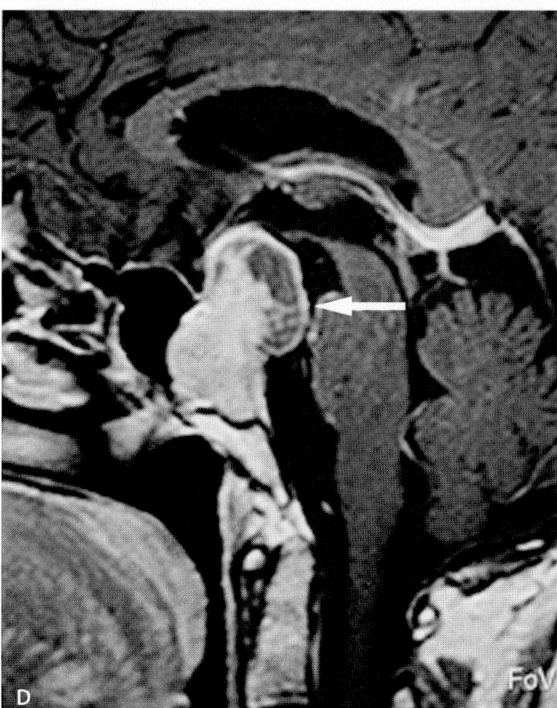

Figure 10.41

Pituitary adenoma (prolactinoma); 50-year-old female with headache and diffuse facial pain, brain tumor detected on routine paranasal sinus scan. **A** coronal CT of paranasal sinuses, almost all scans normal **B** coronal CT, most posterior section shows abnormal sphenoid sinus (*arrow*). **C** coronal CT shows tumor in sella turcica (*arrow*); patient was then referred for neuroradiologic MRI. **D** sagittal T1-weighted post-Gd MRI shows tumor in sella turcica (*arrow*), extending into sphenoid sinus.

Suggested Reading

Barnes L, Verbin R, Gnepp D (1985) Diseases of the nose, paranasal sinuses and nasopharynx. In: Barnes L (ed) Surgical pathology of the head and neck, vol. 1. Marcel Dekker, New York, pp 403–451

De Juan E Jr, Green WR, Lliff NT (1983) Allergic periorbital mycopyocele in children. Am J Ophthalmol 96:299–303

Ericson S (1992) Conventional and computerized imaging of maxillary sinus pathology related to dental problems. In: Westesson P-L (ed) Oral and maxillofacial surgery. Clinics of North America: contemporary maxillofacial imaging. Saunders, Philadelphia, pp 153–181

Farman AG, Nortje C, Wood RE (1993) Diseases of the paranasal sinuses In: Oral and maxillofacial diagnostic imaging. Mosby, St. Louis, pp 379–402

Finn DG, Hudson WR, Baylin G (1981) Unilateral polyposis and mucoceles in children. Laryngoscope 91:1444–1449

Forno AD, Borgo CD, Turriziani A, Ottaviani F, Antinori A, Fantoni M (1998) Non-Hodgkin's lymphoma of the maxillary sinus in a patient with acquired immunodeficiency syndrome. J Laryngol 112:982–985

Larheim TA, Kolbenstvedt A, Lien HH (1984) Carcinoma of maxillary sinus, palate and maxillary gingiva: occurrence of jaw destruction. Scand J Dent Res 92:235–240

Moser FG, Panush D, Rubin JS, Honigsberg RM, Spryregen S, Eisig SB (1991) Incidental paranasal sinus abnormalities on MRI of the brain. Clin Radiol 43:252–254

Rak KM, Newell JD 2nd, Yakes WF, Damiano MA, Luethke JM (1991) Paranasal sinus on MR images of the brain: significance of mucosal thickening. AJR Am J Roentgenol 156:381–384

Rao VM, Sharma D, Madan A (2001) Imaging of frontal sinus disease: concepts, interpretation, and technology. Otolaryngol Clin North Am 34:23–39

Som PM, Brandwein MS (2003) Sinonasal cavities: inflammatory diseases. In: Som PM, Curtin HD (eds) Head and neck imaging, 4th edn. Mosby, St. Louis, pp 193–259

Som PM, Shugar J (1980) The CT classification of ethmoid mucoceles. J Comput Assist Tomogr 4:199–203

Suri A, Mahapatra AK, Gaikwad S, Sarkar C (2004) Giant mucoceles of the frontal sinus: a series and review. J Clin Neurosci 11:214–218

Zizmor J, Noyek AM (1973) Cyst, benign tumors and malignant tumors of the paranasal sinuses. Otolaryngol Clin North Am 6:487–508

Maxillofacial Soft Tissues

In collaboration with A. Kolbenstvedt

Introduction

This chapter is a collection of heterogeneous cases of soft-tissue abnormalities in the masticator space, the oral cavity, and the submental, sublingual, submandibular, and oropharyngeal spaces.

Traditionally, maxillofacial imaging has focused mainly on the osseous structures of the facial skeleton. This is due to the great importance of bony abnormalities for those working in dentistry. It is also a reflection of the fact that traditional maxillofacial imaging relied on plain film and dental imaging techniques that only depict the skeletal structures. With contemporary imaging techniques such as CT, MRI and ultrasound the soft tissue can also be visualized in great detail. From a clinical point of view the differential diagnosis of many conditions in the maxillofacial area includes soft-tissue lesions that would not been seen on traditional skeletal imaging. For instance, in the evaluation of swellings in spaces around the jaws, skeletal imaging is often insufficient.

This chapter has been included to illustrate the value of applying advanced contemporary imaging of the maxillofacial soft-tissue structures. We present a variety of conditions, congenital or acquired, in which CT and/or MRI was necessary or improved the diagnostic assessment.

Infection (Abscess)

Definition

Localized collection of pus.

Clinical Features

- Swelling, pain, redness, warmth, dysfunction
- Fever, malaise

Imaging Features

- Single or multiloculated low-density area surrounded by rim enhancement
- T2-weighted and STIR MRI: high-signal area surrounded by low-signal rim
- T1-weighted post-Gd MRI: no contrast enhancement except in peripheral rim
- Cellulitis or phlegmon will spread diffusely and enhance accordingly

See also Chapters 5 and 12.

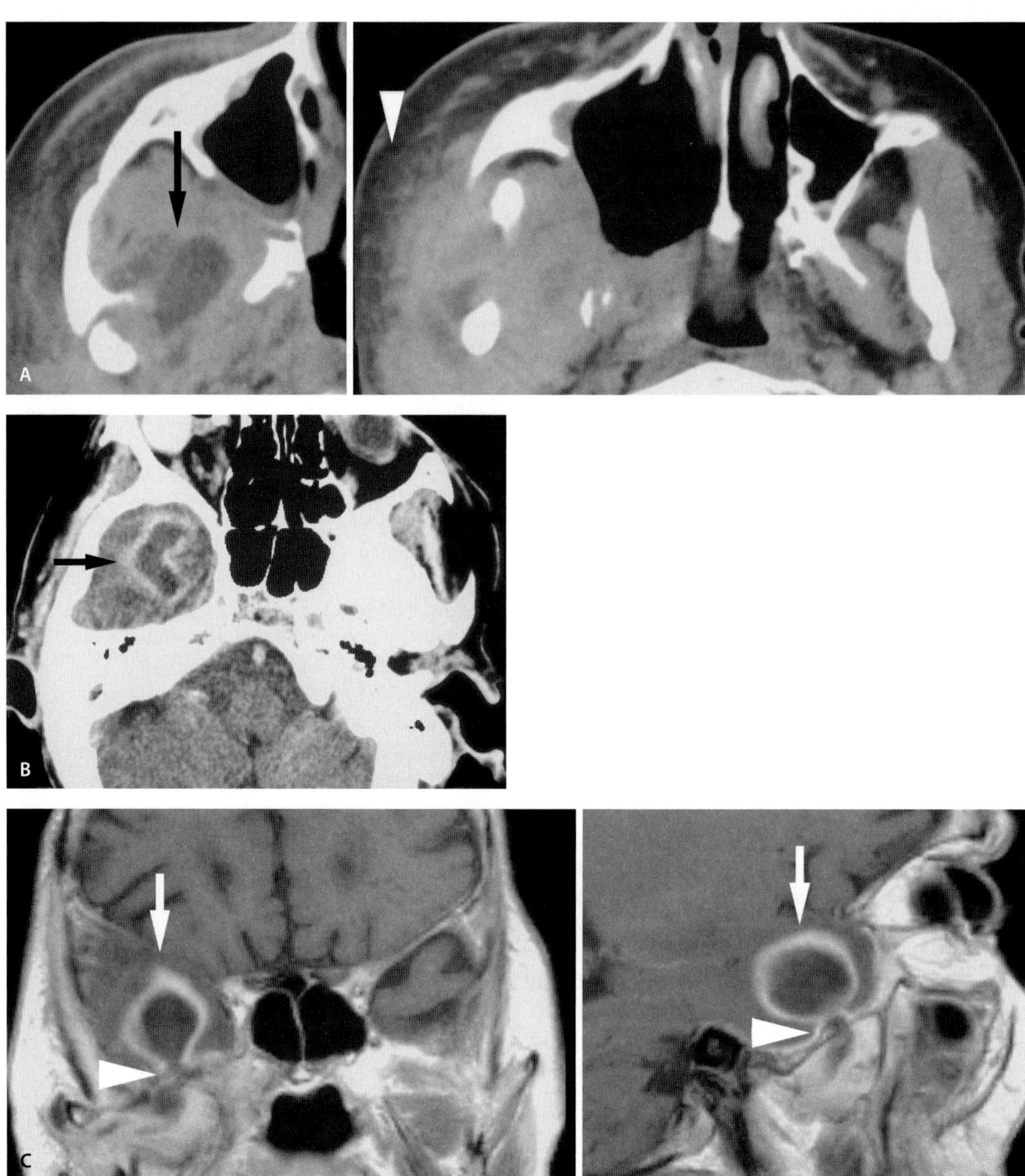

Figure 11.1

Abscess in masticator space with intracranial spread; 85-year-old male with history of right-sided maxillary sinus squamous cell carcinoma, now with right-sided facial swelling, fever and chewing problems. **A** Axial post-contrast CT image shows (*left*) low-density area with peripheral rim enhancement consistent with abscess in masticator space (*arrow*) and (*right*) cellulitis; soft-tissue swelling, loss of fat planes between muscles and streaking (reticulation pattern) of cheek fat (*arrowhead*). **B** Axial post-contrast CT image shows abscess in middle cranial fossa (*arrow*). **C** Coronal T1-weighted post-Gd MRI (*left*) and sagittal view (*right*) demonstrate intracranial abscess (*arrows*) through oval foramen (*arrowheads*)

Muscular Hypertrophy, Atrophy and Dehiscence

Definition

Abnormally thick muscle (hypertrophy), abnormally thin muscle (atrophy), usually with fatty infiltration, or muscle defect (dehiscence).

Clinical Features

- Painless swelling, usually firm
- Benign masseteric hypertrophy; males more often than females, about half of cases bilateral; all muscles of mastication may be involved

Imaging Features

- Muscle hypertrophy, otherwise normal appearance
- Muscle asymmetry, functional abnormalities
- Muscle atrophy, fatty replacement
- Muscle dehiscence allowing herniation

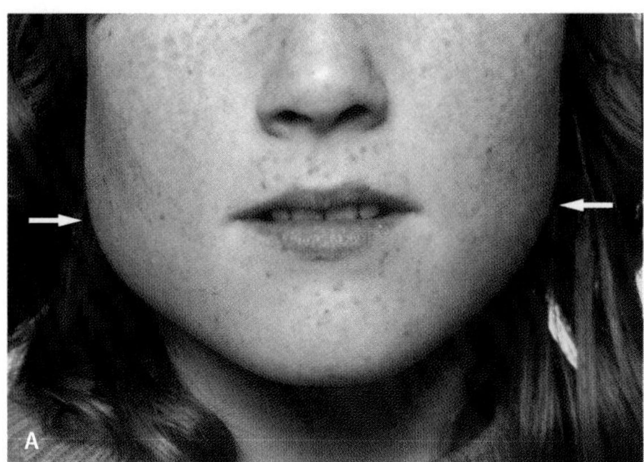

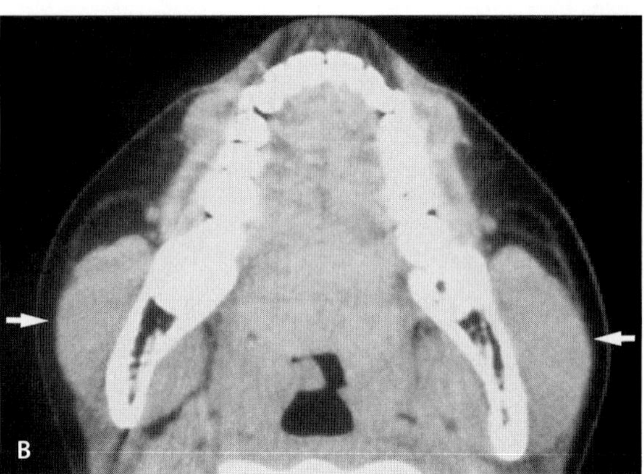

Figure 11.2

Masseteric hypertrophy; 12-year-old female with bilateral painless swelling of mandibular angles. A Clinical photograph shows bilateral swelling of mandibular angles (*arrows*). B Axial CT image shows bilaterally enlarged masseter muscles (*arrows*); bone structures including temporomandibular joints were normal

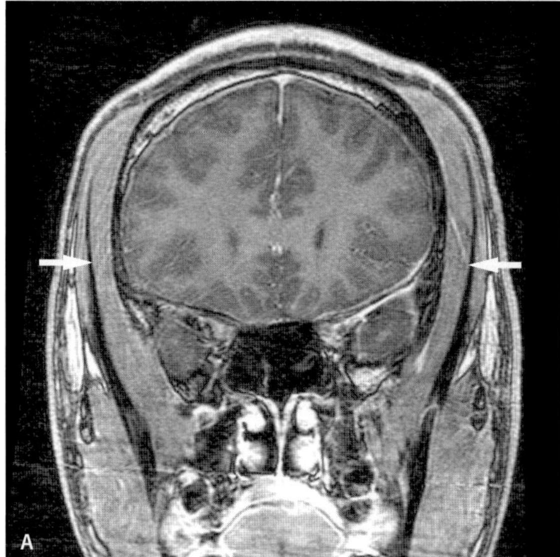

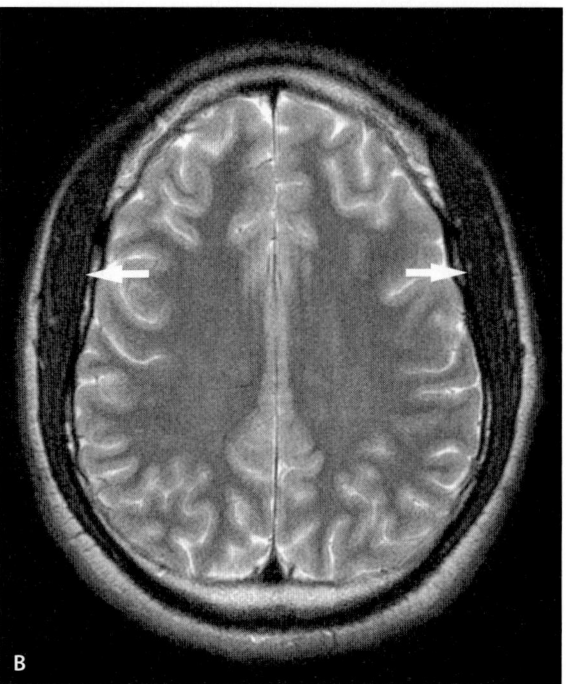

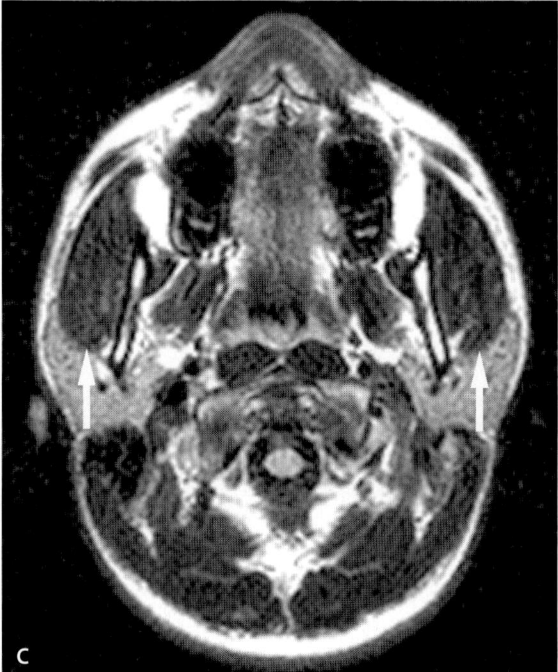

Figure 11.3

Temporalis hypertrophy and masseteric hypertrophy; 17-year-old male with history of psychosis; no organic causes for his symptoms were found. **A** Coronal T1-weighted MRI shows bilaterally thickened temporalis muscles (*arrows*). **B** Axial T2-weighted MRI confirms thickened temporalis muscles (*arrows*). **C** Axial T2-weighted MRI shows bilaterally thickened masseter muscles (*arrows*)

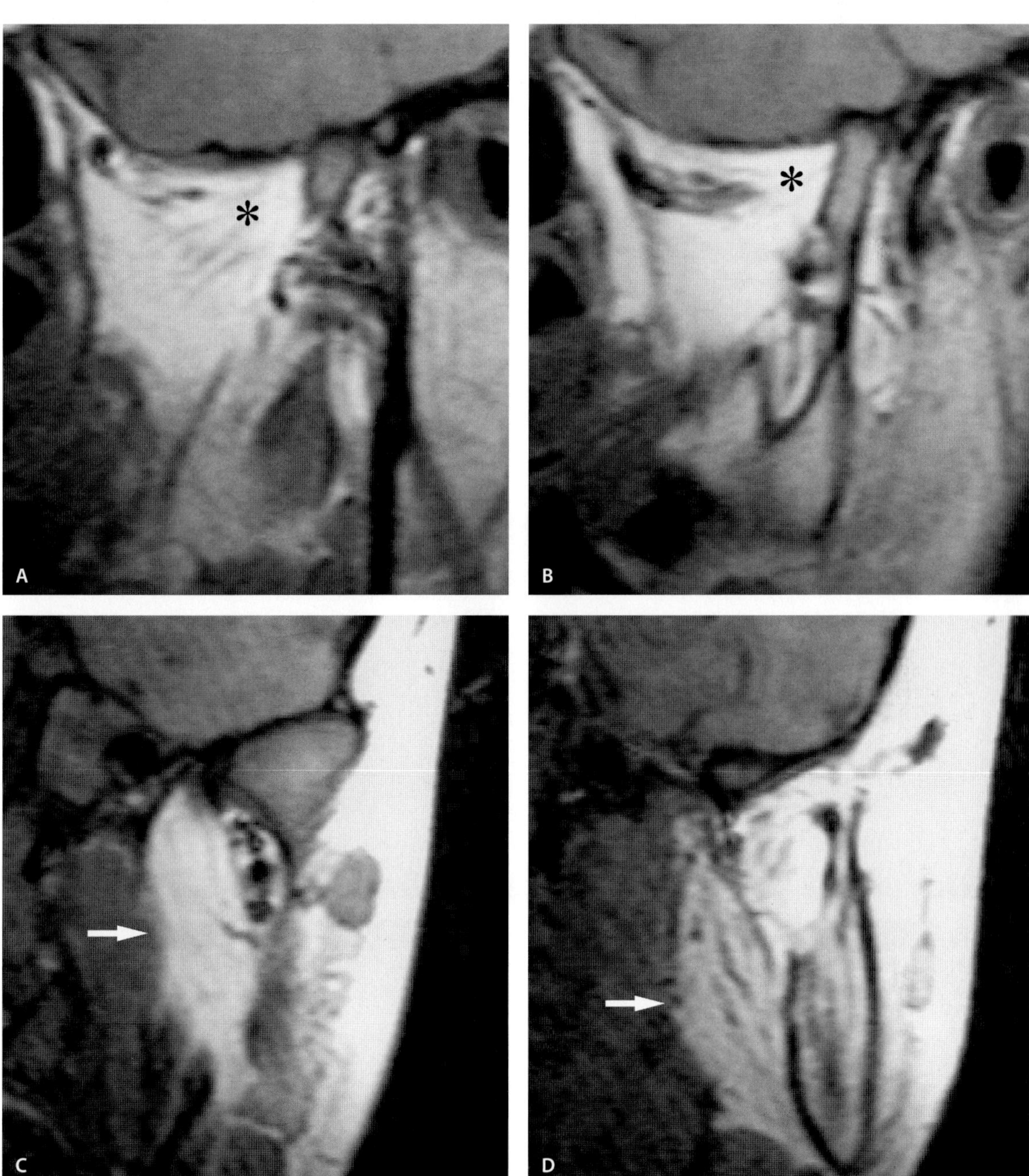

Figure 11.4

Arthrogryposis multiplex congenita; 9-year-old male with micrognathic growth, anterior open bite, and severely limited mandibular motion with chewing and articulation problems. **A** Oblique sagittal T1-weighted MRI, medial aspect of mandibular condyle, shows lateral pterygoid muscle atrophy with fatty replacement (*asterisk*). **B** Oblique sagittal T1-weighted MRI, mid section of mandibular condyle, confirms atrophy with fatty replacement of most of the lateral pterygoid muscle (*asterisk*). **C** Oblique coronal T1-weighted MRI through mandibular condyle shows medial pterygoid muscle atrophy with fatty replacement (*arrow*). **D** Oblique coronal T1-weighted MRI anterior to condyle confirms atrophy with fatty replacement of medial pterygoid muscle (*arrow*)

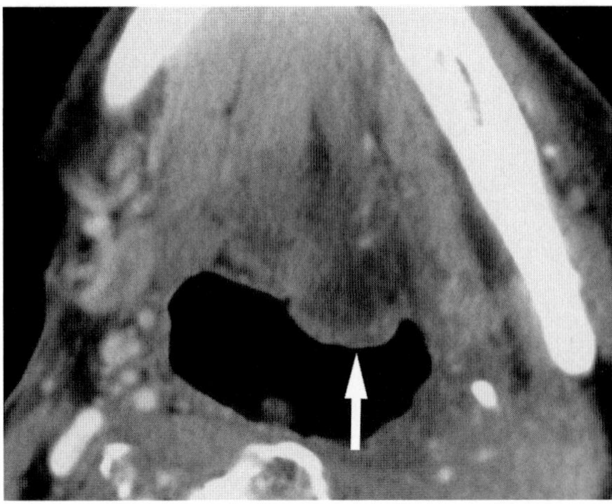

Figure 11.5

Hypoglossal nerve denervation atrophy; 68-year-old male with history of larynx carcinoma and laryngectomy, now with suprahyoid recurrence. Axial CT image shows atrophy and fatty replacement of left lingual muscles with prolapse of left hemi-tongue into oropharynx (*arrow*)

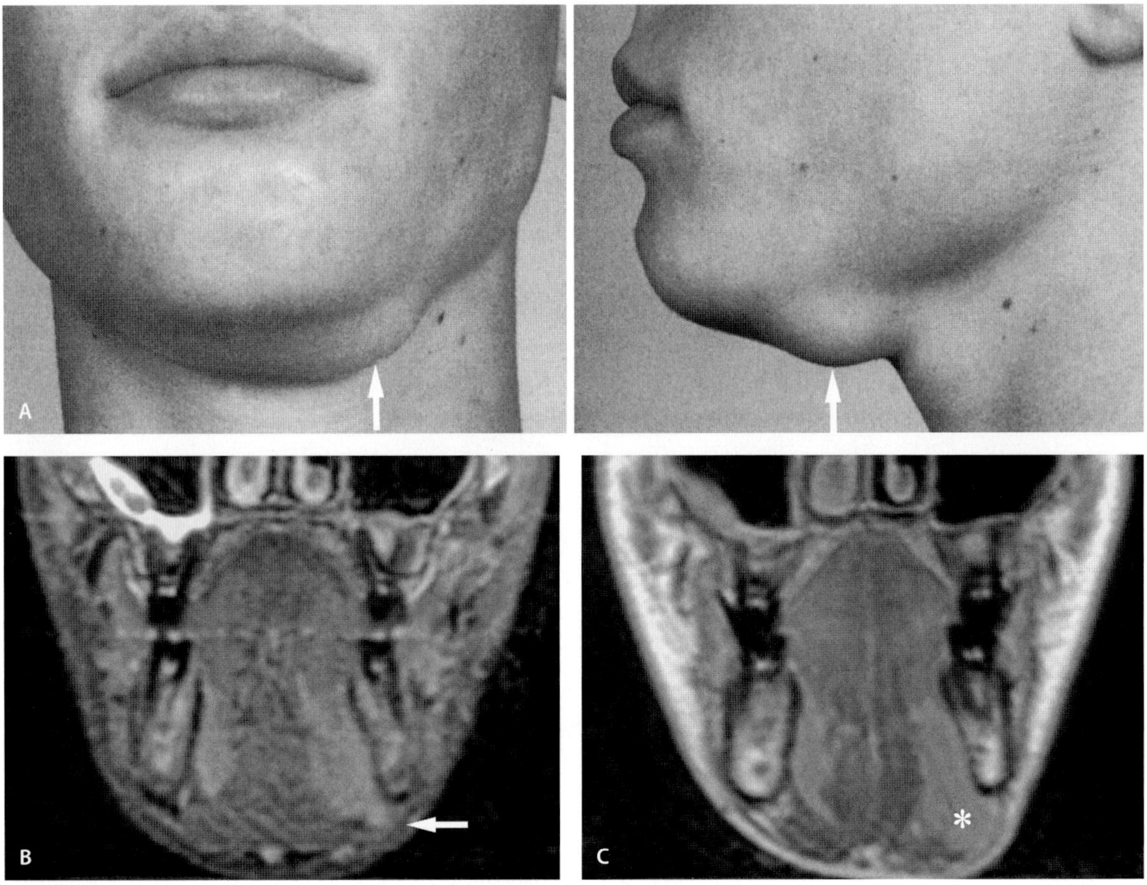

Figure 11.6

Mylohyoid herniation of sublingual gland; 14-year-old male with left-sided nontender, intermittent submandibular swelling. **A** Clinical photographs, en face view (*left*) and side view (*right*) show submandibular swelling (*arrows*) while patient is pressing his tongue down. **B** Coronal STIR MRI shows left mylohyoid dehiscence with small sublingual protrusion (*arrow*). **C** Coronal T1-weighted post-Gd MRI shows sublingual gland herniation (*asterisk*) while patient is provoking swelling by tongue pressing movement (reproduced with permission from Hopp et al. 2004)

Calcifications

Definition
Calcium deposits in soft-tissue structures.

Clinical Features
- Incidental finding on routine examinations such as panoramic radiography and paranasal sinus films
- Pain, limited motion (tendinitis)

Imaging Features
- Calcified tissue, highly variable in size
- May be found many places; tonsils, vessels, tendons, salivary glands and ducts, paranasal sinuses and nose, ossification of stylohyoid ligament, myositis ossificans

See also the sections "Vascular Malformations" and "Cysts".
See also Chapters 10 and 12.

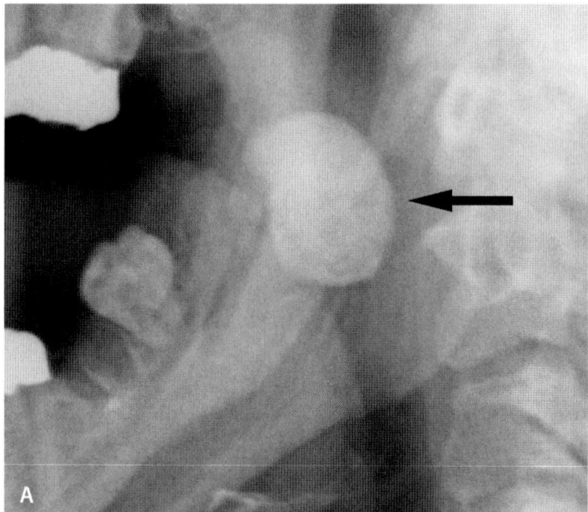

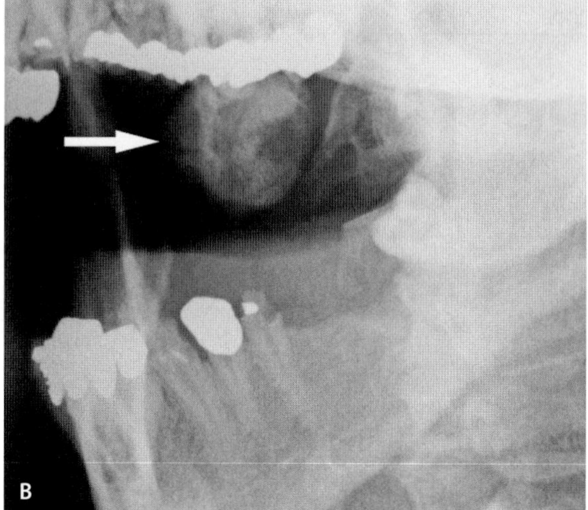

Figure 11.7

Calcification in palatine tonsil; 31-year-old female with prominent, hard mass in right tonsil region. **A** Lateral view shows large calcification (*arrow*). **B** Oblique lateral view shows calcification freely projected from skeleton (*arrow*) (**A** reproduced with permission from Aspestrand and Kolbenstvedt 1987)

Figure 11.8

Calcification in lingual tonsil; 74-year-old female with painless swelling in posterior part of tongue. Axial CT image shows calcified mass in posterior part of asymmetric tongue (*arrow*)

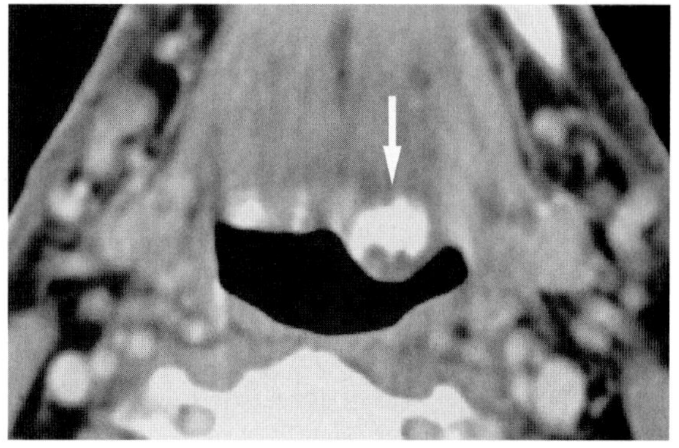

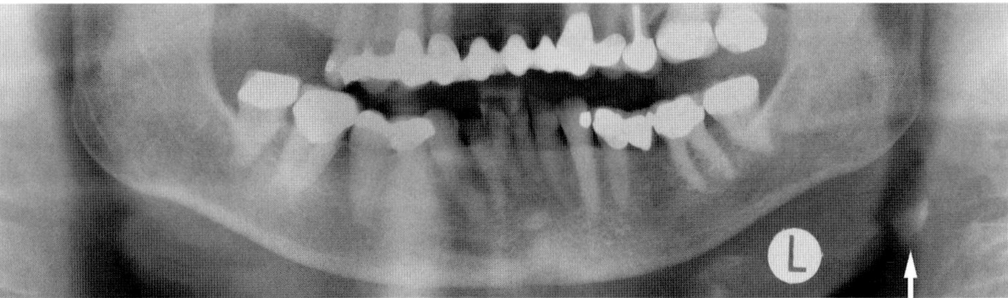

Figure 11.9

Carotid artery calcification; 82-year-old female with incidental finding. Panoramic view shows calcified plaque close to hyoid bone in area of carotid bifurcation (*arrow*) (courtesy of Dr. D.M. Almog, Rochester, NY)

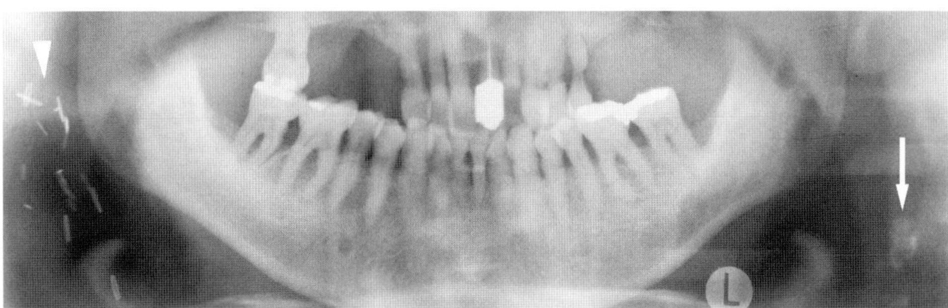

Figure 11.10

Carotid artery calcification; patient with previous endarterectomy on right side. Panoramic view shows calcified plaque in area of carotid bifurcation (*arrow*) and surgical clips used for hemostasis during surgery (*arrowhead*) (courtesy of Dr. D.M. Almog, Rochester, NY)

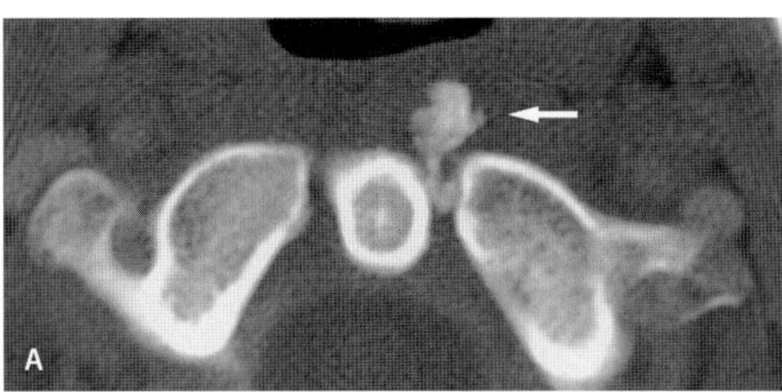

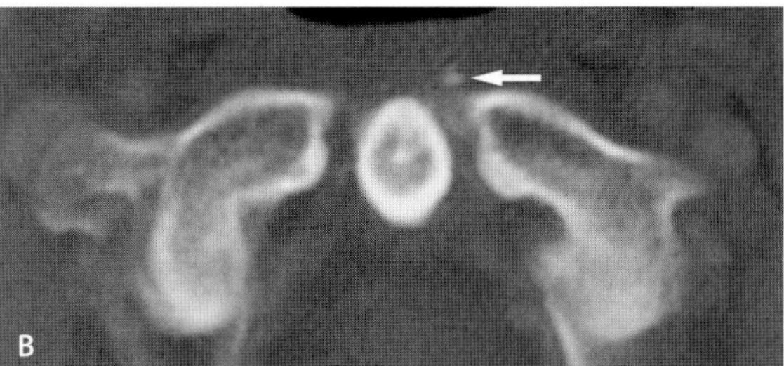

Figure 11.11

Retropharyngeal tendinitis; 56-year-old male with pain on swallowing and restricted head movement, reexamined after 6 weeks. **A** Axial CT image shows prevertebral calcification corresponding to tendon of longus colli muscle (*arrow*). **B** Axial CT image 6 weeks later shows marked reduction of calcification (*arrow*)

Vascular Malformations

Definition

Congenitally malformed vascular channels; arterial, venous, capillary, lymphatic or mixed.

Clinical Features

- High-flow lesions: arteriovenous malformations or fistulae:
  - Present at birth.
  - May be detected in later life.
  - May worsen during puberty or pregnancy.
  - May cause increased cardiac output and strain.
  - Palpable pulse in veins.
- Slow-flow lesions: venous, capillary, lymphatic and mixed malformations:
  - Often affect head and neck region.
  - Venous and lymphatic lesions may become large and interfere with swallowing and respiratory function.
  - May invade bone.
  - No spontaneous regression.
  - Capillary malformations are usually diagnosed clinically as port-wine stains.

Imaging Features

- High-flow lesions: arteriovenous malformations or fistulae:
  - Heterogeneous.
  - May contain varicose dilatations with turbulent flow, with variable signal strength.
  - Afferent and efferent blood vessels dilated.
  - Well or poorly defined.
  - T1-weighted MRI: round and linear flow-voids.
- Slow-flow lesions (venous):
  - Calcified phleboliths.
  - Gradual contrast medium enhancement from periphery to center.
  - T1-weighted MRI: iso- or hypointense to muscle.
  - T2-weighted MRI: high signal ("light bulb" sign).
  - Phleboliths may cause round but not linear flow voids.
  - T1-weighted post-Gd MRI: gradually increasing enhancement from periphery to center.
- Slow-flow lesions (lymphatic):
  - Low-density (fluid-filled) soft-tissue mass without phleboliths.
  - Single, multilobulated or microcystic.
  - Poorly or well defined.
  - No enhancement of fluid zone.
  - T1-weighted MRI: iso-or hypointense to muscle.
  - T2-weighted MRI: high signal.
  - T1-weighted post-Gd MRI: no enhancement except in septa or walls.

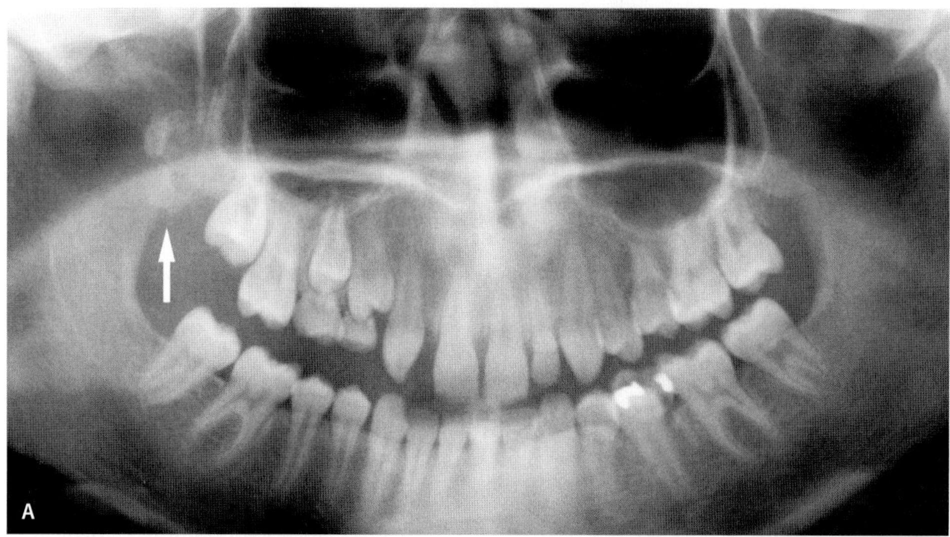
A

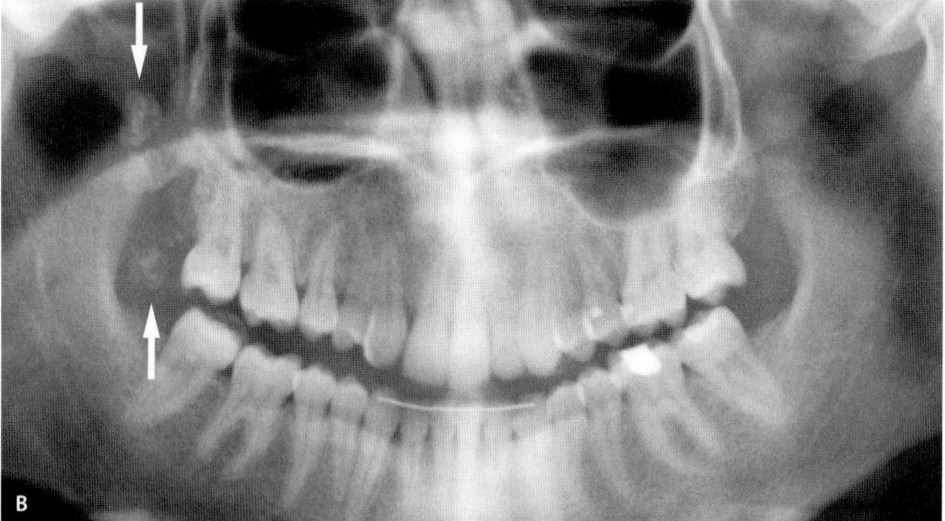
B

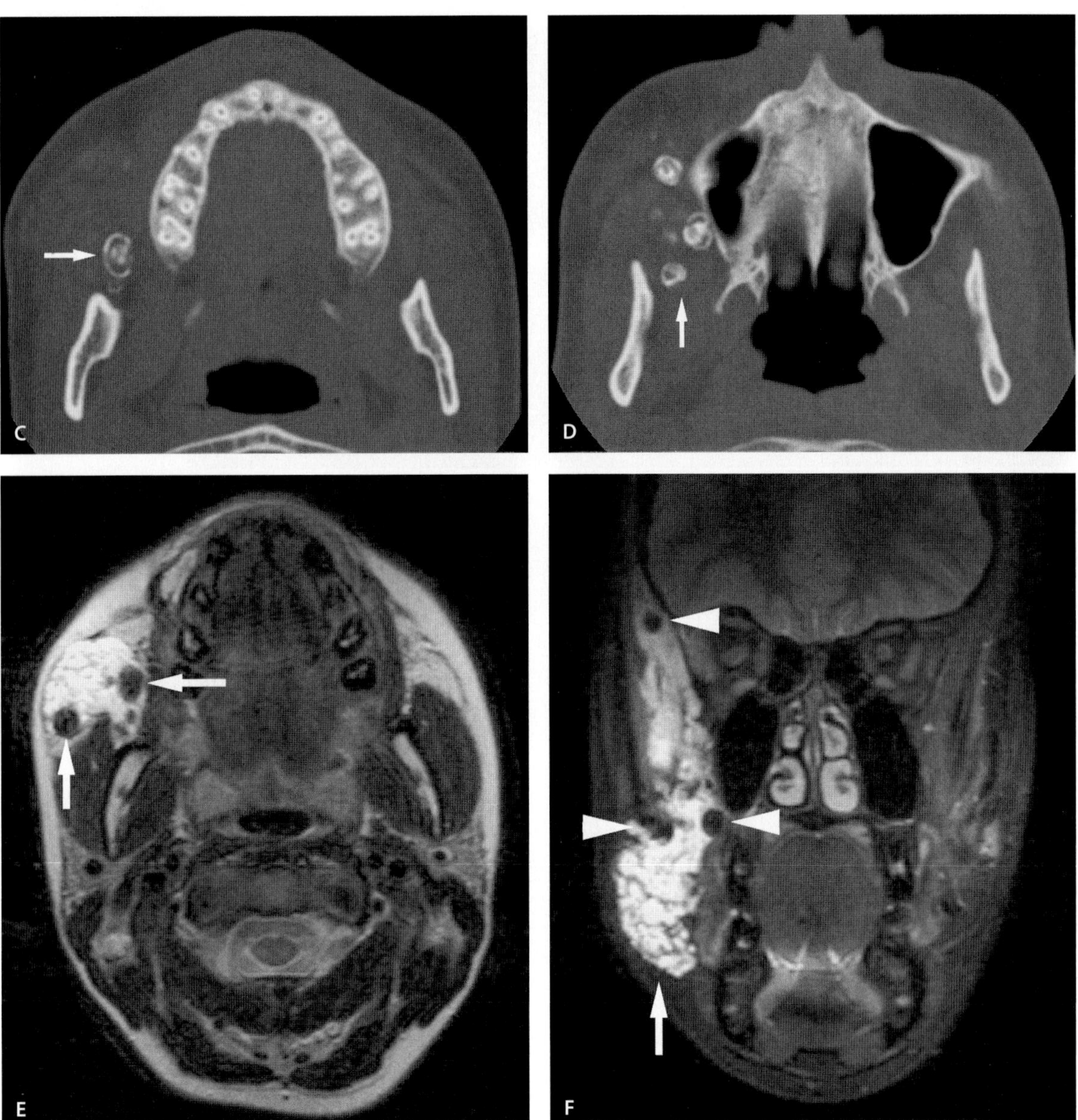

Figure 11.12

Venous malformation of cheek; 19-year-old female with incidental finding of calcifications on panoramic view that showed progression during a 5-year period. **A** Panoramic view shows calcifications (*arrow*) when the patient was 14 years old. **B** Panoramic view 5 years later shows larger and multiple calcifications (*arrows*). **C** Axial CT image shows large calcification just anterior to mandibular ramus characteristic of a phlebolith (*arrow*). **D** Axial CT image shows multiple calcifications, including three large ones (*arrow*) consistent with phleboliths. **E** Axial T2-weighted MRI shows high signal area with signal voids of phleboliths (*arrows*). **F** Coronal STIR MRI shows high signal area (*arrow*) with signal voids of phleboliths including some large ones (*arrowheads*)

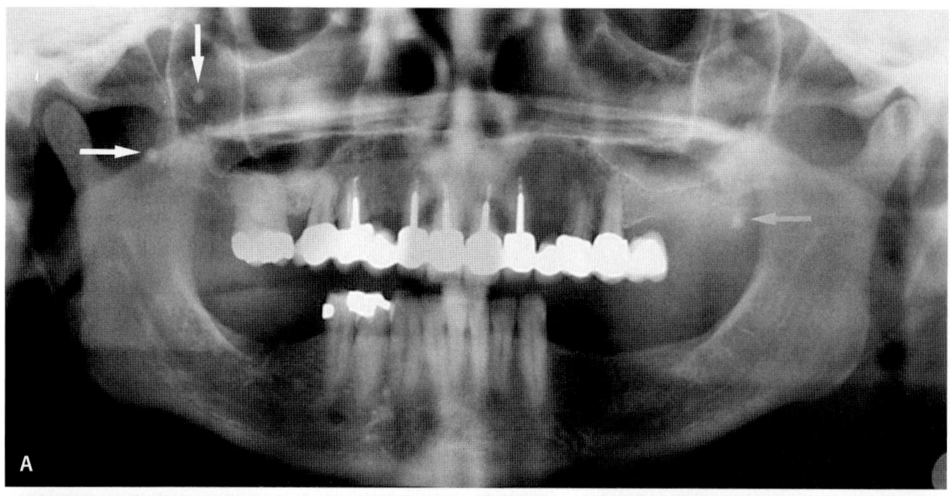

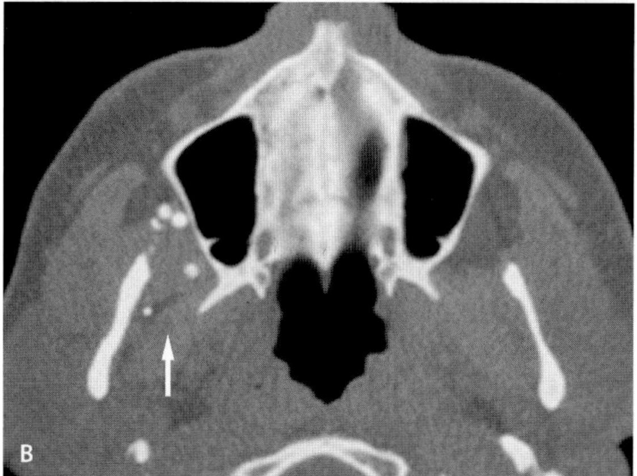

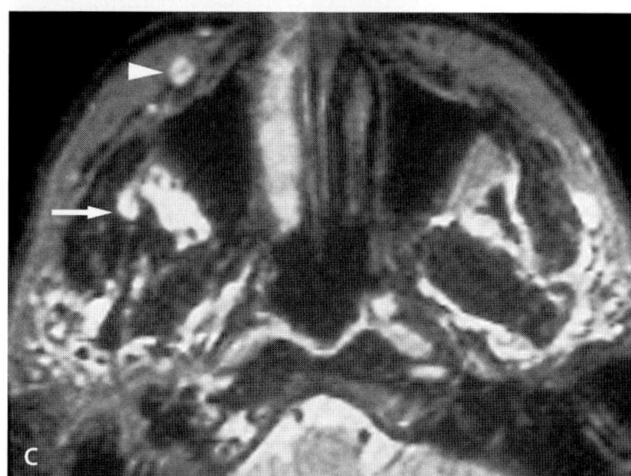

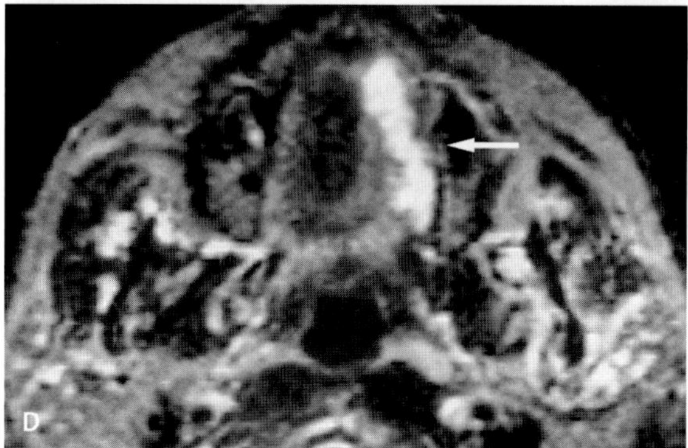

Figure 11.13

Venous malformations of cheek and hard palate; 44-year-old female with painless swelling in hard palate that was believed to be a dental abscess, but on incision did not show any pus collection. **A** Panoramic view shows tiny calcifications (*arrows*). **B** Axial CT image shows multiple small, dense calcifications (*arrow*). **C** Axial T2-weighted MRI shows area of high signal with tiny voids of signal (*arrow*), including a smaller similar area anterior to maxillary sinus (*arrowhead*). **D** Axial T2-weighted MRI of hard palate shows high signal from left side, corresponding to area of incision (*arrow*)

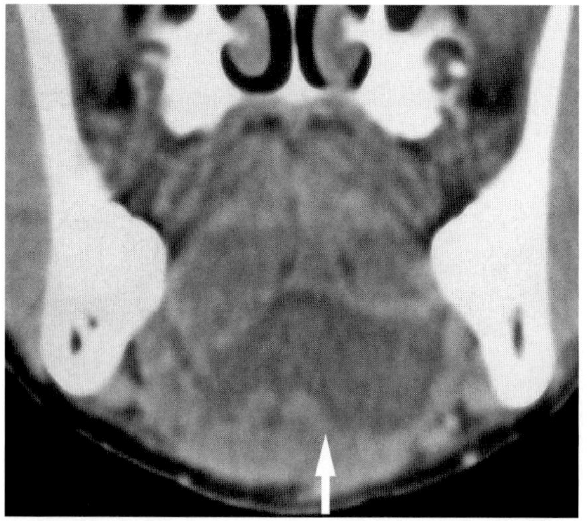

Figure 11.14

Cystic lymphatic malformation; 14-year-old female with submental swelling. Coronal post-enhanced CT image shows well-defined mass in sublingual space crossing midline (*arrows*), hypodense with enhanced border

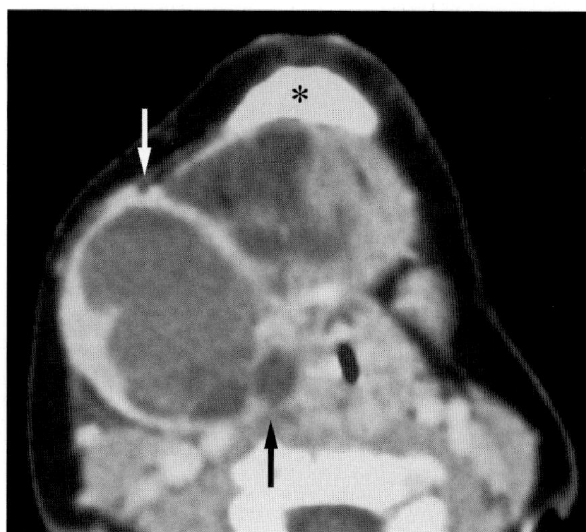

Figure 11.15

Cystic lymphatic malformation; 10-month-old female with swelling of floor of mouth and upper neck. Axial CT image shows well-defined hypodense, lobulated mass (*arrows*) in submandibular space; note mandible (*asterisk*)

Cysts

Definition

Epithelial-lined fluid-filled cavity with thin fibrous wall.

Clinical Features

- Painless swelling (if not infected).
- Thyroglossal duct cyst:
  - Most common of congenital neck lesions (about 70%); may occur anywhere from foramen cecum to thyroid gland; majority at hyoid bone level.
  - Commonly in midline when suprahyoid; seldom in floor of mouth; only 1–2% in tongue.
- Second branchial cleft cyst:
  - Far the most common of all branchial anomalies.
  - Typically located in lateral neck ventral to anterior edge of sternocleidomastoid muscle, dorsal to submandibular gland, and superficial to carotid sheath; usually caudal to angle of mandible.
- Dermoid or epidermoid cyst:
  - Least common of congenital neck lesions (only about 7%), but floor of mouth particularly involved; about half in sublingual space; midline or asymmetric; may contain fat globules or calcifications.
  - Terms used interchangeable, but dermoid cyst may have hair follicles and sebaceous glands.

Imaging Features

- Well-defined unilocular, hypodense area with thin, enhancing peripheral rim
- T1-weighted MRI: usually low signal, but occasionally high (dermoid)
- T2-weighted MRI or STIR: high signal
- T1-weighted post-Gd MRI: no enhancement, occasionally in thin peripheral rim

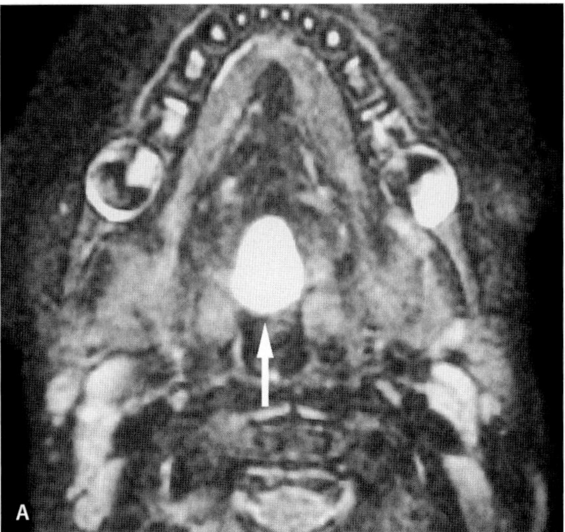

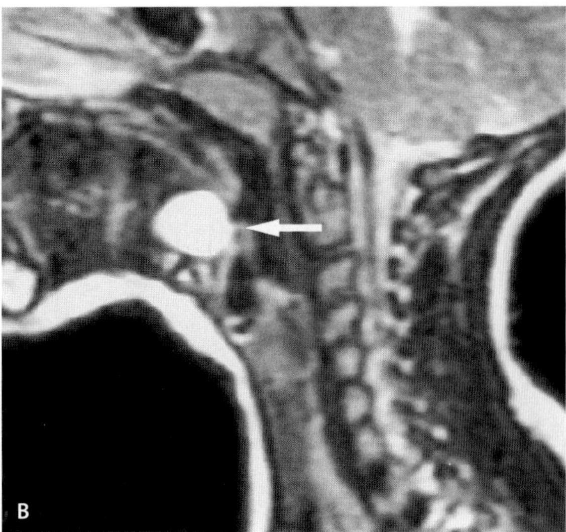

Figure 11.16

Thyroglossal duct cyst; 3-year-old female with mass in midline of base of tongue, **A** Axial T2-weighted MRI shows well-defined high-signal mass in base of tongue (*arrow*). **B** Sagittal T2-weighted MRI confirms high-signal mass in tongue (*arrow*)

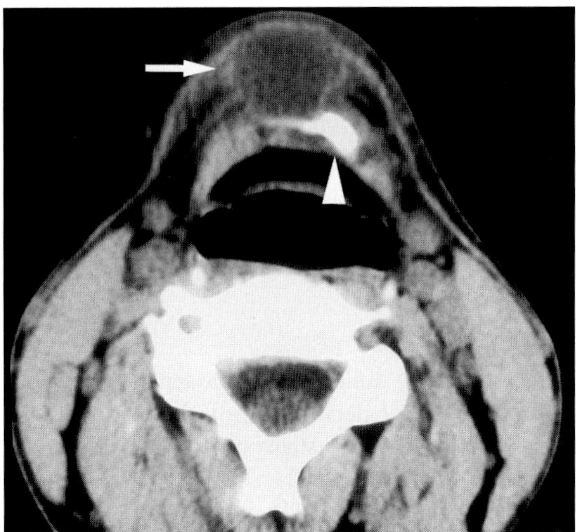

Figure 11.17

Thyroglossal duct cyst; 29-year-old male with lump in midline of neck, anterior to hyoid bone. Axial post-contrast CT image shows well-defined hypodense area with enhancing peripheral rim in midline (*arrow*) anterior to hyoid bone (*arrowhead*)

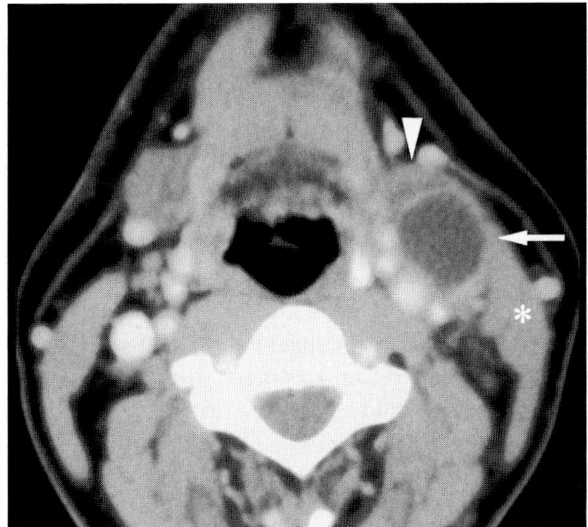

Figure 11.18

Second branchial cleft cyst; 38-year-old male with soft submandibular tumor at anterior border of sternocleidomastoid muscle; cyst confirmed by surgery. Axial post-contrast CT image shows well-defined low-density mass with enhancing peripheral rim in submandibular space (*arrow*), just dorsal to submandibular gland (*arrowhead*), lateral to carotid sheath and ventral to sternocleidomastoid muscle (*asterisk*)

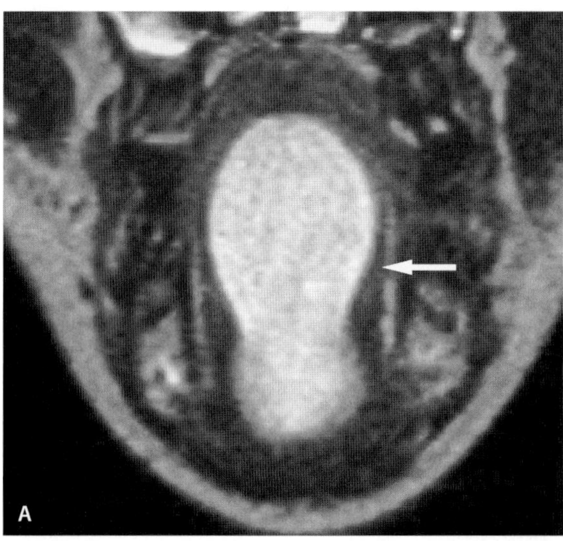

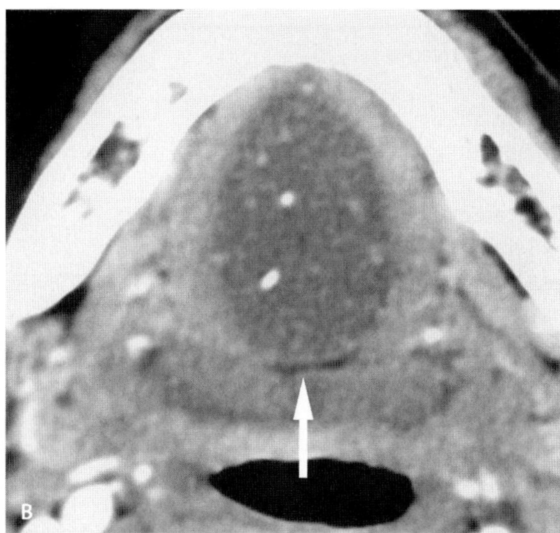

Figure 11.19

Dermoid cyst in sublingual space and in tongue; 25-year-old female with sublingual swelling. **A** Coronal STIR MRI shows high-signal mass with smooth delineation (*arrow*). **B** Axial CT image shows cyst (*arrow*) with multiple calcifications

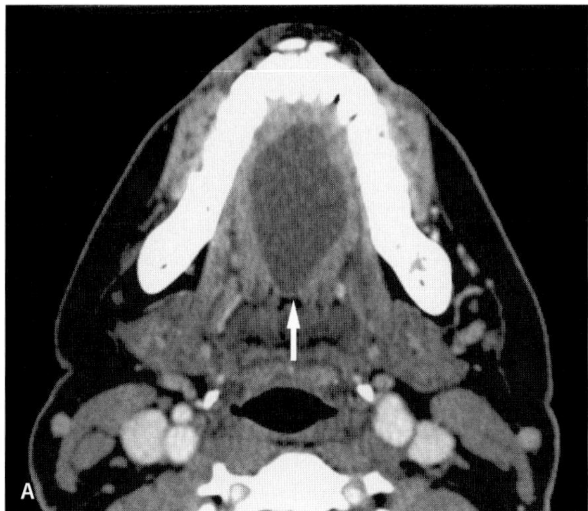

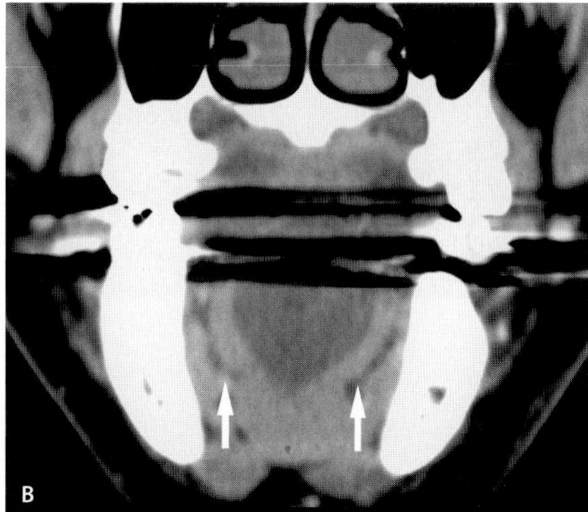

Figure 11.20

Dermoid cyst of tongue; 34-year-old female with mass in tongue. **A** Axial post-contrast CT image shows hypodense mass without calcifications in floor of mouth (*arrow*). **B** Coronal post-contrast CT image shows deviation of both genioglossus muscles laterally (*arrows*)

Lingual Thyroid

Definition

Ectopic thyroid tissue in tongue.

Clinical Features

- Incidental finding.
- Usually painless mass in tongue base; dysphagia or other symptoms may occur.
- Ectopic thyroid tissue may occur along entire - thyroglossal duct tract; 90% in base of tongue, usually in midline.
- Majority have no other functioning thyroid present.
- Female predominance.

Imaging Features

- Hyperdense mass compared to muscle; post-contrast enhancement
- T1-weighted and T2-weighted MRI: iso- or hyperintense to muscle
- T1-weighted post-Gd MRI: homogeneous contrast enhancement

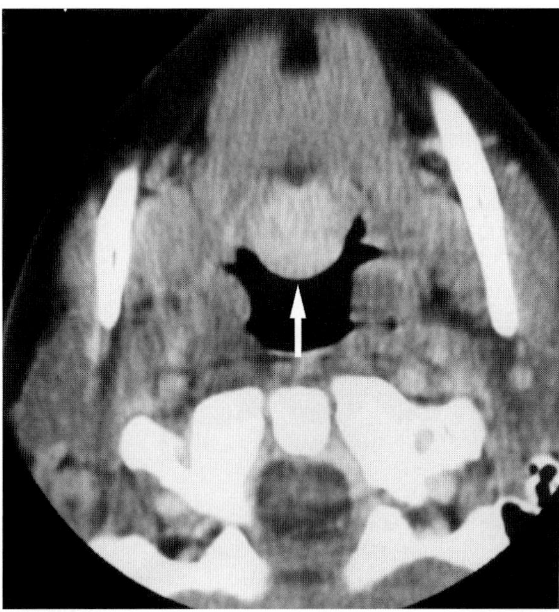

Figure 11.21
Lingual thyroid gland; 16-year-old female with lump in tongue base. Axial CT shows soft-tissue mass in posterior part of tongue (*arrow*)

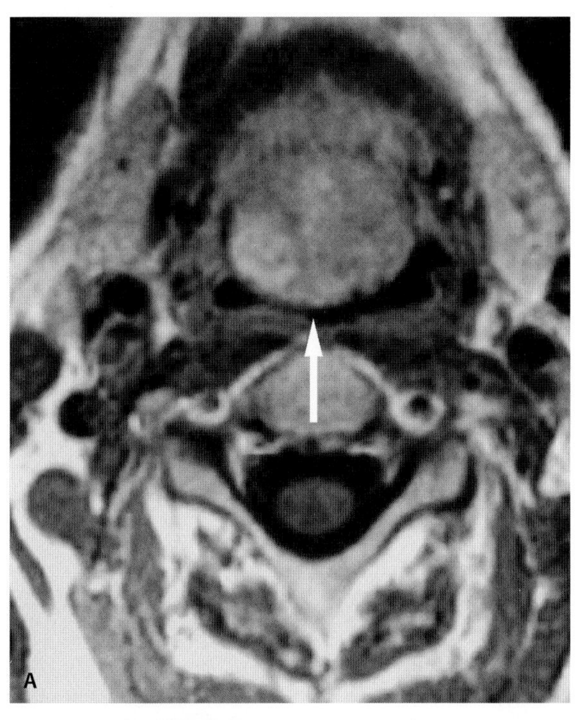

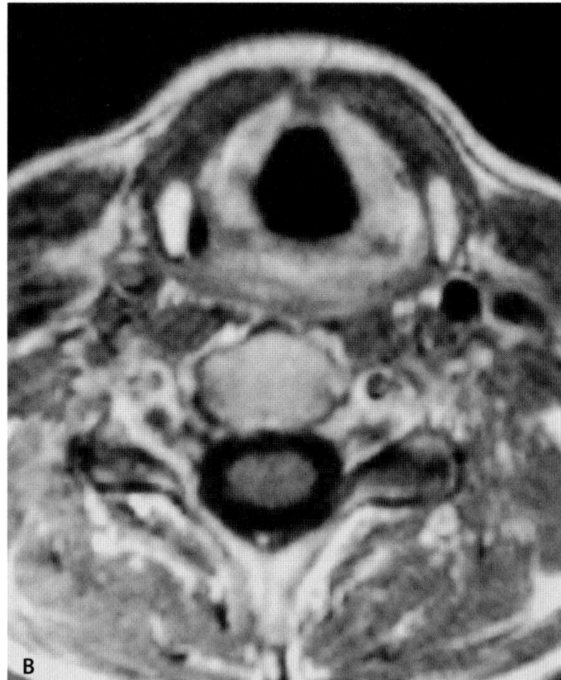

Figure 11.22

Lingual thyroid gland; 42-year-old male with lump in tongue base. A Axial T1-weighted MRI shows soft-tissue mass in posterior part of tongue (*arrow*). B Axial T1-weighted MRI shows absence of normal thyroid gland. C Sagittal T1-weighted post-Gd MRI shows thyroid mass in posterior part of tongue (*arrow*)

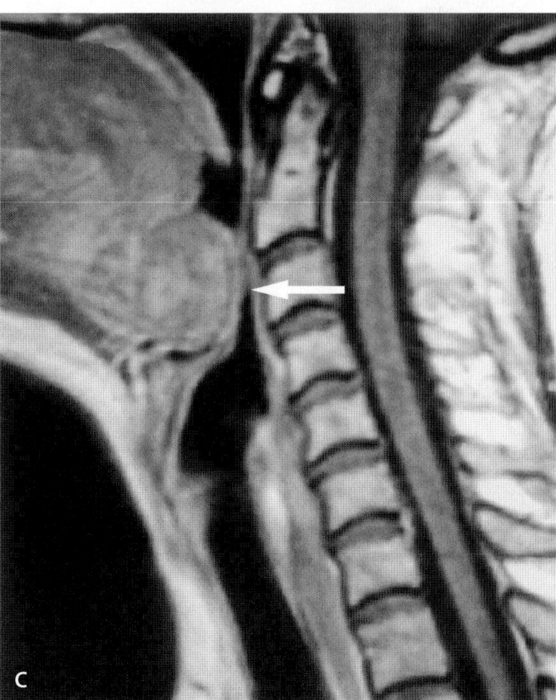

Benign Tumors

Lipoma

Definition

Benign tumor consisting of mature fat arranged in lobules, separated by fibrous tissue septa, usually surrounded by thin, fibrous capsule.

Clinical Features

- Painless swelling
- Most common mesenchymal tumor but only 13% in head and neck; most located in posterior cervical region
- Within oral cavity only 1–4% of all benign tumors

Imaging Features

- Well-defined homogeneous low-density mass; no contrast enhancement
- T1-weighted MRI: homogeneous high signal as subcutaneous fat
- T1-weighted fat-suppressed MRI: homogeneous reduced signal
- T1-weighted post-Gd MRI: no contrast enhancement

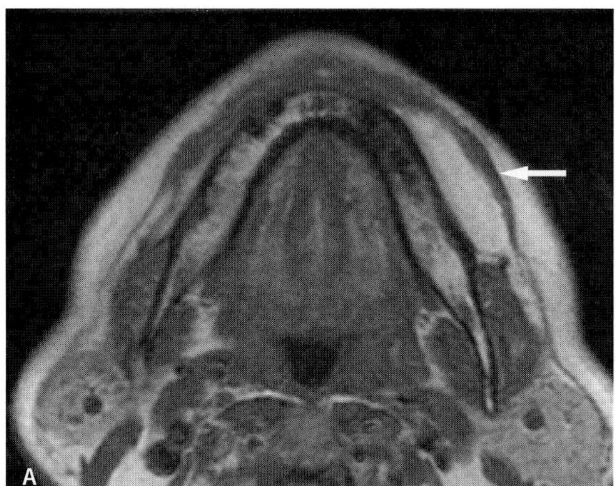

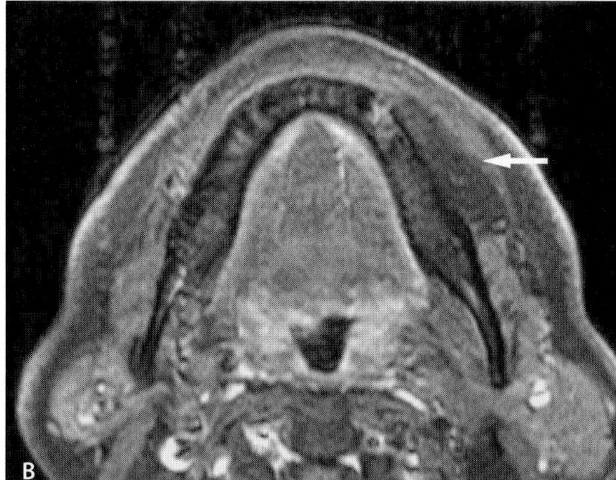

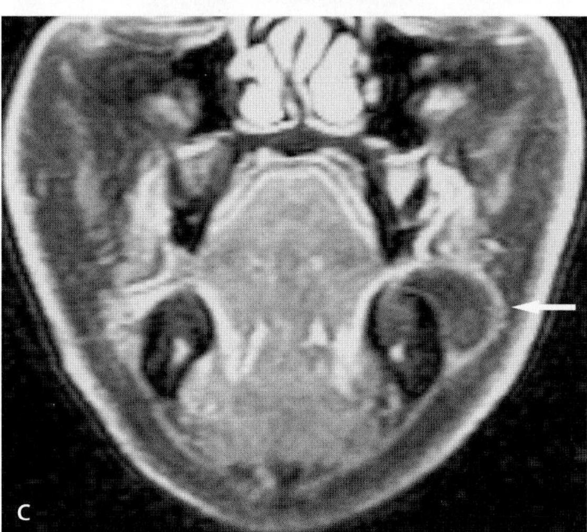

Figure 11.23

Lipoma of lower gingivobuccal sulcus; 67-year-old male with fullness of left lower gingivobuccal sulcus with clinical suspicion of being fatty. **A** Axial T1-weighted MRI shows well-defined area of homogeneous high signal along left mandible (*arrow*). **B** Axial T1-weighted fat-suppressed MRI shows reduced signal in entire area (*arrow*). **C** Coronal T1-weighted fat-suppressed post-Gd MRI shows no enhancement of mass except in periphery (*arrow*)

Schwannoma

Definition

Benign nerve sheath tumor emanating from Schwann cells. (The terminology is confusing. The following terms have been used for the same tumor: schwannoma, neuroma, neurinoma, neurolemmoma, perineural fibroblastoma.)

Clinical Features

- Asymptomatic mass.
- About 13% of schwannomas are found in head and neck, most in the lateral cervical region.
- Almost half of oral schwannomas reported to occur in the tongue.

Imaging Features

- Well-defined homogeneous soft-tissue mass, enhancement, but variable appearance because of cystic and solid components. Schwannoma is often cystic, as opposed to neuroma, which is seldom cystic.
- Enlarged foramina.
- Atrophy of muscles.
- Associated with neurofibromatosis.
- T1-weighted MRI: isointense with muscle.
- T2-weighted MRI: hyperintense, homogeneous, both cystic and solid components, or heterogeneous.
- T1-weighted post-Gd MRI: cystic nature with rim enhancement.

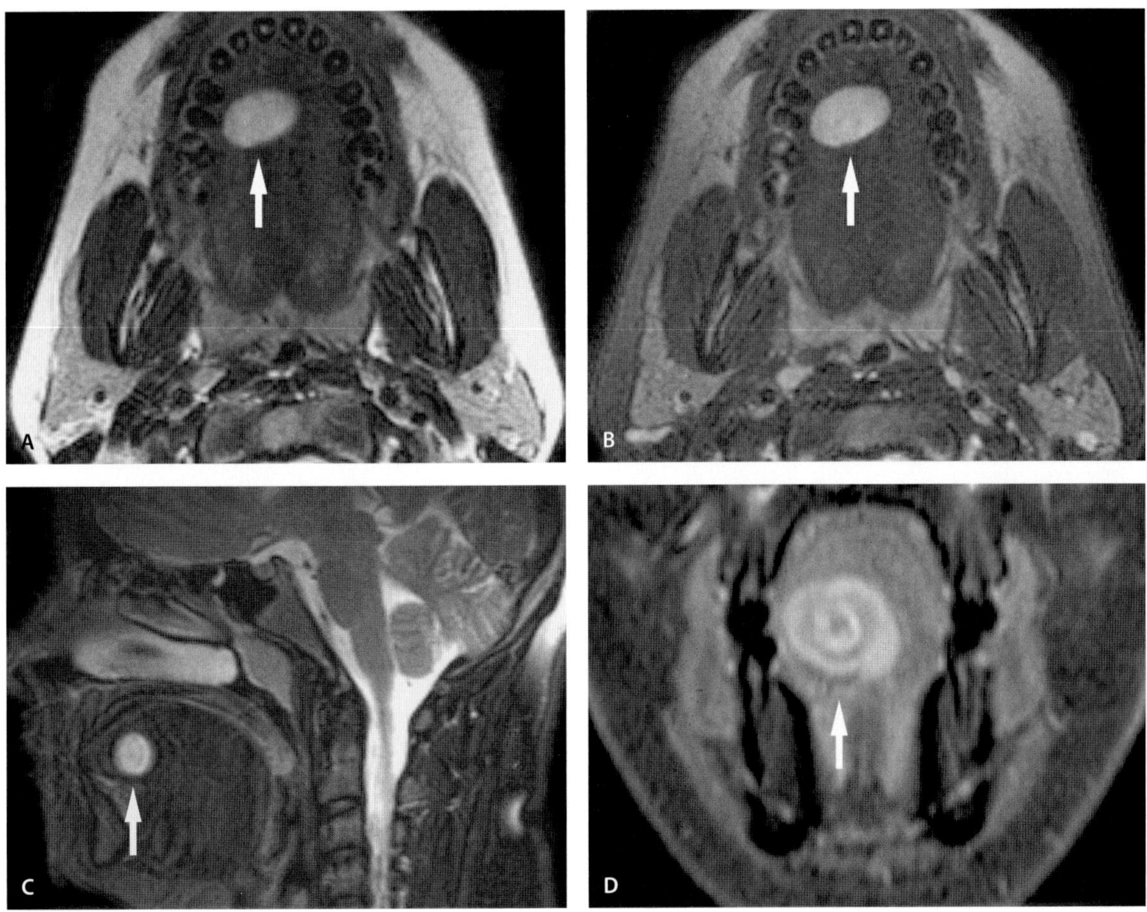

Figure 11.24

Schwannoma of tongue; 13-year-old with slowly growing mass of tongue. A Axial T2-weighted MRI shows well-defined high-signal mass in right anterior tongue (*arrow*). B Axial T2-weighted fat-suppressed MRI shows high-signal mass (*arrow*), indicating no evident fatty component. C Sagittal T2-weighted fat-suppressed MRI confirms high-signal mass in anterior part of tongue (*arrow*). D Coronal T1-weighted fat-suppressed post-Gd MRI shows serpentine onion-type contrast enhancement of mass (*arrow*)

Malignant Tumors

Oropharyngeal Carcinomas

Definition

Malignant epithelial tumor.

Clinical Features (Oral Carcinomas)

- Painless mass
- Most frequent malignant tumor in oral cavity, predominantly squamous cell type
- Predilection areas: floor of mouth, ventrolateral tongue, and soft palate complex (soft palate proper, anterior tonsillar pillar, retromolar trigone)
- Typically males, 50–70 years, drinking smokers
- Lymph node involvement in 30–65% when diagnosed; single most important prognostic factor
- Somewhat less aggressive than oropharynx carcinomas
- Oral Carcinomas

Imaging Features (Oral Carcinomas)

- Isodense to muscle, moderate contrast enhancement
- Surrounding structures invaded
- T1-weighted MRI; isointense to muscle signal
- T2-weighted MRI: inhomogeneous increased signal
- T1-weighted post-Gd MRI: moderate enhancement
- Non-contrast T1-weighted MRI reported most useful sequence to assess tumor extent
- Oral Carcinomas

See also Chapter 4.

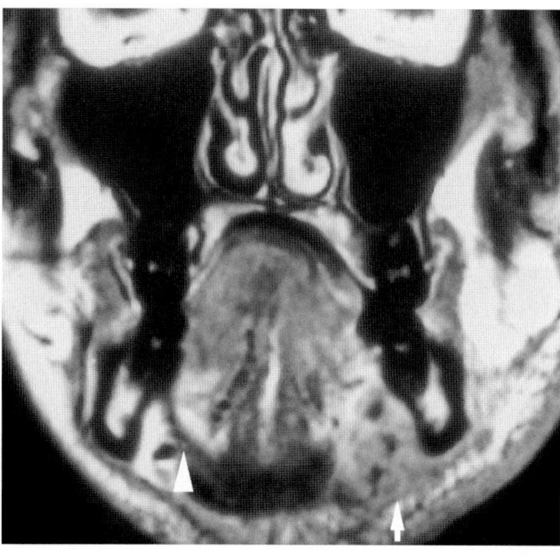

Figure 11.25

Squamous cell carcinoma of tongue invading floor of mouth; 22-year-old male with history of tongue cancer, now with recurrence. Coronal T1-weighted post-Gd MRI shows moderately contrast-enhanced tumor penetrating mylohyoid muscle and platysma (*arrow*). Note normal mylohyoid muscle on contralateral side (*arrowhead*)

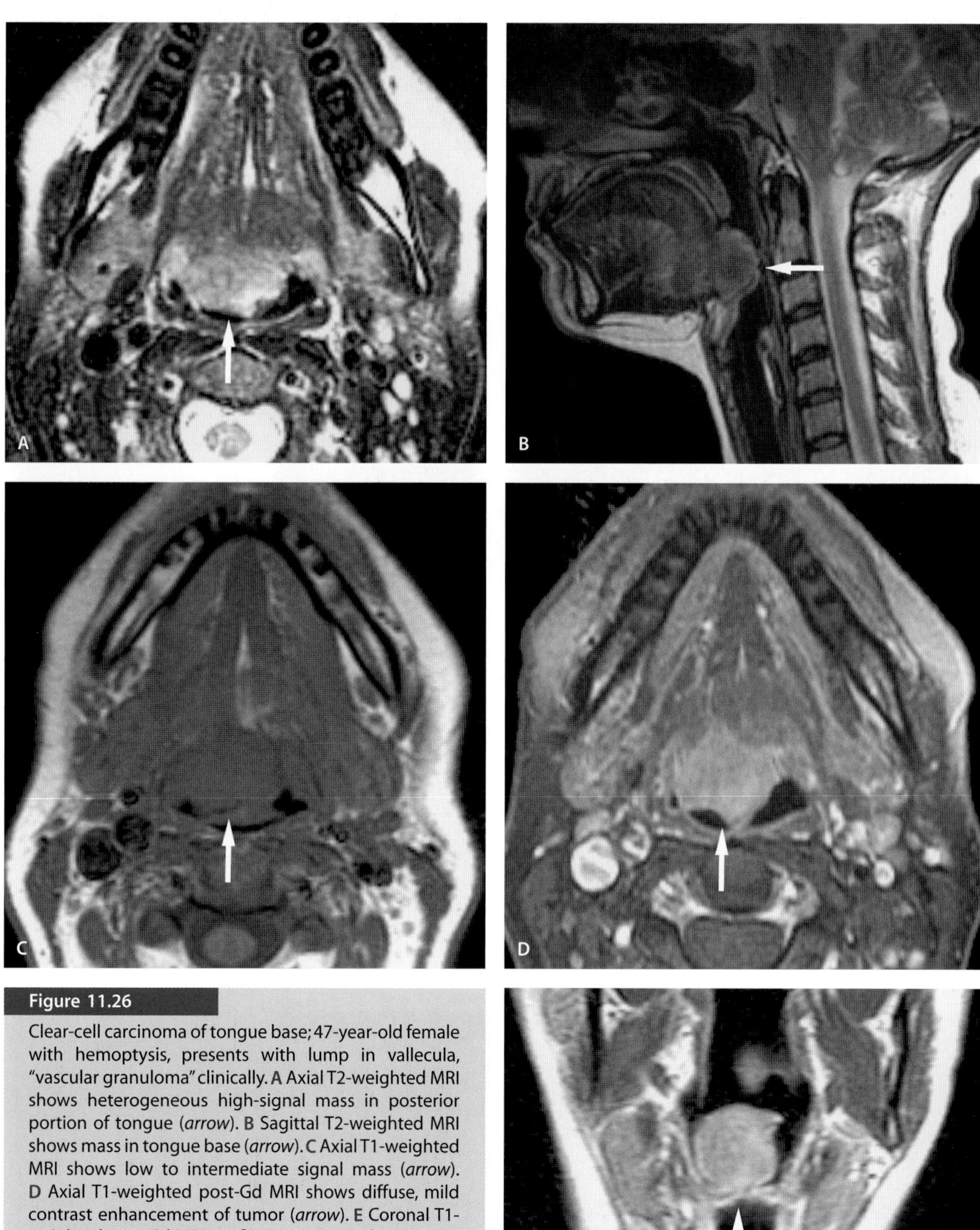

Figure 11.26

Clear-cell carcinoma of tongue base; 47-year-old female with hemoptysis, presents with lump in vallecula, "vascular granuloma" clinically. **A** Axial T2-weighted MRI shows heterogeneous high-signal mass in posterior portion of tongue (*arrow*). **B** Sagittal T2-weighted MRI shows mass in tongue base (*arrow*). **C** Axial T1-weighted MRI shows low to intermediate signal mass (*arrow*). **D** Axial T1-weighted post-Gd MRI shows diffuse, mild contrast enhancement of tumor (*arrow*). **E** Coronal T1-weighted post-Gd MRI confirms contrast enhancement of tumor (*arrow*)

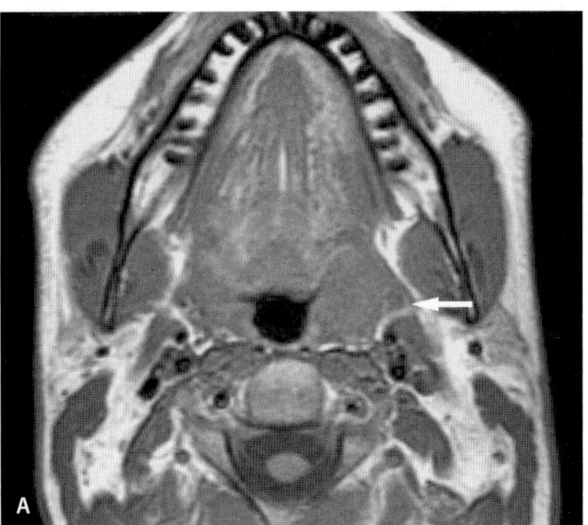

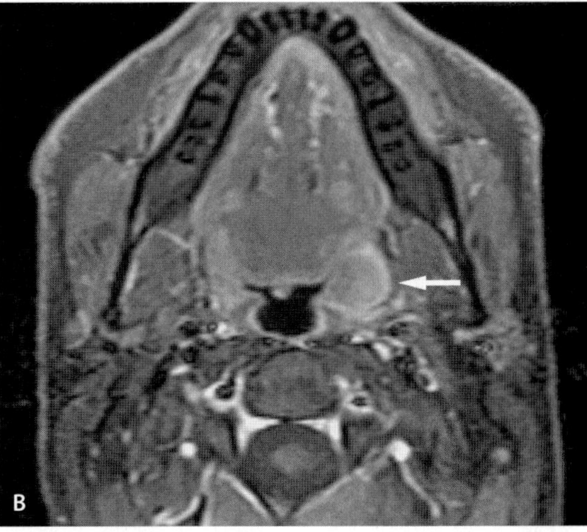

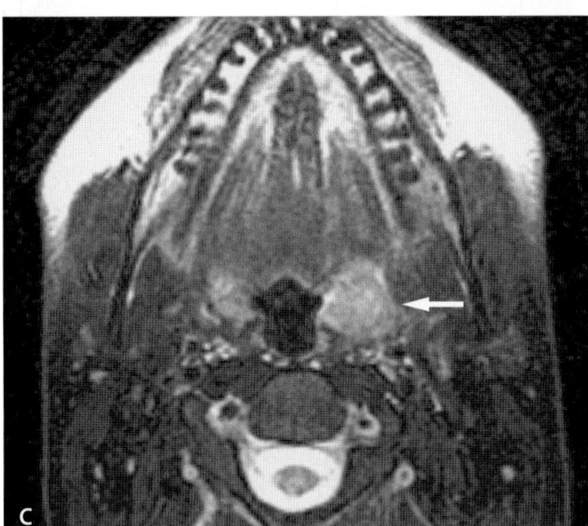

Figure 11.27

Squamous cell carcinoma of tonsil; 43-year-old male with known multiple sclerosis and a history of squamous cell carcinoma of left palatine tonsil. **A** Axial T1-weighted MRI shows low to intermediate signal mass in left palatine tonsil (*arrow*). **B** Axial T1-weighted fat-suppressed post-Gd MRI shows moderately contrast-enhanced mass (*arrow*). **C** Axial T2-weighted fat-suppressed MRI shows high-signal mass (*arrow*)

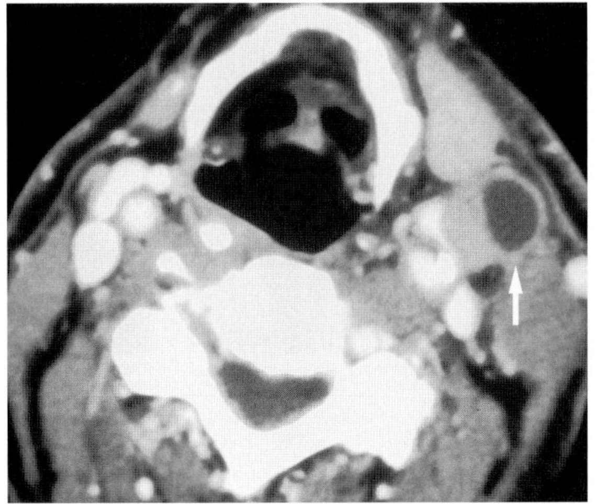

Figure 11.28

Lymph node metastasis; 65-year-old male with squamous cell carcinoma of left palatine tonsil, metastasizing. Axial post-contrast CT image shows well-defined mass in submandibular space, hypodense with enhanced border (*arrow*). Note similarity with branchial cleft cyst in Fig. 11.18

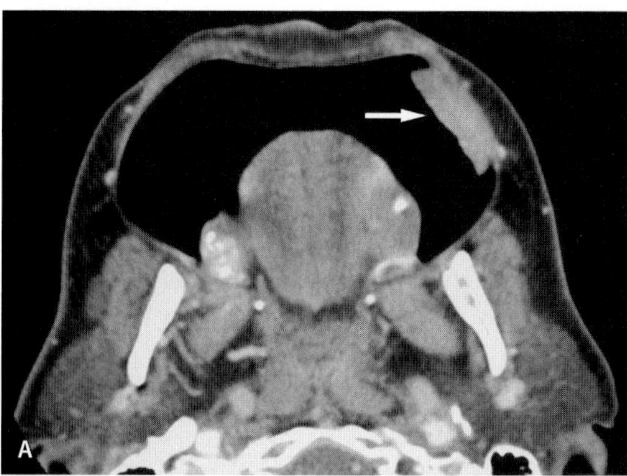

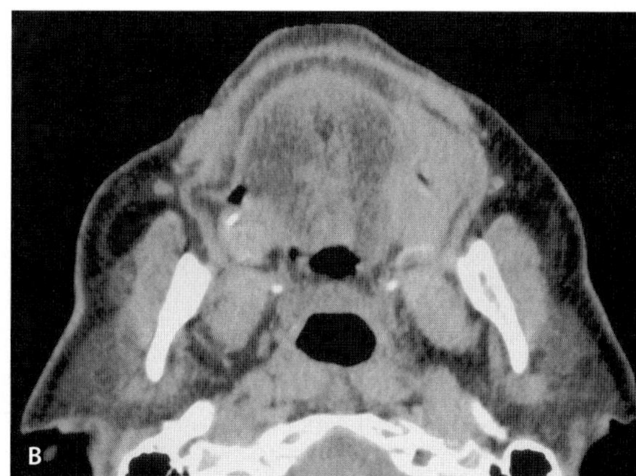

Figure 11.29

Squamous cell carcinoma of cheek with and without blowing cheek; 74-year-old male with lump in cheek. **A** Axial CT image with blowing cheek shows soft-tissue tumor in buccal mucosa (*arrow*). **B** Axial CT without blowing cheek cannot reveal origin of tumor

Adenoid Cystic Carcinoma

Definition

Malignant epithelial tumor with various histologic features showing three growth patterns: glandular (cribriform), tubular or solid.

Clinical Features

- Painless mass, slowly growing
- Seldom regional lymph node metastases, in contrast to squamous cell carcinoma
- In oral cavity usually in palate (minor salivary glands)

Imaging Features

- Cannot be distinguished from squamous cell carcinoma
- Perineural tumor extension is however typical

See also Chapter 4.

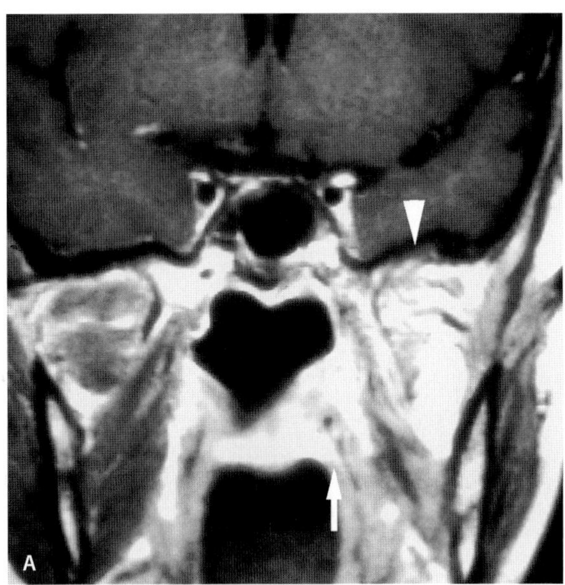

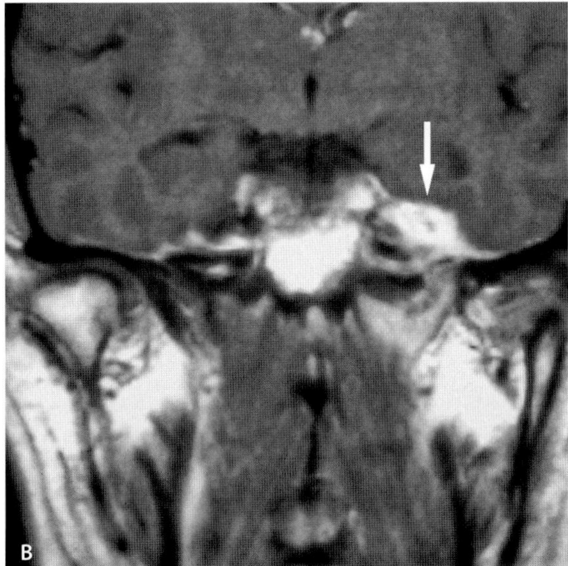

Figure 11.30

Adenoid cystic carcinoma of epipharynx with intracranial spread; 50-year-old female treated with irradiation 5 years previously, now with recurrence. **A** Coronal T1-weighted post-Gd MRI shows contrast-enhancing tumor recurrence in epipharynx wall (*arrow*) and atrophy of medial and lateral pterygoid muscles (*arrowhead*). **B** Coronal T1-weighted post-Gd MRI shows tumor growing intracranially (*arrow*) through oval foramen, compressing mandibular nerve

Lymphoma

Definition

Malignant tumor of lymphatic tissue; a number of different types.

Clinical Features

- Both Hodgkin's and non-Hodgkin's lymphoma occur in the maxillofacial area, most frequently presenting with lymph node enlargement.
- Non-Hodgkin's lymphoma more frequently involves extranodal sites.

Imaging Features

- Cannot distinguish non-Hodgkin's and Hodgkin's disease in head and neck area based on imaging findings of lymph nodes.
- Well-defined or ill-defined unspecified mass, either enhancing or not.

See also Chapter 4.

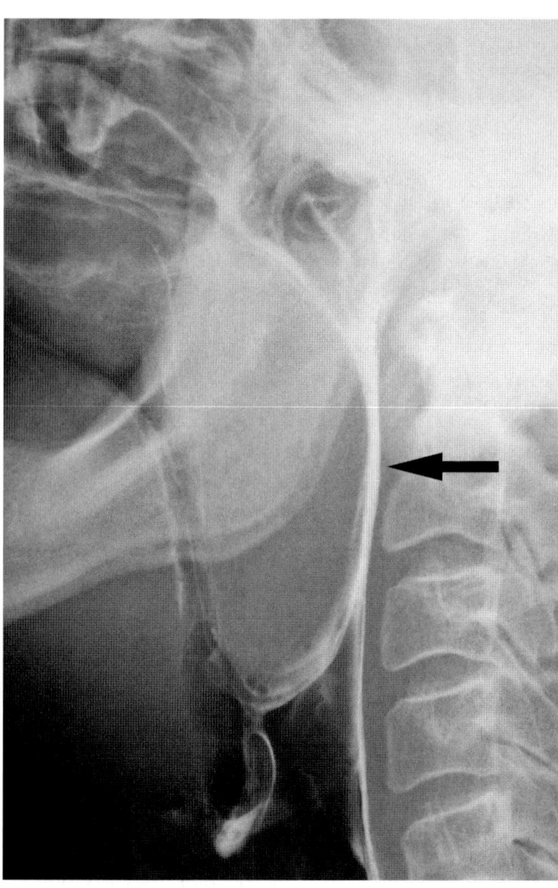

Figure 11.31

Oropharyngeal non-Hodgkin's lymphoma; 62-year-old male with swallowing and breathing problems. Lateral view with contrast material in nose shows large soft palate mass (*arrow*) extending downward to level of top of epiglottic cartilage

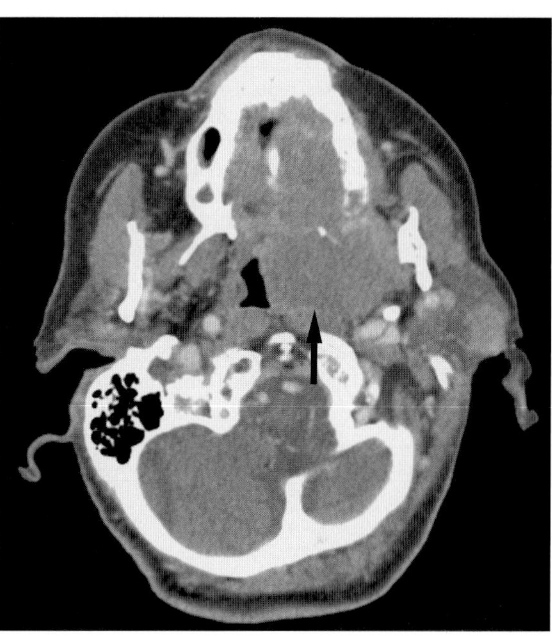

Figure 11.32

Oral and parapharyngeal non-Hodgkin's lymphoma; 88-year-old female with 3-year history of lymphoma with radiation therapy to neck and right axilla; metastatic disease suspected to oral cavity. **A** Axial post-contrast CT image shows large lobulated nonenhancing parapharyngeal mass that occludes most of the pharynx and oral cavity (*arrow*). Imaging cannot determine if the intraparotid lymph node is involved with lymphoma

Suggested Reading

Al-Ghambi S, Black MJ, Lafond G (1992) Extracranial head and neck schwannomas. J Otolaryngol 21:186–188

Allard RHB (1982) The thyroglossal duct cyst. Head Neck Surg 5:134–146

Aspestrand F, Kolbenstvedt A (1987) Calcifications of the palatine tonsillary region: CT demonstration. Radiology 165:479–480

Braun IF, Hoffman JC Jr, Reede D, et al (1984) Computed tomography of the buccomasseteric region: 2. Pathology. AJNR Am J Neuroradiol 5:611–616

Bredesen K, Aalokken TM, Kolbenstvedt A (2001) CT of the oral vestibule with distended cheeks. Acta Radiol 42:84–87

Dolata J (1994) Thyroglossal cyst in the floor of mouth: an unusual location. Otolaryngol Head Neck Surg 110:580–583

Flickinger FW, Lozano RL, Yuh WT, et al (1989) Neurilemmoma of the tongue: MR findings. J Comput Assist Tomogr 13:886–888

Fujimura N, Enomoto S (1992) Lipoma of tongue with cartilaginous changes: case report and review of literature. J Oral Maxillofac Surg 50:1015–1017

Gallo WJ, Moss M, Shapiri DN, et al (1977) Neurilemmoma: review of the literature and report of five cases. J Oral Surg 35:235–236

Hopp E, Mortensen B, Kolbenstvedt A (2004) Mylohyoid herniation of the sublingual gland diagnosed by magnetic resonance imaging. Dentomaxillofac Radiol 33:351–353

Johnson JT (1990) A surgeon looks at cervical lymph nodes. Radiology 145:607–610

King RC, Smith BR, Burk JL (1994) Dermoid cysts in the floor of the mouth. Oral Surg Oral Med Oral Pathol 78:567–576

Lindberg R (1972) Distribution of cervical lymph node metastases from squamous cell carcinoma of the upper respiratory and digestive tracts. Cancer 29:1446–1449

Mukherji SK (2003) Pharynx. In: Som PM, Curtin HD (eds) Head and neck imaging, 4th edn. Mosby, St. Louis, pp 1466–1520

New GB (1947) Congenital cysts of the tongue, the floor of the mouth, the pharynx and the larynx. Arch Otolaryngol 45:145–158

Schellhas KP (1989) MR imaging of muscles of mastication. AJR Am J Roentgenol 153:847–855

Smoker WRK (2003) The oral cavity. In: Som PM, Curtin HD (eds) Head and neck imaging, 4th edn. Mosby, St. Louis, pp 1377–1464

Som PM (1987) Lymph nodes of the neck. Radiology 165: 593–600

Som PM, Scherl MP, Rao VM, et al (1986) Rare presentations of ordinary lipomas of head and neck: a review AJNR Am J Neuroradiol 7:657–664

Thomas JR (1979) Thyroglossal duct cysts. Ear Nose Throat J 58:512–514

Tryhus MR, Smoker WRK, Harnsberger HR (1990) The normal and diseased masticator space. Semin Ultrasound CT MR 11:476–485

Worley CM, Laskin DM (1993) Coincidental sublingual and submental epidermoid cysts. J Oral Maxillofac Surg 51:787–790

Yasumoto M, Shibuya H, Takeda M, Korenaga T (1995) Squamous cell carcinoma of the oral cavity: MR findings and value of T1- versus T2-weighted fast spin-echo images. AJR Am J Roentgenol 164:981–987

Salivary Glands

In collaboration with A. Kolbenstvedt

Introduction

Salivary gland conditions are probably more diverse than those of any other organ system: congenital, obstructive, infectious, inflammatory, systemic, and neoplastic. The frequency of tumors is however less than 3% of all tumors. On the other hand, although advanced soft-tissue imaging with CT and MRI are used, the radiologic differentiation between benign and malignant diseases remains difficult. The more common obstructive conditions are of particular interest for those working in the dental field, because conventional film examination should be the initial radiologic evaluation for patients with suspected stones. Those working in the environments of saliva should also be the first to notice any reduced salivation that may have many causes, and a significant impact on teeth conditions.

This chapter illustrates a number of different conditions, some common and others rare. The intention is not to be complete, but rather to show a variety of salivary gland conditions of relevance to the maxillofacial radiologist.

Nonneoplastic Conditions

Infection/inflammation

Definition

Sialoadenitis: infection/inflammation of the gland.

Sialodochitis: infection/inflammation of the duct.

Clinical Features

- Acute sialoadenitis:
  - Painful swelling, with or without pus
  - Most common in parotid gland, bilateral or unilateral
  - Neonates or elderly in particular
  - Regional lymphadenopathy, fever, malaise
  - Acute exacerbation of chronic sialoadenitis
  - Bacterial infection; *Staphylococcus aureus* most common, local, unilateral, suppurative, diffuse (cellulitis) or localized (abscess)
  - Retrograde, calculus etiology
  - Viral infection; systemic, bilateral (mumps)
- Chronic sialoadenitis:
  - Parotid or submandibular gland; rarely in sublingual gland
  - Intermittent swelling and tenderness
  - Vague or no symptoms
  - Recurrent bacterial infection
  - Autoimmune diseases
  - Prior radiation therapy
  - Treatment of thyroid cancer with radioactive iodine
  - Retrograde, calculus etiology

Imaging Features

- Sialoadenitis:
  - Enlargement (diffuse) of gland, increased density, enhancing with contrast
  - Associated cellulitis; streaking (stranding) in subcutaneous fat, thickened platysma
  - Abscess; localized density area surrounded by enhanced rim
  - Sialolithiasis
  - T1-weighted MRI: enlarged gland, low signal, diffuse or localized (abscess)
  - T2-weighted MRI: enlarged gland, high signal, diffuse or localized (abscess); may also be low depending on whether edema or cellular infiltration dominates
  - T1-weighted post-Gd MRI: moderate, diffuse contrast enhancement or only enhanced peripheral rim (abscess)
- Sialodochitis:
  - Dilated duct, usually with single or multiple strictures ("string of sausages")
- Sialography:
  - Conventional technique superior to other imaging methods to demonstrate subtle anatomy of salivary duct system

- MR sialography can be done with heavily T2-weighted images without injection of contrast medium. This visualizes the main parotid duct with secondary ducts and submandibular duct but not finer ducts as seen with conventional sialography. However, MR sialography may be useful in cases in which cannulation of the duct cannot be performed

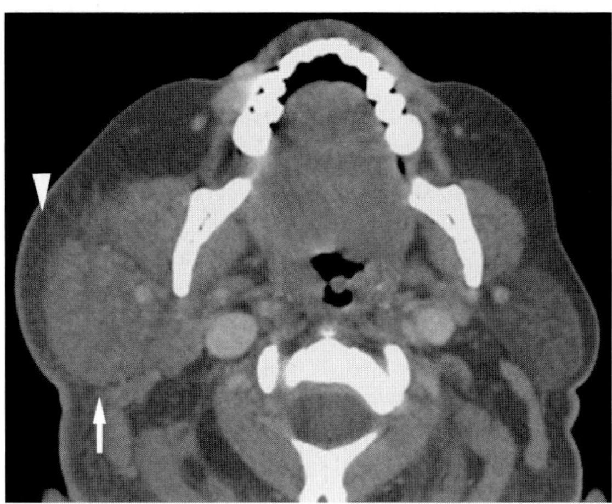

Figure 12.1

Acute suppurative parotitis: 61-year-old female with past history of diabetes mellitus, chronic renal failure, coronary artery disease status after myocardial infarction and PTCA, stroke, hypertension, hyperlipidemia, hypothyroidism, congestive heart failure; now presenting with an acute swelling of right side of face in the setting of known *Staphylococcus* bacteremia. Axial post-contrast CT image shows enlarged right parotid gland with increased density (*arrow*), with streaking opacities in overlying fat (*arrowhead*)

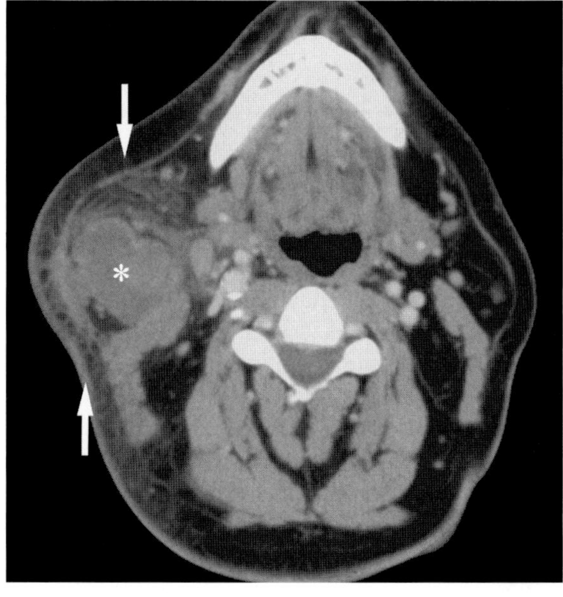

Figure 12.2

Parotid abscess; 52-year-old male with non-resolving right parotitis. Axial post-contrast CT image shows homogeneous density with contrast-enhancing rim consistent with abscess in parotid gland (*asterisk*) with streaking in fat (*arrows*)

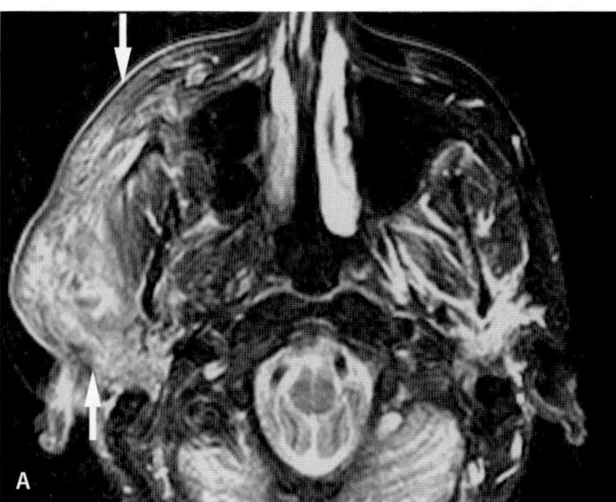

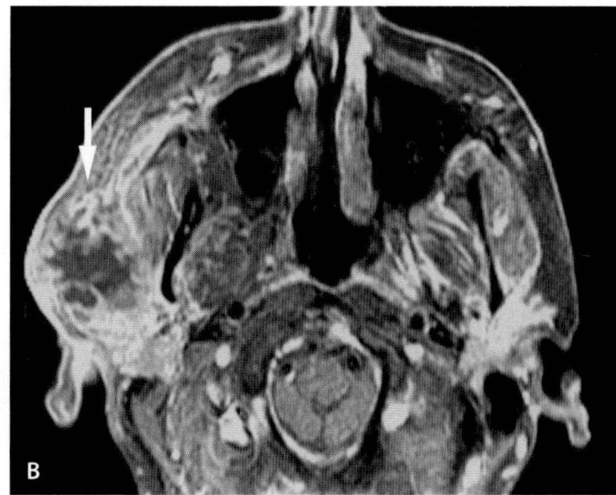

Figure 12.3

Abscess and cellulitis in parotid region; 52-year-old female with right parotid swelling and pain, and clinical suspicion of abscess. A Axial T2-weighted fat-suppressed MRI shows diffuse high signal in right lateral half of face consistent with subcutaneous edema and cellulitis (*arrows*). B Axial T1-weighted fat-suppressed post-Gd MRI shows low signal area surrounded by irregular contrast-enhancing rim consistent with abscess (*arrow*). Note also diffuse enhancement in subcutaneous fat extending to anterior portion of maxilla. Abscess was surgically drained

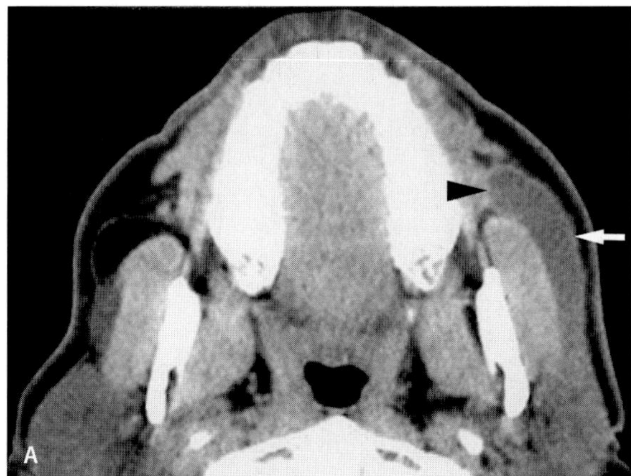

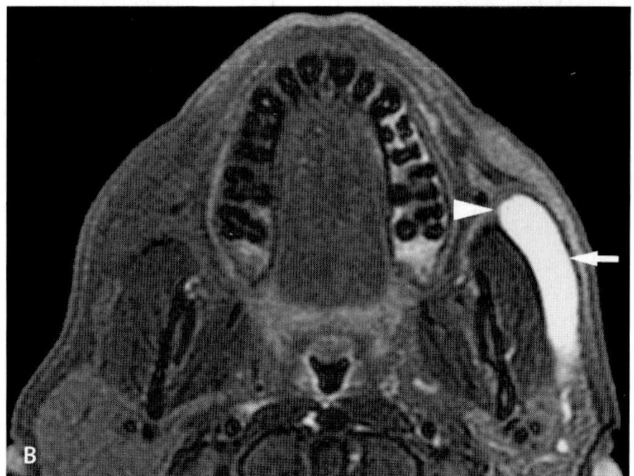

Figure 12.4

Stenosis and dilatation of Stensen's duct but no stones; 56-year-old male with a remote history of injury to left cheek after which he developed intermittent swelling (gland itself was not enlarged or abnormal on CT or MRI imaging). On clinical examination there was scarring at orifice of left Stensen's duct. A Axial post-contrast CT shows dilated Stensen's duct (*arrow*) with closed orifice (*arrowhead*). B Axial T2-weighted fat-suppressed MRI confirms dilated duct (*arrow*) and closed orifice (*arrowhead*). C Axial T1-weighted fat-suppressed post-Gd MRI shows no contrast enhancement of dilated duct (*arrow*)

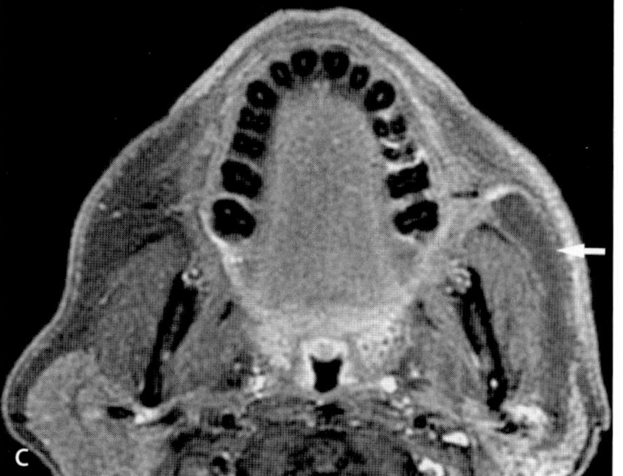

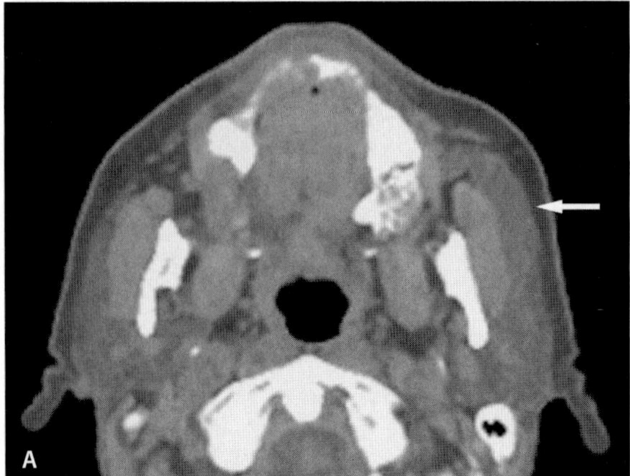

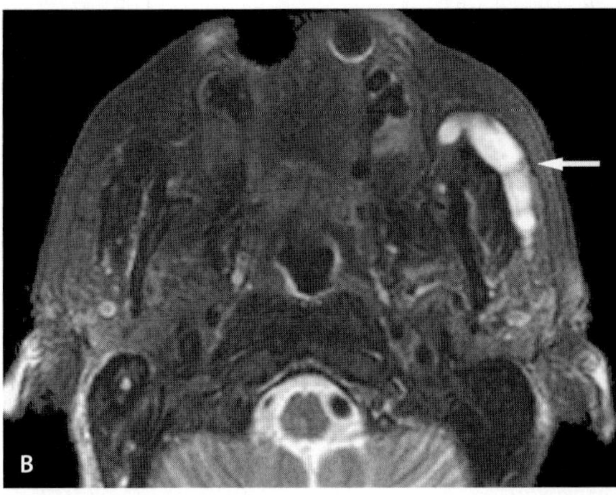

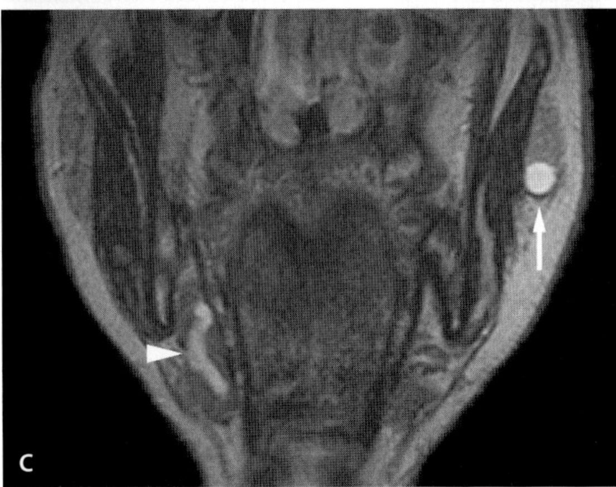

Figure 12.5

Dilated Stensen's duct and Wharton's duct; 76-year-old male with enlarged right submandibular salivary gland and question of possible tumor (no calculi or gland abnormalities except slightly enlarged right submandibular gland found on CT and MRI imaging). A Axial post-contrast CT image shows dilated left Stensen's duct (*arrow*). B Axial T2-weighted MRI confirms dilated duct (*arrow*). C Coronal T2-weighted MRI confirms dilated Stensen's duct (*arrow*) and shows prominent right Wharton's duct as well (*arrowhead*)

Sialolithiasis

Definition

Formation of sialoliths (calculi, stones) in ducts or secretary portions of the salivary glands.

Clinical Features

- Small stones may disappear spontaneously
- Small stones may be symptomatic, large stones may be asymptomatic
- Leads to reduced salivary flow, hyposalivation
- May result in retrograde infection; an abscess or more commonly, a chronic recurrent sialoadenitis with intermittent swelling and tenderness/pain, usually at meals
- Total obstruction will eventually lead to parenchyma atrophy

Imaging Features

- Round or oval calcifications typical; 10–20% are radiolucent
- Most stones are solitary; about 25% multiple
- 80–90% in submandibular gland or Wharton's duct; about 85% in duct

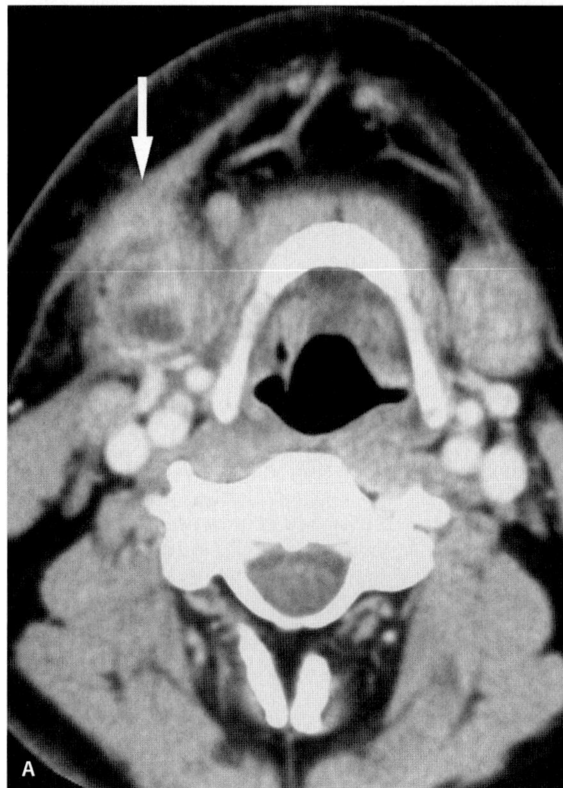

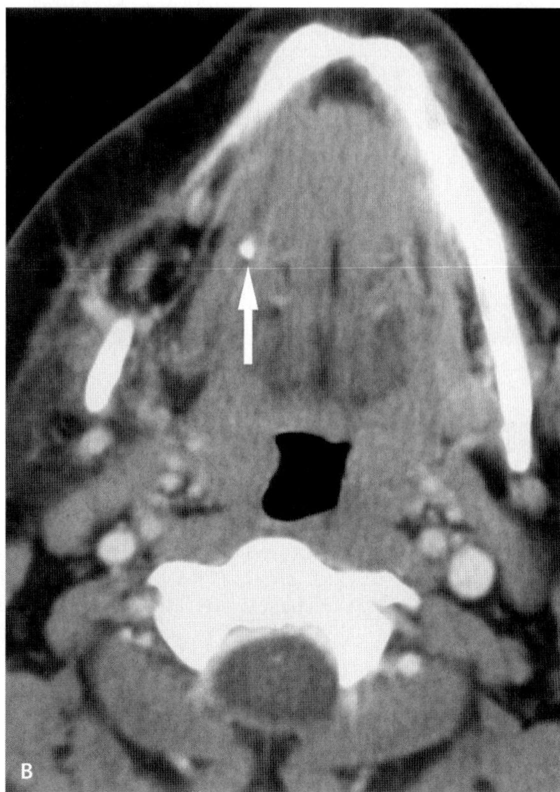

Figure 12.6

Submandibular gland multilocular abscess due to stone in Wharton's duct; 69-year-old male with intermittent submandibular swelling and tenderness. A Axial post-contrast CT shows enlarged submandibular gland with abscess (*arrow*). B Axial post-contrast CT image shows stone in submandibular duct (*arrow*)

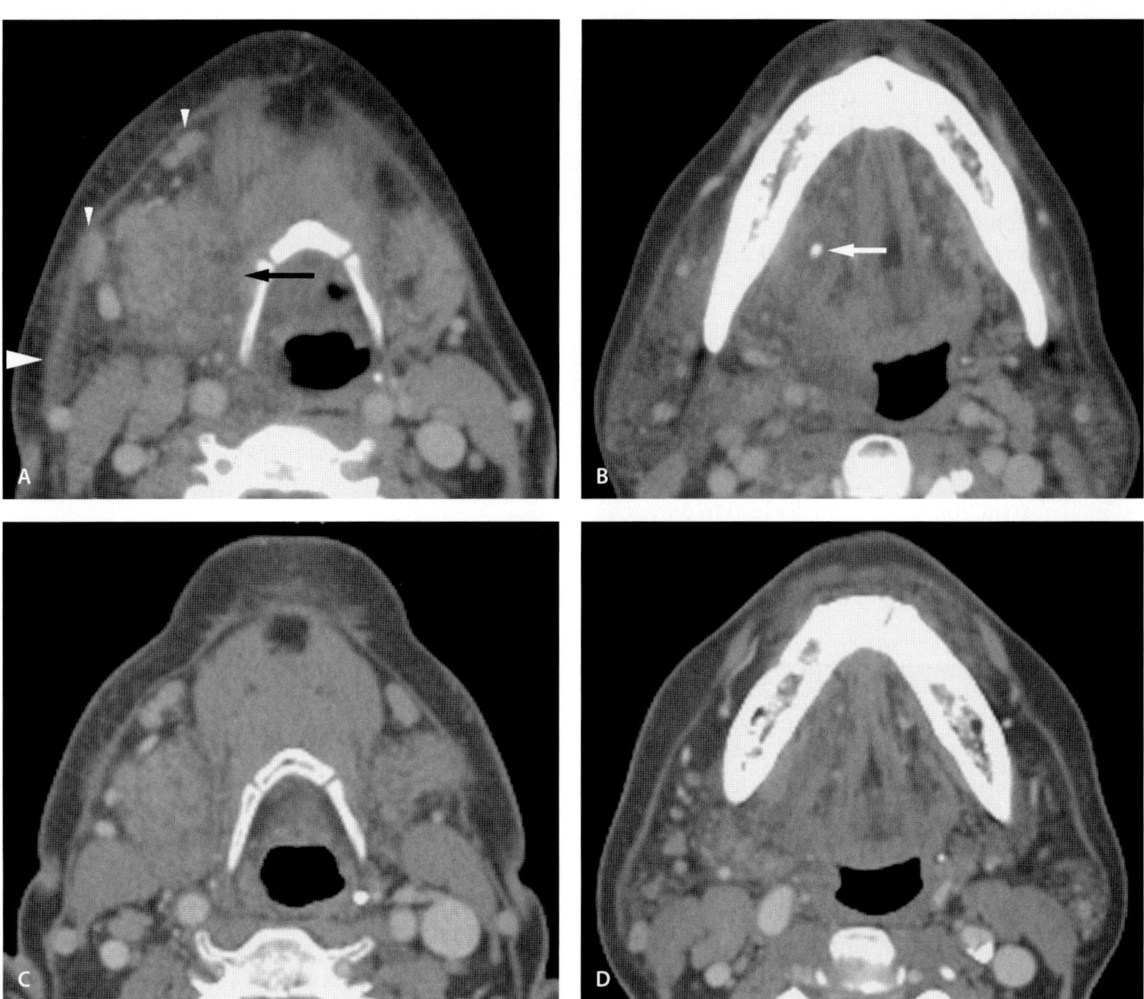

Figure 12.7

Submandibular sialoadenitis with cellulitis due to Wharton's duct stone that was released within 2 days; 59-year-old female with right mandibular swelling and pain that reduced significantly after 2 days. **A** Axial post-contrast CT image shows diffuse enlargement of right submandibular gland (*arrow*) with thickened platysma (*large arrowhead*) streaking in overlying fat, and right submandibular lymphadenopathy (*small arrowheads*). **B** Axial post-contrast CT image shows small stone in Wharton's duct (*arrow*). **C** Axial post-contrast CT image 2 days later shows significantly reduced swelling. **D** Axial post-contrast CT image 2 days later shows no evidence of stone

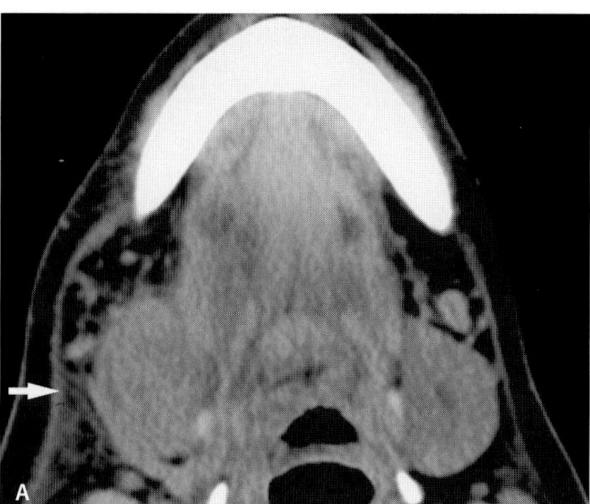
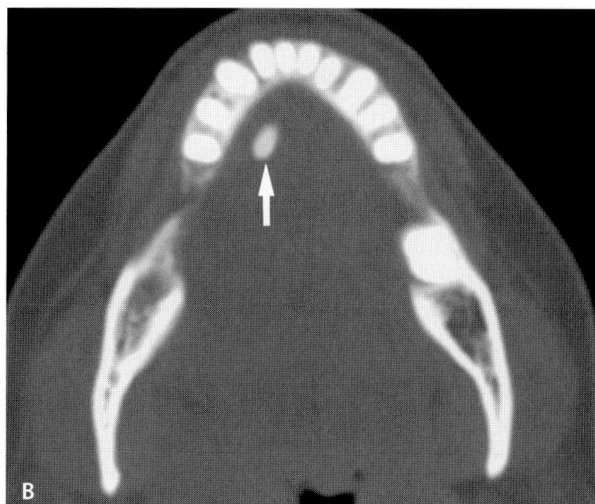

Figure 12.8

Submandibular sialoadenitis due to duct stone; 59-year-old female with right submandibular swelling. **A** Axial post-contrast CT image shows enlarged submandibular gland with stranding and reticulation of periglandular fat (*arrow*). **B** Axial CT image shows stone in anterior part of Wharton's duct (*arrow*)

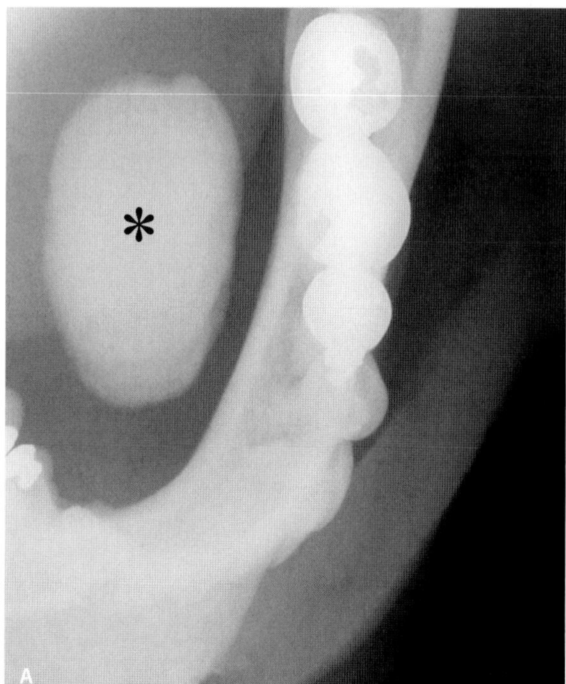
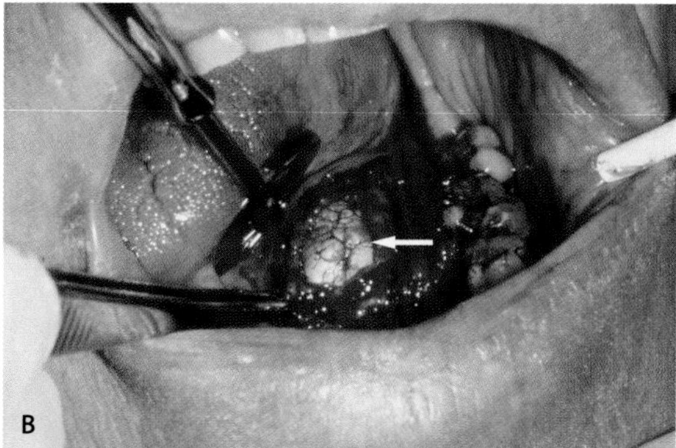
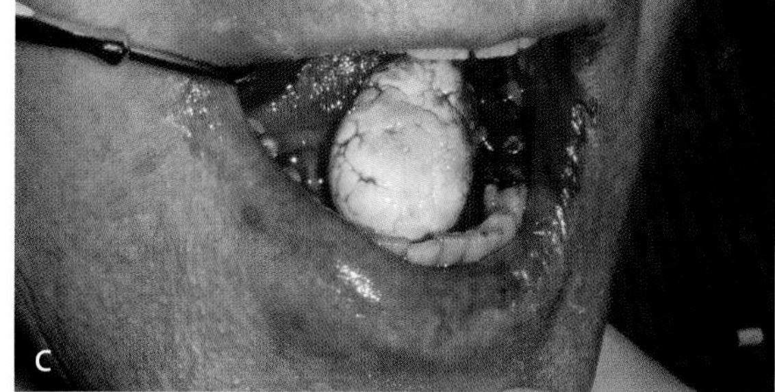

Figure 12.9

Submandibular duct stone; 55-year-old male with incidental finding of painless swelling in floor of mouth, and no history of pain or variable swelling. **A** Intraoral occlusal view shows large stone in Wharton's duct (*asterisk*). **B** Clinical photograph during surgery shows stone after surgical incision (*arrow*). **C** Clinical photograph of "released" stone (about 28 mm long)

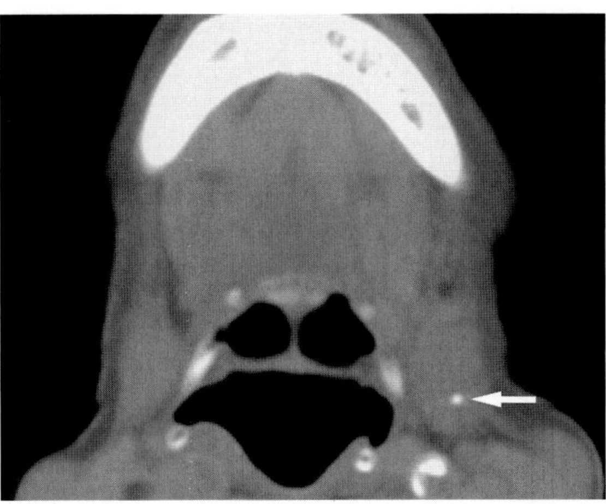

Figure 12.10

Submandibular gland stone; 86-year-old female with submandibular pain. Axial post-contrast CT image shows small stone in hilum of submandibular gland (*arrow*)

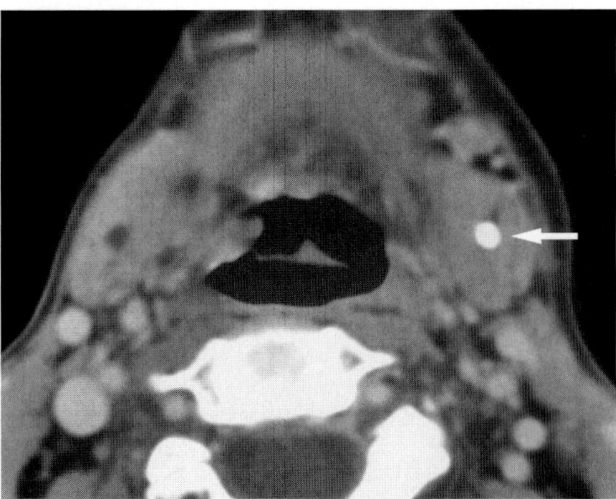

Figure 12.11

Submandibular gland stone; 79-year-old female with left submandibular mass for about 2 months. Axial post-contrast CT image shows stone in hilum of submandibular gland (*arrow*)

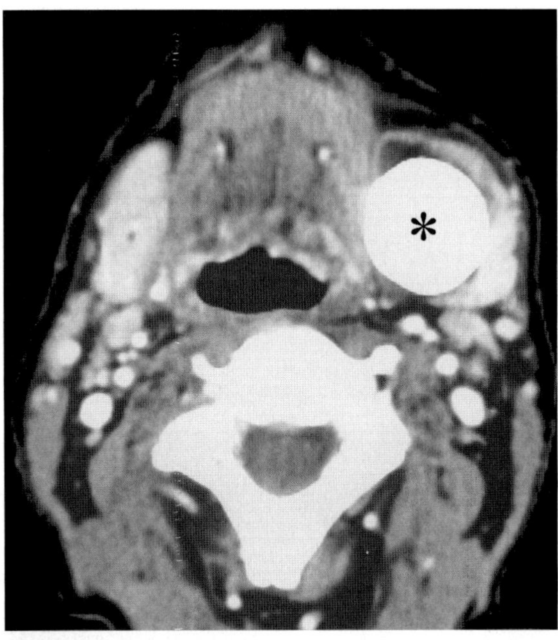

Figure 12.12

Submandibular gland stone; 61-year-old male, heavy drinking smoker, with incidental finding of a hard submandibular mass, which had been painless for more than 10 years; question of oral cancer in soft palate. Axial post-contrast CT image shows large stone in submandibular gland (*asterisk*)

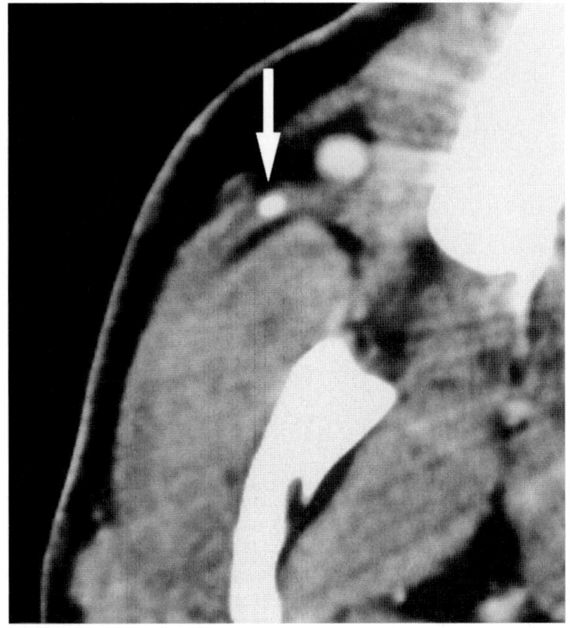

Figure 12.13

Parotid duct stone; 59-year-old with intermittent parotid gland swelling for about 6 months; question about parotitis or tumor. Axial post-contrast CT image shows stone in dilated Stensen's duct (*arrow*), and some enlarged and irregularly (scattered) enhanced gland consistent with chronic sialoadenitis

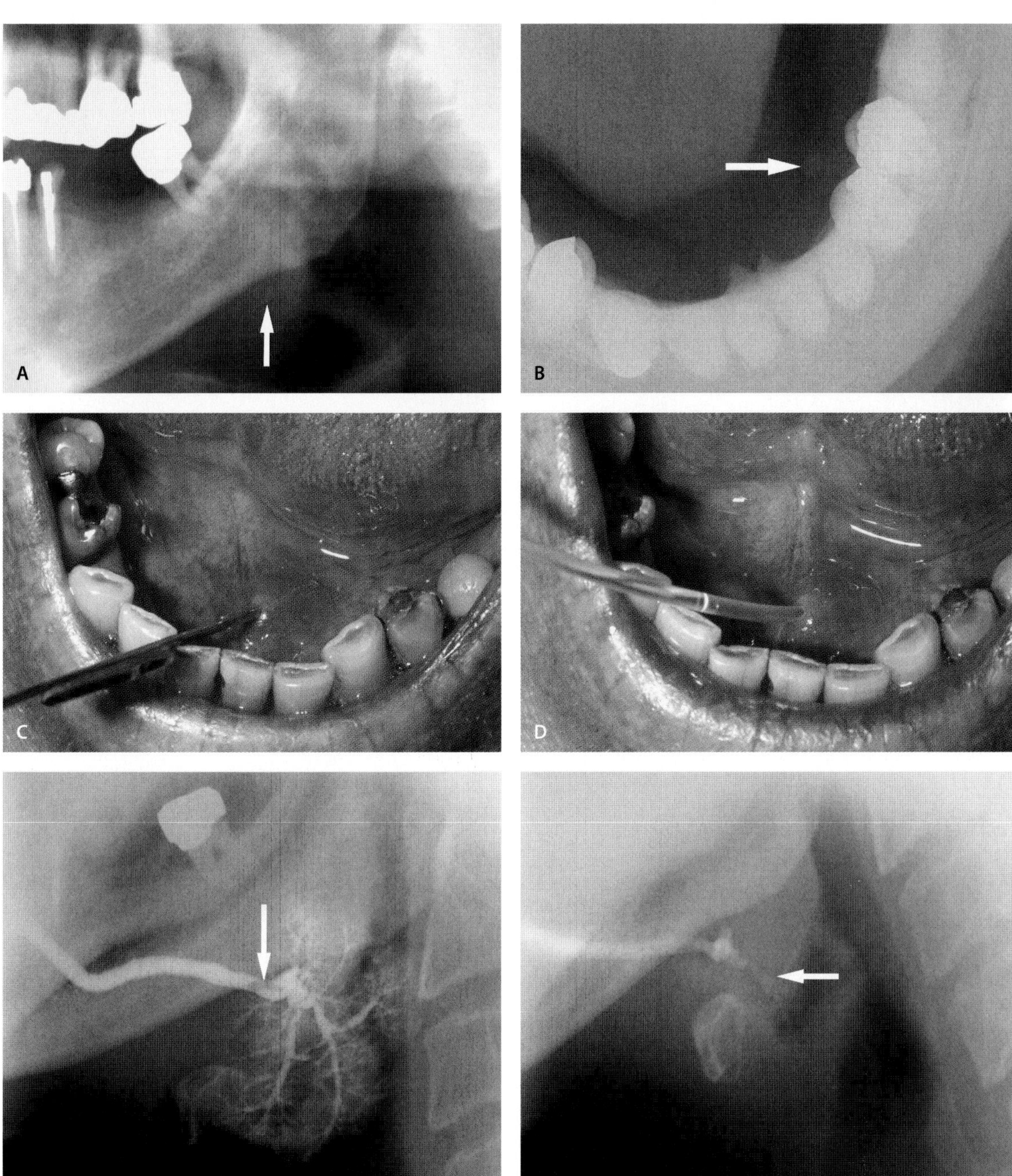

Figure 12.14

Sialolithiasis and reduced salivary flow, but normal submandibular parenchyma and Wharton's duct sialogram; 72-year-old male with intermittent swelling related to meals for about 2 weeks. **A** Panoramic view shows a small stone in posterior part of Wharton's duct (*arrow*). **B** Occlusal view shows another small stone in anterior part of submandibular duct (*arrow*). **C** Clinical photograph shows silver probe to widen submandibular duct. **D** Clinical photograph shows cannula into submandibular duct. **E** Submandibular sialogram shows normal parenchymatous filling with void of filling at stone (*arrow*) but otherwise normal Wharton's duct. **F** Retention of contrast medium (*arrow*) after 15 min confirms reduced salivary flow

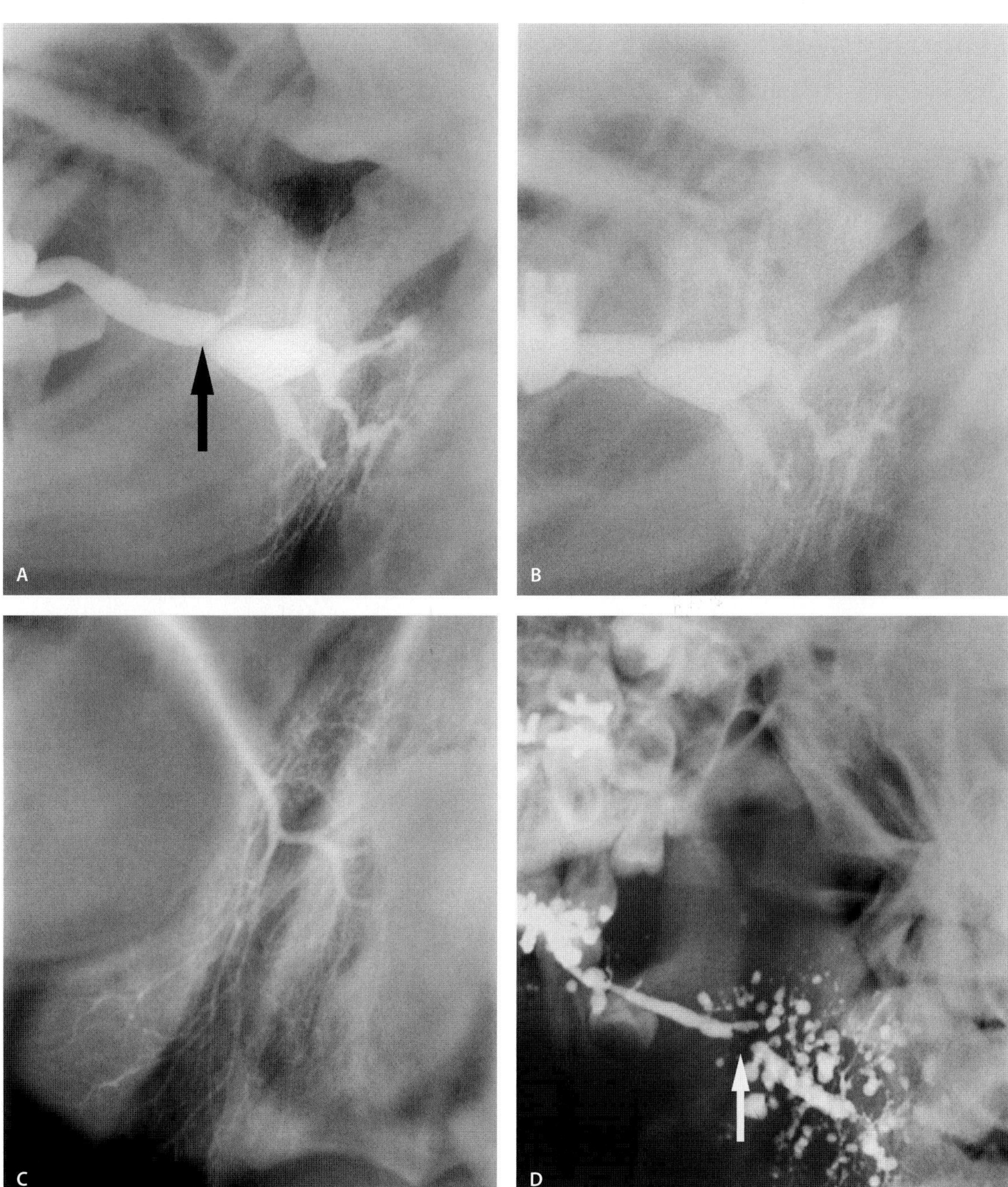

Figure 12.15

Stenosis of Stensen's duct with reduced salivary flow, with sialodochitis and sialoadenitis; 47-year-old female with intermittent parotid swelling and discharge of mucus. A Parotid sialogram shows severely dilated duct with one stricture (*arrow*), and dilated intraglandular ducts with degenerated parenchyma (most of it not visualized); no calculi were detected. B Parotid sialogram after 5 min shows severe retention of contrast medium, confirming reduced salivary flow. C Normal sialogram (another patient for comparison). D Advanced chronic sialoadenitis (another patient for comparison), with multiple scattered non-uniform collections of contrast medium (sialectasias) due to radiolucent stone, void of contrast filling (*arrow*)

Sjögren Syndrome

Definition

Chronic, systemic autoimmune disease of exocrine glands characterized by periductal lymphocytic aggregates that extend into and destroy salivary and lacrimal parenchyma primarily, but also other exocrine glands.

May produce a localized parenchymal mass; benign lymphoepithelial lesion.

Diagnosis is based on a set of criteria: subjective symptoms of dry mouth and eyes, confirmation of xerostomy and xerophthalmia by clinical tests, serologic evidence of autoantibodies, and histologic evidence of salivary lymphocytic infiltration by labial or parotid biopsy.

Clinical Features

- Primary Sjögren syndrome or secondary; associated with a connective tissue disease, usually rheumatoid arthritis
- Second in frequency to rheumatoid arthritis of all autoimmune diseases
- Predominantly women, 40–60 years of age
- Tender glandular swelling; recurrent episodes
- Nonpainful glandular enlargement
- Xerostomia and keratoconjunctivitis sicca
- Higher risk of developing non-Hodgkin's lymphoma, extranodal in particular

Imaging Features

- Parotid glands involved, but occasionally also submandibular glands.
- Lymphadenopathy typically absent.
- Earliest sialographic signs: multiple peripheral punctate collections (1 mm or less) of contrast medium with conventional sialography ("leafless fruit-laden tree") uniformly distributed in the gland, later with larger globular collections of contrast medium due to parenchyma destruction but characteristically with normal central duct system; contrast medium drains from main ducts but remains in punctate and globular collections.
- With reduced salivary flow, ascending superimposed sialoadenitis and sialodochitis will develop.
- CT and MRI images normal in early disease, then variable enlargement.
- T1-weighted MRI: multiple punctate changes of low density uniformly distributed in the gland earliest signs, diagnostic for Sjögren syndrome.
- T2-weighted MRI: multiple punctate changes have high signal reflecting watery saliva.
- Punctuate changes will progress to globular, cavitary and destructive abnormalities.
- At end-stage a honeycomb appearance may develop, with multiple cystic lesions and abnormally dense parenchyma.
- MR sialography has been found to correlate with conventional sialography and with labial biopsy findings.

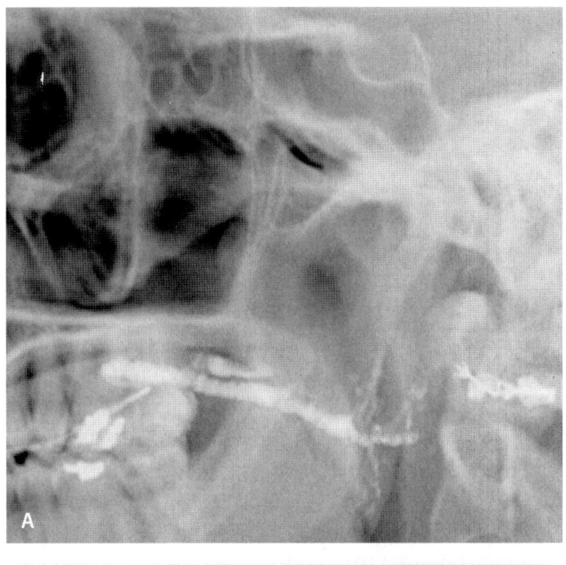

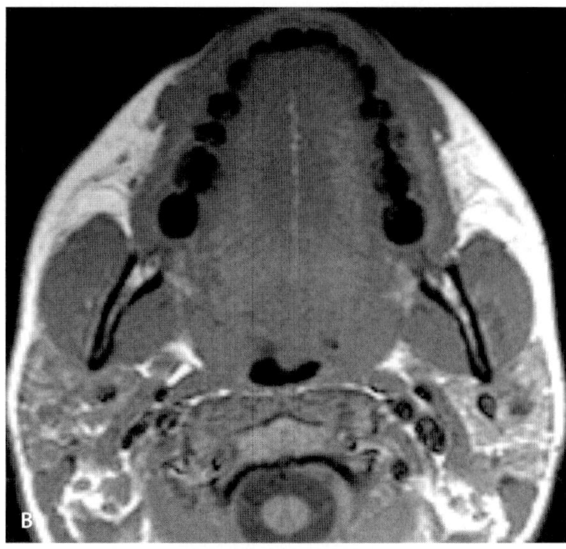

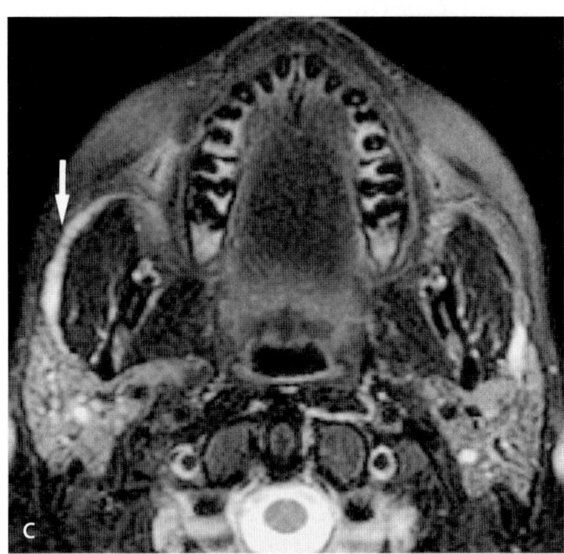

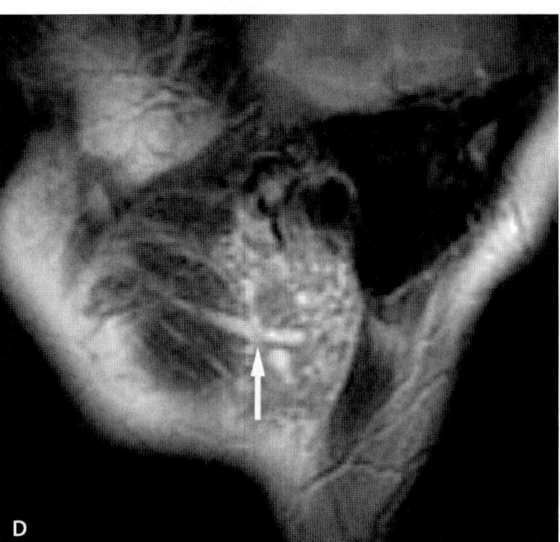

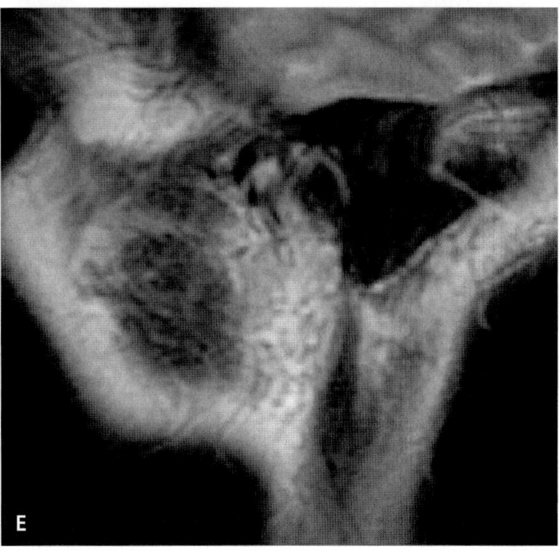

Figure 12.16

Sjögren syndrome; 31-year-old female with 2-year history of swelling, mostly of right parotid gland but also of left. A Conventional sialography shows multiple strictures and dilatations consistent with sialodochitis and poor filling of parenchyma, with some punctate contrast medium collections. B T1-weighted MRI shows some swelling of right parotid gland which has a little less signal than left gland, and with multiple small irregularities. C T2-weighted MRI shows small cystic fluid-filled irregularities consistent with chronic sialoadenitis. Note dilated parotid duct along masseter muscle (*arrow*). D Sagittal T2-weighted MRI of right side shows dilated parotid duct (*arrow*). E Sagittal T2-weighted MRI of left side shows no dilated duct for comparison

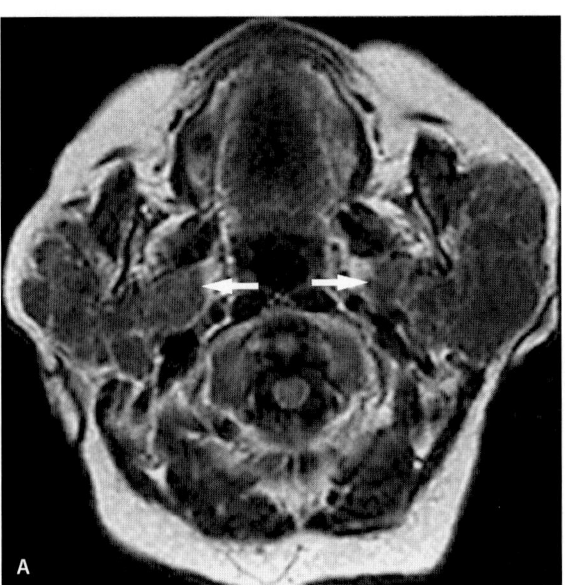

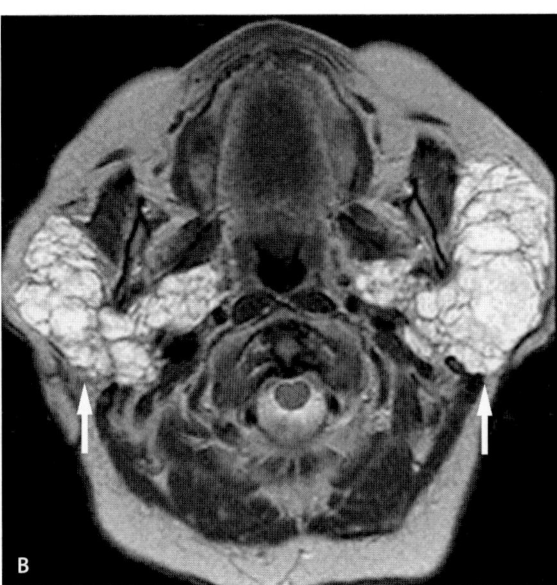

Figure 12.17

Sjögren syndrome, advanced stage; 64-year-old female with history of Sjögren syndrome and multiple sclerosis presents with enlargement of both parotid glands. **A** Axial T1-weighted MRI shows enlarged parotid glands with multiple low-signal cystic changes (*arrows*). **B** Axial T2-weighted MRI shows honeycomb areas of high-signal watery saliva in parotid glands (*arrows*), both superficial and deep lobes

Figure 12.18

Sjögren syndrome, advanced stage; 32-year-old female with recurrent parotitis for years, finally diagnosed with Sjögren syndrome. Axial post-contrast CT image shows bilaterally enlarged parotid glands with multiple cystic lesions surrounded by heterogeneously enhanced tissue (*arrows*)

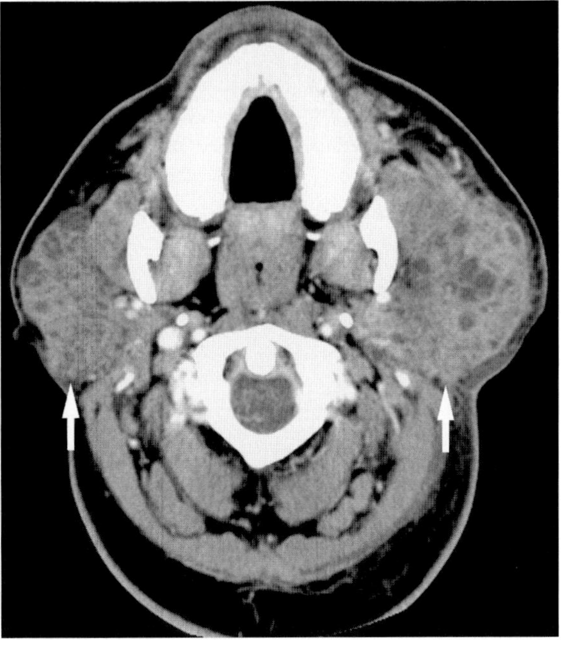

Benign Lymphoepithelial Cysts Associated with HIV-AIDS

Definition

Mixed cystic and solid intraglandular masses in HIV-AIDS.

Clinical Features

- Bilaterally enlarged parotid glands
- Rarely in submandibular or sublingual glands
- Reactive adenoid, tonsils, and lymphadenopathy

Imaging Features

- Bilateral multiple cystic and solid masses
- T1-weighted MRI: low signal
- T2-weighted MRI: high (cyst) or low (solid mass) signal
- T1-weighted post-Gd MRI: rim enhancement of cysts, heterogeneous or homogeneous enhancement of solid masses

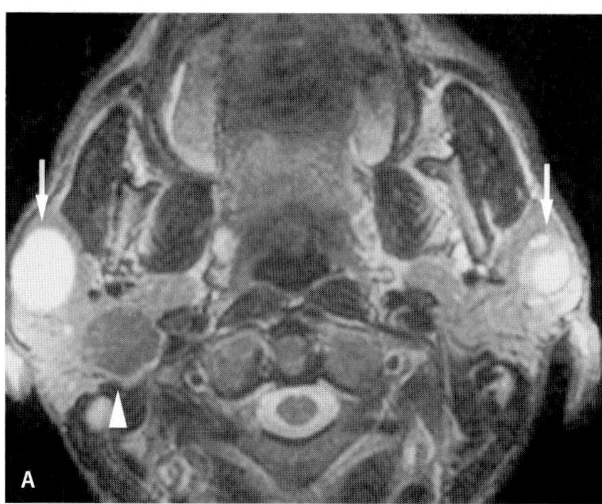

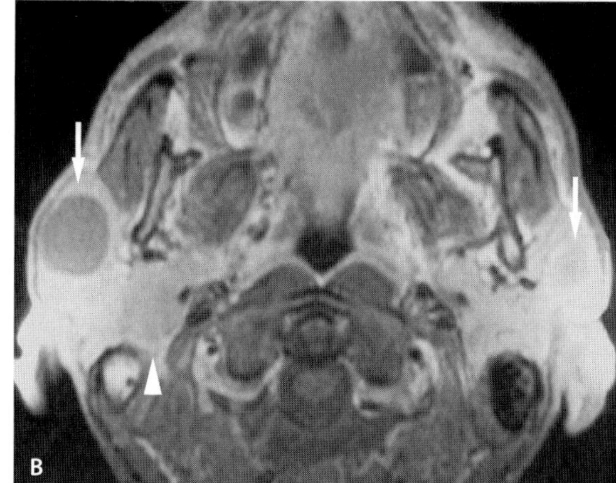

Figure 12.19

Benign bilateral lymphoepithelial cysts; 53-year-old male with AIDS presents with bilaterally enlarged parotid glands. **A** Axial T2-weighted MRI shows bilateral fluid-filled cysts (*arrows*) and a solid lesion (*arrowhead*). **B** Axial T1-weighted post-Gd MRI shows rim enhancement of cysts but contrast enhancement of solid lesion (*arrowhead*)

Ranula

Definition

Mucous retention cyst, or mucocele, primarily in sublingual gland or its ductal elements.

Simple or plunging (diving) cyst; involves submandibular space with pseudocyst.

Clinical Features

- Painless sublingual soft swelling, probably from trauma or infection

Imaging Features

- Well-defined ovoid low-density cyst with thin wall
- Enhancing wall, thickened if infected
- T1-weighted MRI: low signal
- T2-weighted MRI: high signal
- T1-weighted post-Gd MRI: no enhancement except cyst wall, in particular if infected
- Simple form (most common), and a deep or plunging form that penetrates to submandibular space behind or through mylohyoid muscle because of cyst wall rupture

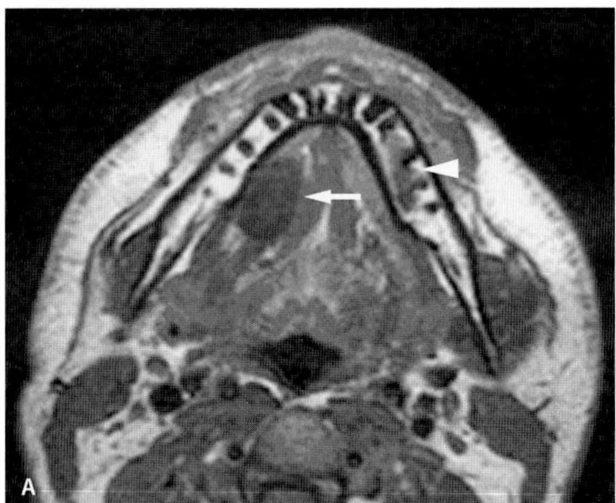

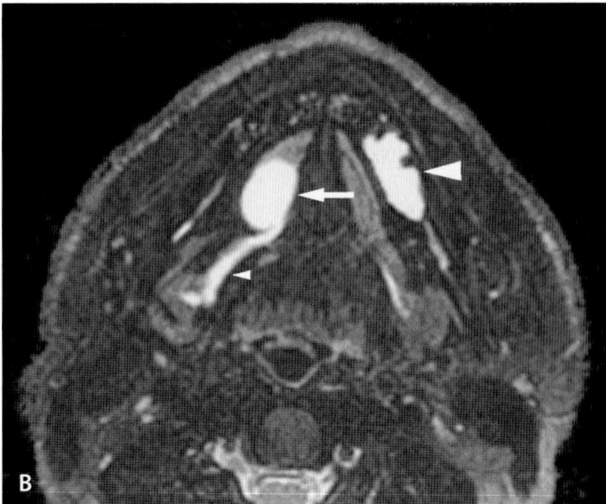

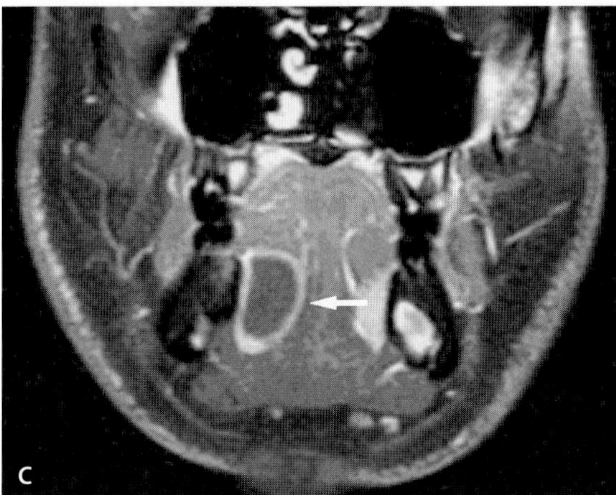

Figure 12.20

Sublingual (simple) ranula; 24-year-old male with a sublingual lump for about 2 months (clinical suspicion of neoplasm in floor of mouth), with incidental finding of a mandibular cyst. **A** Axial T1-weighted MRI shows well-defined oval low-signal area in floor of mouth on right side (*arrow*) and low-signal marrow in a region of left mandible (*arrowhead*). **B** Axial T2-weighted MRI shows high-signal area in floor of mouth (*arrow*) and high-signal area in marrow of mandible (*arrowhead*). Note dilated Wharton's duct on right side (*small arrowhead*). **C** Coronal T1-weighted post-Gd MRI shows no enhancement of ranula except in periphery (*arrow*), probably due to infection/inflammation with capsular hyperemia

Tumors

Clinical Features (in General)

- Usually a painless mass; may be tender.
- Salivary gland tumors represent fewer than 3% of all tumors.
- 75–85% of all salivary gland tumors occur in parotid gland; most are benign; minor salivary glands, palate in particular, and submandibular glands, will have most of the remainder; sublingual tumors very rare.
- However, a mass in submandibular gland, even more so for a mass in sublingual gland, has a greater chance of being malignant than does a mass in parotid gland.
- It has been estimated that for 100 parotid tumors there are 10 submandibular and 10 minor salivary gland tumors and only 1 sublingual tumor.

Imaging Features (in General)

- An ill-defined mass should be suspicious for malignancy.
- However, it may be difficult to differentiate between benign and malignant salivary gland tumors since both types commonly have a benign appearance; well-defined and cystic.

Benign Tumors

Pleomorphic Adenoma (Benign Mixed Tumor)

Definition

Tumor of variable capsulation characterized microscopically by architectural rather than cellular pleomorphism. Epithelial and modified myoepithelial elements intermingle with tissue of mucoid, myxoid or chondroid appearance. Epithelial and myoepithelial components form ducts, strands, sheets or structures resembling a swarm of bees. Squamous metaplasia is found in about 25% of pleomorphic adenomas (WHO).

Clinical Features

- Most frequent salivary gland tumor; 70–80% of all benign tumors of major salivary gland.
- More than 80% in parotid gland, and predominantly lateral to the plane of the facial nerve.
- Most frequent tumor of minor salivary glands as well, although about half of all minor salivary gland tumors, or even more, have been reported as malignant.

Imaging Features

- Well-defined mass, highly variable size, cystic, lobulated
- Small tumors show homogeneous enhancement; large, lobulated tumors show heterogeneous enhancement
- May show calcification
- T1-weighted MRI: small tumors show homogeneous, low signal; large, lobulated tumors show heterogeneous low to intermediate signal
- T2-weighted MRI and STIR: small tumors show homogeneous high signal; large, lobulated tumors show heterogeneous intermediate to high signal
- T1-weighted post-Gd MRI: variable, heterogeneously mild to moderate enhancement

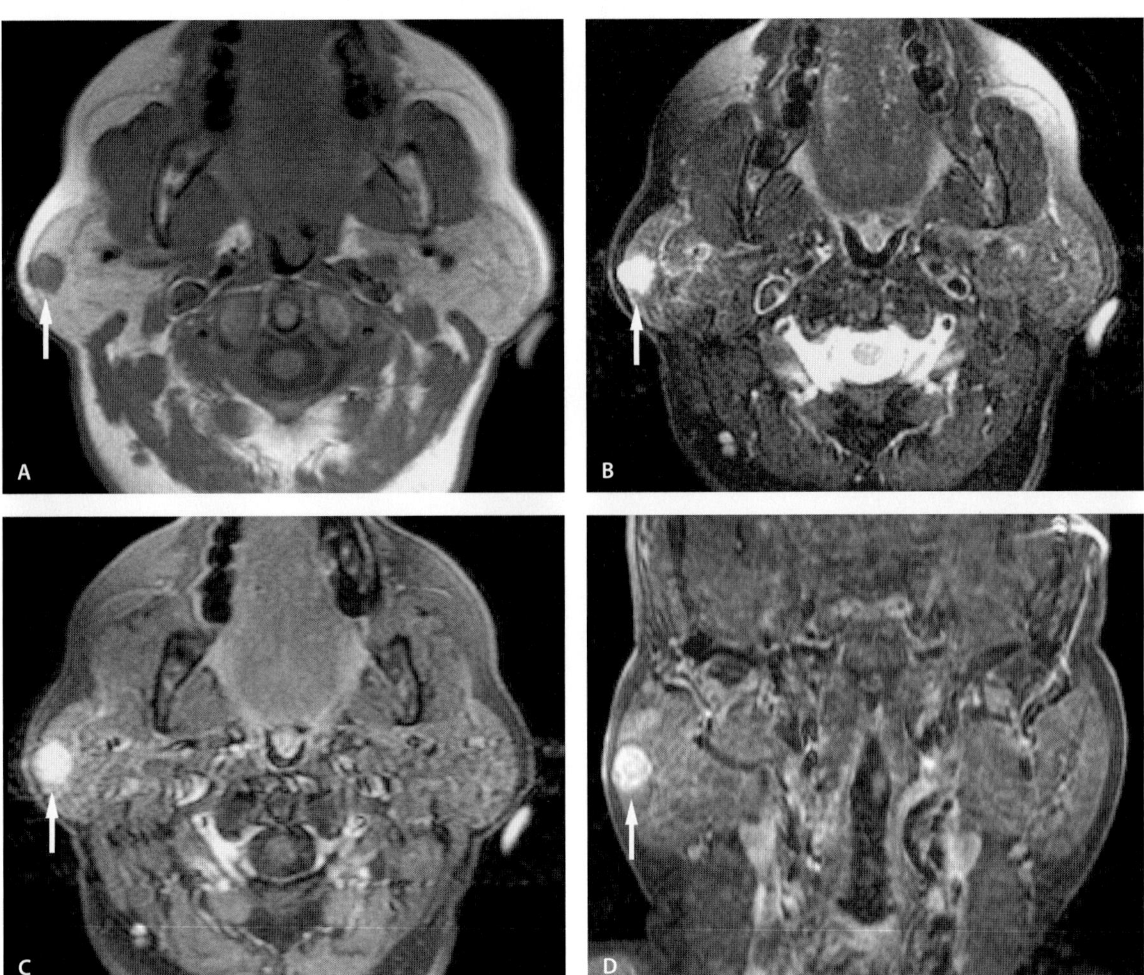

Figure 12.21

Parotid pleomorphic adenoma, superficial lobe, small; 62-year-old female with lump in right parotid gland. A Axial T1-weighted MRI shows rather well defined small low-signal mass superficial in right parotid (*arrow*). B Axial T2-weighted fat-suppressed MRI shows high-signal mass (*arrow*). C Axial T1-weighted fat-suppressed post-Gd MRI shows intense contrast enhancement (*arrow*). D Coronal T1-weighted fat-suppressed post-Gd MRI confirms contrast enhancement of tumor (*arrow*)

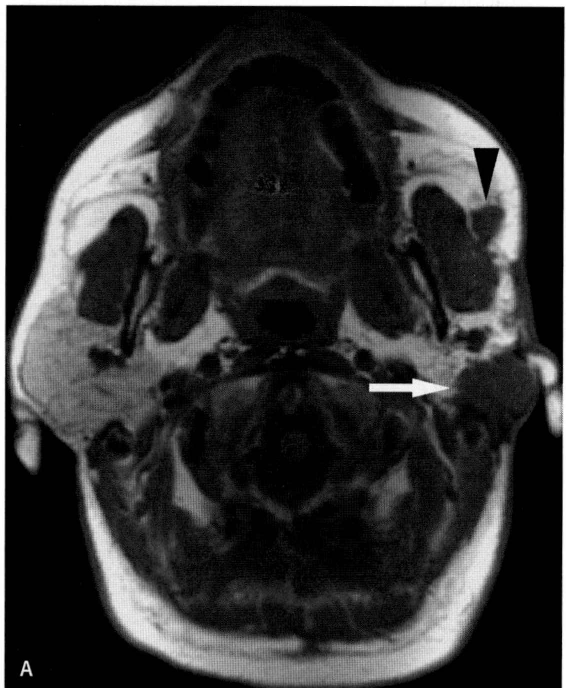

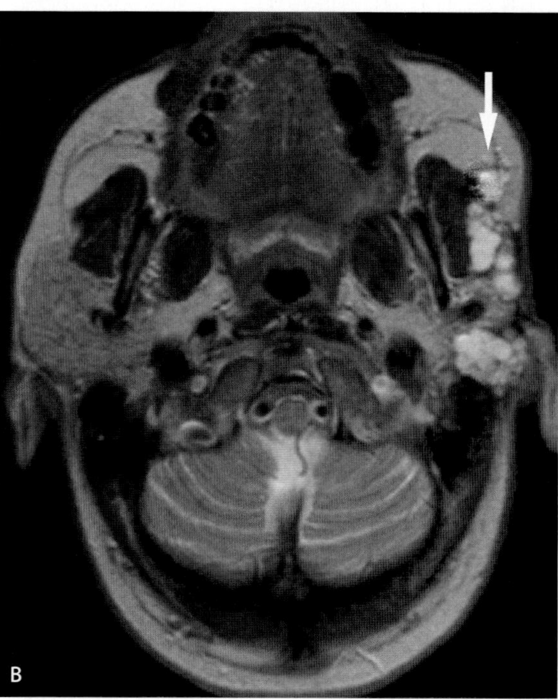

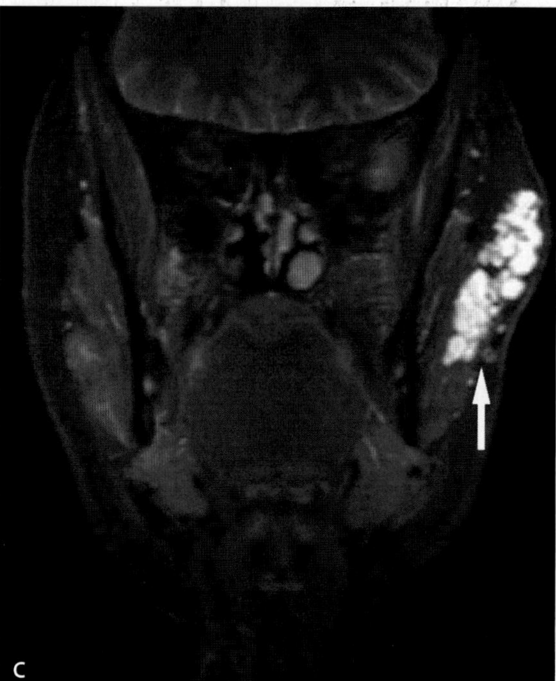

Figure 12.22

Parotid pleomorphic adenoma, superficial lobe; 61-year-old female with history of left parotid tumor surgery, now with multifocal recurrence. **A** Axial T1-weighted MRI shows low-signal mass in posterior portion of left parotid gland (*arrow*) and in accessory gland (*arrowhead*). **B** Axial T2-weighted MRI shows high-signal tumor superficial to masseter muscle in addition to posterior portion of the gland (*arrow*). **C** Coronal STIR MRI shows high-signal cystic tumor masses just beneath skin (*arrow*)

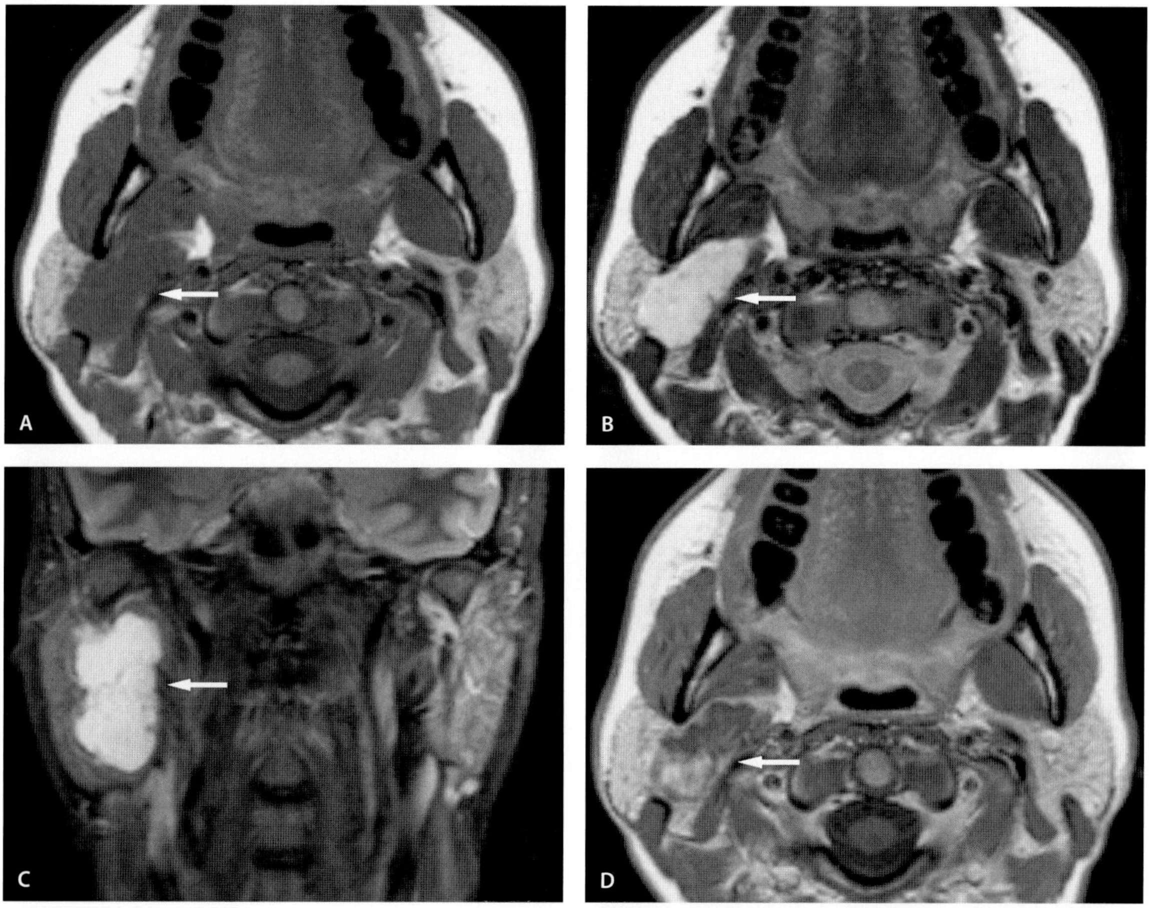

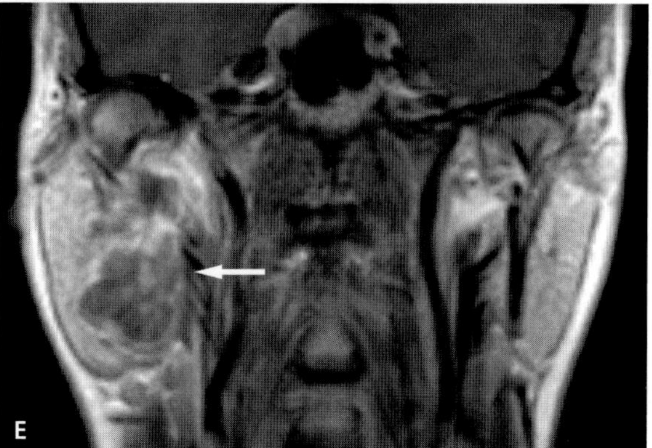

Figure 12.23

Parotid pleomorphic adenoma, deep lobe; 40-year-old female with swelling of right parotid gland. A Axial T1-weighted MRI shows well-defined low-signal mass in deep lobe of right parotid gland (*arrow*). B Axial T2-weighted MRI shows well-defined homogeneous high-signal mass (*arrow*). C Coronal STIR MRI shows well-defined high-signal mass in larger portion of parotid gland (*arrow*). D Axial T1-weighted post-Gd MRI shows contrast enhancement in posterior portion of tumor (*arrow*). E Coronal T1-weighted post-Gd MRI confirms no contrast enhancement in anterior portion of tumor (*arrow*)

Hemangioma

Definition

Benign tumor of proliferating endothelial cells.

Clinical Features

- Most frequent nonepithelial salivary gland tumor; nonepithelial tumors represents fewer than 5% of all salivary tumors.
- Predominantly in parotid gland.
- Most common salivary gland tumor during infancy and childhood; 90% of all parotid tumors in first year of life.
- Premature infants in particular.
- Females more than males.

Imaging Features

- Soft-tissue mass, frequently lobulated, isodense to muscle, contrast-enhancing
- Uni- or bilateral, single or multiple
- T1-weighted MRI: isointense to muscle
- T2-weighted MRI: high signal
- T1-weighted post-Gd MRI: intense contrast enhancement

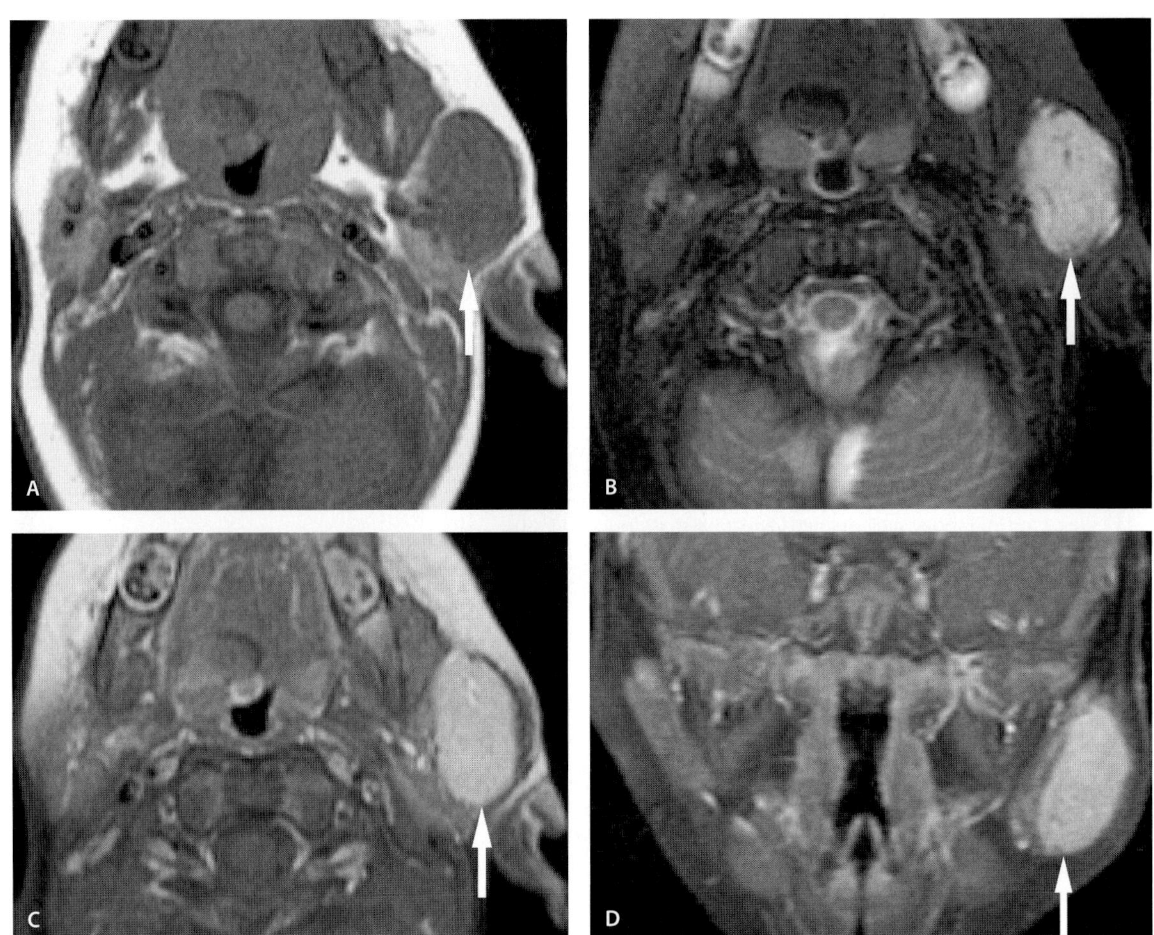

Figure 12.24

Parotid infantile hemangioma; 9-month-old female with soft asymptomatic swelling of left parotid gland (*arrow*). **A** Axial T1-weighted MRI shows well-defined mass isointense to muscle in left parotid gland (*arrow*) with no reaction in surrounding fat. **B** Axial T2-weighted fat-suppressed MRI shows high-signal mass (*arrow*), and linear flow voids. **C** Axial T1-weighted post-Gd MRI shows enhancement of mass (*arrow*) with rim of nonenhancing parotid gland around mass. **D** Coronal T1-weighted post-Gd MRI confirms enhancement of mass (*arrow*) surrounded by nonenhancing parenchyma

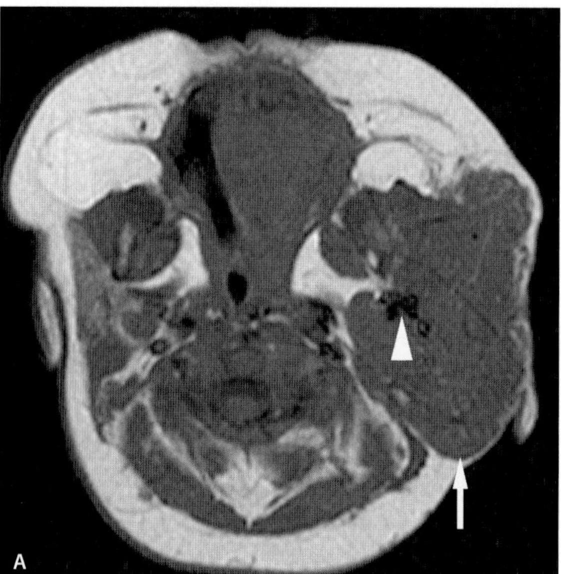

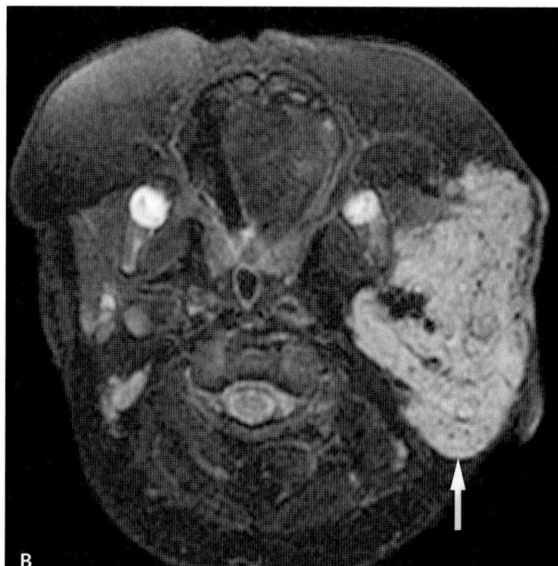

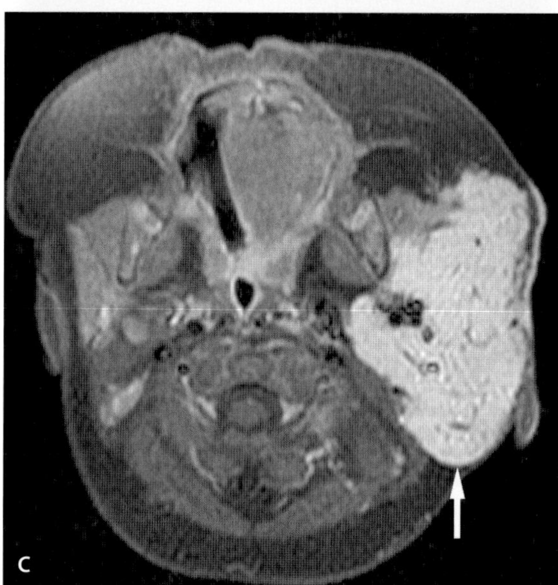

Figure 12.25

Parotid infantile hemangioma; 4-month-old presenting with soft enlargement of the left parotid gland and a "birth mark" on the left cheek. **A** Axial T1-weighted MRI shows enlargement of left parotid gland (*arrow*) with flow voids from large sinusoidal vessels (*arrowhead*). **B** Axial T2-weighted fat-suppressed MRI shows mass with high signal (*arrow*). **C** Axial T1-weighted fat-suppressed post-Gd MRI shows marked homogeneous contrast enhancement (*arrow*)

Malignant Tumors

Mucoepidermoid Carcinoma

Definition

Tumor characterized by presence of squamous cells, mucus-producing cells, and cells of intermediate type (WHO).

Clinical Features

- 3–16% of all salivary gland tumors
- 12–29% of malignant salivary gland tumors
- 7–41% of minor salivary gland tumors; most common malignant minor salivary gland tumor
- About half of cases in major salivary glands; 80% in parotid gland
- Usually in age group 35–65 years
- Most common malignant salivary gland tumor in patients under 20 years of age

Imaging Features

- May look benign with well-defined, smooth borders and cystic areas
- Occasionally focal calcification may be seen
- May have similar appearance to pleomorphic adenomas, in particular low-grade (less aggressive) mucoepidermoid carcinomas

See also Chapter 4.

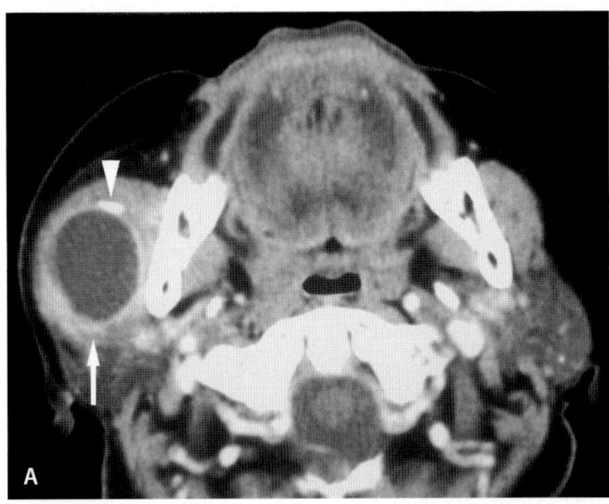

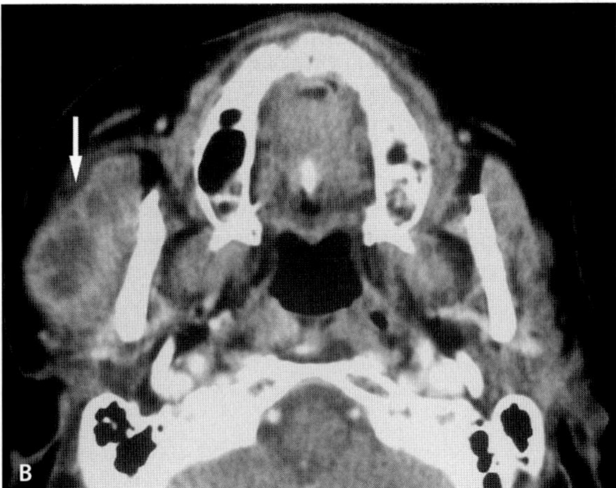

Figure 12.26

Parotid high-grade mucoepidermoid cell carcinoma (with evident inflammatory response); 59-year-old female with tender swelling of right parotid gland. **A** Axial post-contrast CT image shows well-defined expansive, cystic, low-density mass with contrast-enhanced periphery (*arrow*) in superficial lobe, and calcification consistent with sialolith (*arrowhead*). **B** Axial post-contrast CT image (more cranial than image A) shows lobulated, heterogeneously enhanced mass; mostly without enhancement (*arrow*)

Acinic Cell Carcinoma

Definition

Malignant epithelial tumor that demonstrates some cytological differentiation toward acinar cells (WHO).

Clinical Features

- 7–18% of all malignant salivary tumors
- 10–30% of parotid malignancies
- Vast majority in parotid gland, minor salivary glands second most common site
- Most common malignant salivary gland tumor after mucoepidermoid carcinoma in childhood and adolescence

Imaging Features

- Nonspecific, benign appearance, well-defined mass, may be cystic
- May have similar appearance to pleomorphic adenomas
- Recurrent tumors can be multinodular

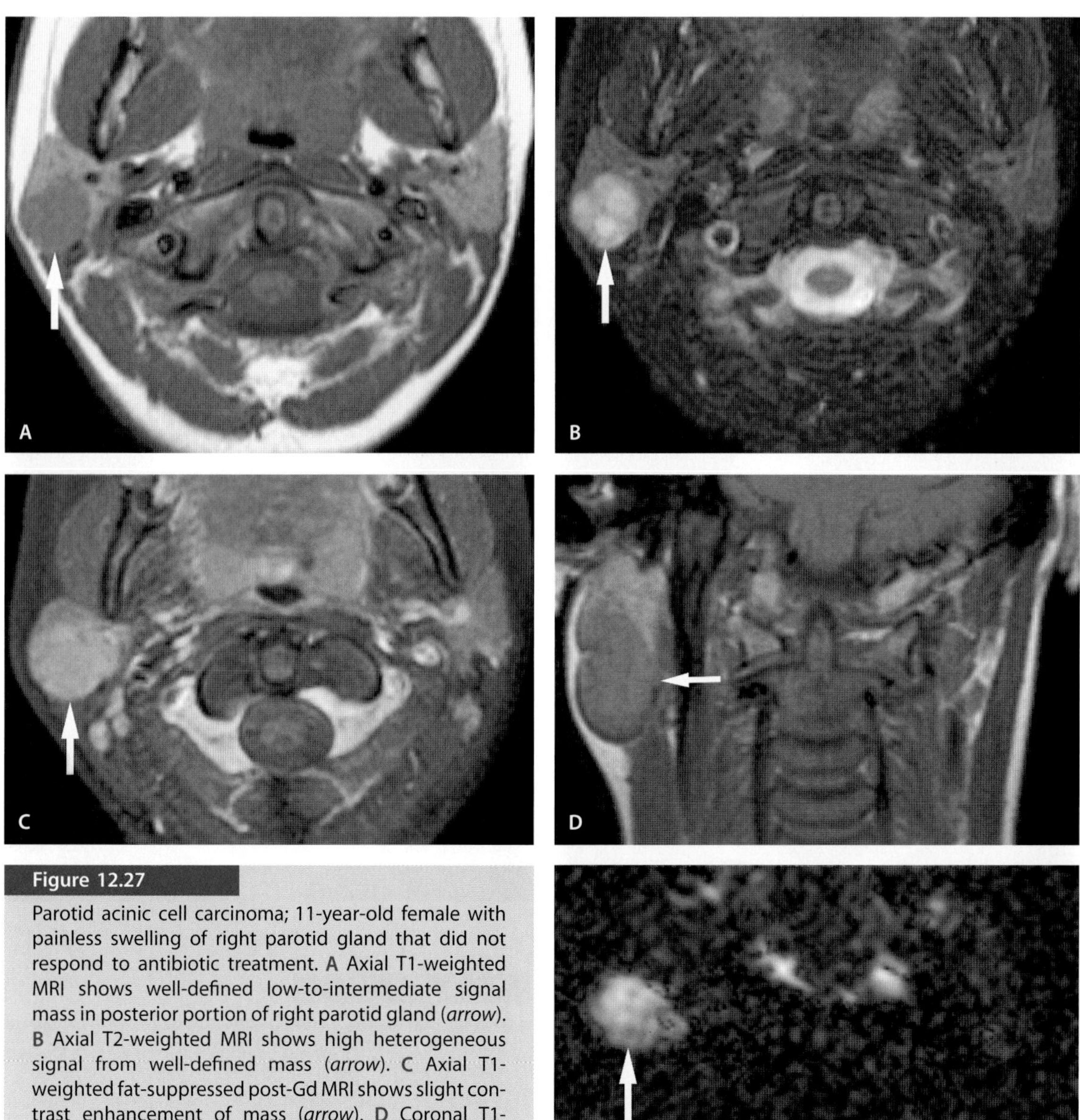

Figure 12.27

Parotid acinic cell carcinoma; 11-year-old female with painless swelling of right parotid gland that did not respond to antibiotic treatment. A Axial T1-weighted MRI shows well-defined low-to-intermediate signal mass in posterior portion of right parotid gland (*arrow*). B Axial T2-weighted MRI shows high heterogeneous signal from well-defined mass (*arrow*). C Axial T1-weighted fat-suppressed post-Gd MRI shows slight contrast enhancement of mass (*arrow*). D Coronal T1-weighted MRI shows well-defined mass occupying large portion of posterior aspect of parotid gland (*arrow*). E Axial diffusion-weighted MRI demonstrates high signal from mass (*arrow*)

Lymphoma

Definition

Malignant neoplasm of cells from the lymphatic system.

Clinical Features

- Rare entity in salivary glands
- About 80% in parotid gland; nearly 20% in submandibular gland
- Majority non-Hodgkin's and B-cell type
- More frequently in patients with autoimmune diseases

Imaging Features (Parotid Gland)

- Most commonly in intraglandular lymph nodes or from mucosa-associated lymphoid tissue (MALT)
- One or more well-defined masses, usually mild, homogeneous contrast-enhancing, but may show heterogeneous contrast enhancement
- MRI: homogeneous intermediate on all imaging sequences; mild contrast enhancement

Adenocarcinoma

Definition

Carcinoma with glandular, ductal or secretory differentiation that does not fit into other categories of carcinoma (WHO).

Clinical Features

- Rare entity in salivary glands
- Minor salivary and parotid glands more common than submandibular and sublingual glands

Imaging Features

- Unspecific mass; variable enhancement

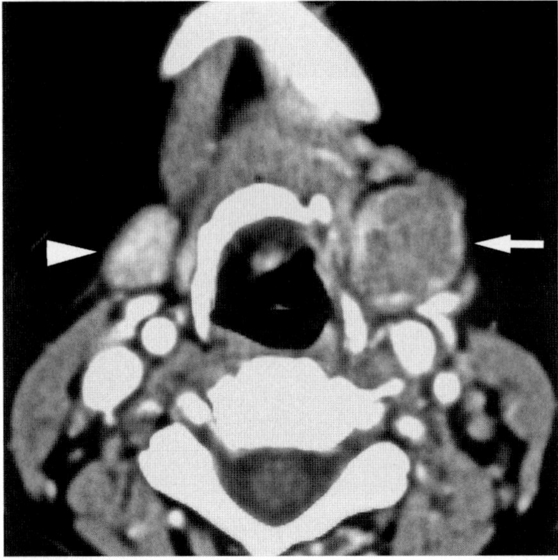

Figure 12.28

Submandibular gland non-Hodgkin's B-cell lymphoma; 56-year-old female with weight loss, poor general condition and lump in submandibular region; no pathologic lymph nodes were found by surgery. Axial post-contrast CT image shows low-density mass with enhancing peripheral rim of remaining parenchyma of left submandibular gland (*arrow*), with normal right gland for comparison (*arrowhead*)

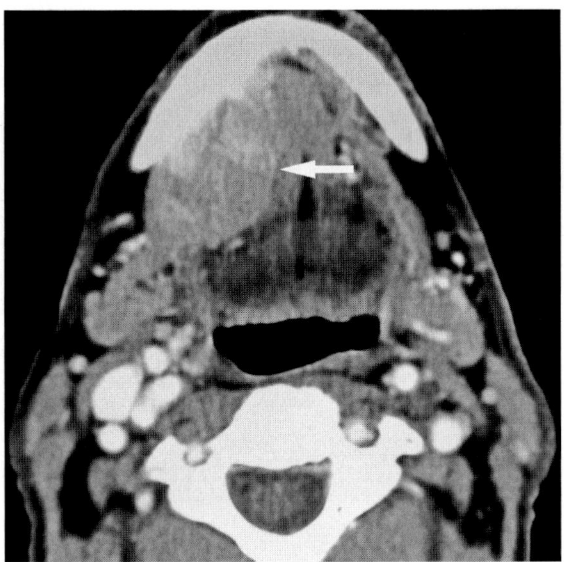

Figure 12.29

Sublingual gland adenocarcinoma; 84-year-old male with Marfan syndrome and aortic insufficiency, presenting with moderately tender sublingual lump. Axial post-contrast CT image shows rather well-defined contrast-enhancing sublingual mass (*arrow*) extending to submandibular gland region, dislocating right genioglossus muscle towards left and mylohyoid muscle laterally and inferiorly

Suggested Reading

Aasen S, Kolbenstvedt A (1992) CT appearances of normal and obstructed submandibular duct. Acta Radiol 33:414–419

Barnes L, Myers E, Prokopakis EP (1998) Primary malignant lymphoma of the parotid gland. Arch Otolaryngol Head Neck Surg 124:573–577

Benson BW (2004) Salivary gland radiology. In: White SW, Pharoah MJ (eds) Oral radiology. Principles and interpretation, 5th edn. Mosby, St. Louis, pp 658–676

Eneroth CM (1971) Salivary gland tumors in the parotid gland, submandibular gland and the palate region. Cancer 27:1415–1418

Farman AG, Nortje C, Wood RE (1993) Salivary gland diseases. In: Oral and maxillofacial diagnostic imaging. Mosby, St. Louis, pp 403–424

Jager L, Menauer F, Holzknecht N, Scholz V, Grevers G, Reiser M (2000) Sialolithiasis: MR sialography of the submandibular duct - an alternative to conventional sialography and US? Radiology 216:665–671

Joe VQ, Westesson PL (1994) Tumors of the parotid gland: MR imaging characteristics of various histologic types. AJR Am J Roentgenol 163:433–438

Ohbayashi N, Yamada I, Yoshino N, Sasaki T (1998) Sjogren syndrome: comparison of assessments with MR sialography and conventional sialography. Radiology 209:683–688

Raine C, Saliba K, Chippindale AJ, McLean NR (2003) Radiological imaging in primary parotid malignancy. Br J Plast Surg 56:637–643

Sakamoto M, Sasano T, Higano S, Takahashi S, Iikubo M, Kakehata S (2003) Usefulness of heavily T2 weighted magnetic resonance images for the differential diagnosis of parotid tumors. Dentomaxillofac Radiol 32:295–299

Seifert G (1991) Histological typing of salivary gland tumors, 2nd edn. WHO. Springer, Berlin, pp 28, 32, 33

Som PM, Brandwein MS (2003) Salivary glands: anatomy and pathology. In: Som PM, Curtin HD (eds) Head and neck imaging, 4th edn. Mosby, St. Louis, pp 2005–2133

Som PM, Shugar J, Train JS, Biller H (1981) Manifestations of parotid gland enlargement: radiologic, pathologic and clinical correlations. Part 1: The autoimmune pseudosialectasias. Radiology 141:415–419

Spiro RH, Huvos AG, Strong EW (1978) Acinic cell carcinoma of salivary origin. A clinicopathologic study of 67 cases. Cancer 41:924–935

Spiro RH, Huvos AG, Strong EW (1982) Adenocarcinoma of salivary origin. Clinicopathologic study of 204 patients. Am J Surg 144:423–431

Tonami H, Ogawa Y, Matoba M, Kuginuki Y, Yokota H, Higashi K, Okimura T, Yamamoto I, Sugai S (1998) MR sialography in patients with Sjogren syndrome. AJNR Am J Neuroradiol 19:1119–120

Adjacent Structures; Cervical Spine, Neck, Skull Base and Orbit

In collaboration with M. Oka · R. Sidhu · N. Kakimoto

Introduction

This chapter contains a selection of cases from structures surrounding the maxillofacial area. It is not the intention to cover all abnormalities in these regions, but instead to give the maxillofacial radiologist a feel and sense for radiographic abnormalities that may occur in areas adjacent to the maxillofacial region. Thus, we have selected characteristic and illustrative cases from the cervical spine, neck, skull base, and orbit that are likely to be seen on maxillofacial imaging studies. The chapter includes chronic and acute conditions, tumors, inflammation, and degenerative changes, and is divided into four parts: cervical spine, neck, skull base and orbit. For a more complete review of imaging findings of these areas we refer the reader to traditional textbooks on head and neck imaging.

Cervical Spine

A portion of the upper cervical spine will in many cases be depicted on regular maxillofacial imaging studies. This pertains to plain films of the jaw, lateral cephalograms, panoramic images, and MRI and CT scans of the maxillofacial region. This short review of cervical spine abnormalities has been done with this in mind. It is not the purpose to present a complete atlas of cervical pathology, but instead to illustrate those cases that the maxillofacial radiologist is likely to encounter. Thus, we have included mostly bony abnormalities but some soft tissue lesions are also illustrated. There are many more conditions affecting the cervical spine than we have illustrated such as demyelinating disease, spondylosis, and nerve root compression to give a few examples.

Calcific Tendinitis Longus Colli

Definition

Recurrent deposits of crystalline calcium compounds within the longus colli muscle.

Clinical Features

- Diagnosis based upon clinical presentation and imaging.
- Cervical pain, dysphagia, and distinctive radiographic appearance.
- Symptoms usually manifest over a few days and often resolve benignly within 2 weeks.
- Often unrecognized cause of acute to subacute neck pain.
- Self-limiting disease which resolves spontaneously with symptomatic treatment.

Imaging Features

- Calcification at C1-C2 level with prominence of prevertebral soft tissues.
- Pathognomonic lateral neck film with prevertebral soft-tissue swelling and amorphous radiodensity anterior to C1-C2 vertebral bodies.
- CT, axial scans, highly reliable for diagnosis.

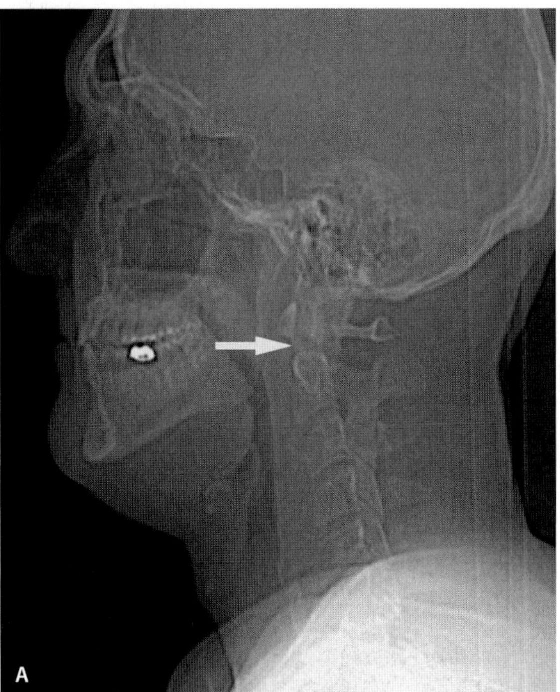

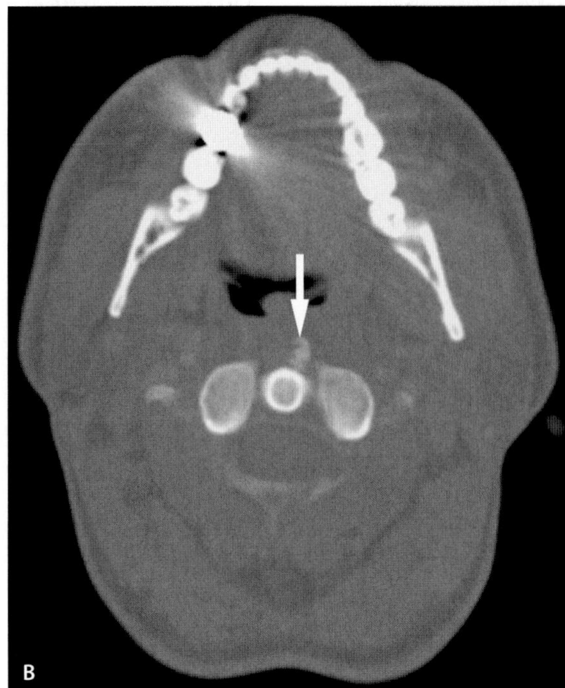

Figure 13.1

Calcific tendinitis longus colli; 47-year-old male with neck pain, clinical question of retropharyngeal abscess or phlegmon in neck. **A** Lateral view shows calcific density anteriorly between C1 and C2 (*arrow*) with slightly prominent soft tissues. **B** Axial CT image shows a prevertebral calcification (*arrow*). No mass or lymphadenopathy

Ossification of Posterior Longitudinal Ligament

Definition

Calcification of posterior longitudinal ligament of spinal column.

Clinical Features

- Histologically this mostly represents ossification rather than amorphous calcification.
- Most commonly affects cervical spine.
- More common in Japan for unknown reasons.
- Often causes neurological symptoms secondary to narrow spinal canal.
- More frequent in males than females.

Imaging Features

- CT highly reliable for diagnosis.
- Often causes significant spinal canal stenosis.
- On axial CT images posterior longitudinal ligament is seen as a "mushroom", "hill", "square", or a mixture of these shapes.
- Four morphologic forms: continuous and segmental forms account for 95%.
- Characteristic sharp radiolucent line separates ossified posterior longitudinal ligament from posterior vertebral margin; about 50% of cases.
- Segmental form of ossified posterior longitudinal ligament needs to be differentiated from calcified discs and posterior osteophytes; neither of these two conditions shows a characteristic sharp radiolucent line and in contrast to ossified posterior longitudinal ligament, osteophytic growth is along a horizontal axis.
- Differential diagnosis:
  - Ankylosing spondylitis, which more commonly affects the lumbar spine with syndesmophytes rather than ossification of posterior longitudinal ligament.
  - DISH (diffuse idiopathic skeletal hyperostosis) which is a more generalized condition with extensive calcification and ossification, particularly in spine.

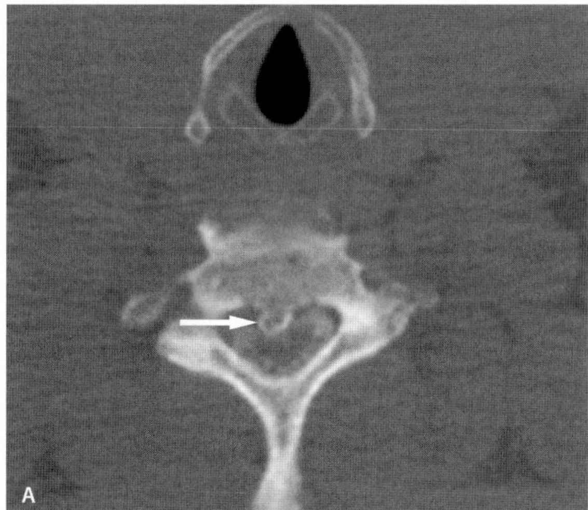

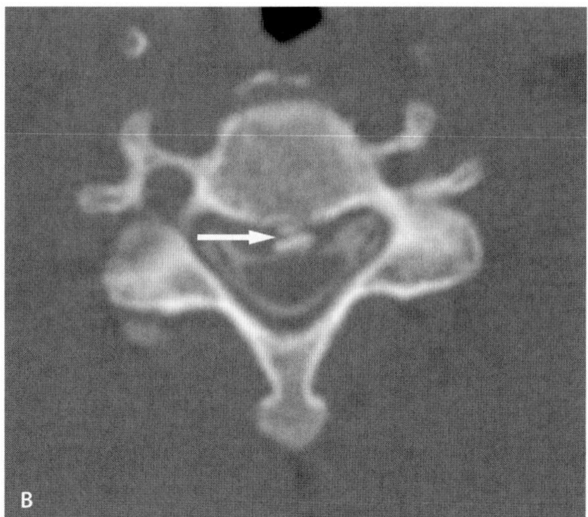

Figure 13.2

Ossification of longus colli ligament; 55-year-old male with a 5-year history of cervical and lumbar radiculopathy; no neurologic deficit on examination. **A** Axial CT-myelography of cervical spine shows ossified posterior longitudinal ligament having a mushroom-shaped appearance at C4-C5 level (*arrow*). **B** Well-appreciated lucent line between posterior margin of vertebral body and ossified ligament (*arrow*), representing connective tissue

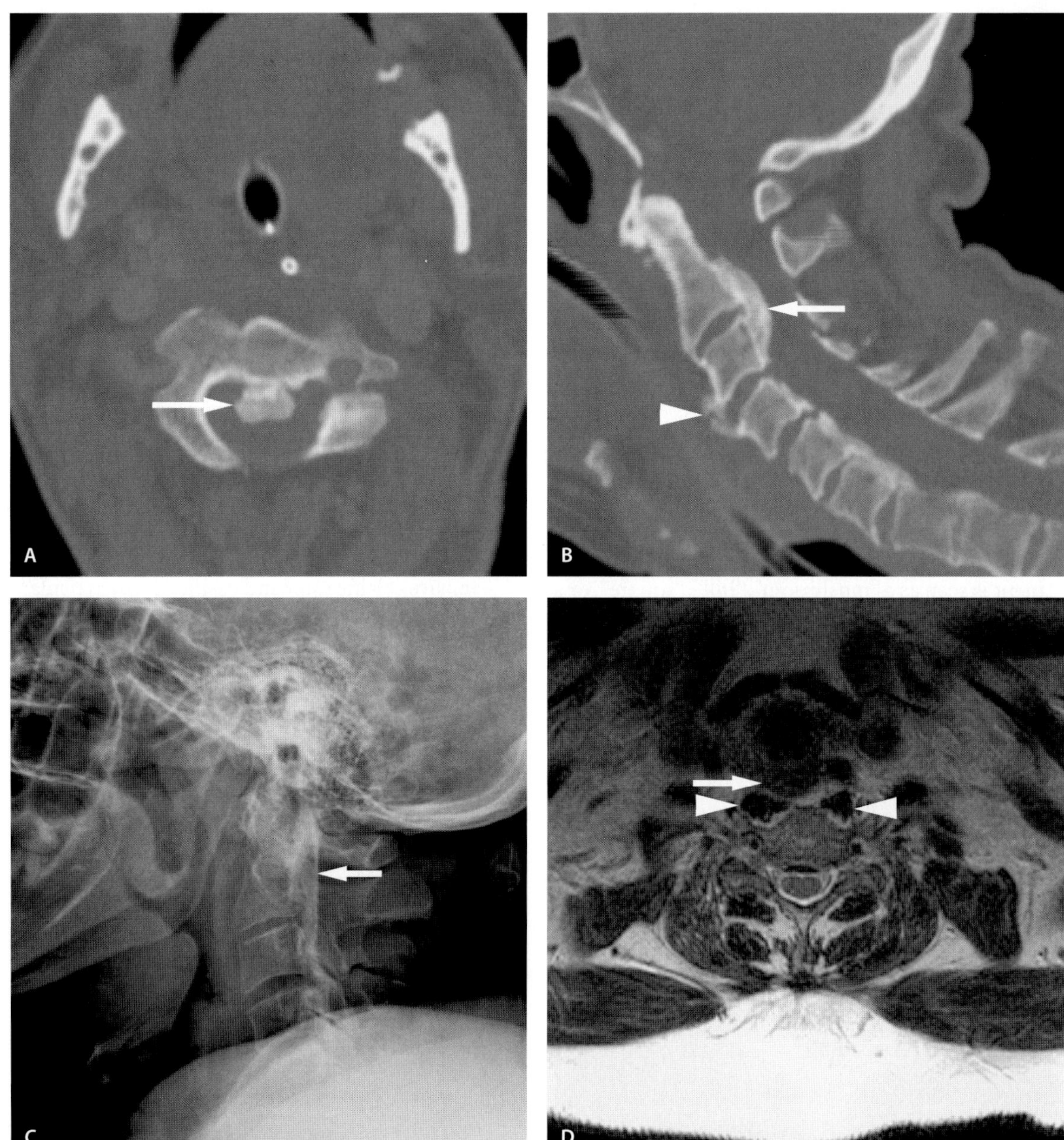

Figure 13.3

Ossification of longus colli ligament; 52-year-old female with a history of left arm pain and clinical suspicion of cervical disc displacement or mass. **A** Axial CT image shows mushroom-shaped ossification (*arrow*) with radiolucent line between ossification and vertebral body. **B** Sagittal CT image shows ossification between C2 and C3 (*arrow*), and segmental ossification at C4-C7, as well as anterior osteophytes C3-C4 consistent with degenerative changes (*arrowhead*). **C** Lateral view of another patient shows severe ossification (*arrow*). **D** Axial T1-weighted MRI, same patient as in **C**, shows evident ossification (*arrow*) anterior to longus colli muscles (*arrowheads*)

Rheumatoid Pannus at Craniocervical Junction

Definition

Hypertrophied synovitis with production of inflammatory joint fluid containing several different types of enzymes.

Clinical Features

- Cervical spine pain and limitation of motion.
- Enlargement of retrodental pannus can induce or aggravate compressive myelopathy.

Imaging Features

- MRI is superior imaging method; shows both inflammatory soft tissue and compression of spinal cord.
- MRI depicts effect of inflammatory process on neural tissue, ligaments, bursae, and fat pads.
- Pannus; often low signal on T1-weighted and high signal on T2-weighted MRI, showing contrast enhancement, depending on activity of inflammation.
- Atlantoaxial dislocation or cranial migration of dens may be seen.

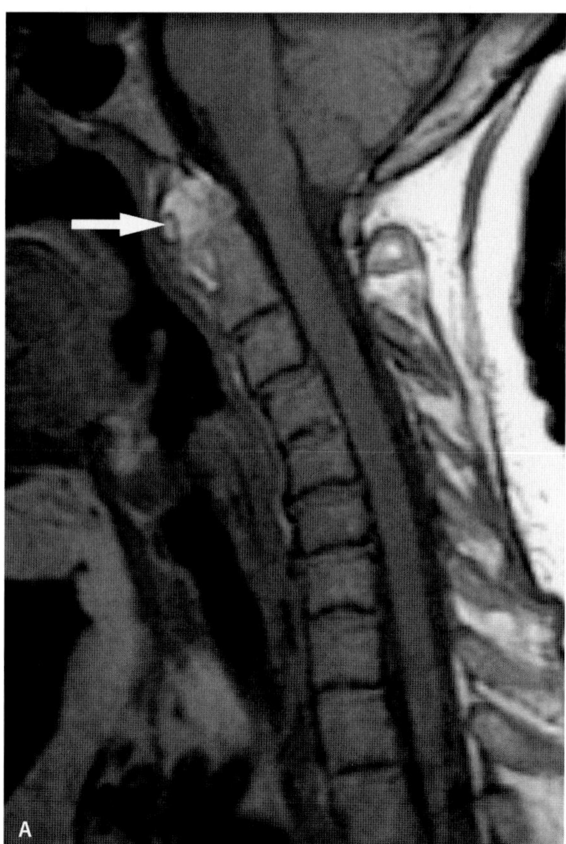

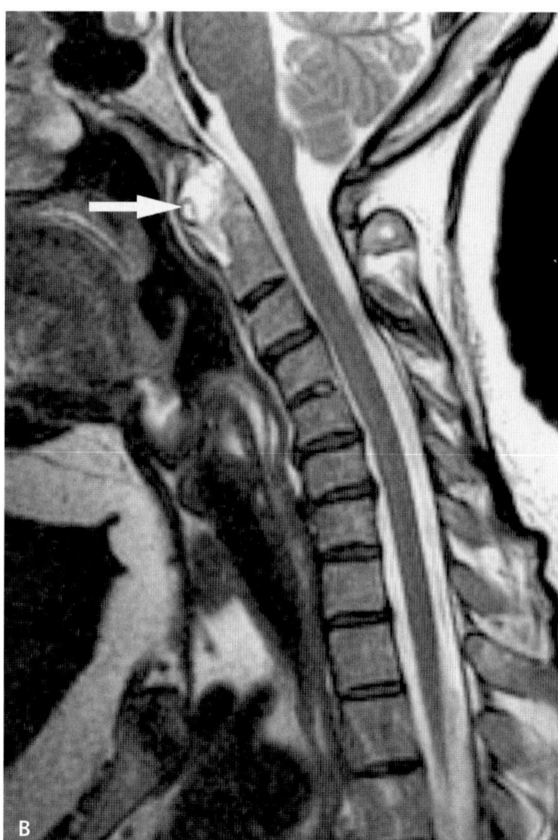

Figure 13.4

Rheumatoid pannus at craniocervical junction; 46-year-old female with long history of rheumatoid arthritis, now with cervical spine pain. **A** Sagittal T1-weighted MRI shows hyperintense mass anterior to eroded dens (*arrow*). **B** Sagittal T2-weighted MRI shows same mass to be markedly hyperintense with a few heterogeneous foci (*arrow*). Kyphotic deformity of mid-cervical spine and degenerative changes at C5–C6 in particular

Tuberculosis at Craniocervical Junction

Definition

Granulomatous or caseous type inflammation caused by *Tuberculum bacilli.*

Clinical Features

- Pain, rigidity, deformity, cold abscess and paraplegia.
- Thoracolumbar commonest site.
- Can occur as paradiscal, central body, subligamentous type, and appendiceal.
- Commonly involves two or three vertebrae.

Imaging Features

- Progressive bone destruction leads to collapse.
- Often paraspinal phlegmon.
- T1-weighted MRI: low signal.
- T2-weighted MRI: high signal, depending on activity of inflammation.
- T1-weighted post-Gd MRI: enhancing of inflammatory granulomatous tissue.

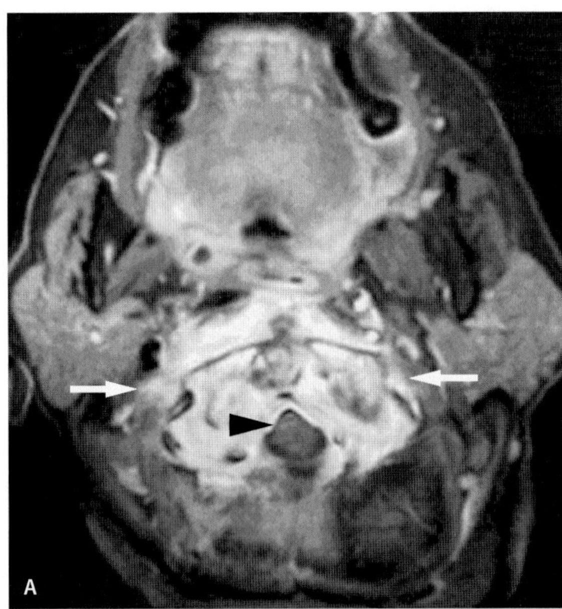

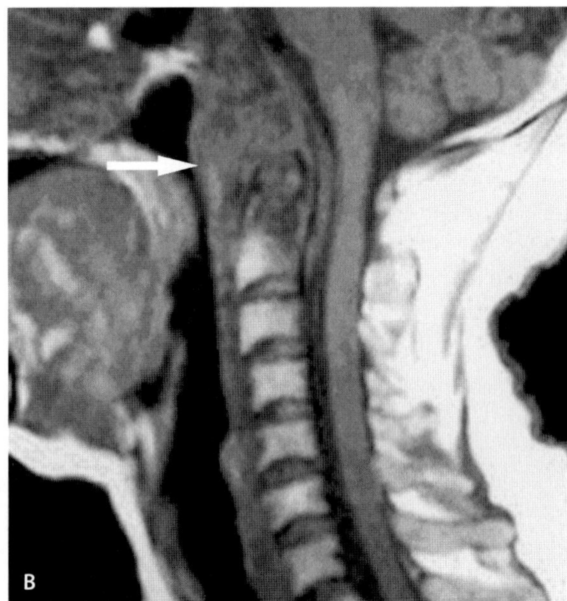

Figure 13.5

Tuberculosis at craniocervical junction; 50-year-old female presented with history of neck ache and low-grade fever for two months. A Axial T1-weighted post-Gd MRI shows destruction and erosion of atlantoaxial joint with an enhancing soft-tissue mass (*arrows*). A small epidural component is seen causing pressure on thecal sac (*arrowhead*). B Sagittal T1-weighted MRI shows destruction of C1 and C2 with a soft-tissue mass (*arrow*) (courtesy of Dr. Humera Ahsan, Aga Khan University, Karachi, Pakistan)

Chiari Malformation Type I

Definition

Herniation of cerebellar tonsils through foramen magnum into cervical spinal canal.

Clinical Features

- Often nonspecific symptoms such as headache, neck pain, dizziness, vertigo, or cranial nerve symptoms.
- Chiari I is often an incidental finding and has no clinical implication in absence of symptoms.

Imaging Features

- Cerebellar tonsil located more than 5 mm inferior to a line between hard palate and posterior lip of foramen magnum.
- More common in children.
- Chiari I is often difficult to see, but a "full" foramen magnum on axial CT images is a good sign.
- There are no osseous abnormalities.
- MRI shows peg-like tonsils below foramen magnum.
- Narrow posterior cranial fossa.
- Associated syringomyelia or syrinx (CSF in center of spinal cord) may be seen.
- Restricted CSF flow due to cerebellar tonsil being displaced inferiorly into foramen magnum.

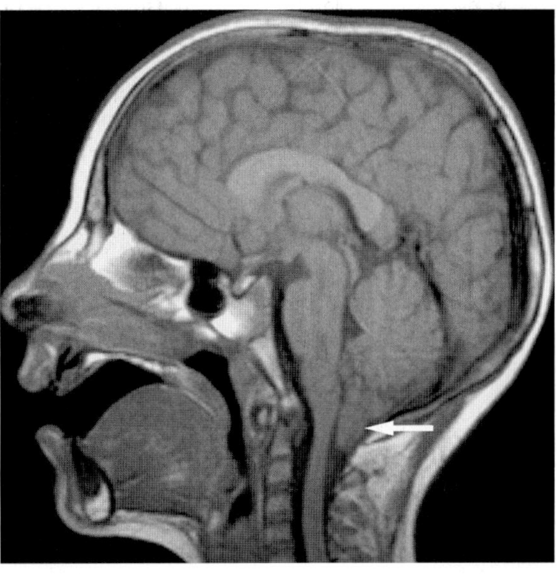

Figure 13.6

Chiari malformation type I; 7-year-old female with Noonan syndrome presents with neck pain. Mid-sagittal T1-weighted MRI shows descent of point of tonsils through foramen magnum (*arrow*) and absence of CSF in cisterna magna

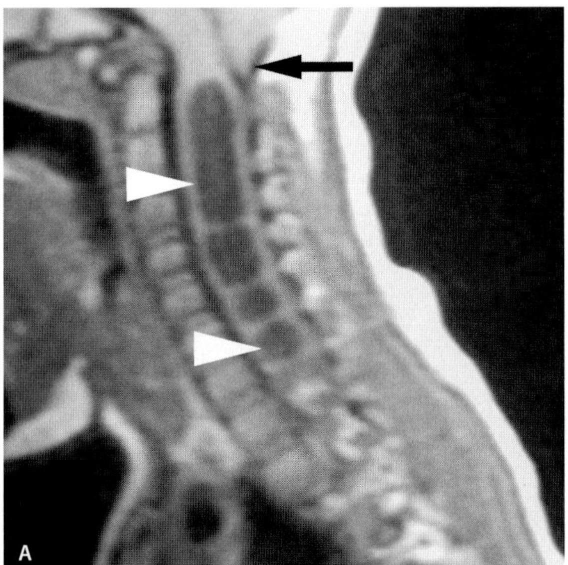

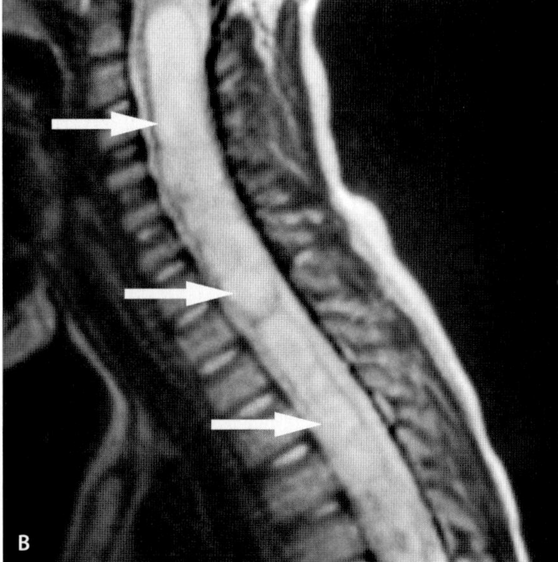

Figure 13.7

Chiari malformation Type I; 5-year-old asymptomatic male. **A** Mid-sagittal T1-weighted MRI demonstrates caudal displacement of cerebellar tonsils (*arrow*). Dark signal in center of cervical cord represents syringo- or hydromyelia with multiple locations (*arrowheads*). **B** Sagittal T2-weighted MRI reveals associated hydromyelia with multiple locations of fluid in center of cord. These are sequelae of decreased CSF dynamics through foramen magnum (*arrows*)

Chordoma at Craniocervical Junction

Definition

Benign but locally aggressive and infiltrating tumor arising from notochordal remnants along neuraxis.

Clinical Features

- Presents with pain and/or neurologic symptoms.
- Commonest location sacrum, followed by clivus, and spinal axis.
- Slow-growing tumor with destruction of adjacent bone.

Imaging Features

- Destructive expansile lesion in spine with surrounding soft-tissue mass.
- Locally aggressive.
- Destruction and calcification better seen on CT images.
- T1-weighted MRI: iso- to hypointense.
- T2-weighted MRI: moderately to extremely hyperintense; extreme T2 hyperintensity is often a hallmark of chordoma, but not seen in our case (Fig. 13.8B).
- T1-weighted post-Gd MRI; variable enhancement.

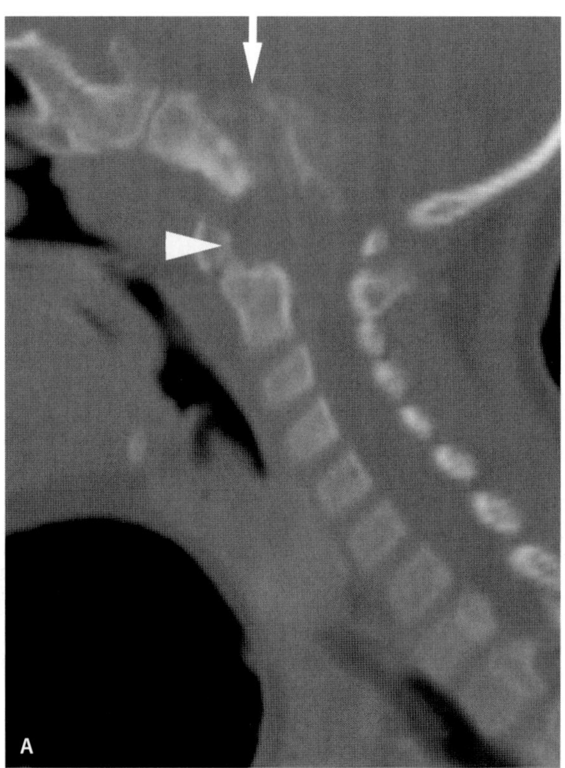

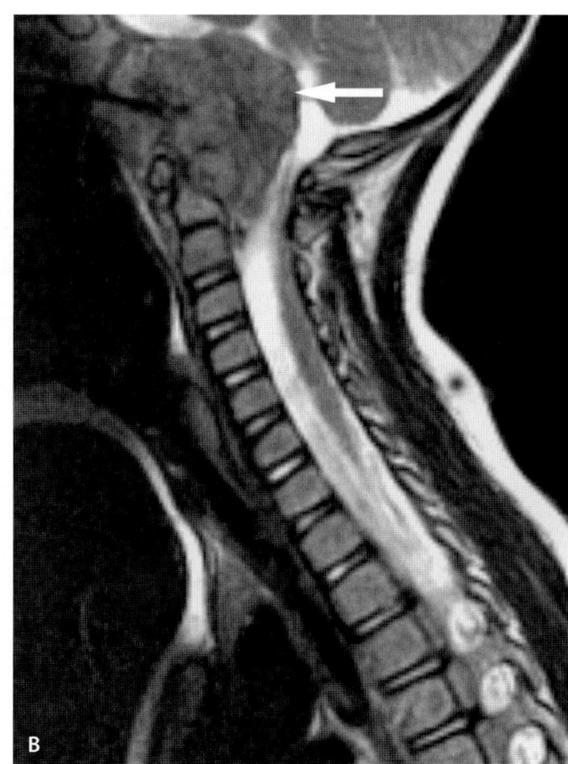

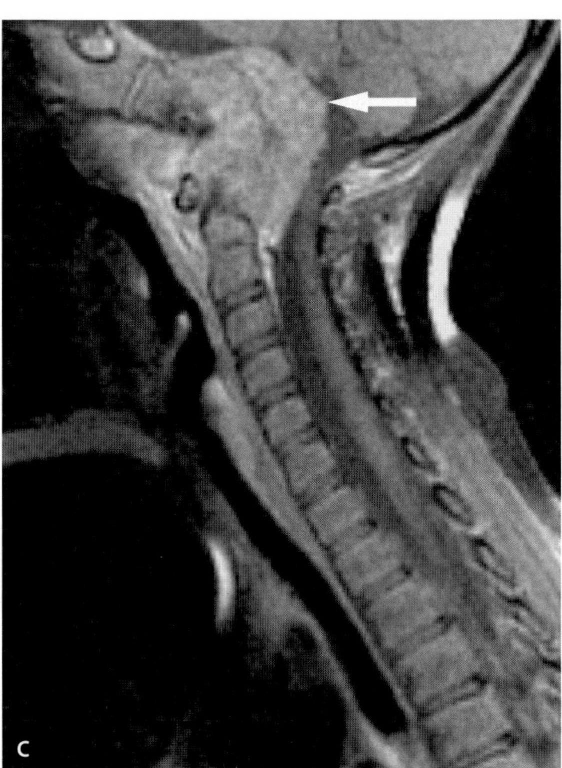

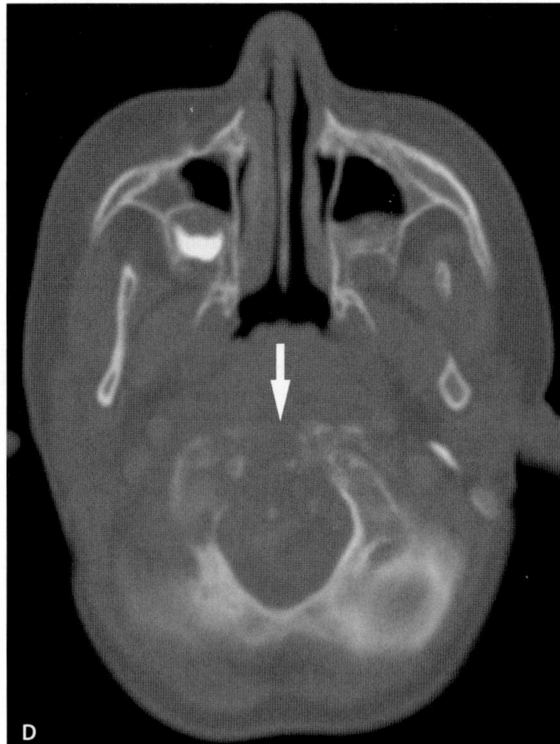

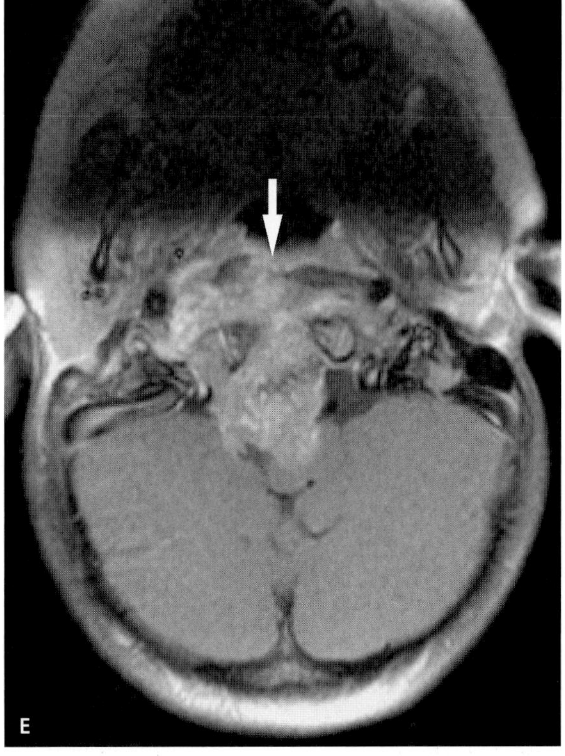

Figure 13.8

Chordoma at craniocervical junction; 3-year-old female with a history of anorexia and lethargy for two months, presenting with mild cervical spine pain. A Sagittal reconstructed CT image shows destruction and bone production in skull base (*arrow*) and C1 area. Top of dens is eroded (*arrowhead*). B Sagittal T2-weighted MRI shows a large hypointense expansile mass emanating from the clivus (*arrow*). C Sagittal T1-weighted post-Gd MRI demonstrates a slight enhancement of mass (*arrow*) involving the clivus, C1 and C2, and extending intracranially and into foramen magnum and nasopharynx. D Axial CT image through foramen magnum illustrates destruction anteriorly (*arrow*) and bone production. E Axial T1-weighted post-Gd MRI demonstrates irregular slightly enhancing destructive mass in foramen magnum (*arrow*) extending into the brain stem, causing brain stem compression

Cervical Spine Teratoma

Definition

True neoplasm consisting of all three embryonic layers.

Clinical Features

- The most common tumors outside of the spinal cord (extra medullary) in cervical spine of newborns are neurofibromas/schwannomas followed by drop metastases and congenital lesions.
- Teratoma is a rare tumor.
- Approximately 10 % associated with other congenital anomalies.

Imaging Features

- Often large relatively well circumscribed lesions.
- Usually well-encapsulated, with both cystic and solid components.
- Fat content is typical.
- T1- and T2-weighted MRI: heterogeneous signal due to difference of cellular components.
- T1-weighted post-Gd MRI: contrast enhancement of solid portions.

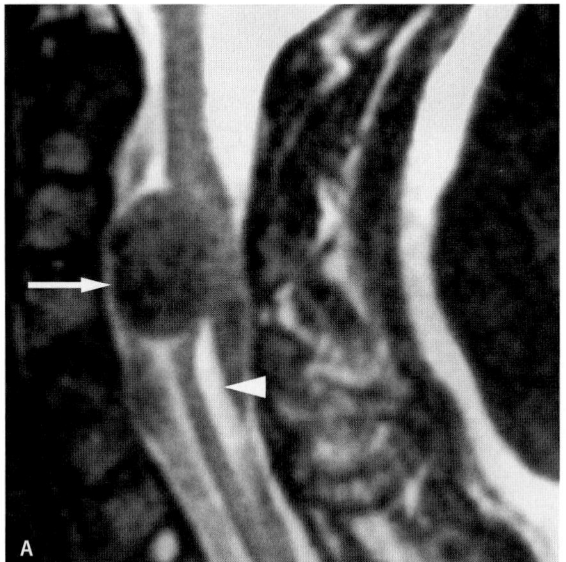

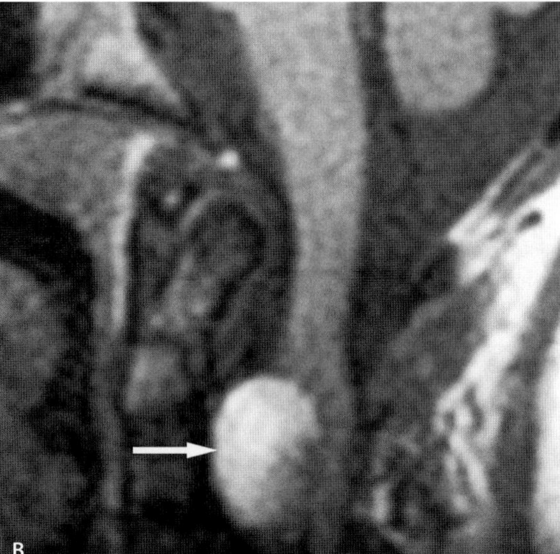

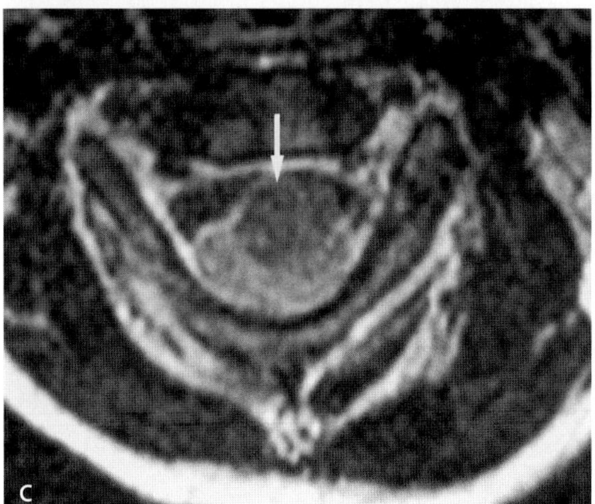

Figure 13.9

Spinal teratoma; 7-year-old female with right hemiparesis. A Sagittal T2-weighted MRI shows enlargement of upper cervical canal. Anterior to cord there is hypointense mass displacing cord (*arrow*). Exophytic mass largely fills spinal canal with almost complete obliteration of CSF space. Only posterior margin appears to infiltrate cord. Syrinx is seen below mass (*arrowhead*). B Sagittal T1-weighted post-Gd MRI shows near homogeneous enhancement (*arrow*), but no cord enhancement. C Axial T2-weighted MRI shows mass (*arrow*) compressing and displacing cord posteriorly

Cervical Spine Cord Astrocytoma

Definition

Tumors derived from the glial cells (astrocytes or "star-shaped" cells).

Clinical Features

- Most common intramedullary (inside spinal cord) spinal cord tumor in children.
- Cervical spine commonest site of involvement.
- Multisegmental involvement usually seen.
- Cysts and syrinx formation common.

Imaging Features

- Expansion of cord.
- Cord edema.
- Cysts are common.
- Relatively short segment involved as opposed to transverse myelitis in which a longer segment of cord is affected.
- T1-weighted MRI: iso- to slightly hypointense.
- T2-weighted MRI: hyperintense.
- T1-weighted post-Gd MRI: patchy contrast enhancement.

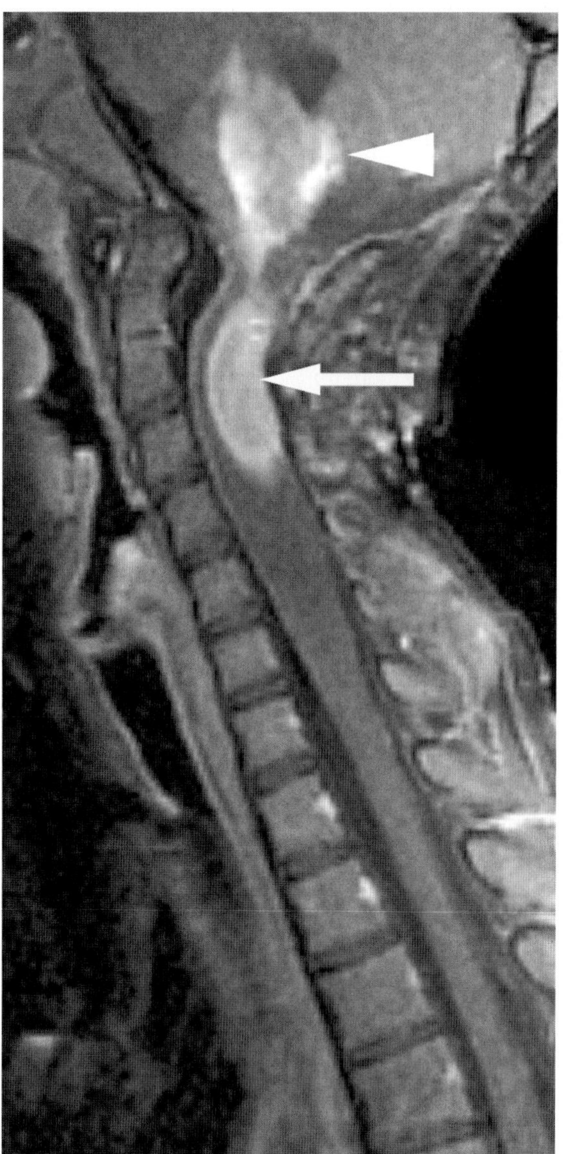

Figure 13.10

Spinal cord astrocytoma; 8-year-old female with known low-grade astrocytoma in cervical cord since age of 18 months when she presented with breathing and swallowing difficulties. Sagittal T1-weighted post-Gd MRI shows intense contrast enhancement in tumor (*arrow*), extending into medulla and lower pons (*arrowhead*)

Extramedullary Cervical Lipoma with Cord Compression

Definition

Benign fatty tumor, usually composed of mature fat cells.

Clinical Features

- Initially asymptomatic mass.
- Presents with symptoms of spinal cord compression.
- Often congenital.
- Most common connective tissue tumor of spine.

Imaging Features

- CT: homogeneous non-enhancing mass with fatty attenuation value.
- T1- and T2-weighted MRI: hyperintense.
- T1-weighted fat-suppressed MRI: hypointense.

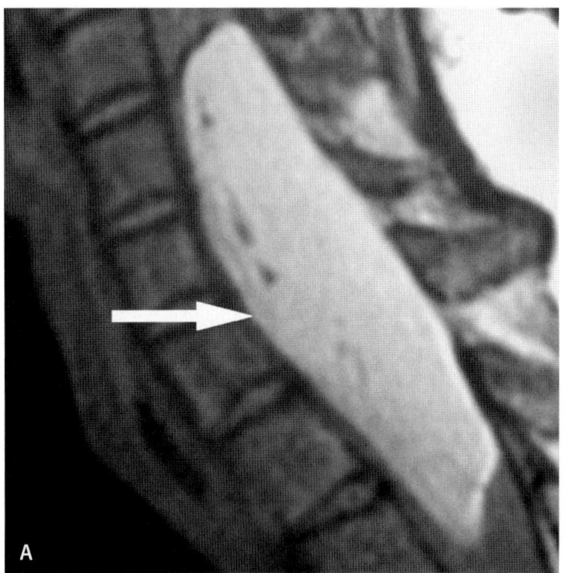

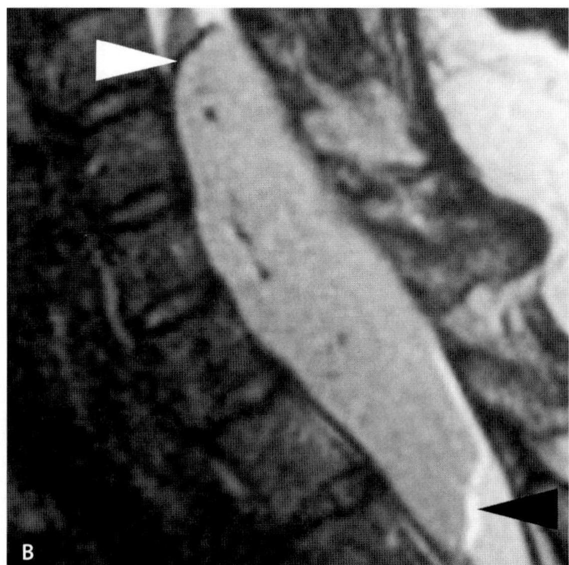

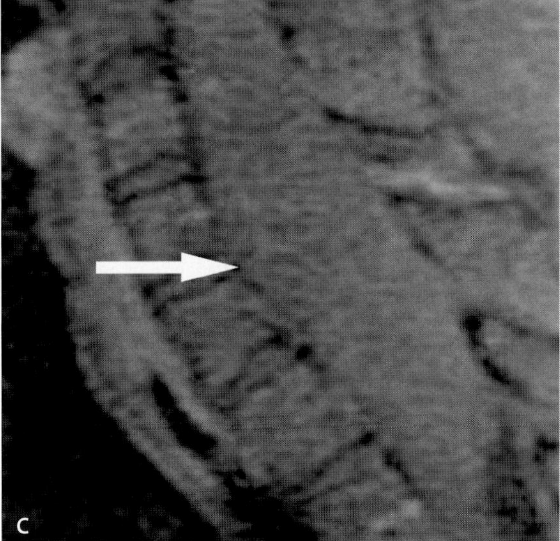

Figure 13.11

Extramedullary cervical lipoma with cord compression; patient had long history of cord compression symptoms. Surgery confirmed the location and fatty nature of the encapsulated tumor. **A** Sagittal proton density MRI shows a large intradural mass (*arrow*), secondarily widened canal to longstanding pressure tumor. **B** Sagittal T2-weighted MRI shows slightly hyperintense mass compared to spinal cord. Note chemical shift misregistration artifact at CSF/lipoma and lipoma/CSF borders (*arrowheads*). **C** Sagittal T1-weighted fat-suppressed MRI shows fatty nature of tumor (*arrow*)

Cervical Spine Meningioma

Definition

Tumor arising in meninges surrounding brain and spinal cord.

Clinical Features

- Peak incidence in fifth to sixth decade with female predominance.
- Thoracic spine commonest followed by cervical spine.
- Majority are intradural extramedullary.
- Patients with neurofibromatosis type 2 (NF-2) can have multiple meningiomas, with intracranial occurrence and along spinal axis; meningiomas originate from meningothelial cells which may be found in spinal arachnoid membranes.

Imaging Features

- Similar characteristics to schwannoma.
- Calcification not uncommon.
- T1-weighted MRI: isointense to cord.
- T2-weighted MRI: hypointense to cord.
- T1-weighted post-Gd MRI: homogeneous and significant contrast enhancement.

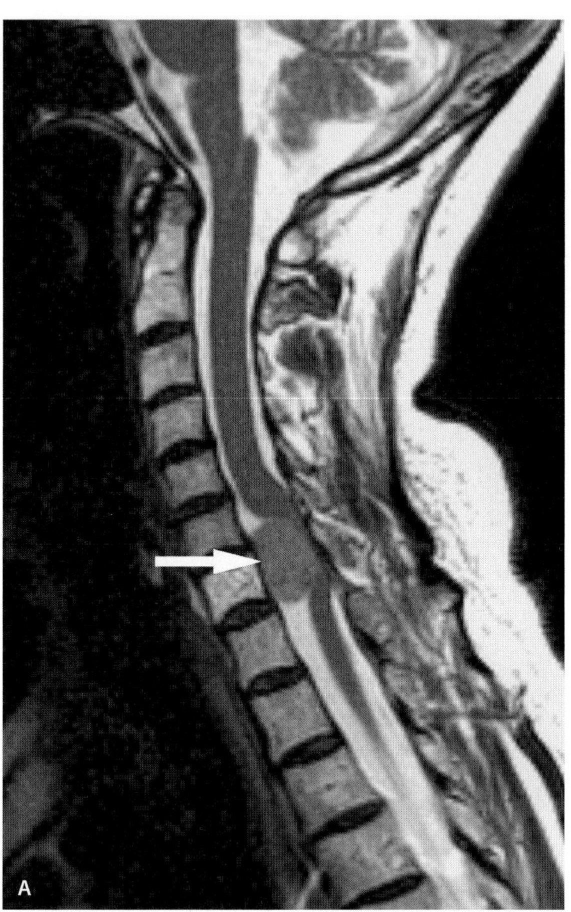

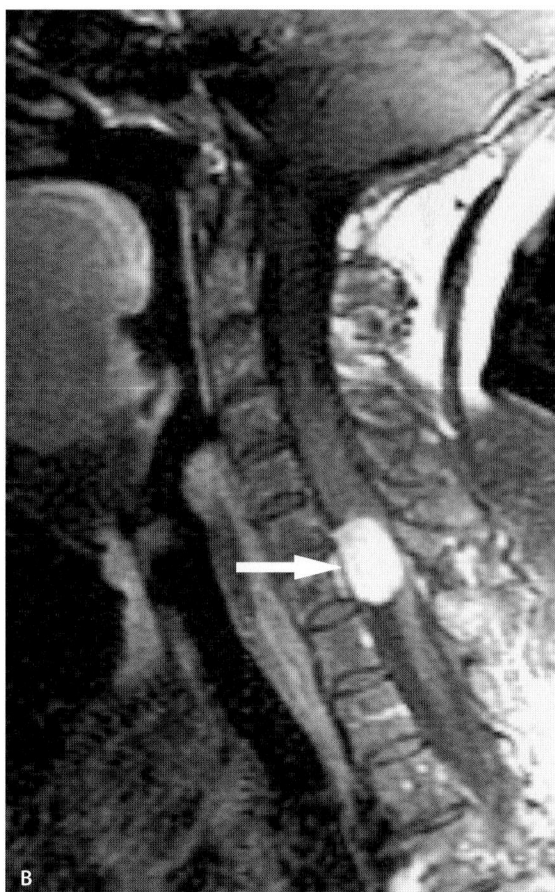

Figure 13.12

Meningioma; 67-year-old woman with progressive weakness in both lower extremities and pain in both arms. Remote history of breast cancer. **A** Sagittal T2-weighted MRI shows well-defined mass with homogeneous signal isointense to cord (*arrow*). **B** Sagittal T1-weighted post-Gd MRI shows intense contrast-enhanced tumor (*arrow*)

Cervical Spine Neurofibromatosis Type 1 (NF-1)

Definition

Tumors arising from nerve sheath of peripheral nerve; Schwann's cells, fibroblasts, and perineural cells.

Clinical Features

- NF-1 the commonest neurocutaneous syndrome.
- Manifestations can arise from any system of body.
- Bony changes usually associated.
- Many patients have neurofibromas in cervical region.

Imaging Features

- Iso- to hypodense to muscle on CT
- Spinal lesions best seen on MRI
- T1-weighted MRI: neurofibromas appear iso- to hypointense.
- T2-weighted MRI: hyperintense
- T1-weighted post-Gd MRI: strong contrast enhancement; may show "target pattern"

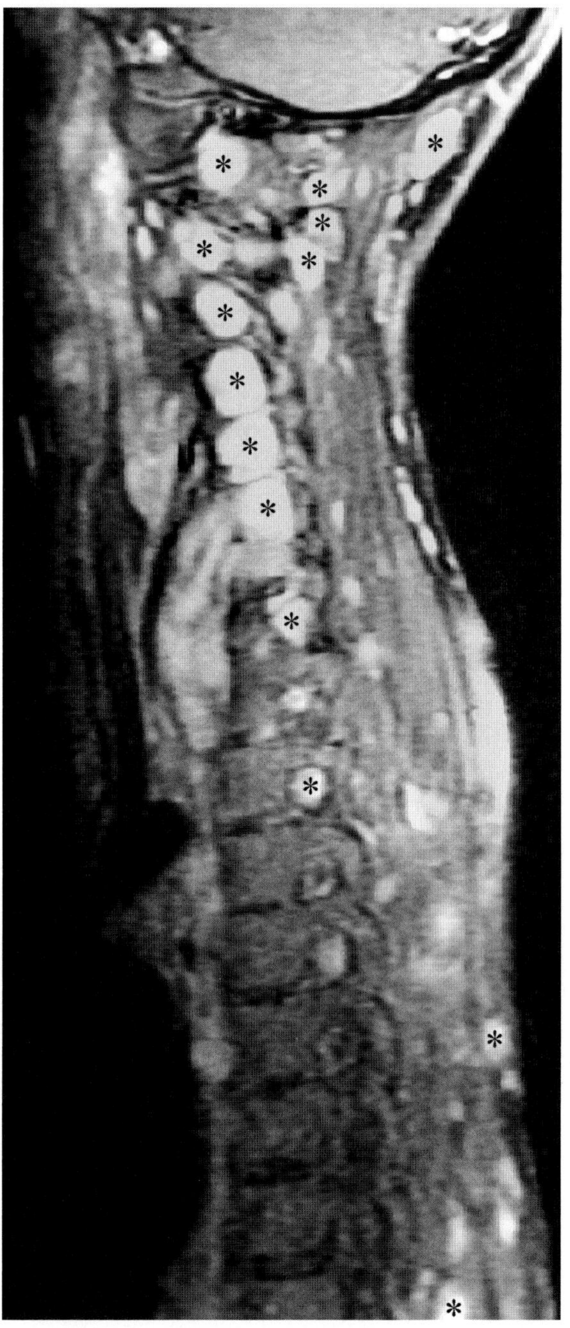

Figure 13.13

Neurofibromatosis type 1 (NF-1); 16-year-old female with known NF-1, presenting with balance and coordination problems. Sagittal T2-weighted fat-suppressed MRI shows enlargement of the neural foramina with multiple rounded neurofibromas (*asteriscs*)

Cervical Spine Fracture

Definition

Fracture and/or dislocation of cervical spine.

Clinical Features

- Presents invariably with cervical spine pain or tenderness.
- More advanced fractures neurologic symptoms.
- Plain films often negative.

Imaging Features

- CT, sagittal and coronal images, best for fracture diagnosis.
- MRI best for cord injury and for ligamentous injuries.
- Burst fracture involves fracture of posterior wall of vertebral body often with retropulsion.
- Compression fracture has intact posterior wall of vertebral body.

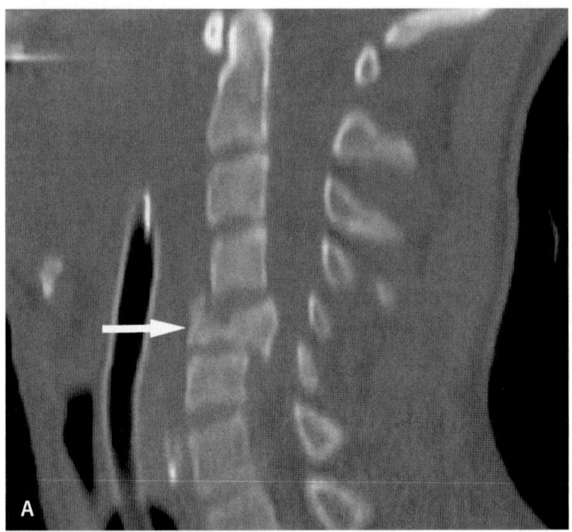

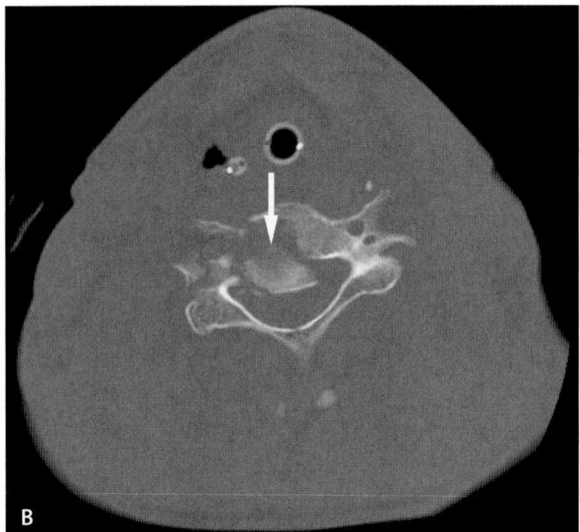

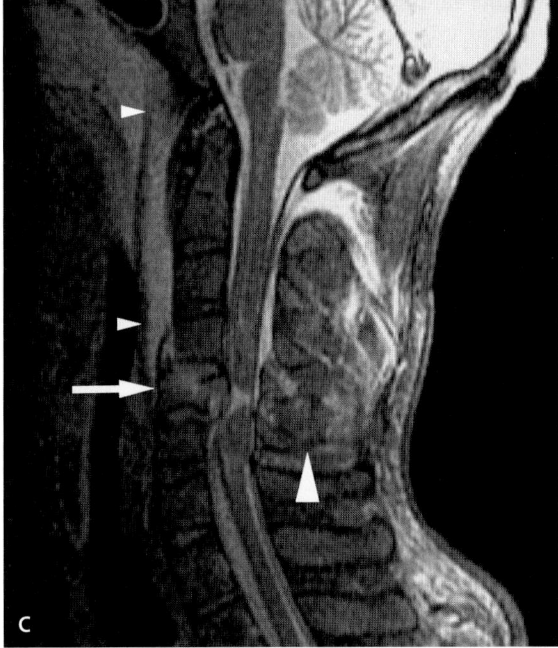

Figure 13.14

C5 burst fracture; 27-year-old male all-terrain vehicle accident. A Sagittally reformatted CT image shows burst fracture of C5 with subluxation and severe central canal narrowing (*arrow*). B Axial CT image demonstrates fragment displaced into central canal (*arrow*). Also fracture through right foramen tranversarium where vertebral artery is located. This injury may cause damage to vertebral artery which could lead to a posterior fossa stroke. C Sagittal STIR MRI shows spinal cord contusion, C5 burst fracture (*arrow*), prevertebral hematoma C1 to C4 (*arrowheads*) and injury to posterior elements (*large arrowhead*)

Neck

Diagnosis of lesions of the suprahyoid neck is primarily not the duty of the maxillofacial radiologist. However, many of the structures of this area will be depicted on regular maxillofacial imaging studies and therefore the maxillofacial radiologist will often have to make a gross evaluation to determine whether there is an abnormality that needs further attention or the structures are normal. Conversely some larger maxillofacial lesions will extend into the suprahyoid neck and the maxillofacial radiologist will have to have a working knowledge of neck anatomy in order to formulate an interpretation of the findings.

This section is included to provide examples of abnormalities in the supra- and infrahyoid neck that may be recognized by the maxillofacial radiologist, such as inflammations, nontumorous expansive masses, muscle paralysis, and benign and malignant tumors with their characteristics.

Hypopharynx Abscess

Definition

Pus collection in pharyngeal/hypopharyngeal soft tissues.

Clinical Features

- Dysphagia
- Neck and oral pain
- Fever
- Stridor
- Odynophagia

Imaging Features

- Soft-tissue swelling
- Ring-enhancing lesion with low attenuation center
- Stranding (lymphedema) and obliteration of adjacent fat planes
- Thickening of platysma
- Lymphadenopathy
- T1-weigted MRI: decreased signal
- T2-weighted MRI: increased signal
- T1-weighted post-Gd MRI: peripheral enhancement

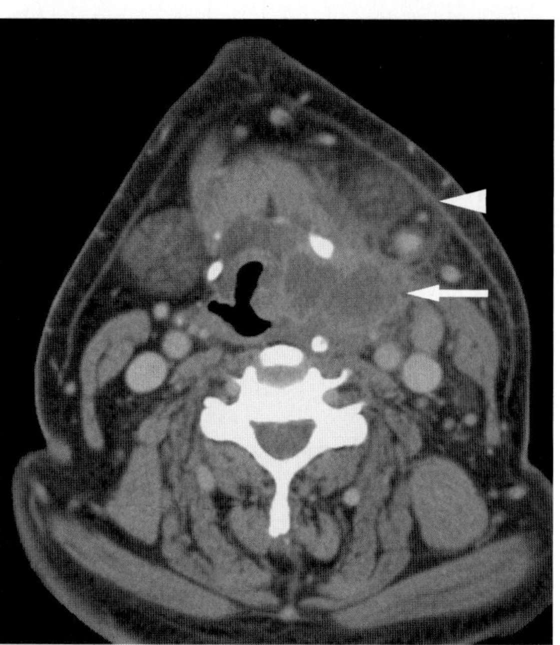

Figure 13.15

Hypopharynx abscess; 48-year-old male presenting with a peripharyngeal soft-tissue swelling, neck pain, fever and stridor. Axial CT image shows multilobulated ring-enhancing mass (*arrow*), consistent with abscess in left hypopharynx with a compression narrowing and deviation of hypopharyngeal airway. Thickening of platysma (*arrowhead*) and stranding of subcutaneous fat

Thyroid Abscess

Definition

Well-circumscribed pus collection within thyroid gland.

Clinical Features

- Swelling, pain, redness.
- Induration (localized hardening of soft tissue).
- Fever.
- Dysphagia/odynophagia.
- Tender gland sometimes with referred pain to pharynx/ear.
- Often occurs in immunocompromised and debilitated patients.
- *Staphylococcus aureus*, *Pneumococcus* common organisms.

Imaging Features

- Ring-enhancing lesion with central area of necrosis within thyroid gland
- Swelling
- Fat stranding
- Lymphadenopathy

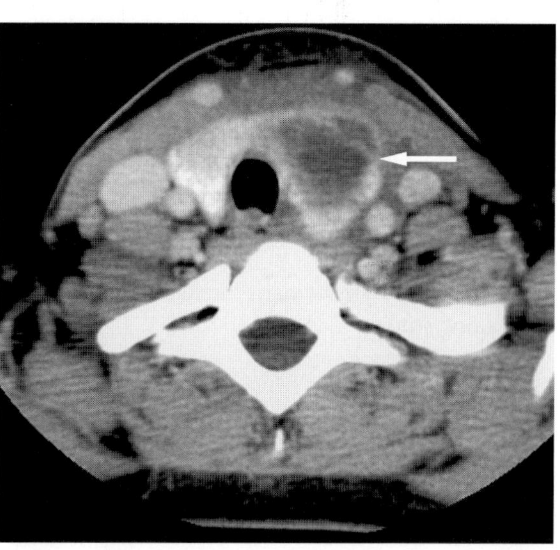

Figure 13.16

Thyroid abscess; 19-year-old female presenting with a 2-week history of a sore throat, left neck pain, and headache. Axial post-contrast CT image shows ill-defined hypodense lesion in left lobe of the thyroid gland with ring enhancement (*arrow*), consistent with abscess and soft-tissue edema. Low dense areas are also noted in oropharynx especially on the left side and inferiorly to the thoracic inlet, and bilateral lymphadenopathy

Tornwaldt's Cyst

Definition

Developmental cyst occurs when pharyngeal bursa ectoderm retracts with the notochord into the clivus. Named after Gustav Ludwig Tornwaldt (1843–1910).

Clinical Features

- Most often asymptomatic incidental finding on imaging study.
- Seen incidentally in up to 3% of healthy adults; usually no treatment need.
- May cause symptoms when infected.
- Infection may spread to mediastinum.

Imaging Features

- Cystic lesion mostly in mid-line of nasopharynx
- Low attenuation
- T1-weighted MRI: low signal intensity
- T2-weighted MRI: high signal
- T1-weighted post-Gd MRI: no contrast enhancement

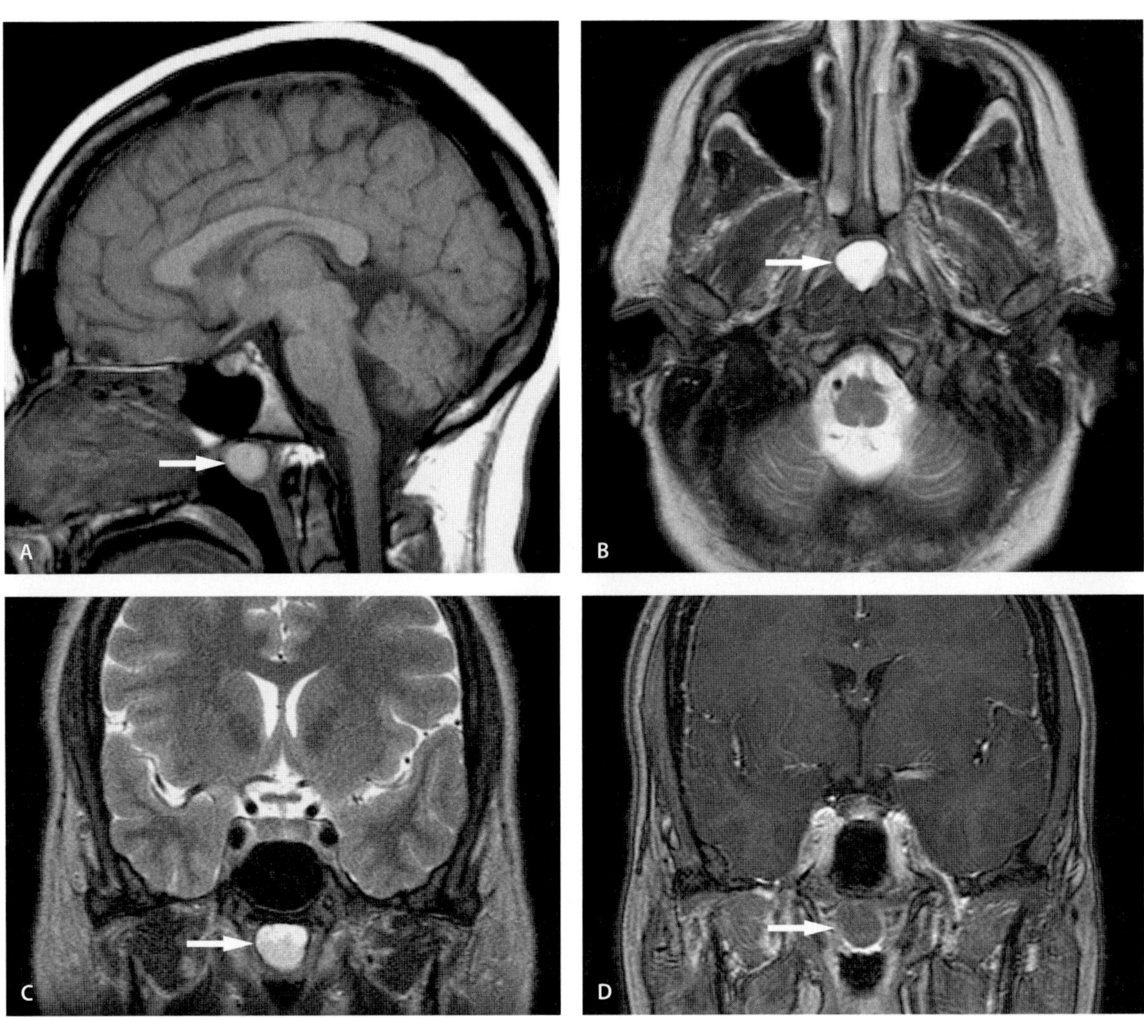

Figure 13.17

Tornwaldt's cyst, large; incidental findings in 30-year-old. A Sagittal T1-weighted MRI shows low-signal cyst (*arrow*) in posterior nasopharynx. B Axial T2-weighted MRI shows bright signal cyst (*arrow*). C Coronal T2-weighted MRI shows bright signal cyst (*arrow*). D Coronal T1-weighted post-Gd MRI shows no enhancement of the cyst (*arrow*)

Dermoid Cyst in Floor of Mouth

Definition
Growth of a piece of skin underneath the surface as result of abnormal development; may contain skin, hair, bone, teeth or embryonal tissue.

Clinical Features
- Most commonly involves floor of mouth; sublingual, submental, or submandibular regions.
- Differential diagnosis includes epidermoid, ranula, thyroglossal duct cyst, and cystic hygroma.
- Soft nonpainful mass.

Imaging Features
- Typically well-circumscribed, thin-walled, unilocular mass
- Low attenuation
- T1-weighted MRI: homogeneous low signal
- T2-weighted MRI: homogeneous high signal
- T1-weighted post-Gd MRI: no contrast enhancement of cyst except wall, in particular if infected

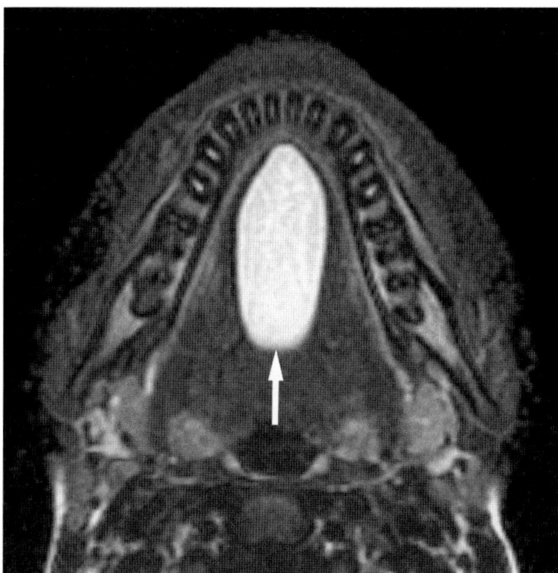

Figure 13.18

Dermoid cyst; 18-year-old male with doughy swelling of floor of mouth clinically considered a thyroglossal duct cyst. Axial T2-weigted fat-suppressed MRI shows well-defined oval mass with high signal in floor of mouth (*arrow*), located in sublingual space depressing mylohyoid muscle down (not shown)

Goiter

Definition
Diffuse or multinodular enlargement of thyroid gland.

Clinical Features
- More common in middle-aged females.
- Often associated with iodine deficiency.
- Midline neck mass.
- Often asymptomatic enlargement of thyroid gland; symptoms depend upon state of hypo- or hyperthyroidism.
- Endemic goiters are prevalent in iodine deficient areas.
- Goiter is a clinical diagnosis that simply implies an enlargement of thyroid gland developing because thyroid gland compensates for inadequate thyroid hormone output.

Imaging Features
- Nodular enlargement of thyroid gland often with cystic lesions.
- Displaces and narrows trachea.
- Multinodular goiter is usually not associated with tumors.
- Substernal or mediastinal extension requires imaging for detection.
- T2-weighted MRI: high signal due to colloid or hemorrhage.
- Nuclear scan with radioactive iodine or Tc-99m pertechnetate is often very helpful (cannot be done for 6 weeks if intravenous contrast has been used).
- Ultrasound is often used to characterize multinodular goiter.

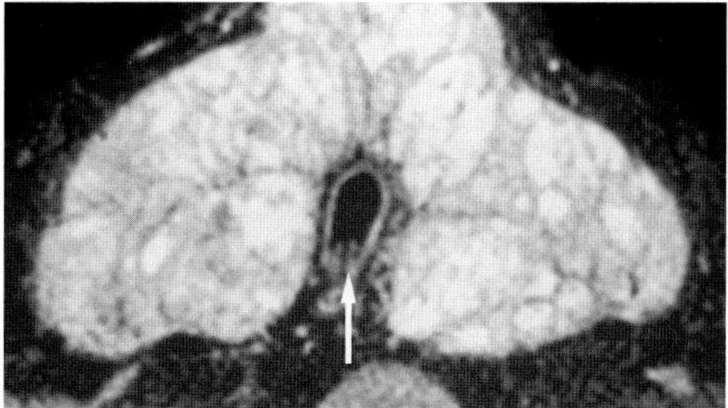

Figure 13.19

Goiter; 18-year-old presenting with hyperthyroidism. Axial T2-weighted fat-suppressed MRI shows large multilobulated thyroid gland compressing and narrowing trachea (*arrow*)

Vocal Cord Paralysis

Definition

Vocal cord does not move to center due to muscle paralysis.

Clinical Features

- Patient presents with hoarseness
- Occasionally a sign of a tumor along the recurrent laryngeal nerve

Imaging Features

- Paralyzed vocal cord is located laterally in larynx; unable to migrate to midline (as normal) due to lack of innervation of muscles.

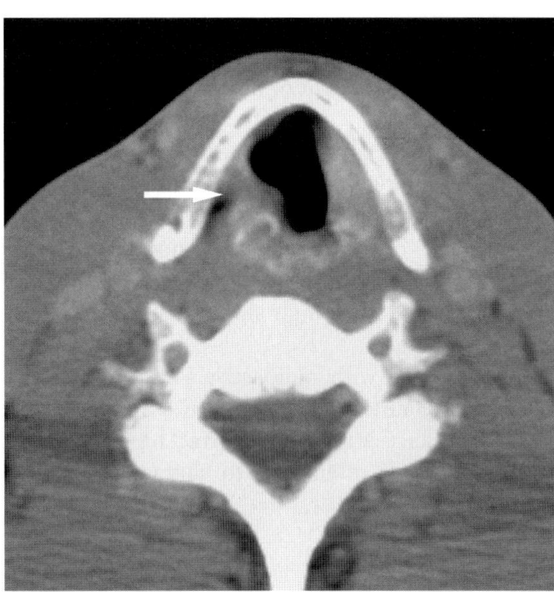

Figure 13.20

Right vocal cord paralysis secondary to lung cancer; 63-year-old man presents with hoarseness. Axial CT image through larynx shows right vocal cord (*arrow*) laterally in larynx

Neck Hemangioma

Definition

Hemangioma or benign neoplasm that exhibits increased blood circulation, endothelial cells, mast cells, and macrophages.

Clinical Features

- Most common tumor in head and neck in infancy and childhood.
- Approximately 7% of all benign soft-tissue tumors.
- Rapidly enlarges.
- Ultimately regresses by adolescence.
- Typically becomes apparent during the first month of life.
- Diffuse skin lesion or soft cystic mass in oral cavity, pharynx, parotid gland, or neck.
- Associated with intracranial arterial vascular malformations.
- Often requires no treatment. Steroids are occasionally used.

Imaging Features

- T1-weighted MRI: intermediate signal with flow void
- T1-weighted post-Gd MRI: dramatic enhancement
- Often extensively infiltrative in nature

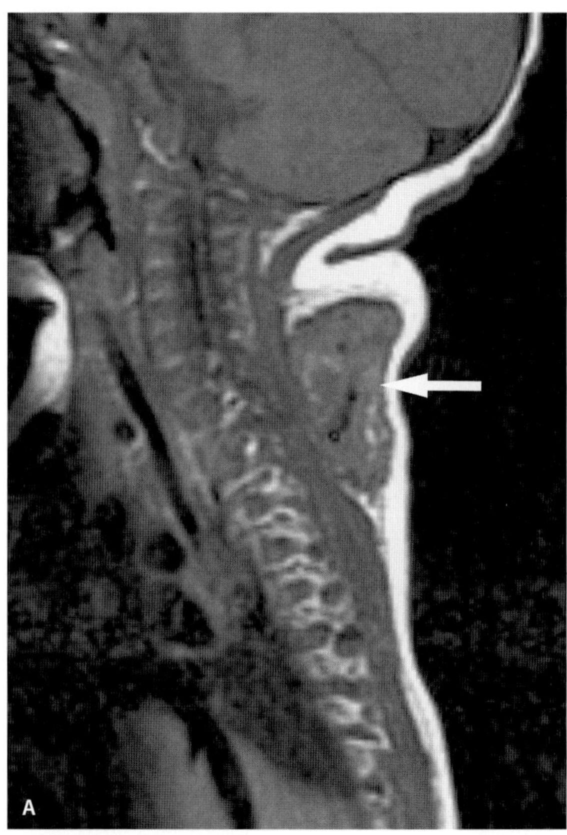

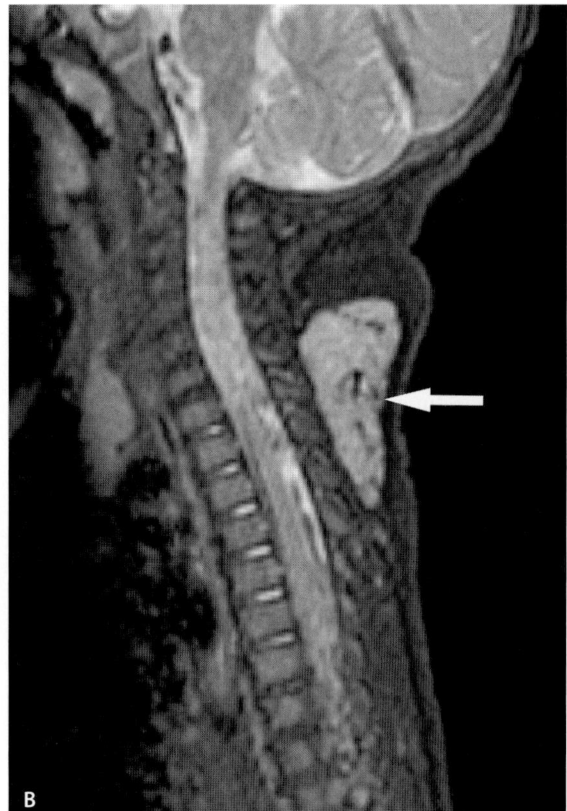

Figure 13.21

Hemangioma; 6-month-old infant twin girl presents with mass in back of neck. The mass has been observed for only a few days. **A** Sagittal T1-weighted MRI shows a well-circumscribed large mass in posterior neck with flow voids (*arrow*). **B** Sagittal STIR MRI shows intermediate high signal intensity also with flow voids (*arrow*). **C** Sagittal T1-weighted post-Gd MRI shows dramatic enhancement (*arrow*).

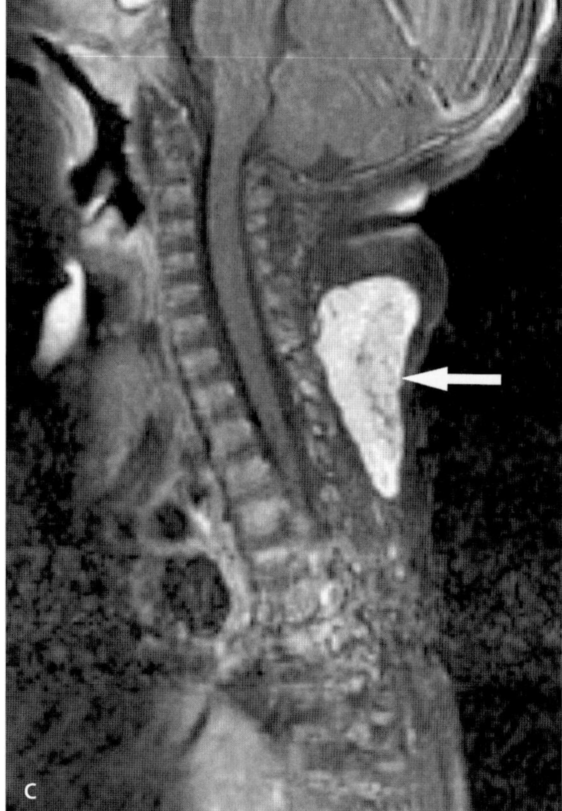

Neck Lipoma

Definition

Benign fatty neoplasm.

Clinical Features

- Often occurs in posterior neck.
- Soft benign neoplasm, usually does not enlarge in size.

Imaging Features

- Low attenuation
- Well-circumscribed
- T1-weighted MRI: high signal
- T2-weighted MRI: intermediate signal
- T1-weighted fat-suppressed MRI: low signal

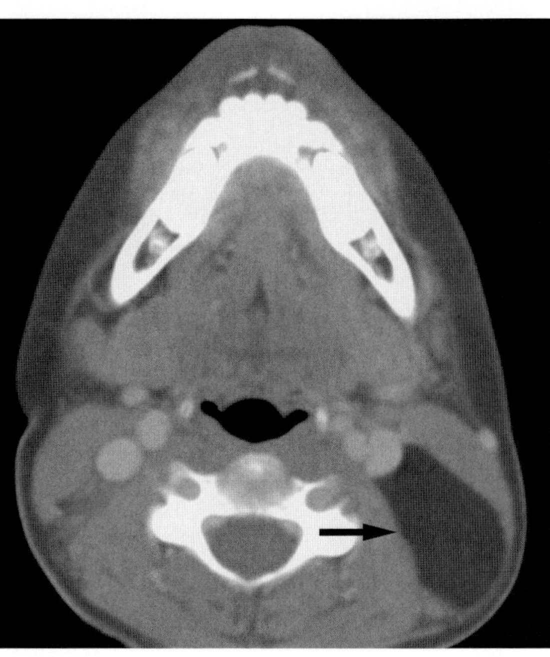

Figure 13.22

Lipoma; 8-year-old female with a 3-week history of left posterior neck mass. No redness, no fever and no tenderness. Axial CT image shows low-attenuation well-circumscribed fatty appearing mass in posterior triangle of left neck (*arrow*), deep to sternocleidomastoid muscle

Neck Plexiform Neurofibroma

Definition

Benign neoplasm consisting of Schwann cells and fibroblasts.

Clinical Features

- Malignant transformation in 5% to 10%.
- Unique to neurofibromatosis type 1 (from von Recklinghausen's disease).
- Common in the scalp, neck, mediastinum, retroperitoneum, cranial nerve five, and orbits.
- Masses are soft and elastic.
- Accounts for elephantiasis, seen in neurofibromatosis.
- Sarcomatous transformation in about 5% of patients.

Imaging Features

- Infiltrated aggressive appearing tumors along cranial nerves
- Multilobulated masses along nerves with low to intermediate attenuation.
- T1-weighted MRI: intermediate signal.
- T2-weighted MRI: high signal. Sometimes target sign: low signal intensity centrally with ring of high signal in periphery
- T1-weighted post-Gd MRI: often dramatic enhancement
- Three types: localized, diffused, plexiform.

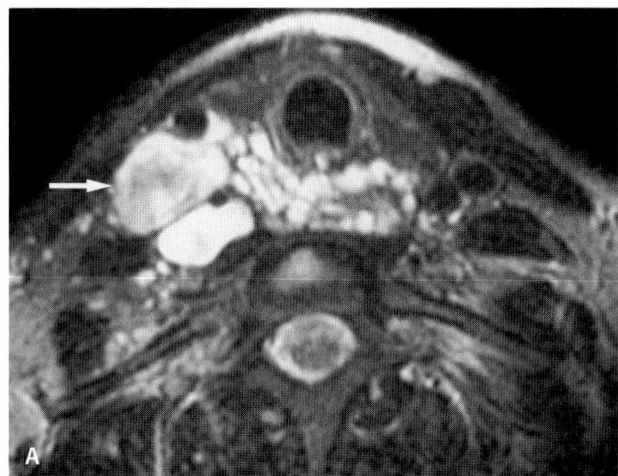

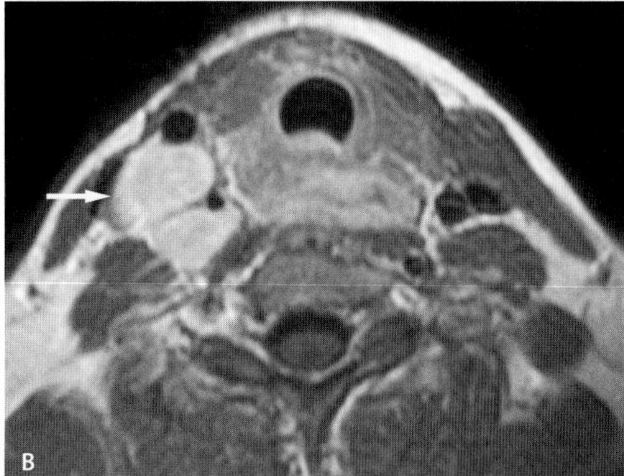

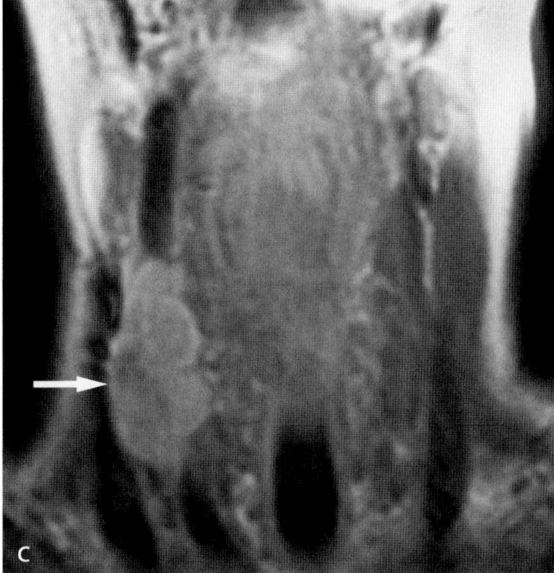

Figure 13.23

Plexiform neurofibromatosis; 9-year-old female presents with a painless swelling of right lower neck. A Axial T2-weighted fat-suppressed MRI shows multilobulated complex mass in right lower neck extending across midline (*arrow*), and separating common carotid artery and jugular vein, and abutting spine. B Axial T1-weighted post-Gd MRI shows enhancing mass separating carotid artery and jugular vein (*arrow*). C Coronal T1-weighted post-Gd MRI shows contrast-enhanced multilobulated mass in carotid sheath (*arrow*).

Pharynx Rhabdomyosarcoma

Definition

Malignant tumor of striated muscles, primarily affecting children and young adults.

Clinical Features

- Most common malignant orbital tumor in childhood
- Mean age 7 years
- Often metastasizes to lung or cervical nodes

Imaging Features

- Large, aggressive soft-tissue mass.
- Ill-defined inhomogeneous large soft-tissue mass which erodes and infiltrates surrounding structures including bones.
- MRI is best to characterize the soft tissue and extent.
- T1-weighted MRI: intermediate signal.
- T2-weighted MRI: hyperintense.
- T1-weighted post-Gd MRI: variable enhancement

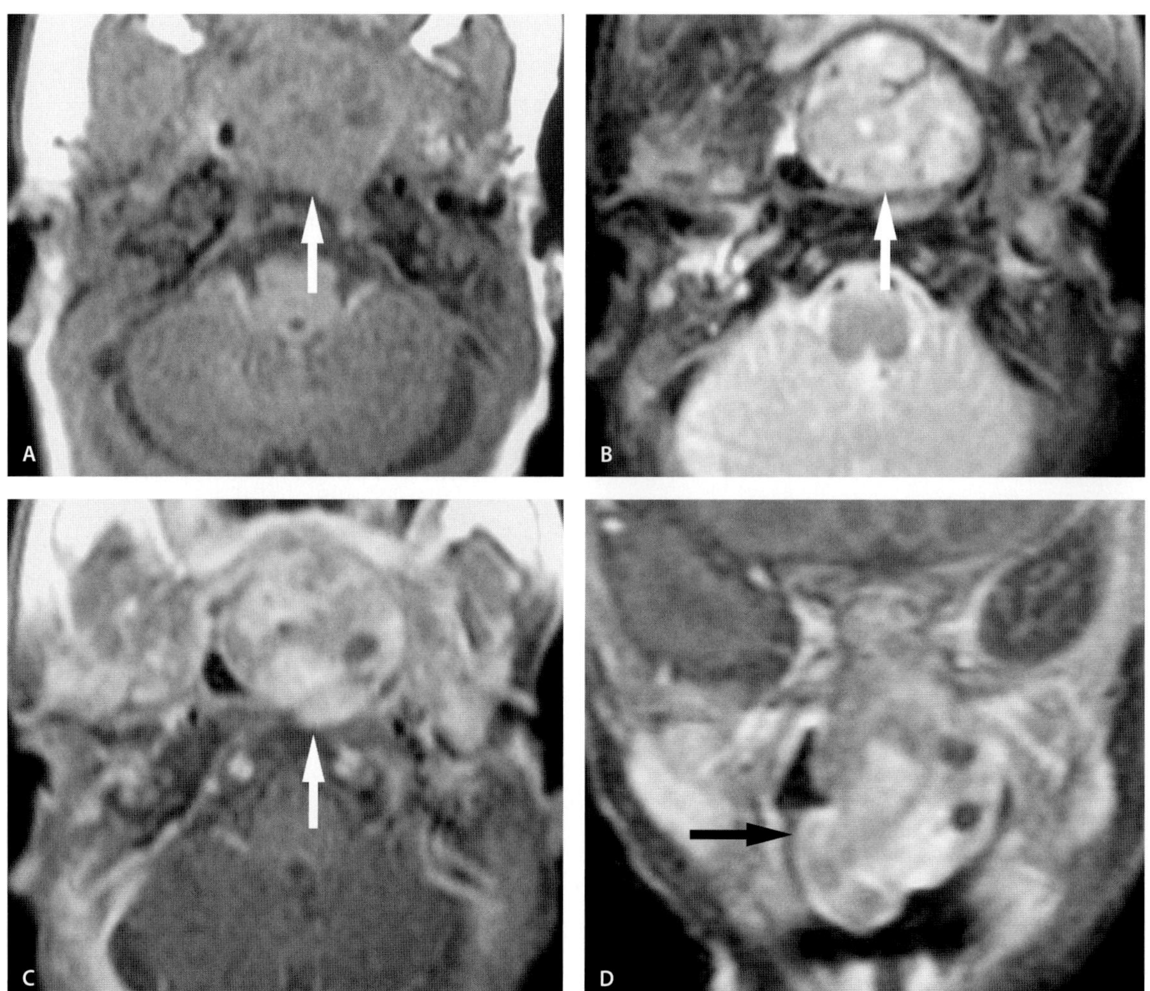

Figure 13.24

Rhabdomyosarcoma; 5-week-old female with stridor and a posterior pharyngeal mass. A Axial T1-weighted MRI shows a large right pharyngeal mass isointense to muscle (*arrow*). B Axial T2-weighted MRI shows a well-circumscribed mass (*arrow*) in nasopharynx with linear and punctate areas of low attenuation representing vascular structure. C Contrast-enhanced T1-weighted MRI shows enhancement and flow voids (*arrow*). D Contrast-enhanced T1-weighted fat-suppressed MRI shows large enhancing lesion in nasopharynx (*arrow*)

Tongue Base Carcinoma

Definition

Squamous cell malignant neoplasm of the tongue.

Clinical Features

- Infiltrating lesion often on lateral or posterior aspect of tongue.
- Painless swelling and/or induration.
- Risk factors for oral cavity squamous carcinoma: smoking, alcohol abuse, chewing tobacco, chewing betel nuts.

Imaging Features

- T2-weighted fat-suppressed image often delineates tumor best.
- Sagittal, coronal axial images are essential to as precisely as possible outline the extent of the tumor.
- Crossing the midline is important for surgical planning (generally not resectable if cross midline).
- T1-weighted MRI: intermediate signal.
- T2-weighted MRI: intermediate to high signal.
- T1-weighted post-Gd MRI: some enhancement.

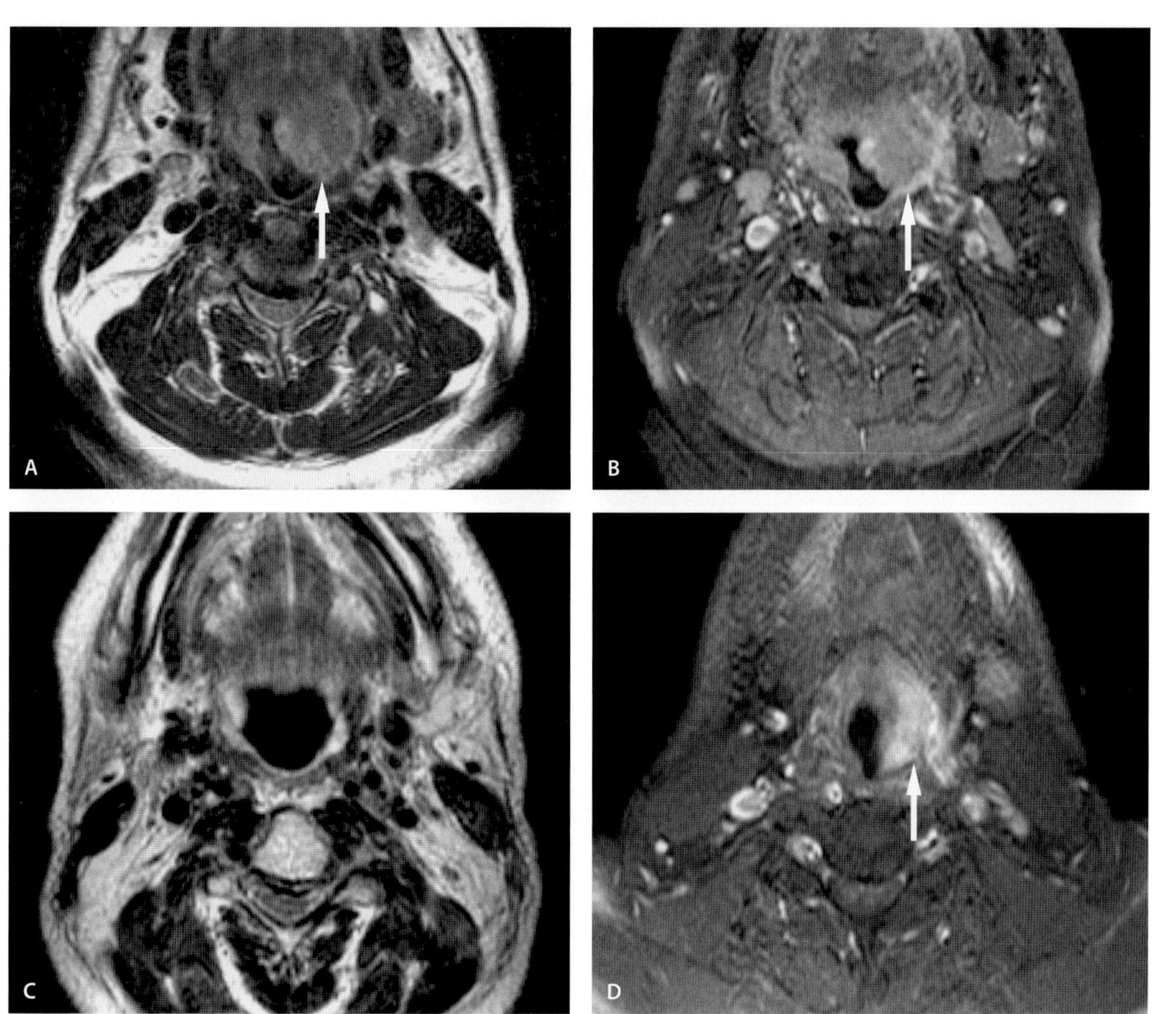

Figure 13.25

Tongue base carcinoma; 64-year-old man presents with left throat pain. A Axial T2-weighted MRI shows a large low intensity mass in left tongue base extending to hypopharynx (*arrow*). The signal is higher than muscle but still not bright. B Axial T1-weighted fat-suppressed post-Gd MRI shows slight enhancement of mass (*arrow*). C Axial T2-weighted MRI, more caudal section, shows no lymphadenopathy. D Axial T1-weighted fat-suppressed post-Gd MRI, more caudal section, shows extension to left hypopharynx (*arrow*)

Hypopharynx Carcinoma

Definition

Squamous cell malignant neoplasm of pharynx.

Clinical Features

- Infiltrating lesion in wall of pharynx
- Painless
- Often associated with swallowing problems
- Risk factors for hypopharynx squamous carcinoma: smoking, alcohol abuse

Imaging Features

- Soft-tissue mass in hypopharynx
- Asymmetry of hypopharynx, supraglottic area, false and true vocal cords
- Obliteration of piriform sinus

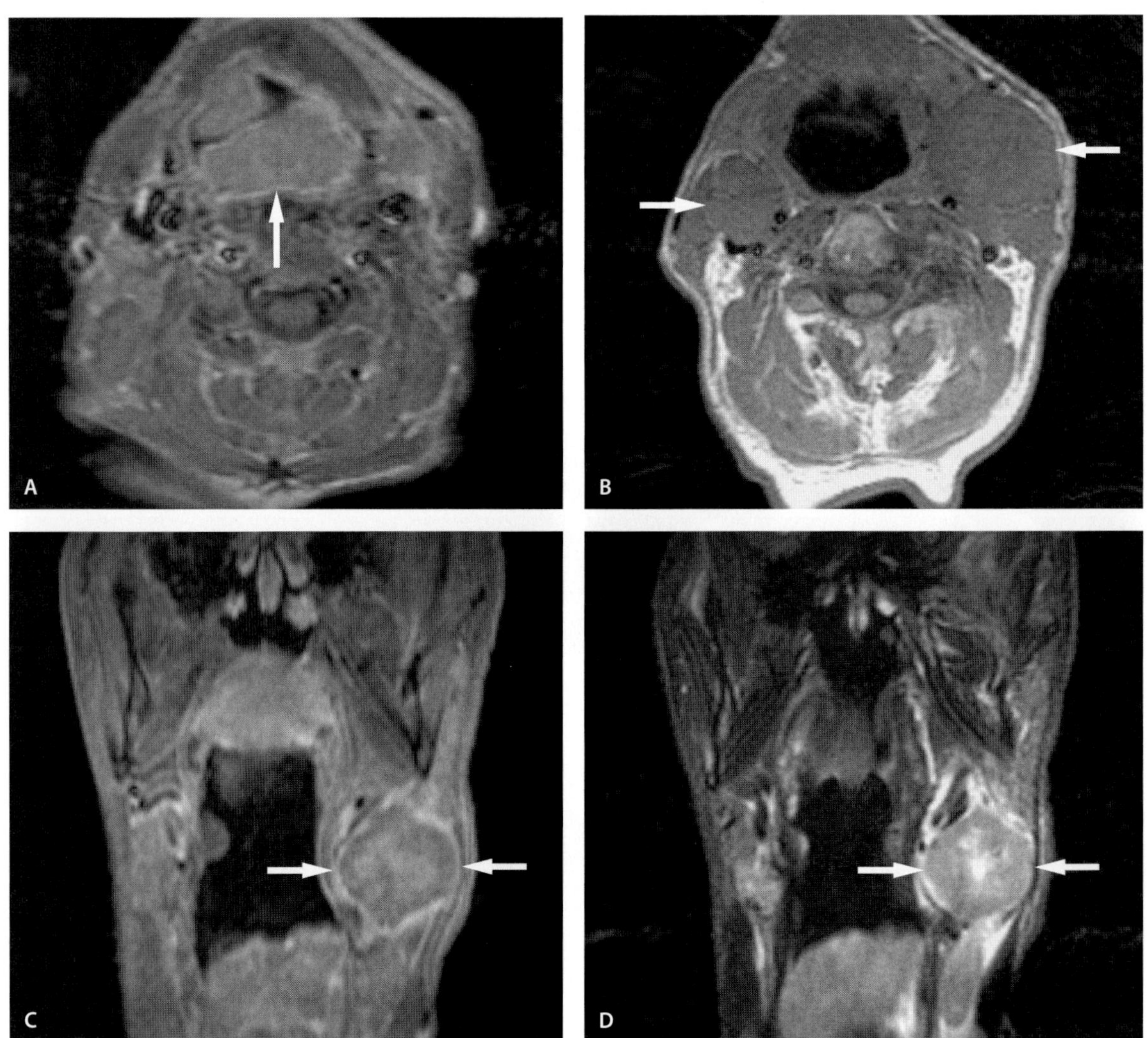

Figure 13.26

Hypopharynx carcinoma; 60-year-old female with a feeling of a lump in the throat. **A** Axial T1-weighted post-Gd fat-suppressed MRI shows a large almost circumferential hypopharyngeal mass (*arrow*). **B** Axial T1-weighted MRI shows bilateral enlarged lymph nodes (*arrows*). **C** Coronal T1-weighted post-Gd MRI shows left-sided enlarged lymph node (*arrows*). **D** Coronal T2-weighted post-Gd MRI shows left-sided enlarged lymph node (*arrows*)

Burkitt's Lymphoma

Definition

Stem cell non-Hodgkin's lymphoma.

Clinical Features

- Most commonly seen in children
- Most common malignant disease of children in tropical Africa
- Involvement of jaw characteristic
- Related to Epstein-Barr virus

Imaging Features

- Rapidly growing soft-tissue mass
- Destruction of bone

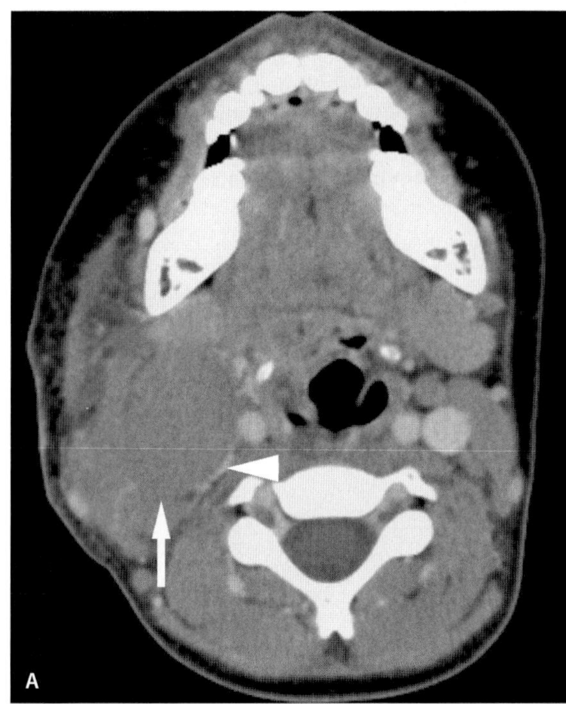

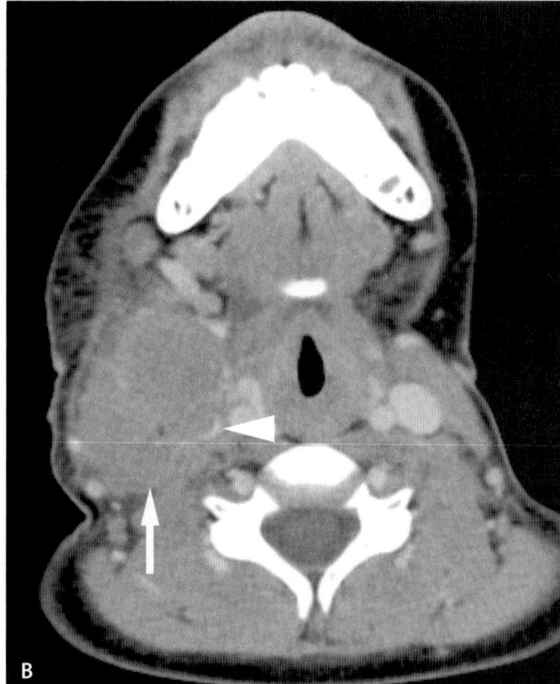

Figure 13.27

Burkitt's lymphoma; 7-year-old female with a 2-week history of large nontender neck mass. Axial post-contrast CT images (B more caudal than A) show a large soft-tissue mass (*arrows*) severely compressing internal jugular vein (*arrowheads*) and pushing midline structures towards other side. This appearance is nonspecific and the enlarged lymph node could be from any type of lymphoma or metastasis

Castleman's Disease

Definition

Benign lymph-node disease; angiofollicular hyperplasia.

Clinical Features

- 70% of cases present in chest, 10% in head and neck
- Often asymptomatic

Imaging Features

- Often intense enhancement due to hypervascular stroma.
- No central necrosis as seen in malignant lymph nodes.
- Differential diagnoses are mononucleosis, cat scratch disease and lymphoma.

Lymphadenopathy

Definition

Benign or malignant enlargement of lymph nodes.

Clinical Features

- Palpable nodal masses in neck.
- Often bilateral.
- Often painless unless infected.
- May be idiopathic or due to infection; other differential diagnoses: lymphoma, mononucleosis, cat scratch disease, Castleman's disease, HIV.
- Proportionally enlarged lymph nodes are often normally seen in young children.

Imaging Features

- Enlarged lymph nodes.
- No central necrosis if benign, but occasionally seen in malignant lymph nodes.
- Cannot separate specific etiology on imaging studies.

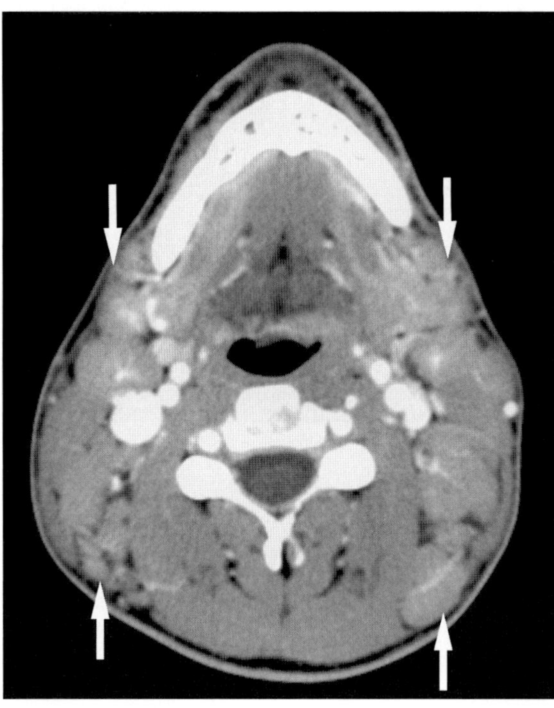

Figure 13.28

Castleman's disease in 19-year-old male with relapsing/remitting symptoms. Axial post-contrast CT image shows multiple slightly enlarged lymph nodes bilaterally (*arrows*). From an imaging point of view these are nonspecific, and Castleman's disease is not an imaging diagnosis

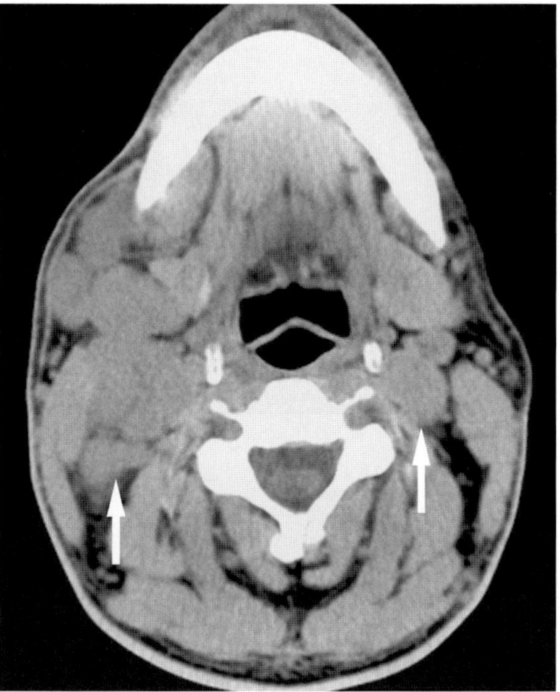

Figure 13.29

Lymphadenopathy; 40-year-old HIV-positive male. Axial CT image shows enlarged lymph nodes bilaterally (*arrows*)

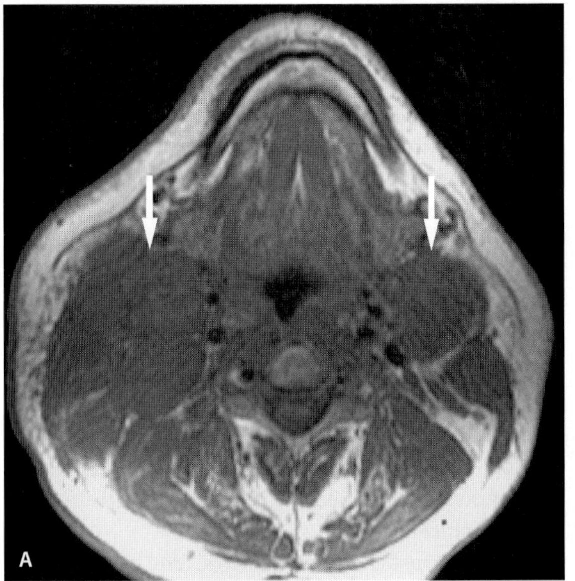

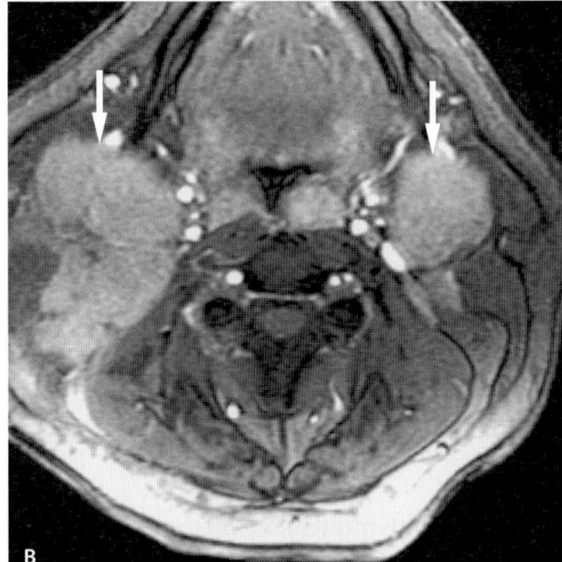

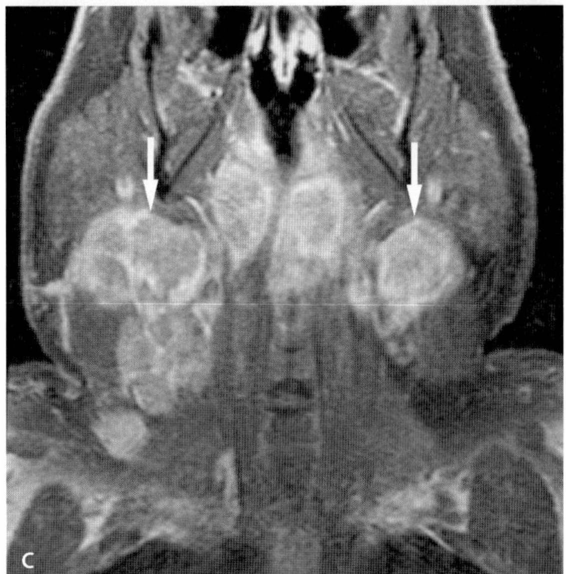

Figure 13.30

Lymphadenopathy; 42-year-old female with a history of nasopharyngeal carcinoma. A Axial T1-weighted MRI shows bilateral enlarged upper cervical lymph nodes (*arrows*). B Axial T1-weighted post-Gd MRI with fat suppression shows enhancement of enlarged lymph nodes (*arrows*). C Coronal T1-weighted post-Gd MRI with fat suppression shows many enhancing enlarged lymph nodes bilaterally (*arrows*)

Skull Base

The skull base is the superior and posterior neighbor to the maxillofacial region. It involves the base of the skull with its foramina, muscles, nerves, and vascular structures. As in the other sections of this chapter, it is not the intention to give a full and complete description of skull-base abnormalities, but rather to illustrate conditions that are likely to be depicted on the images that the maxillofacial radiologist is asked to interpret, but still not in the true maxillofacial area. We have included characteristic infections, tumor-like and vascular lesions, and neoplasms.

Mastoiditis with Intracranial Abscess

Definition

Intracranial encapsulated pus collection due to pyogenic infection secondary to mastoiditis.

Clinical Features

- Intracranial complications result from uncontrolled coalescent mastoiditis.
- Intracranial complications of acute mastoiditis: sigmoid sinus thrombosis, meningitis and abscess (subdural, epidural and parenchymal).
- Subperiosteal abscess can be seen.
- Common signs of mastoiditis: otalgia, postauricular swelling and fever.
- Intracranial abscess may present with headache, seizure, fever, altered mental status, or focal neurologic deficits.

Imaging Features

- Non-contrast CT imaging: middle ear and mastoid completely opacified and mastoid air cells become confluent.
- Post-contrast CT imaging is first-line modality and shows rim-enhancing hypodense fluid collection.
- T1-weighted post-Gd MRI is best to diagnose sinus thrombosis and intracranial complications (venous infarct, meningitis and abscess).
- On diffusion-weighted MR imaging, abscesses are bright indicating restricted diffusion.

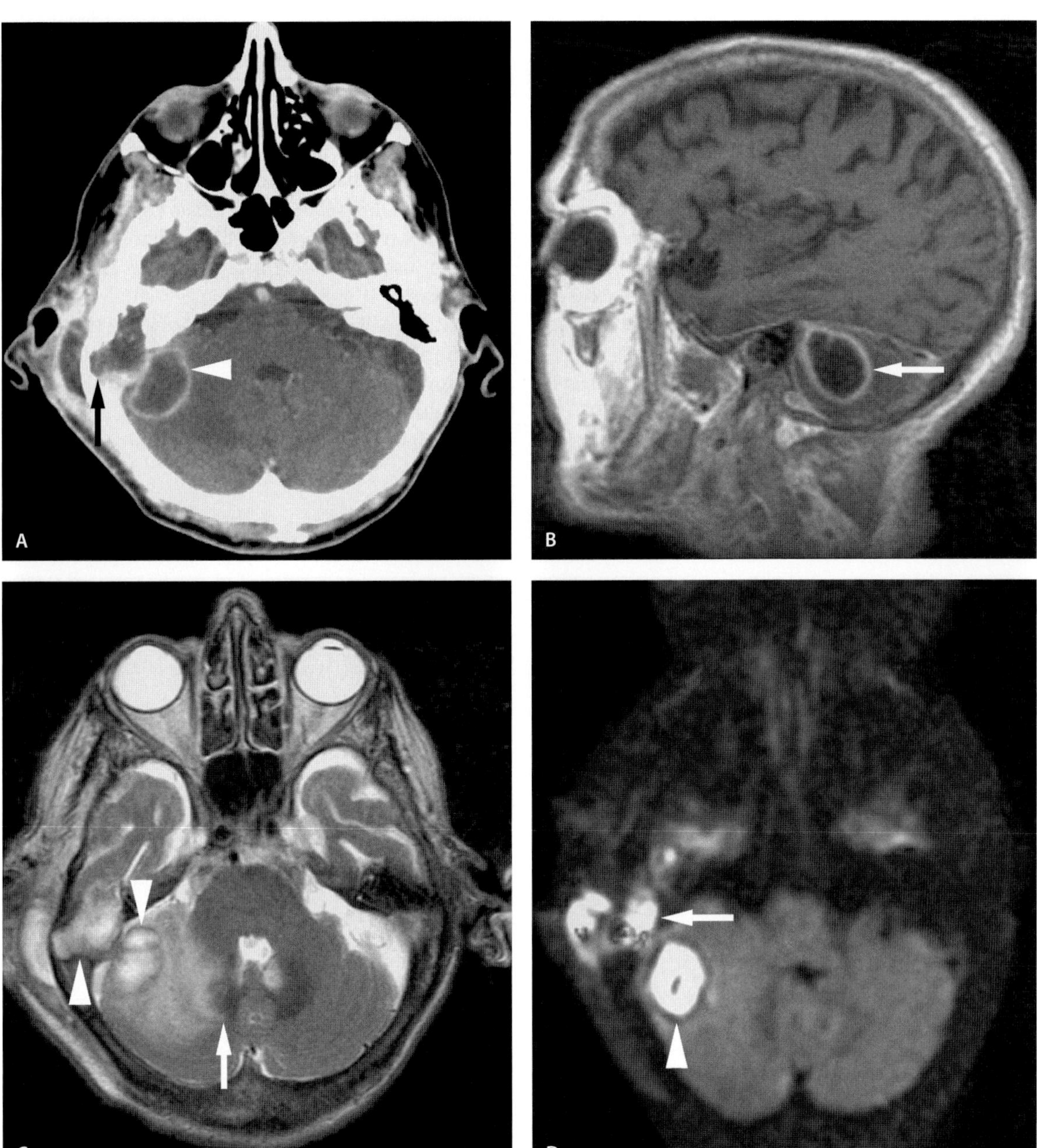

Figure 13.31

Mastoiditis with intracranial abscess; 94-year-old female presented with a 1-week history of fever and mental status change. Patient treated with antibiotics for two episodes of right otitis media. **A** Post-contrast axial CT image demonstrates right mastoiditis with erosion of right petrous temporal bone (*arrow*), involvement of adjacent dura, and ring-enhancing lesion in right cerebellar hemisphere indicating abscess (*arrowhead*). **B** Sagittal T1-weighted post-Gd MRI shows hypointense lesion in right cerebellar hemisphere with ring enhancement (*arrow*). **C** Axial T2-weighted image demonstrates high intensity signal in right mastoid sinus and right cerebellar hemisphere with surrounding edema (*arrowheads*) and mass effect on fourth ventricle (*arrow*). **D** Diffusion-weighted imaging shows an area of hyperintensity in right mastoid sinus (*arrow*) and cerebellar hemisphere (*arrowhead*)

Mastoiditis with Sigmoid Thrombosis

Definition

Clot formation in sigmoid sinuses as a result of mastoiditis.

Clinical Features

- Mastoiditis is a known cause of lateral venous sinus thrombosis.
- Sinus thrombosis may occur via direct extension or be the result of erosive osteitis and retrograde thrombophlebitis.
- Symptoms due to sinus thrombosis are variable: asymptomatic to coma or death.
- May present with headache, nausea/vomiting or seizure.
- Hemorrhagic venous infarct may develop secondary to poor venous drainage.

Imaging Features

- Non-contrast CT images: middle ear and mastoid completely opacified and mastoid air cells become confluent. May show hyperdense sigmoid sinuses.
- Post-contrast CT images: filling defect in sigmoid sinus, useful to diagnose intra- or extracranial abscess.
- Contrast MRI and MR venography are best to diagnose sinus thrombosis and intracranial complications (venous infarct, meningitis and abscess).
- On diffusion-weighted imaging, abscesses show hyperintensity with restricted diffusion.

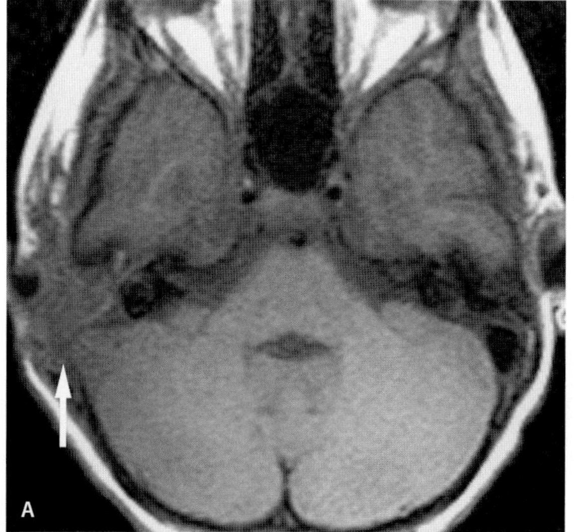

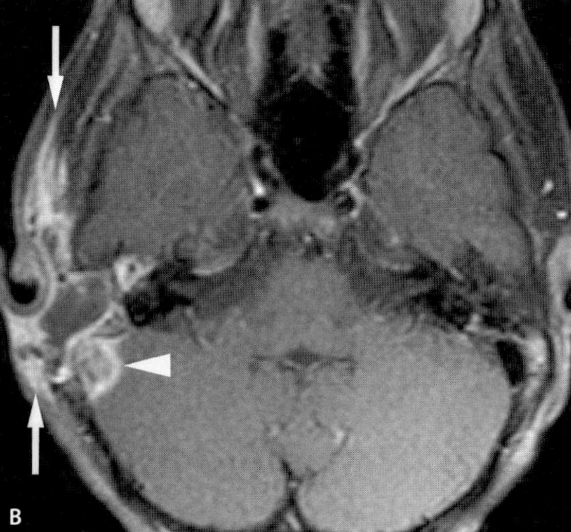

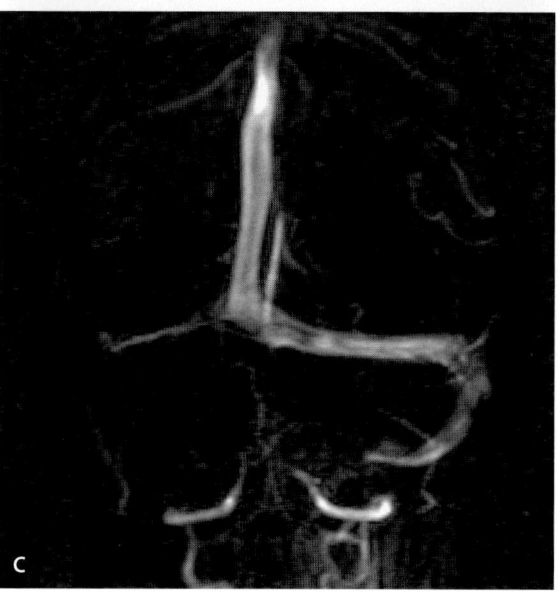

Figure 13.32

Mastoiditis with sigmoid thrombosis; 7-year-old female with a chronic right draining ear. A Axial T1-weighted MRI shows soft-tissue mass in right temporal bone (*arrow*). There is no flow void in sigmoid sinus on this side. B Axial T1-weighted fat-suppressed post-Gd MRI demonstrates abnormal contrast enhancement in area of right temporal bone (*arrows*). In sigmoid sinus there is contrast enhancement in periphery but a central filling defect suggesting a clot (*arrowhead*). C Coronal MR venogram demonstrates lack of flow in right sigmoid sinus

Osteoradionecrosis Involving Skull Base

Definition

Nonvital bone in a site of radiation injury.

Clinical Features

- Serious complication of radiation therapy for neoplasms of the parotid gland, oral cavity, oropharynx, and nasopharynx.
- Predominantly in mandible.
- The risk is greatest during the first 6 to 12 months after radiation therapy, but osteoradionecrosis may develop several years later.
- Clinical diagnosis of mandibular osteoradionecrosis is primarily based on clinical symptoms and signs of ulceration or necrosis of the overlying mucous membrane with exposure of necrotic bone.
- Pathologic fracture and orocutaneous fistula may be seen.

Imaging Features

- CT image with bone window shows cortical disruption and fragmentation.
- T1-weighted MRI: decreased marrow signal.
- T2-weighted MRI: increased marrow signal.
- Can be associated with significant soft-tissue thickening and enhancement in adjacent masticator muscles

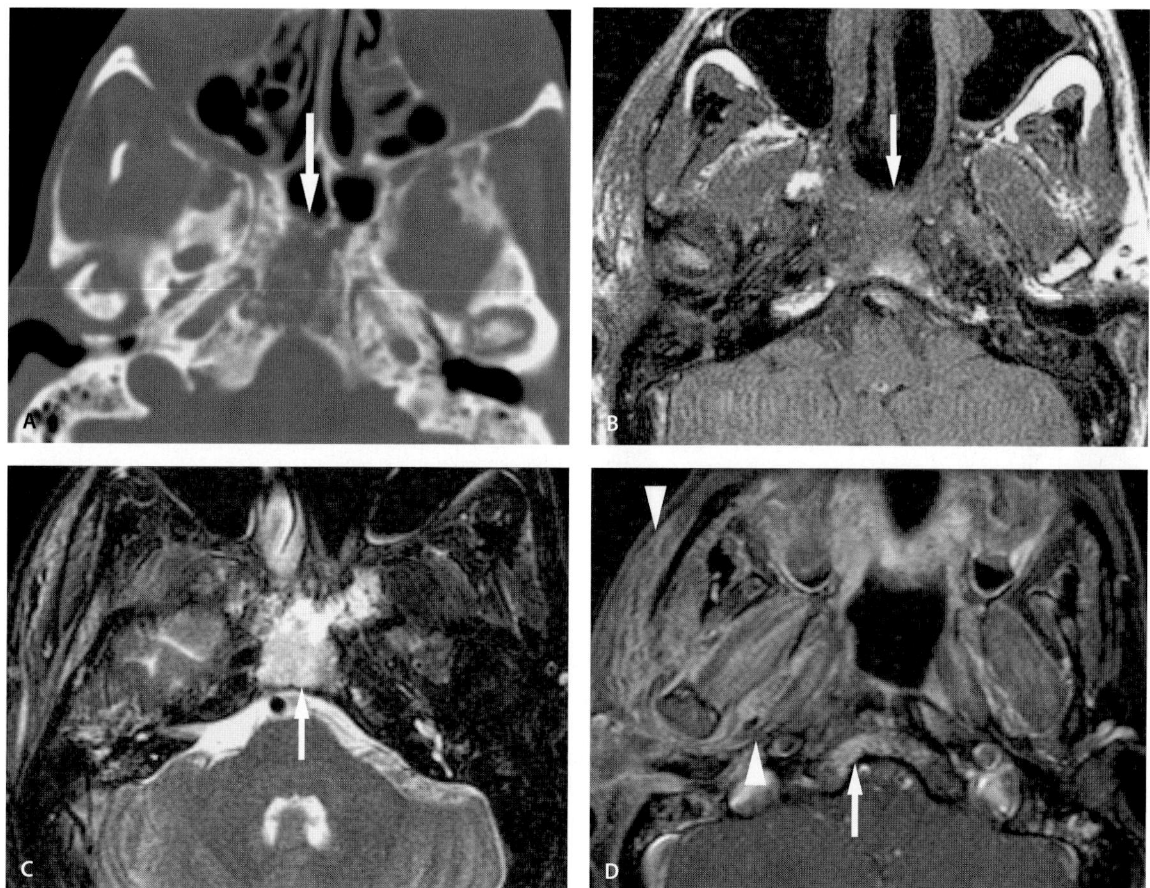

Figure 13.33

Osteoradionecrosis; 42-year-old male status postradiation treatment for nasopharyngeal cancer. **A** Axial CT image shows lytic and osteosclerotic changes of skull base bone (*arrow*). **B** Axial T1-weighted MRI shows hypointense lesion (*arrow*). **C** Axial T2-weightd fat-suppressed MRI shows hyperintensity (*arrow*). **D** Axial T1-weighted fat-suppressed post-Gd MRI shows diffuse enhancement within clivus (*arrow*) and right masticator and buccal space (*arrowheads*)

Langerhans Cell Histiocytosis

Definition

A spectrum of disorders with histiocytic proliferation involving bone and soft tissue.

Clinical Features

- Classified according to sites of involvement into single or multisystem disease.
- Usually presents in first decade.
- Bony involvement is seen in 78% of cases and often includes skull (49%), innominate bone, femur, orbit (11%), and ribs.
- Infiltration in temporal bone presents with conductive hearing loss and draining ear.
- Frequently diagnosed only after treatment with antibiotics fails to cure a suspected middle ear or mastoid infection.

Imaging Features

- External auditory canal and mastoid are common locations.
- Bone margins are geographic and moderately well defined. "Punched-out" borders also may be found.
- Early imaging findings mimic inflammatory disease.
- Post-contrast CT or MRI help to differentiate inflammatory mastoid lesions.
- On CT images or MRI, enhancement within lesion may be homogeneous or may occur only in periphery.

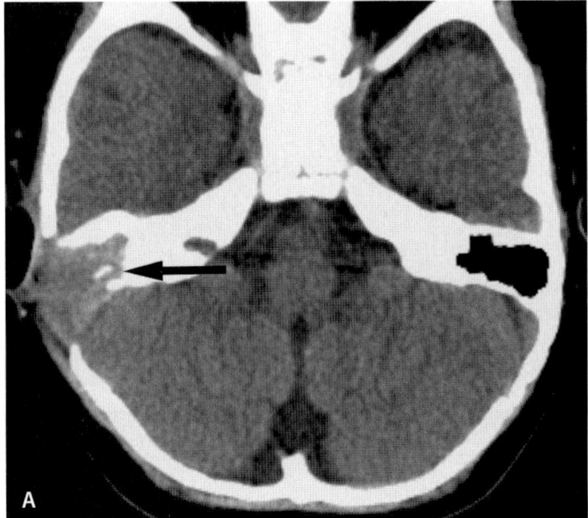

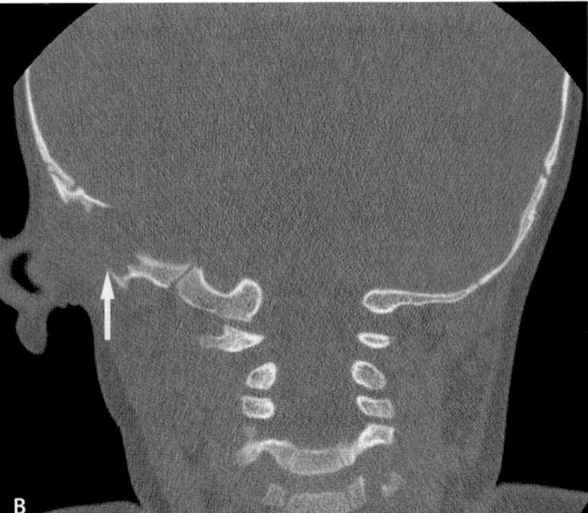

Figure 13.34

Langerhans cell histiocytosis; 1-year-old male who has had two episodes of otitis media and a recent onset of right auricular swelling. **A** Axial CT image shows soft-tissue mass with opacification and destruction of right mastoid air cells (*arrow*). **B** Coronal CT image with bone window shows irregular "geographic" border with complete loss of portions of mastoid cortex (*arrow*)

Fibrous Dysplasia

Definition

Progressive replacement of normal cancellous bone by poorly organized fibro-osseous tissue.

Clinical Features

- Usually seen in young age group (<30 years old).
- Symptoms depended on the lesion location.
- Monostotic: 70% of cases, single osseous site is affected.
- Polyostotic: 25% of cases, involves more than two separated sites.
- Usually self-limiting, often does not progress after third decade of life.
- McCune-Albright syndrome: a variant that consists of polyostotic fibrous dysplasia, skin pigmentation and sexual precocity.

Imaging Features

- Affects any bone including skull, skull base and facial bones.
- Bone CT imaging is best for diagnosis showing expansile lesion centered in medullary space with variable attenuation.
- Ground-glass matrix in expansile bone lesion is typical.
- Abrupt or gradual transition zone between lesion and normal bone.
- T1- and T2-weighted MRI: low signal.
- T1-weighted post-Gd MRI: variable enhancement of internal matrix

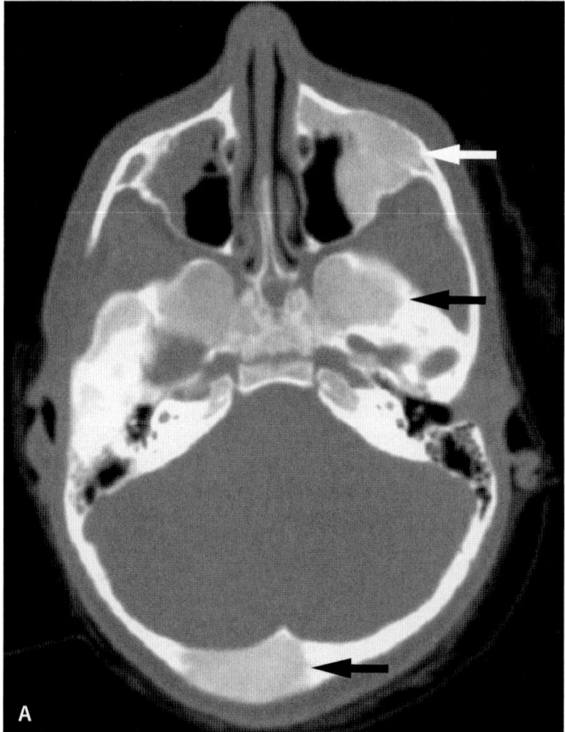

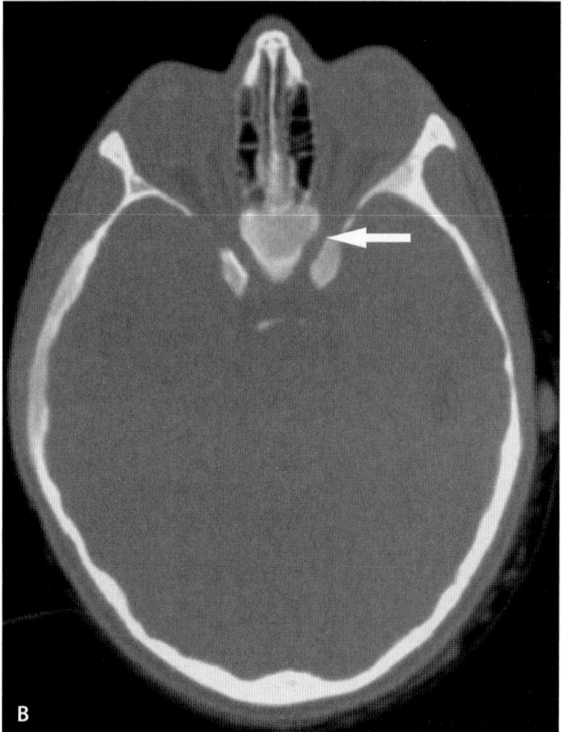

Figure 13.35

Fibrous dysplasia; 4-year-old female with facial deformity. A Axial CT image with bone window shows ground-glass appearance of left maxillary sinus (*white arrow*), left skull base (*black arrow*) and right occipital bone (*posterior black arrow*). B Axial CT image with bone window, more cranial, shows ground-glass appearance of sphenoid bone with mild narrowing of left optic canal (*arrow*)

Giant Aneurysm of Skull Base

Definition

Aneurysms involving the skull base.

Clinical Features

- Most aneurysms are acquired and spontaneous; some occur after infection, trauma or local surgery. There is a small genetic predisposition.
- Pressure on the nerves in the cavernous sinus can lead to ophthalmoplegia or facial pain.
- Hemorrhage is unusual.
- Can rupture into the sphenoid sinus, into the subarachnoid space or into the cavernous sinus.

Imaging Features

- Large aneurysms may erode the skull base.
- Imaging of large aneurysms is varied and depends on the patency of the lumen and the presence of thrombosis.
- A dynamic scan's arterial phase may help separate the aneurysm from the normal cavernous sinus.
- Calcification can be present in the aneurysm's wall.

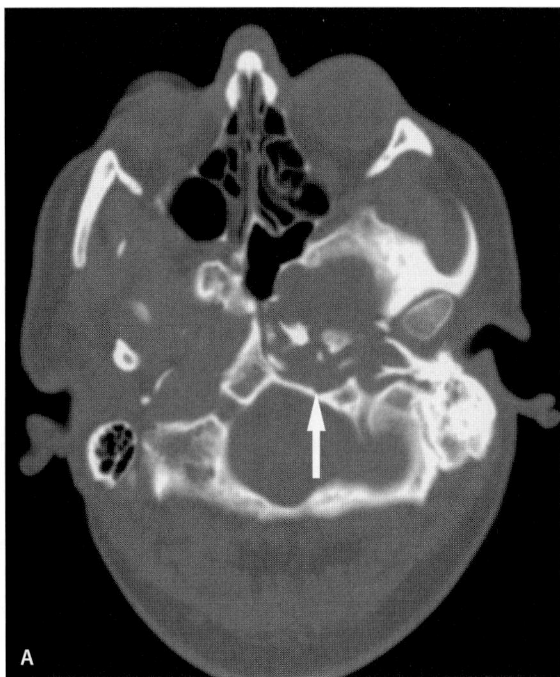

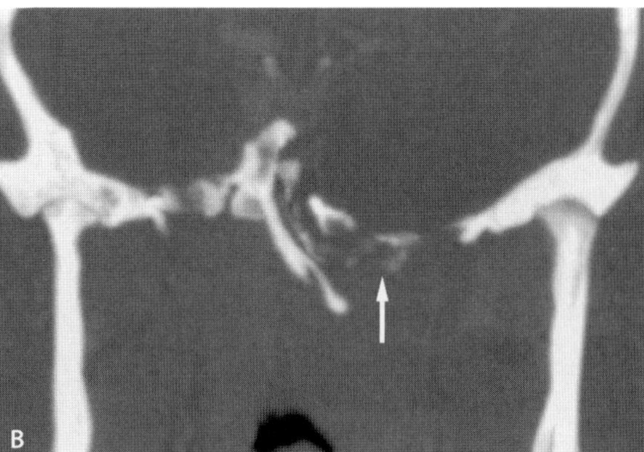

Figure 13.36

Giant aneurysm in skull base; 33-year-old male with history of carotid aneurysm treated using balloon and coils with complete occlusion of left internal carotid artery. A Axial CT image, bone window, shows erosion of left middle cranial fossa due to a large aneurysm (*arrow*). Lumen of aneurysm is completely occluded. B Coronal CT image confirms severe bone destruction (*arrow*)

Glomus Vagale Paraganglioma

Definition

Benign vascular tumor arising from neural crest paraganglion cells associated with nodose ganglia of vagus nerve.

Clinical Features

- Depending on the location of the paraganglioma, the tumor is named carotid body tumor, glomus vagale, glomus jugulare, or glomus tympanicum.
- Usually fourth to fifth decade; slight female dominance.
- Can occur sporadically or as autosomal dominant familial tumor.
- Presents with vagal neuropathy, hoarseness, Horner syndrome (glomus vagale).

Imaging Features

- Located in nasopharyngeal carotid space.
- Displace parapharyngeal fat anteriorly and internal carotid artery anteromedially.
- Usually solitary lesions at one site.
- Highly vascular and intensely enhancing mass.
- May contain areas of hemorrhage and necrosis.
- T1-weighted MRI: characteristic salt and pepper appearance due to flow (pepper) and hyperintensity due to hemorrhage (salt).

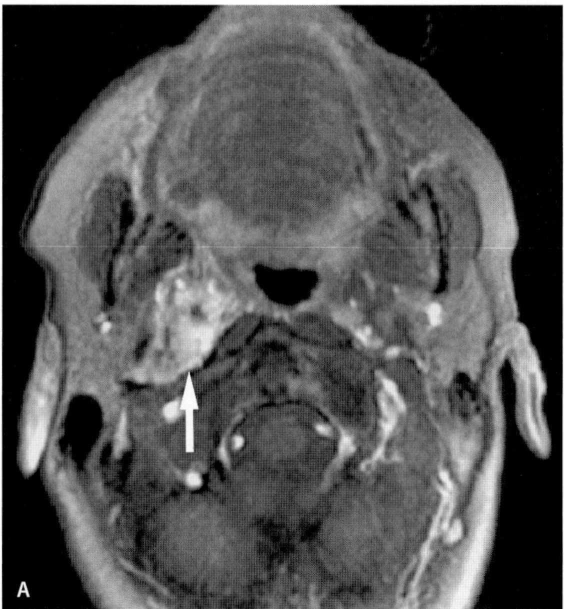

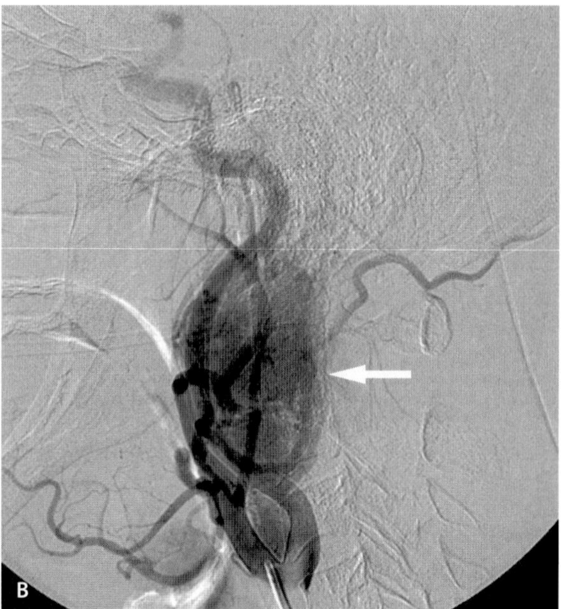

Figure 13.37

Glomus vagale paraganglioma; 54-year-old female with symptoms of dysphagia. There was a palpable mass on the right side of the neck. **A** Axial T1-weighted post-Gd MRI demonstrates enhancing mass in right carotid space (*arrow*), consistent with paraganglioma. **B** Right common carotid angiogram demonstrates large vascular mass (*arrow*)

Craniopharyngioma

Definition

Benign tumor derived from remnants of Rathke's pouch.

There are two types: adamantinomatous and papillary.

Clinical Features

- Bimodal age distribution (peak 5–15 years; papillary type >50 years).
- Pediatric patient with morning headache, visual defect, short stature.
- Endocrine disturbances.
- Hydrocephalus.

Imaging Features

- Typically found in suprasellar location.
- Heterogeneous appearance with calcification and cystic component.
- T1-weighted MRI: signal varies with cyst contents.
- T1-weighted post-Gd MRI: solid portions are enhanced heterogeneously.

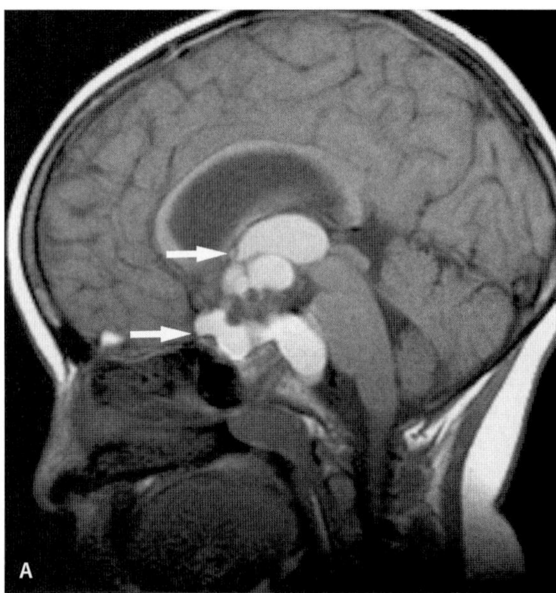

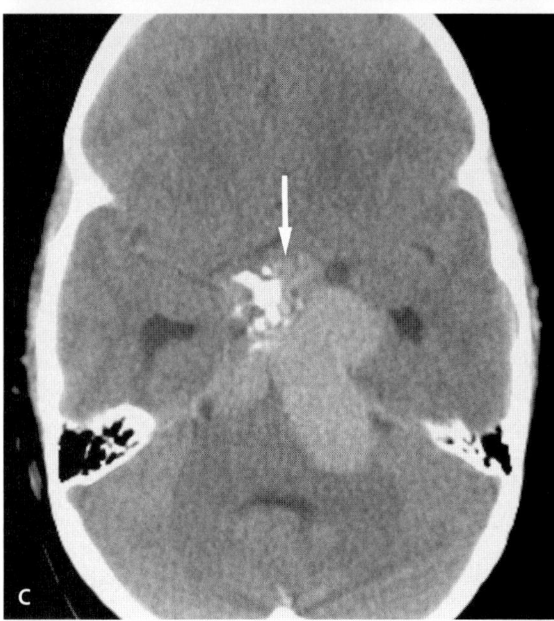

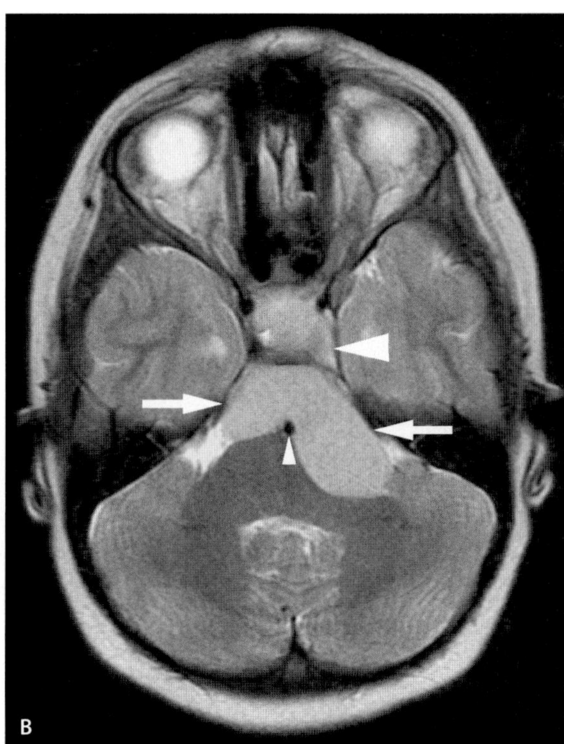

Figure 13.38

Craniopharyngioma; 7-year-old female with history of longstanding headache. A Sagittal T1-weighted MRI shows a large lobulated sellar/suprasellar mass extending upwards to third ventricle and posteriorly into prepontine cistern (*arrows*). Most cysts show hyperintensity. B Axial T2-weighted MRI shows extension into cerebellopontine angles more to left (*arrows*) with left parasellar extension (*arrowhead*) and encasement of basilar artery (*small arrowhead*). C Axial CT shows eccentrically located calcification within a hyperdense lobulated mass at suprasellar region (*arrow*)

Pituitary Macroadenoma Invading Skull Base

Definition

Pituitary macroadenoma with inferior extension to sphenoid sinus and clivus.

Clinical Features

- Pituitary hormonal abnormality
- Visual field defect and cranial nerve palsy
- Benign and slow-growing

Imaging Features

- Expansion of sella with invasion of surrounding adjacent structures.
- Bony margins are usually smooth.
- On MRI, sellar-infrasellar mass invading basisphenoid and basiocciput.
- May extend into cavernous sinus and encase internal carotid artery.
- Enhancement is necessary to evaluate the tumor extension.

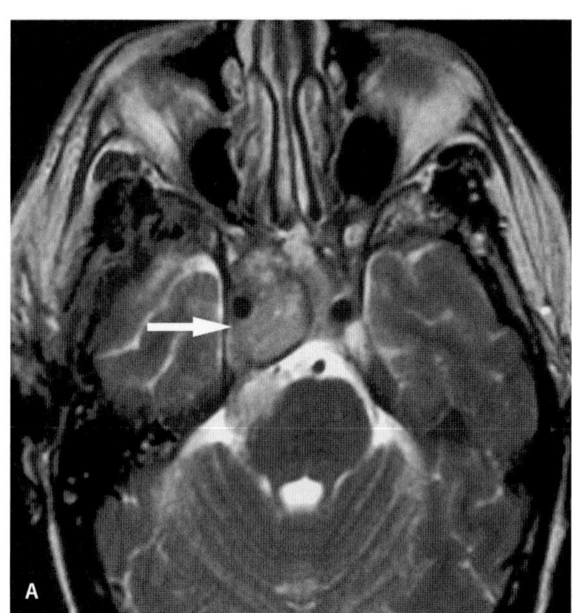

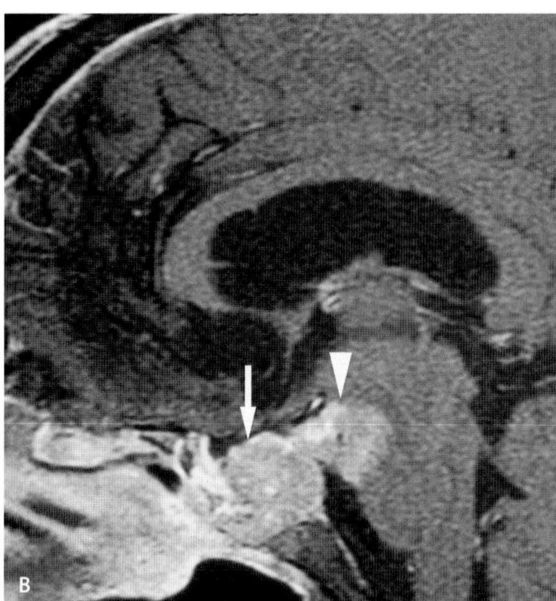

Figure 13.39

Pituitary macroadenoma; 53-year-old male with visual disturbance. A Axial T2-weighted MRI shows heterogeneous large mass in sella and right cavernous sinus (*arrow*). Mass extends posteriorly into brainstem causing compression of brainstem. B Sagittal T1-weighted post-Gd MRI shows mass expanding sella and extending up to superior portion of sphenoid sinus and clivus (*arrow*). Posteriorly mass extends into brainstem causing compression of brainstem (*arrowhead*). C Coronal T1-weighted post-Gd MRI shows mass extending into right cavernous sinus (*arrow*) with encasement of internal carotid artery (*arrowhead*)

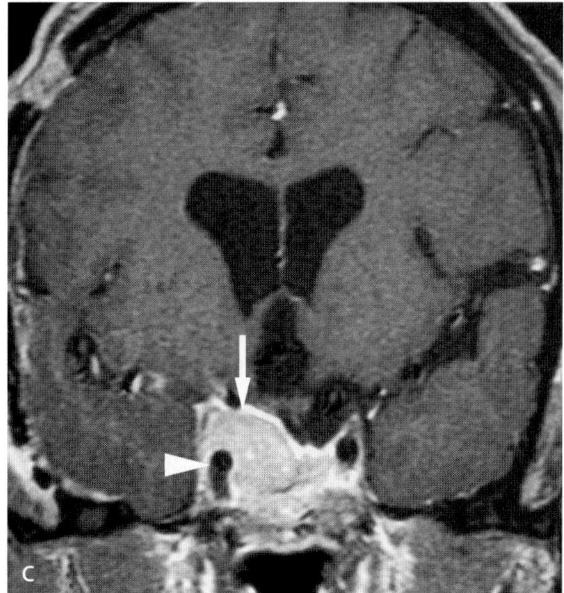

Trigeminal Schwannoma

Definition

Benign encapsulated tumor of Schwann cell arising from trigeminal nerve.

Clinical Features

- Trigeminal nerve is most commonly affected in central skull base.
- Asymptomatic mass in deep facial soft tissue.
- May present with facial pain, decreased sensation and masticator muscle weakness and/or atrophy.
- Predominantly third or fourth decade.

Imaging Features

- Arises in Meckel's cave or in cistern along course of nerve.
- Rarely arises below skull base.
- Extension is common through foramen ovale and foramen rotundum, and CT imaging with bone window is best to see smooth margin of an expanded foramen.
- May have a dumbbell shape with components enlarging cavernous sinus and protruding into posterior cranial fossa.
- Cystic changes or necrosis typical of larger lesions.
- T1-weighted post-Gd fat-suppressed MRI, axial and coronal, are best to see tumor extension.

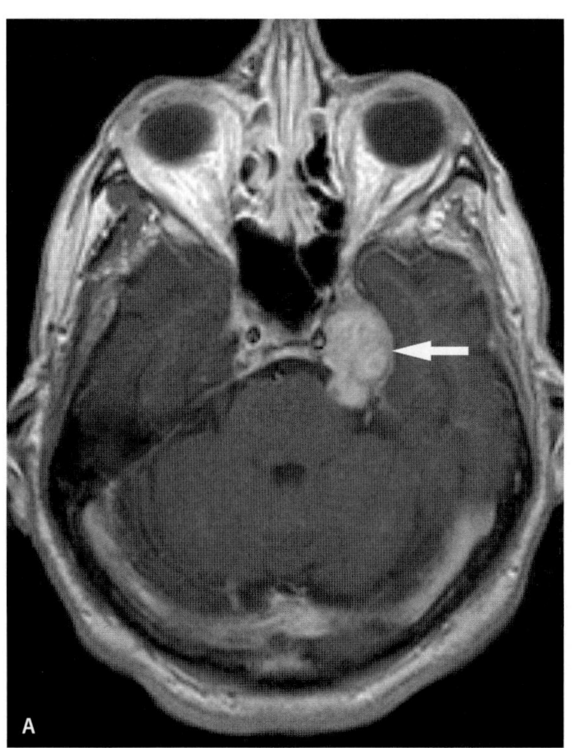

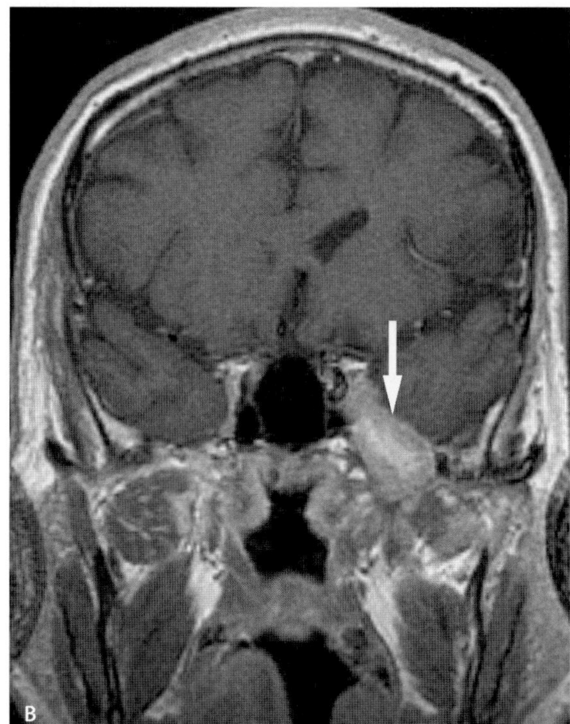

Figure 13.40

Trigeminal schwannoma; 70-year-old male with memory loss and seizures. A Axial T1-weighted post-Gd MRI shows enlarged mass (*arrow*) in wall of left cavernous sinus. B Coronal T1-weighted post-Gd MRI shows mass extending through foramen ovale (*arrow*)

Metastatic Disease to Hypoglossal Canal and Clivus

Definition

Metastatic disease from extracranial primary tumor to skull base.

Clinical Features

- Skull base tumor can be primary or metastatic.
- Hematogenous metastasis from primary tumors in lung, kidney, breast, prostate, and a variety of other rare locations.
- Neurologic symptoms depend on location of metastatic tumor.
- If the hypoglossal canal is affected, symptoms may be difficulty in swallowing (dysphagia) and speech (dysarthria).
- Treatments for skull base tumors can be divided into medical, radiation, and surgical.

Imaging Features

- CT with bone window most useful to evaluate bone destruction.
- Sclerotic changes may be present in prostate metastasis.
- T1-weighted MRI is sensitive for bone metastasis.
- T1-weighted post-Gd MRI: fat saturation necessary to distinguish enhancement from normal hyperintense marrow or fat.

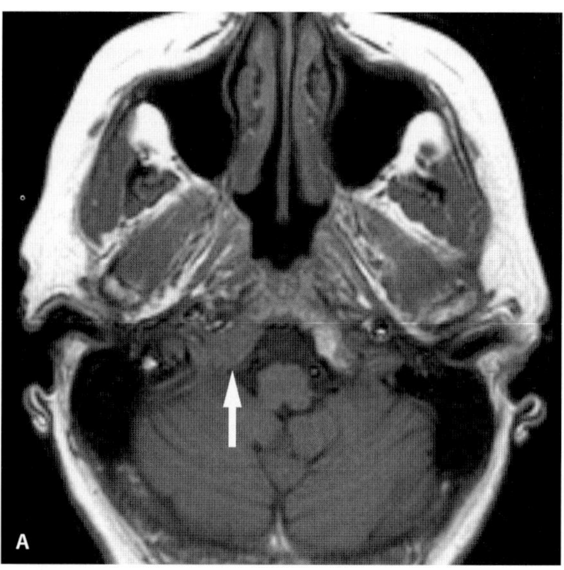

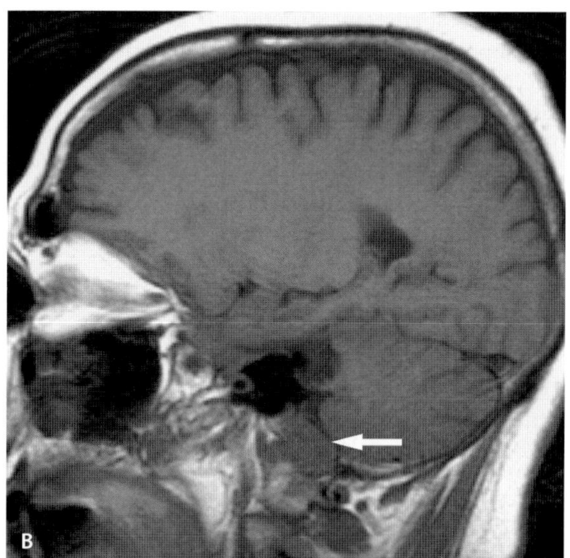

Figure 13.41

Metastatic disease; 55-year-old female with breast cancer presented with swallowing difficulties. A Axial T1-weighted MRI demonstrates well-circumscribed hypointense lesion involving right clivus and hypoglossal canal (*arrow*). B Sagittal T1-weighted MRI confirms well-circumscribed mass (*arrow*). C Axial T1-weighted post-Gd MRI demonstrates evident enhancement of tumor (*arrow*)

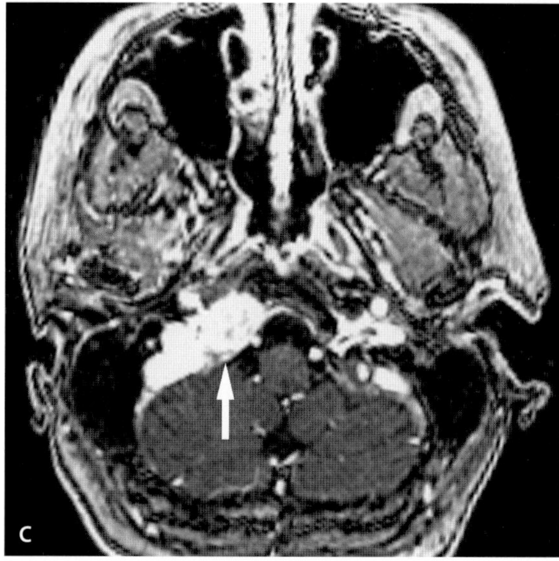

Orbit

Orbital pathology is in many respects completely different from that seen in the maxillofacial area. Imaging of the orbit is done after a thorough clinical examination. The clinical examination can diagnose conditions of the globe with high accuracy, but anything that is posterior to the globe is difficult to diagnosis clinically, often prompting imaging of the orbit. Both CT and MR imaging are used and in general CT imaging is the first choice for trauma and bony pathology whereas MR imaging is the superior technique for soft-tissue abnormalities. Again, it is not the intention in this section of this chapter on adjacent structures to give a full description of orbital conditions, but rather to alert the maxillofacial radiologist as to what may be going on in the orbit which is the closest adjacent structure to the maxillofacial area superiorly and laterally.

Orbital Infectious Disease

Definition

Orbital bacterial infection.

Clinical Features

- Orbital bacterial infection include retention edema of the eyelid, preseptal cellulitis, preseptal abscess, orbital cellulitis, orbital abscess, subperiosteal abscess and cavernous sinus thrombosis.
- The majority are of paranasal sinus origin.
- May develop from infectious processes of face or pharynx, trauma, foreign bodies, or septicemia.
- Presents with orbital edema and painful proptosis with fever.
- Rapidly progressive, potentially blinding diseases.

Imaging Features

- Post-contrast CT imaging is first-line modality and shows inflammation and rim-enhancing hypodense fluid collection.
- Post-contrast MRI is best to assess intracranial complications (meningitis, subdural empyema, cerebritis, or brain abscess).
- On diffusion-weighted imaging, abscess shows hyperintensity.

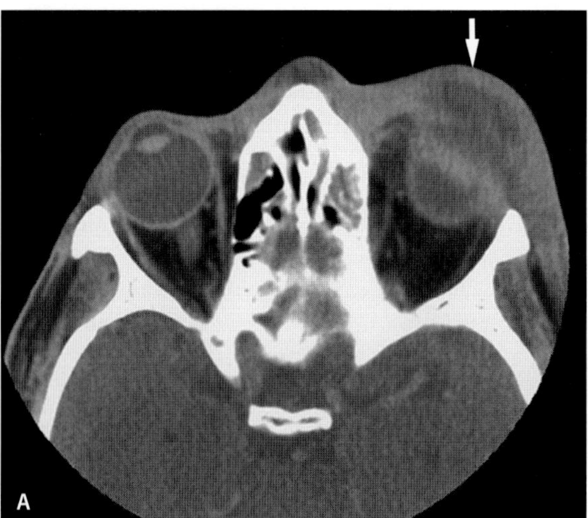

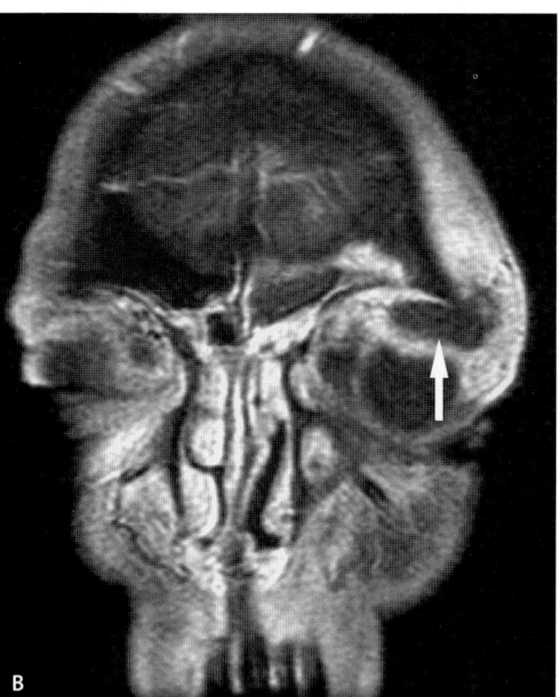

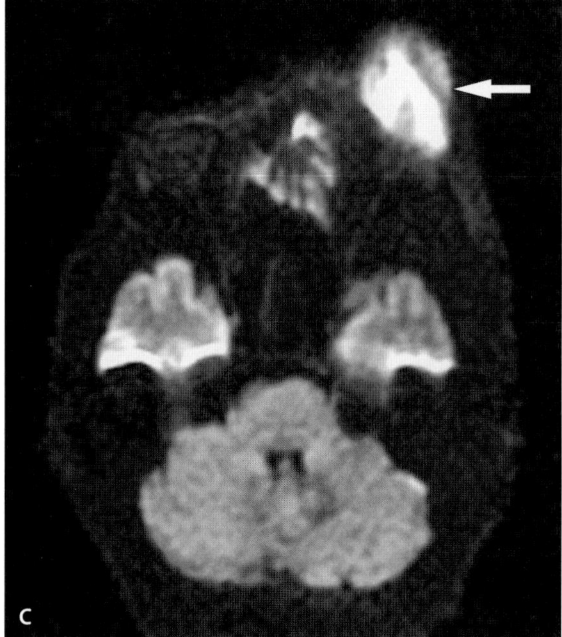

Figure 13.42

Orbital abscess; 26-year-old male with periorbital pain and swelling. A Axial post-contrast CT image demonstrates soft-tissue thickening and inflammatory changes in left periorbital region with a rounded nonenhancing soft-tissue lesion in left upper eyelid (*arrow*) consistent with abscess. Mucosal thickening of ethmoid sinus is also present and may be the source of this abscess. B Coronal T1-weighted fat-suppressed post-Gd MRI shows diffuse enhancement within soft tissue of left periorbital region and nonenhanced fluid collection (*arrow*). Mucosal thickening of frontal sinus is also observed. C On diffusion-weighted imaging, abscess shows very high signal intensity (*arrow*) due to restricted diffusion

Dacryocystocele, Nasolacrimal Duct

Definition

Cystic dilatation of nasolacrimal apparatus resulting from stenosis of the nasolacrimal duct.

Clinical Features

- Present in adults (congenital dacryocystocele is seen in infancy).
- History of dacryocystitis or neoplastic stenosis, prior nasoorbital/nasoethmoidal trauma or surgery.
- Intranasal mass representing inferior extension of cystocele.

Imaging Features

- Medial canthus cyst on CT images
- Enlarged osseous nasolacrimal canal
- Intranasal mass representing inferior extension of cystocele.

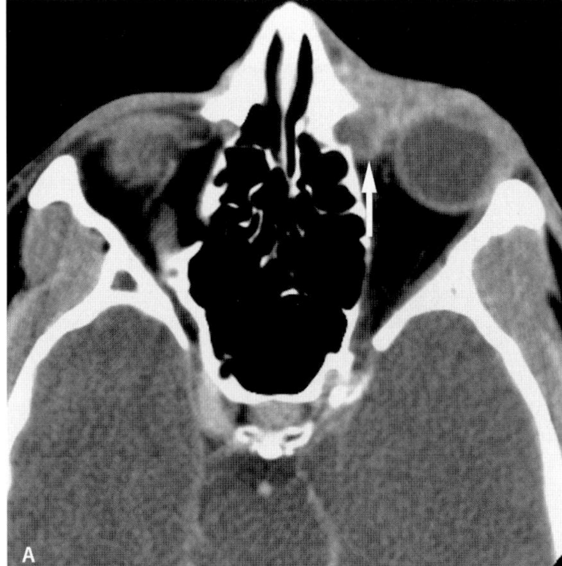

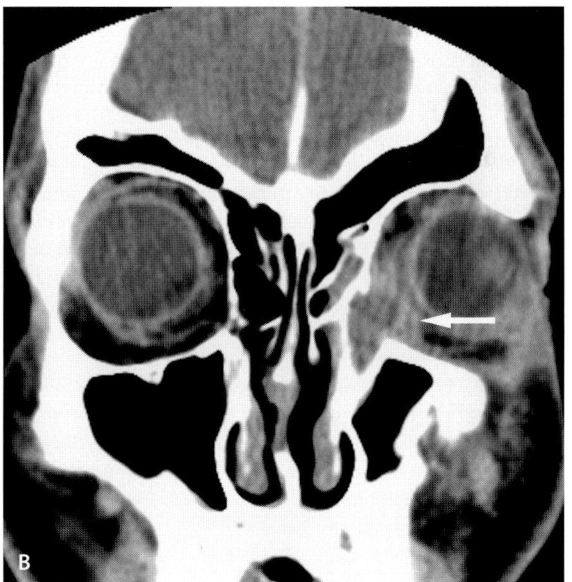

Figure 13.43

Dacrocystocele; 43-year-old female with periorbital recurrent swelling. Axial (**A**) and coronal (**B**) post-contrast CT images show left periorbital soft-tissue swelling representing orbital cellulitis. Osseous nasolacrimal canal is enlarged and rim-enhancing cystic mass is observed in medial canthus which is an infected nasolacrimal cystocele (*arrows*)

Dermoid

Definition

Cystic lesion of orbit resulting from inclusion of ectodermal elements during closure of neural tube.

Dermoid: epithelial elements plus dermal substructures.

Epidermoid: epithelial elements only.

Clinical Features

- Most common developmental cysts involving orbit and periorbital structures.
- Painless firm subcutaneous mass.
- Diplopia if larger.
- Childhood presentation more common than adult.
- Sudden growth or change may occur following rupture.

Imaging Features

- Cystic, well-demarcated, extraconal mass.
- Commonest location is superior temporal aspect of orbit at frontozygomatic suture, but can occur anywhere in orbit.
- On CT images, both epidermoid and dermoid cysts appear as a nonenhancing, low-density mass.
- Calcifications may be seen.
- May have a fat density.
- T1- weighted MRI: usually low signal, but may be hyperintense if fat containing
- T2-weighted MRI: high signal
- Diffusion-weighted imaging: typically high intensity.

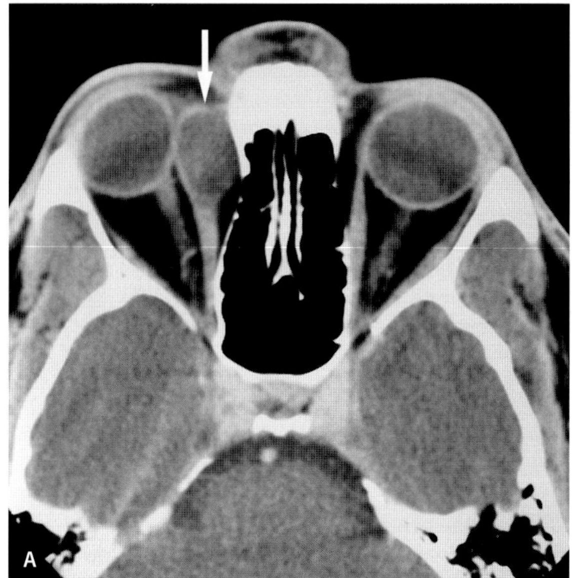

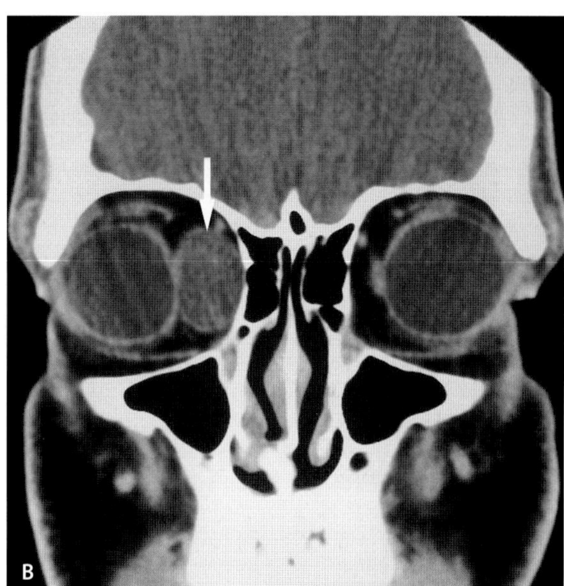

Figure 13.44

Dermoid; young male with palpable lesion over nasal bridge. Axial (A) and coronal (B) non-contrast CT images show well-demarcated, thin-walled mass (*arrows*) in supranasal wall of right orbit

Fibrous Dysplasia

Definition

Progressive replacement of normal cancellous bone by poorly organized fibro-osseous tissue.

Clinical Features

- Usually seen in young age group (<30 years).
- Orbital lesion: optic neuropathy due to optic nerve compression in optic canal.
- Monostotic: 70% of cases, single osseous site is affected.
- Polyostotic: 25% of cases, involves more than two separated sites.
- Usually self-limiting and often does not progress after third decade of life.
- McCune-Albright syndrome is a variant that consists of polyostotic fibrous dysplasia, skin pigmentation and sexual precocity.
- Surgical treatment for optic nerve decompression and for limited cosmetic debulking and re-contouring of bone.

Imaging Features

- Affects any bone including skull, skull base and facial bones.
- Bone CT imaging is best for diagnosis showing expansile lesion centered in medullary space with variable attenuation.
- Ground-glass matrix in expansile bone lesion is typical.
- Abrupt or gradual transition zone between lesion and normal bone.
- T1- and T2-weighted MRI: usually low signal.
- T2-weighted MRI: occasionally high signal simulating a tumor.
- T1-weighted post-Gd MRI: variable enhancement of internal matrix.

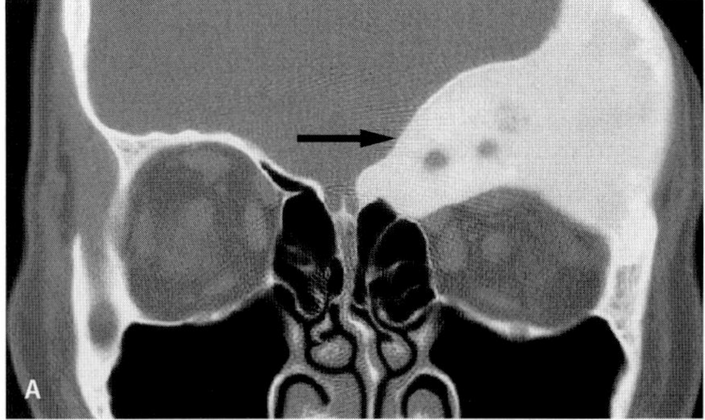

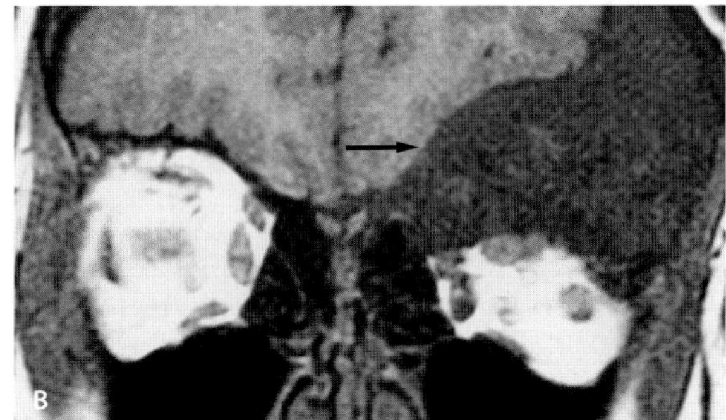

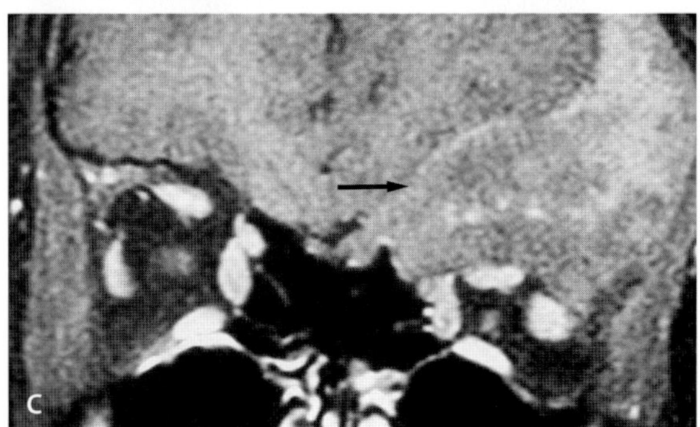

Figure 13.45

Fibrous dysplasia; 17-year-old presents with painless prominence in left supraorbital region. A Coronal CT image shows dense expansile greater wing of sphenoid bone on left side. Orbital cavity is compressed (*arrow*). B T1-weighted MRI shows low signal intensity from fibrous lesion in greater wing of sphenoid bone on left side consistent with fibrous dysplasia (*arrow*). C T1-weighted post-Gd MRI shows heterogeneous enhancement in expanded greater wing of sphenoid bone (*arrow*)

Langerhans Cell Histiocytosis

Definition

A benign spectrum of disorders with histiocytic proliferation involving the orbit.

Clinical Features

- Unifocal Langerhans cell histiocytosis.
- Presents with orbital pain, swelling and proptosis.
- Usually presents in first decade.
- Management is usually conservative, and spontaneous healing may occur.

Imaging Features

- Most common orbital manifestation is a solitary osseous lesion.
- Orbital soft-tissue involvement without an obvious bony defect is rare.
- On CT images, homogeneously hyperdense enhancing mass with bony erosion or destruction.
- T1-weighted MRI: isointense.
- T2-weighted MRI: minimally to moderately hyperintense.
- T1-weighted post-Gd MRI: enhancement.
- Differential diagnosis includes lacrimal gland tumors, rhabdomyosarcomas, metastatic neuroblastoma and lymphoproliferative disease.

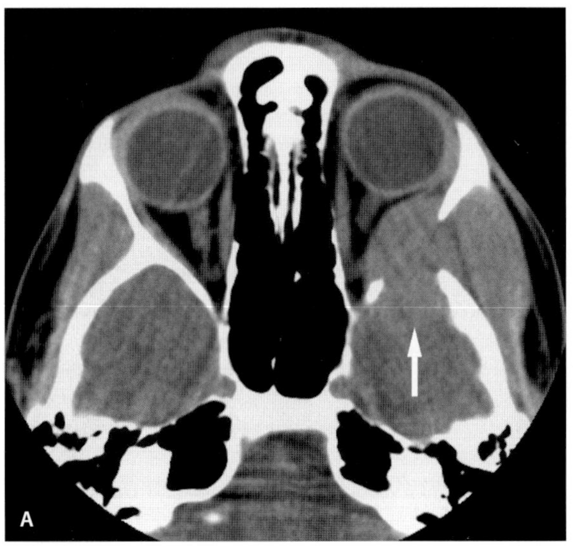

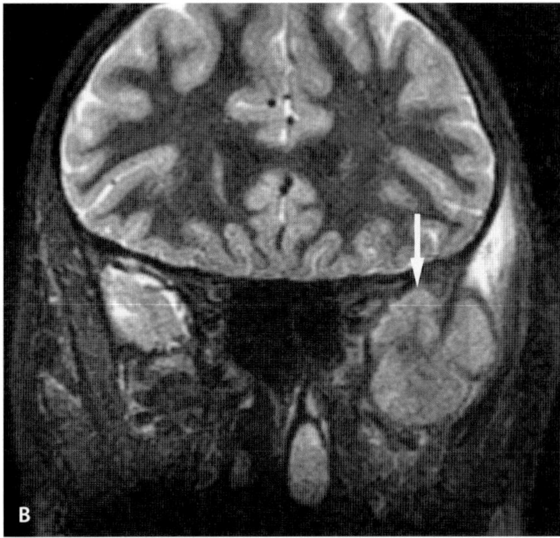

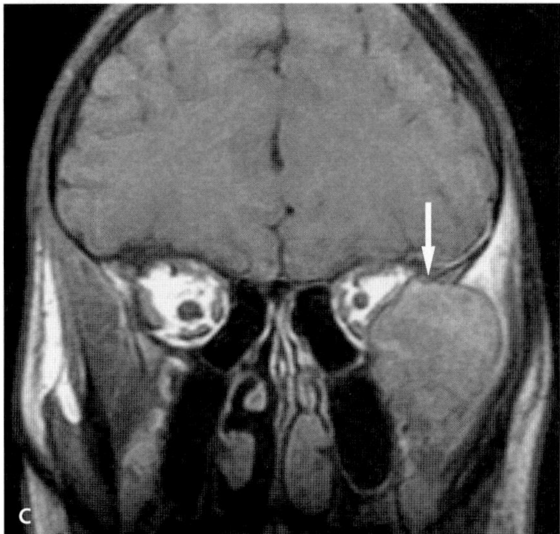

Figure 13.46

Langerhans cell histiocytosis of orbit; 14-year-old male with two weeks of headache, now with periorbital swelling. Clinical question of infection or mass. A Axial CT image shows homogeneous soft-tissue mass (*arrow*) without calcification in retroorbital and greater sphenoid space. There is a punched-out bony lesion involving sphenoid wing and posterior wall of left orbit. B Coronal STIR MRI image demonstrates a well-defined hyperintense mass (*arrow*) in left lateral wall of orbit. The mass extends into left orbit and deviates left lateral rectus muscle. C Coronal T1-weighted post-Gd MRI (*arrow*) shows diffuse enhancement of mass

Neurofibromatosis

Definition

Orbital manifestations associated with neurofibromatosis type 1 (NF-1).

Clinical Features

- Plexiform neurofibroma and optic nerve glioma are typical orbital manifestations in NF-1.
- Café-au-lait spots are earliest sign and noted during first year and tumors begin to appear in childhood.
- Presents with eyelid, periorbital and facial soft-tissue masses, proptosis and ptosis.
- Malignant transformation uncommon.

Imaging Features

- Plexiform neurofibromas are nonencapsulated infiltrative masses involving cranial nerve, muscle, optic nerve sheath, and sclera.
- T1-weighting MRI: signal intensity of plexiform neurofibromas similar to that of muscle
- T2-weighted MRI: often high
- T1-weighted post-Gd MRI: contrast enhancement usually intense.
- May be associated with sphenoid dysplasia, buphthalmos and optic canal and/or orbital fissure enlargement.
- Optic nerve glioma.

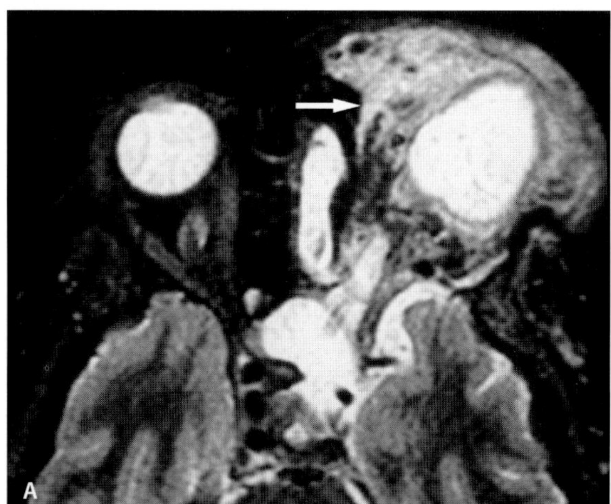

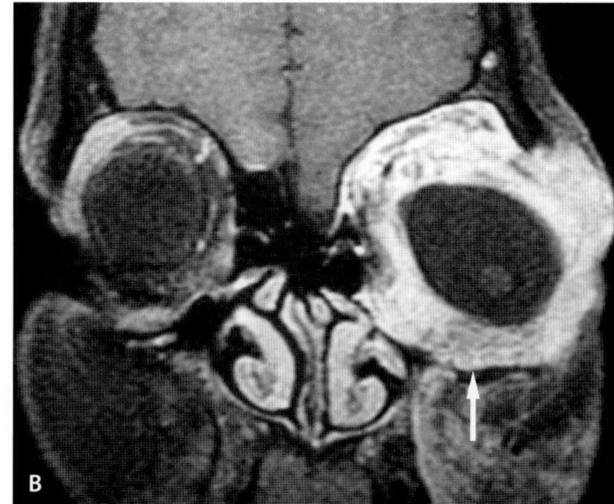

Figure 13.47

Plexiform neurofibroma; 30-year-old with known neurofibromatosis presenting with periorbital swelling. A Axial T2-weighted MRI shows a large infiltrative mass in left orbit deforming globe and extending into retro-orbital area. There are large flow voids in this highly vascular mass (*arrow*). B Coronal T1-weighted post-Gd MRI shows enhancing mass encasing and deforming globe (*arrow*)

Hemangioma

Definition

Benign angioma consisting of a mass of blood vessels.

Clinical Features

- Most common vascular tumor seen in infancy.
- Most prevalent in head and neck region and constitutes 18–38% of head and neck tumors.
- Diagnosis of hemangioma is made by a combination of medical history, physical examination and imaging including ultrasound, CT and MRI.
- Typical hemangiomas are red, raised and bosselated.
- Deep hemangiomas have normal overlying skin and may mimic other vascular malformations.
- Congenital hemangiomas typically show rapid growth and may involute completely.

Imaging Features

- On CT images, hemangiomas are seen as lobulated solid masses that are isodense with muscle and show intense enhancement.
- T1-weighted MRI: usually intermediate signal intensity
- T2-weighted MRI: high signal intensity
- T1-weighted post-Gd MRI: diffuse intense enhancement.
- Hemangiomas need to be differentiated from arteriovenous malformations which are also associated with prominent vascularity.

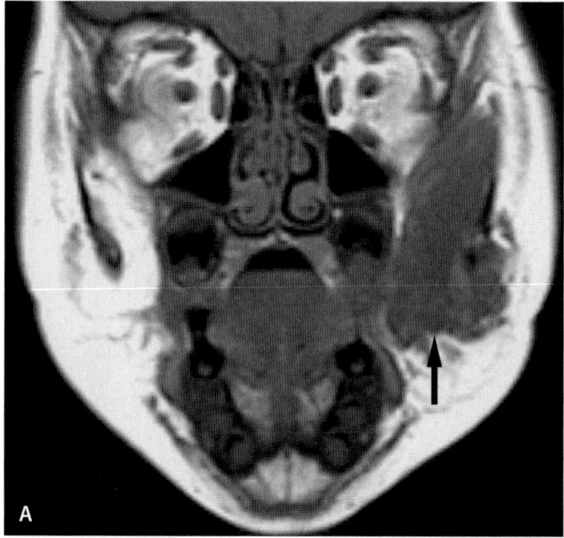

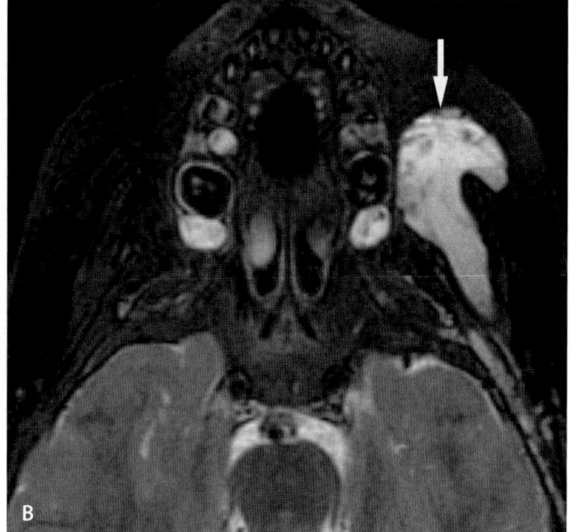

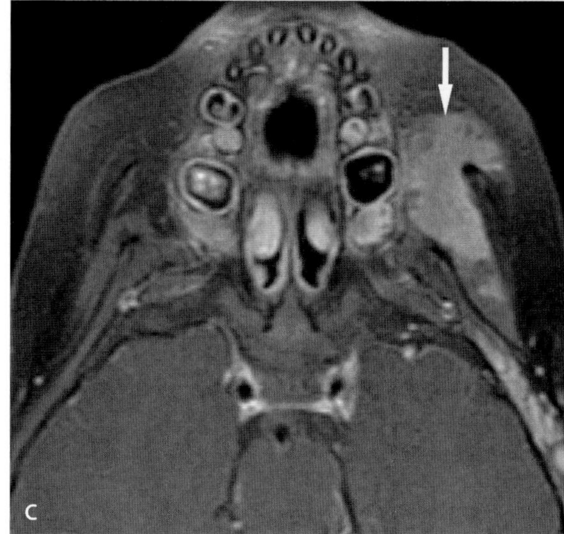

Figure 13.48

Hemangioma; 4-month old presenting with periorbital mass. A Coronal T1-weighted MRI shows left periorbital and cheek soft-tissue mass (*arrow*). B Axial T2-weighted fat-suppressed MRI shows hyperintensity-demonstrating precise outline of mass and left facial structures (*arrow*). C Axial T1-weighted fat-suppressed post-Gd MRI shows diffuse enhancement of soft-tissue hemangioma (*arrow*)

Meningioma

Definition
Meningioma of the intraorbital optic nerve sheath.

Clinical Features
- Slow, painless progressive unilateral visual loss and proptosis.
- Usually middle age. Younger age patients may be associated with NF-2.
- Female predominance.
- Treatment includes stereotactic radiotherapy or surgery.

Imaging Features
- Enhancing mass surrounding intraorbital optic nerve.
- Linear or punctate calcification is characteristic.
- T1-weighted MRI: isointense.
- T2-weighted MRI: hyper- to hypointense.
- T1-weighted post-Gd MRI: best with fat suppression to see extension of tumor and to characterize tumor relative to adjacent orbital structures.
- May extend along optic nerve, making "tram-tracking" appearance on contrast-enhanced MRI.

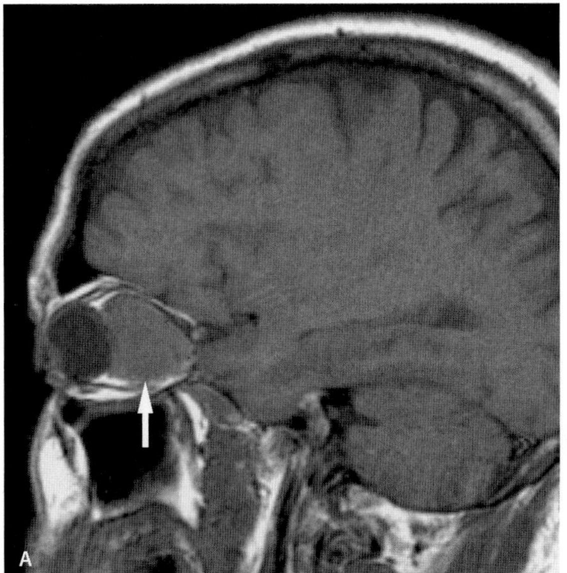

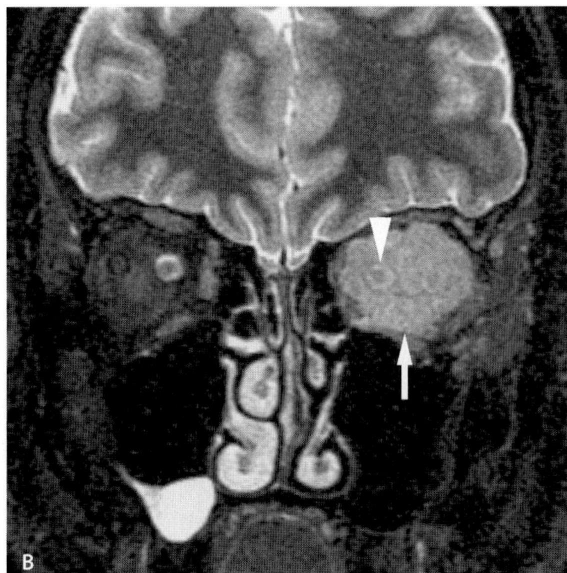

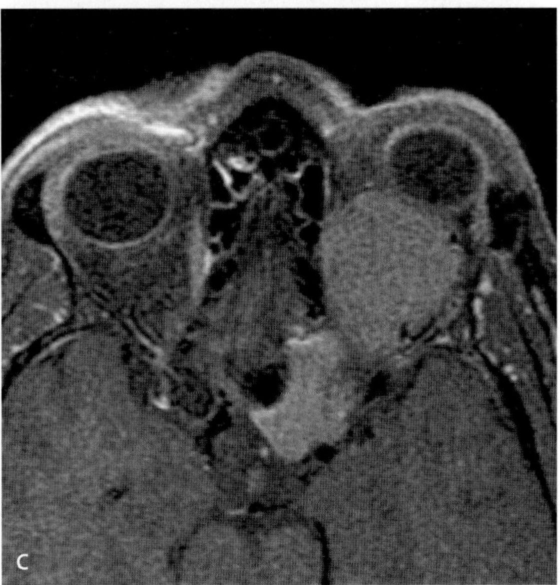

Figure 13.49

Orbital meningioma; 41-year-old male with history of left orbital meningioma resected 12 years ago, now with left proptosis and question of recurrent meningioma or glioma. **A** Sagittal T1-weighted MRI shows a large isointense mass (*arrow*) in the orbit compressing globe anteriorly. **B** On coronal T2-weighted fat-suppressed MRI, mass (*arrow*) shows hyperintensity and optic nerve is seen in center of mass (*arrowhead*). **C** Axial T1-weighted post-Gd MRI shows intracranial extension of mass through optic foramen. Tumor is deforming posterior surface of globe and causing proptosis with displacement of extraocular muscles peripherally

Rhabdomyosarcoma

Definition

Primary mesenchymal tumor arising from a primitive muscle cell known as a rhabdomyoblastoma.

Clinical Features

- Most common primary malignant tumor of orbit in children.
- Often seen in children and young adults under 20 years of age.
- Rapidly developing proptosis and displacement of globe.
- Typically occurs as a unilateral solid mass in supranasal part of orbit.

Imaging Features

- On CT images, rhabdomyosarcoma is seen as a soft-tissue mass with moderately well defined margins.
- Bony destruction is common if larger.
- Calcification and cavitation are uncommon.
- T1-weighted MRI: signal similar to muscle.
- T2-weighted post-Gd MRI: higher than muscle.
- T1-weighted post-Gd MRI: moderate to marked heterogeneous enhancement.

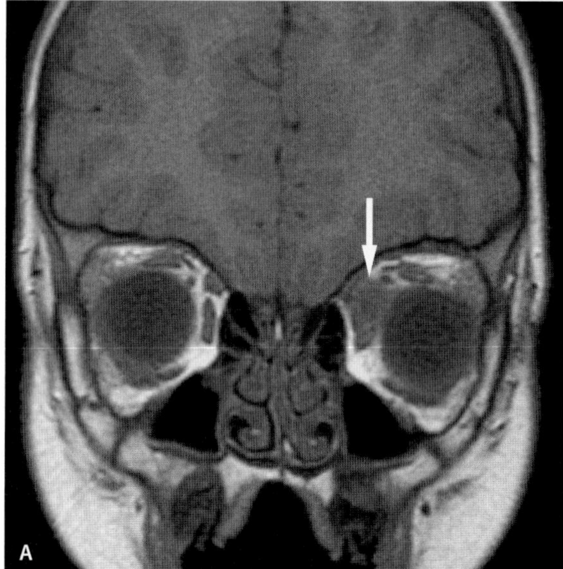

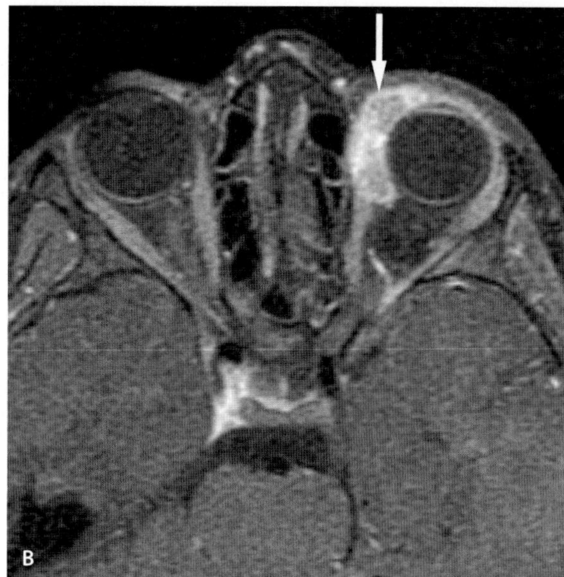

Figure 13.50

Orbital rhabdomyosarcoma; 4-year-old male with history of left eyelid swelling for one week and low-grade fever. **A** Coronal T1-weighted MRI shows a well-defined mass, isointense to extraocular muscles, in medial aspect of left orbital cavity (*arrow*). **B** T1-weighted fat-suppressed post-Gd MRI shows a heterogeneously enhanced mass (*arrow*)

Lymphoblastic Leukemia

Definition
Malignancy of hematopoietic stem cells.

Clinical Features
- Primarily a disease of children and young adults.
- Peak incidence at 4 years of age.
- About 1800 new cases per year in the US, 80% under 15 years of age.

Imaging Features
- On CT images, soft tissue and/or bony mass.
- Bony destruction may occur.
- Calcification and cavitation are uncommon.
- T1-weighted MRI: signal intensity similar to muscle.
- T2-weighted MRI: generally higher signal than muscle but may be low in tumors with high cellular density.
- T1-weighted post-Gd MRI: moderate to marked heterogeneous enhancement.

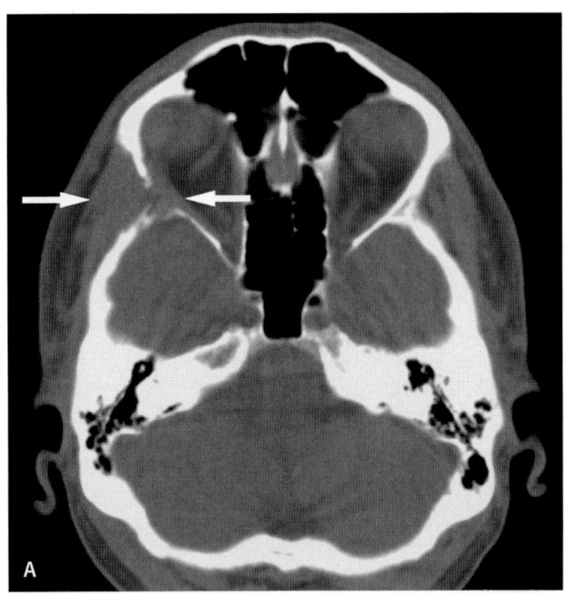

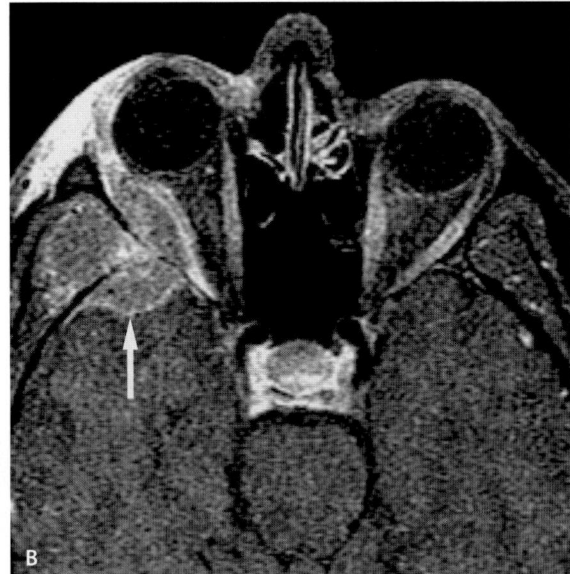

Figure 13.51

Lymphoblastic leukemia; 34-year-old male presenting with right eye proptosis, pain and vision loss. Clinical suspicion of orbital cellulitis. A Axial CT image shows mass (*arrows*) in right infratemporal fossa with bony destruction. B Axial T1-weighted fat-suppressed post-Gd MRI shows dramatic enhancement and intracranial extension of mass (*arrow*)

Suggested Reading

Atlas SW (1989) Magnetic resonance imaging of the orbit: current status. Magn Reson Q 5:39–96

Benitez WI, Sartor KJ, Angtuaco EJ (1988) Craniopharyngioma presenting as a nasopharyngeal mass: CT and MR findings. J Comput Assist Tomogr 12:1068–1072

Castellote A, Vazquez E, Vera J, et al (1999) Cervicothoracic lesions in infants and children. Radiographics 19:583–600

Chung CJ, Armfield KB, Mukherji SK, et al (1999) Cervical neurofibromas in children with NF-1. Pediatr Radiol 29:353–356

Daffner RH, Kirks DR, Gehweiler JA Jr, et al (1982) Computed tomography of fibrous dysplasia. AJR Am J Roentgenol 139:943–948

Dvorak J, Grob D, Baumgartner H, et al (1989) Functional evaluation of the spinal cord by magnetic resonance imaging in patients with rheumatoid arthritis and instability of upper cervical spine. Spine 14:1057–1064

Dworkin HJ, Meier DA, Kaplan M (1995) Advances in the management of patients with thyroid disease. Semin Nucl Med 25:205–220

Enzman DR, Delapza RL, Rubin JB (1990) Magnetic resonance imaging of the spine. Mosby-Year Book, St. Louis

Epstein N (1993) The surgical management of ossification of the posterior longitudinal ligament in 51 patients. J Spinal Disord 6:432–455

Eustic HS, Mafee MF, Walton C, et al (1998) MR imaging and CT of orbital infections and complications in acute rhinosinusitis. Radiol Clin North Am 36:1165–1183

Fagerlund M, Bjornebrink J, Ekelund L, et al (1992) Ultra low field MR imaging of cervical spine involvement in rheumatoid arthritis. Acta Radiol 33:89–92

Fink JN, McAuley DL (2002) Mastoid air sinus abnormalities associated with lateral venous thrombosis: cause or consequence? Stroke 33:290–292

Flickinger FW, Sanal SM (1994) Bone marrow MRI: techniques and accuracy for detecting breast cancer metastases. Magn Reson Imaging 12:829–835

Fries JW (1957) The roentgen features of fibrous dysplasia of the skull and facial bones; a critical analysis of thirty-nine pathologically proven cases. Am J Roentgenol Radium Ther Nucl Med 77:71–88

Fuchshuber S, Grevers G, Issing WJ (2002) Dermoid cyst of the floor of the mouth – a case report. Eur Arch Otorhinolaryngol 259:60–62

Glew D, Watt I, Dieppe PA, et al (1991) MRI of the cervical spine: rheumatoid arthritis compared with cervical spondylosis. Clin Radiol 44:71–76

Go C, Bernstein JM, de Jong AL, et al (2000) Intracranial complications of acute mastoiditis. Int J Pediatr Otorhinolaryngol 52:143–148

Ho MW, Crean SJ (2003) Simultaneous occurrence of sublingual dermoid cyst and oral alimentary tract cyst in an infant: a case report and review of the literature. Int J Paediatr Dent 13:441–446

Huysmans DA, Hermus AR, Corstens FH, et al (1994) Large, compressive goiters treated with radioiodine. Ann Intern Med 121:757–762

Janssen AG, Mansour K, Bos JJ, et al (2000) Abscess of the lacrimal sac due to chronic or subacute dacryocystitis: treatment with temporary stent placement in the nasolacrimal duct. Radiology 215:300–304

Karcioglu ZA, Hadjistilianou D, Rozans M, et al (2004) Orbital rhabdomyosarcoma. Cancer Control 11:328–333

Kaufman LM, Villablanca JP, Mafee MR (1998) Diagnostic imaging of cystic lesions in the child's orbit. Radiol Clin North Am 36:1149–1163

Leeds N, Seaman WB (1962) Fibrous dysplasia of the skull and its differential diagnosis. A clinical and roentgenographic study of 46 cases. Radiology 78:570–582

Mafee MF, Pai E, Philip B (1989) Rhabdomyosarcoma of the orbit. Evaluation with MR imaging and CT. Radiol Clin North Am 36:1215–1227

Maroldi R, Farina D, Palvarini L, et al (2001) Computed tomography and magnetic resonance imaging of pathologic conditions of the middle ear. Eur J Radiol 40:78–93

McCormick PC, Bello JA, Post KD (1988) Trigeminal schwannoma. Surgical series of 14 cases with review of the literature. J Neurosurg 69:850–860

Miyahara H, Matsunaga T (1994) Tornwaldt's disease. Acta Otolaryngol Suppl 517:36–39

Mukherji SK (2003) Pharynx. In: Som PM, Curtin DH (eds) Head and neck imaging, 4th edn. Mosby, St. Louis, pp 1507–1509

Noma S, Kanaoka M, Minami S, et al (1988) Thyroid masses: MR imaging and pathologic correlation. Radiology 168: 759–764

Petito CK, DeGirolami U, Earle KM (1976) Craniopharyngiomas: a clinical and pathological review. Cancer 37: 1944–1952.

Resnick D (1996) Bone and joint imaging, 2nd edn. WB Saunders, Philadelphia, pp 378–387

Robinson DR, Tashjian AH Jr, Levine L (1975) Prostaglandin-stimulated bone resorption by rheumatoid synovia. A possible mechanism for bone destruction in rheumatoid arthritis. J Clin Invest 56:1181–1188

Soo MY, Rajaratnam S (2000) Symptomatic ossification of the posterior longitudinal ligament of the cervical spine: pictorial essay. Australas Radiol 44:14–18

Spiegel JH, Lustig LR, Lee KC, et al (1998) Contemporary presentation and management of a spectrum of mastoid abscesses. Laryngoscope 108:822–828

Terayama K (1989) Genetic studies on ossification of the posterior ligament of the spine. Spine 14:1184–1191

Tetsumura A, Yoshino N, Yamada I, et al (1999) Head and neck hemangiomas: contrast-enhanced three-dimensional MR angiography. Neuroradiology 41:140–143

Visrutaratna P, Oranratanachai K, Singhavejsakul J (2004) Clinics in diagnostic imaging (96). Plexiform neurofibromatosis. Singapore Med J 45:188–192

Weber AL, Montandon C, Robson CD (2000) Neurogenic tumors of the neck. Radiol Clin North Am 38:1077–1090

Weiner HL, Wisoff JH, Rosenberg ME, et al (1994) Craniopharyngiomas: a clinicopathological analysis of factors predictive of recurrence and functional outcome. Neurosurgery 35:1001–1010

Williams LS, Schmalfuss IM, Sistrom CL, et al (2003) MR Imaging of the trigeminal ganglion, nerve, and the perineural vascular plexus: normal appearance and variants with correlation to cadaver specimens. AJNR Am J Neuroradiol 24:1317–1323

Yousem DM (1998) Case review: head and neck imaging. Mosby, St. Louis

Yuh WT, Simonson TM, Wang AM, et al (1994) Venous sinus occlusive disease: MR findings. AJNR Am J Neuroradiol 15:309–316

Interventional Maxillofacial Radiology

Introduction

Interventional radiology or, as it is sometimes called, minimally invasive surgery has evolved from traditional diagnostic radiology over the last 20 years. Thus today many procedures can be done with image guidance that in the past required an open approach. The morbidity, risks and complications can often be reduced significantly by image-guided minimally invasive percutaneous techniques as compared to open surgical procedures. There are many examples of successful interventional radiology performed today: TIPS, in which the portal vein is connected to the hepatic vein bypassing the liver in patients with liver failure, aspiration biopsies in deep locations that were not accessible without an open approach in the past, recanalization of the fallopian tubes for infertility, and maintenance of vascular access in patients with renal disease, to mention a few.

Interventional maxillofacial radiology is in its infancy. Only a few minimally invasive procedures have been applied to this area, but it is quite obvious that the percutaneous approach with needles is much preferred in the maxillofacial region as compared to an open procedure. In this chapter we have collected a few diagnostic and interventional procedures that have been applied to the maxillofacial and related areas. Of these procedures temporomandibular joint (TMJ) arthrography and sialography are those which most typically have been performed by maxillofacial radiologists. It is also our opinion that image-guided biopsies of soft-tissue masses or bone, being good alternatives to open surgery biopsies, should be within the working area of these specialists. Although orbital biopsies and embolizations are beyond their scope, we have also illustrated such procedures to show the maxillofacial radiologist what is indeed possible to safely perform.

TMJ Arthrography

Definition

Radiographic study where contrast material has been injected into lower joint compartment or lower and upper compartments to visualize soft tissues such as articular disc and joint capsule.

Clinical Features

- Initially, developed in the 1940s but gained popularity in the 1980s when internal derangement was discovered as a frequent finding in patients with facial pain and mandibular dysfunction.
- Initially, single contrast arthrography either in lower joint compartment or in both joint compartments with plain films or conventional tomography (arthrotomography); later developed into double-contrast arthrotomography with air as a supplement to the contrast material.
- Fell out of favor with the development of high quality MRI and rarely performed today.

Imaging Features

- Excellent for dynamic studies of the articular disc.
- Gold standard for determining disc or posterior attachment perforations; normal joint has no communication between compartments.
- Double-contrast studies show more exquisite detail but the diagnostic accuracy on a one-to-one comparison is the same as for single-contrast studies.

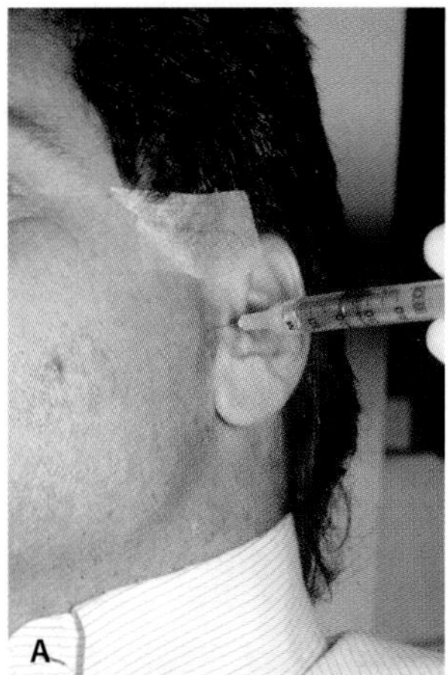

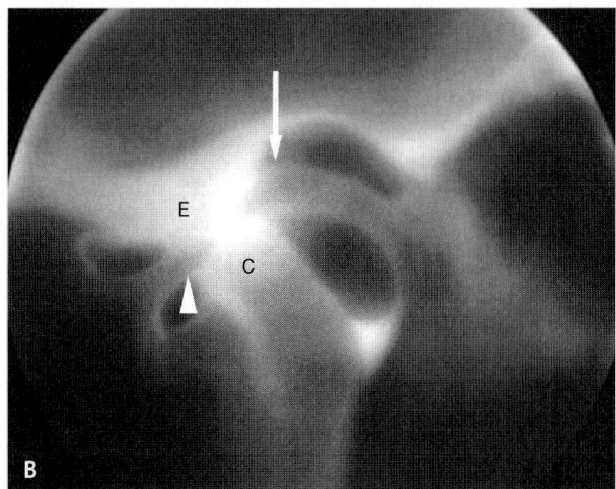

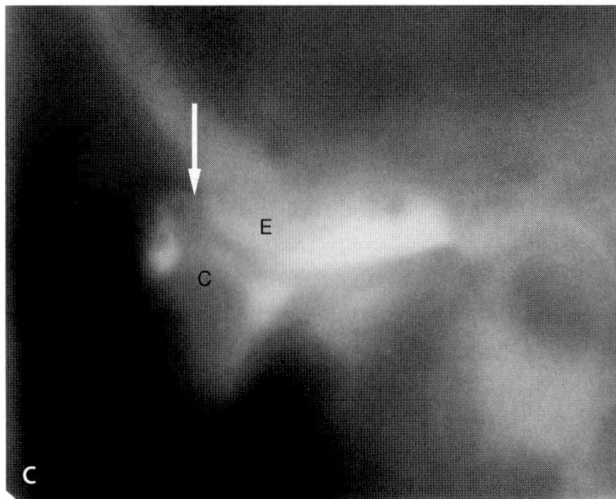

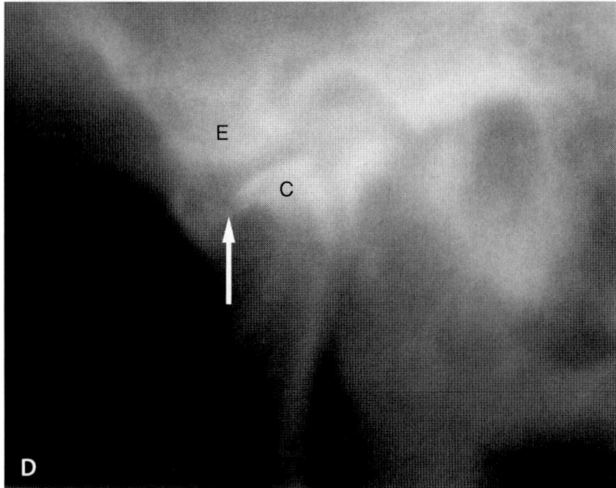

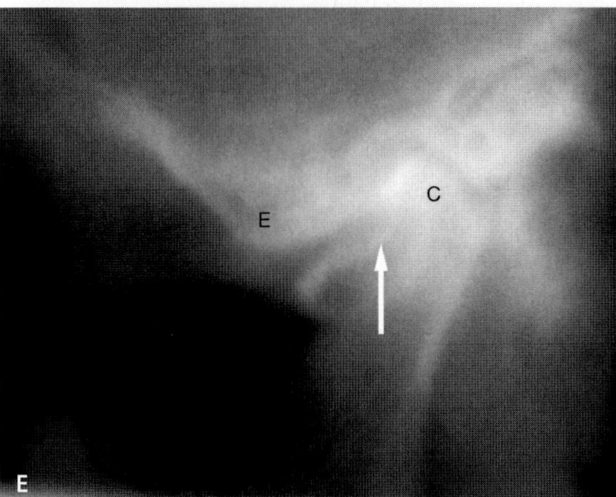

Figure 14.1

TMJ arthrotomography; normal and abnormal. **A** Local anesthesia before contrast injection. **B** Double-contrast dual space arthrotomography, i.e., both joint compartments injected separately; normal disc position in half-open mouth view as indicated by anterior band (*arrowhead*) anterior to condyle (*C*) and posterior band (*arrow*) posterior to condyle; joint spaces also filled with air and thus appear radiolucent. Articular eminence indicated (*E*). **C** Single-contrast dual space arthrotomography; upper space filled through perforation (not seen) in area of disc/posterior attachment, open mouth view; disc anteriorly displaced without reduction as indicated by its posterior band (*arrow*) in front of condyle (*C*). Articular eminence indicated (*E*). **D** Single-contrast lower space arthrotomography; open mouth view shows contrast material in front of condyle (*C*) demonstrating anteriorly displaced disc (*arrow*) without reduction. Articular eminence indicated (*E*). **E** Same joint, closed mouth view; contrast material in extended anterior recess showing lower surface of posterior band (*arrow*) of anteriorly displaced disc in front of condyle (*C*). Articular eminence indicated (*E*)

TMJ Arthroscopy

Definition

Inspection of joint surfaces by performing minimally invasive surgical procedures percutaneously using an arthroscope.

Clinical Features

- Gained popularity in early 1980s when thin (2 to 3 mm diameter) arthroscopic instruments became available.

Imaging Features

- Often difficult to diagnose disc position since no cross-sectional view is obtained.
- Multiple minimally invasive surgical procedures have been performed with limited morbidity and success rates similar to those of open surgical procedures.
- Can be done under general or local anesthesia.
- Diagnosis of adhesions and synovitis are the main applications for arthroscopy.
- Usually only upper joint compartment examined/ treated

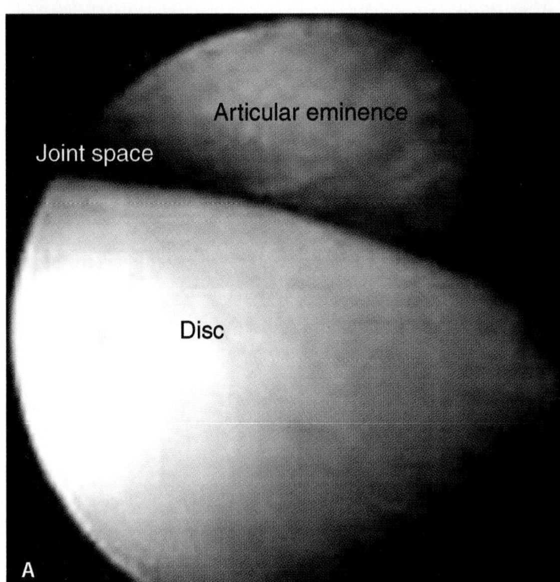

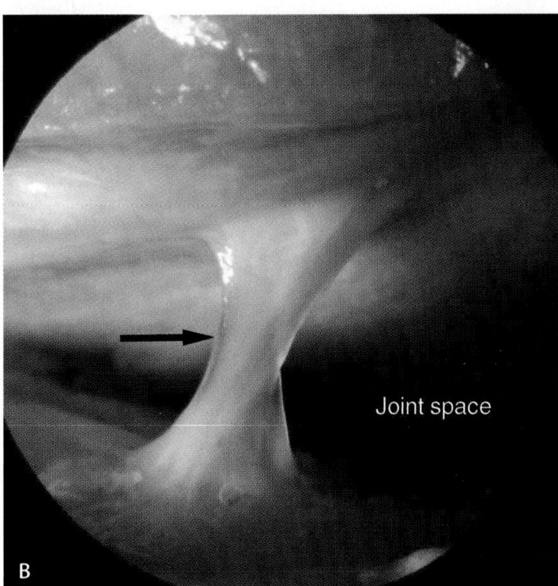

Figure 14.2

TMJ arthroscopy; normal and abnormal. **A** Upper joint compartment; normal joint as indicated by smooth surfaces of both disc and eminence. **B** Upper joint compartment; fibrous adhesion between disc and eminence (*arrow*)

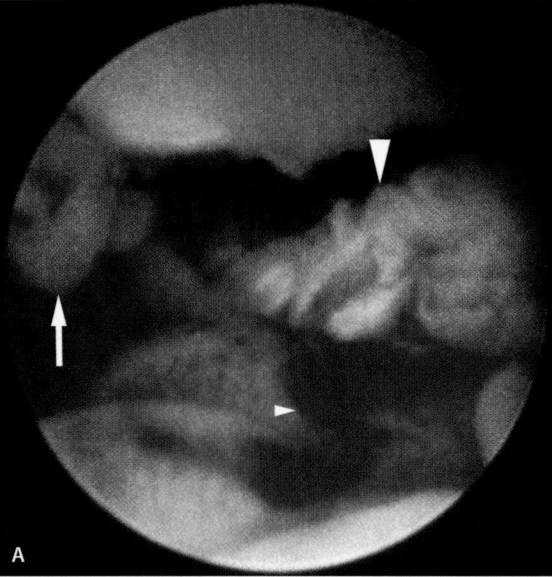

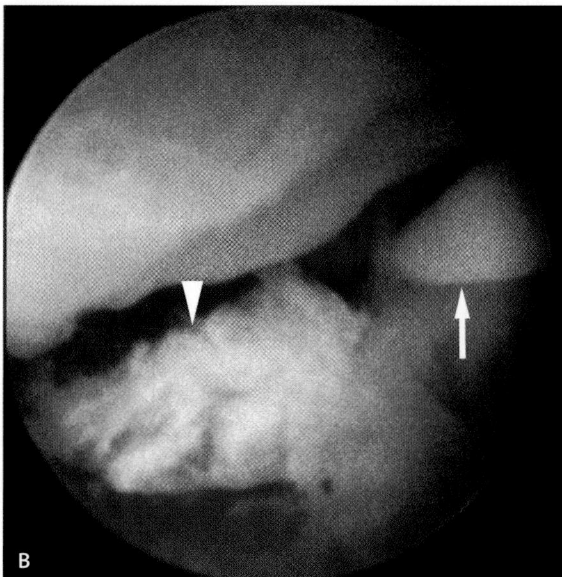

Figure 14.3

TMJ arthroscopy; rheumatoid arthritis. **A** Upper joint compartment; synovial proliferation (*arrowhead*) in disc perforation area, hyperemia (*small arrowhead*), and part of disc (*arrow*). **B** Same joint; synovial proliferation (*arrowhead*) in disc perforation area, and part of disc (*arrow*)

Sialography

Definition

Radiographic studies of salivary glands after injection of contrast material.

Clinical Features

- Sialography is primarily done to image ducts and, if conventional radiography or CT image is normal, to detect salivary stones.
- Also used in the treatment of strictures (ballooning) and removal of stones (fluoroscopically guided basket retrieval).

Imaging Features

- Inflammation, strictures; stones are often better seen on sialography than on MRI or CT images.
- In the late 1970s CT sialography was popularized but this procedure has fallen out of favor because conventional sialography is superior for duct imaging and quality of MR sialography is improving.
- MRI is primary modality for salivary gland masses.

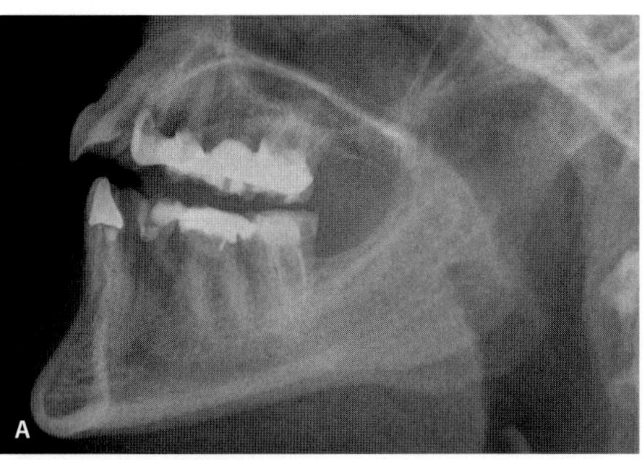

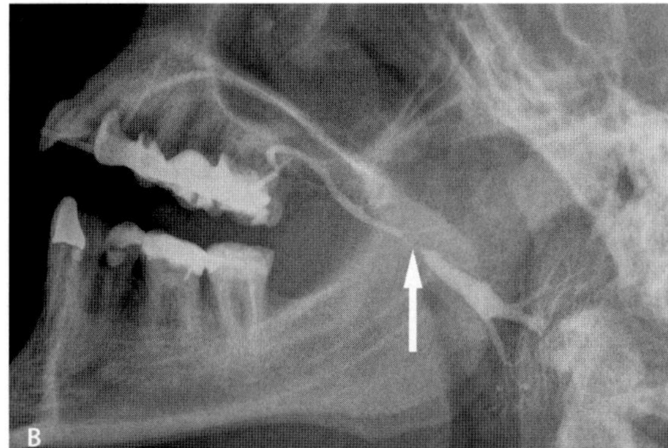

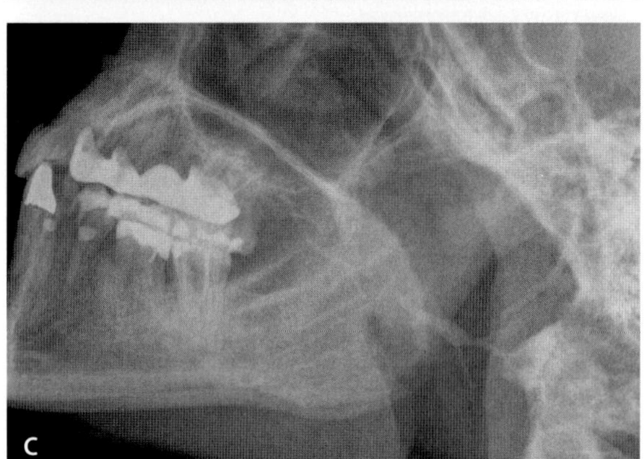

Figure 14.4

Parotid sialography; sialodochitis, normal parenchyma. A Side view shows no signs of stone in Stensen's duct. B Plain film sialography shows stricture (*arrow*), and dilatation proximal duct. C Plain film shows retention of contrast material; only parenchyma is without contrast material after 5 minutes (courtesy of Dr. B. Svensson, Skövde Hospital, Sweden)

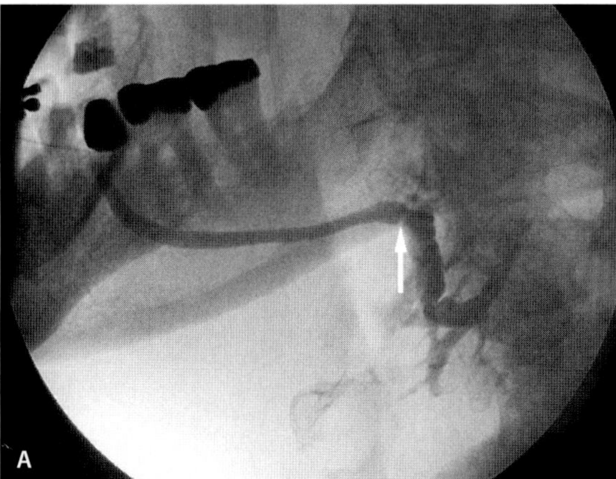

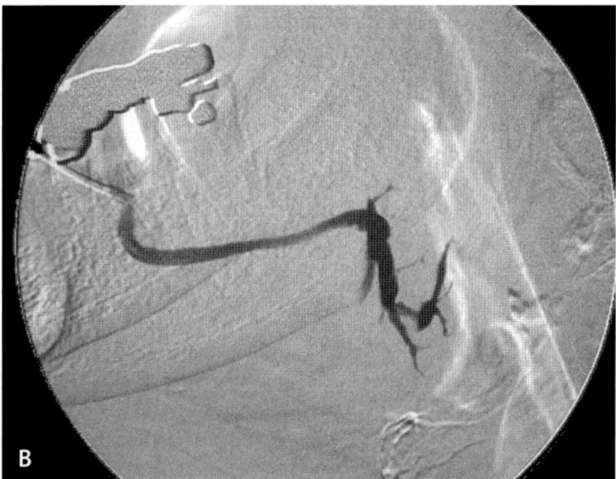

Figure 14.5

Submandibular sialography; sialoadenitis, rather normal Wharton's duct. A Plain film sialography (fluoroscopy) shows mostly a normal duct but with one stricture (*arrow*) and dilatation of intraglandular ducts with abnormal filling of parenchyma. B Digital subtraction sialography of same patient does not show stricture but more clearly lack of parenchyma filling

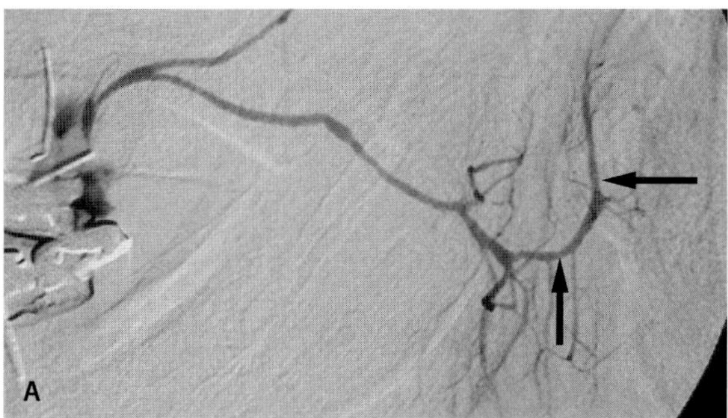

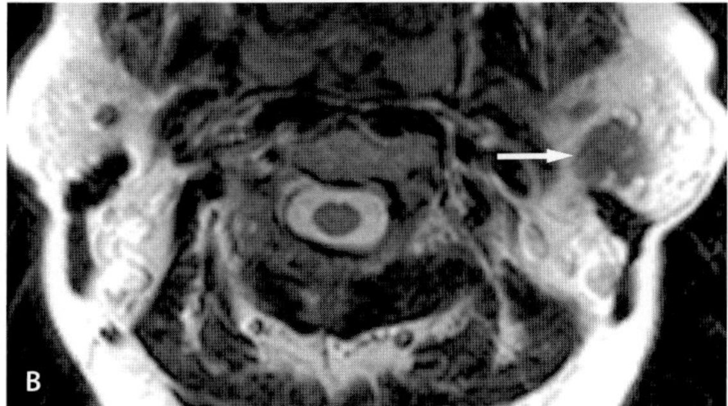

Figure 14.6

Parotid sialography; normal filling of Stensen's duct and gland parenchyma but duct displacement because of tumor. **A** Digital subtraction sialography shows normal caliber duct and normal filling of intraglandular ducts, but displacement (*arrows*) due to tumor; difficult to appreciate. **B** Axial T1-weighted MRI performed same day shows tumor (*arrow*) in left parotid gland

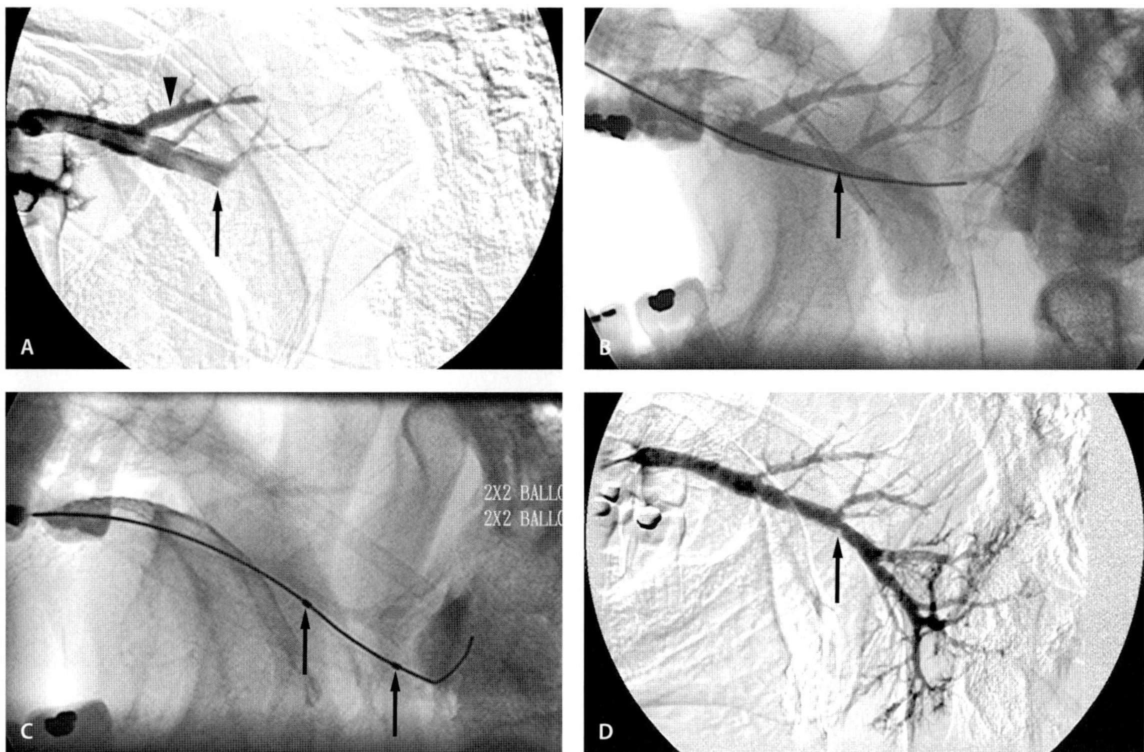

Figure 14.7

Parotid sialography; abnormal filling of Stensen's duct and no filling of parenchyma before successful duct ballooning. **A** Digital subtraction sialography shows abrupt blockage of mid Stensen's duct (*arrow*), and filling of secondary ducts (*arrowhead*) and third ducts more enhanced than usual. **B** Plain film sialography (fluoroscopy) after probing with a guide wire (*arrow*) shows that blockage could be passed with contrast material. **C** Plain film sialography (fluoroscopy) shows that symmetry 2 mm by 2 cm balloon has been inserted (*arrows*) and expanded to dilate stricture. **D** Digital subtraction sialography after procedure shows small residual stricture (*arrow*), but filling of gland; inflammatory changes

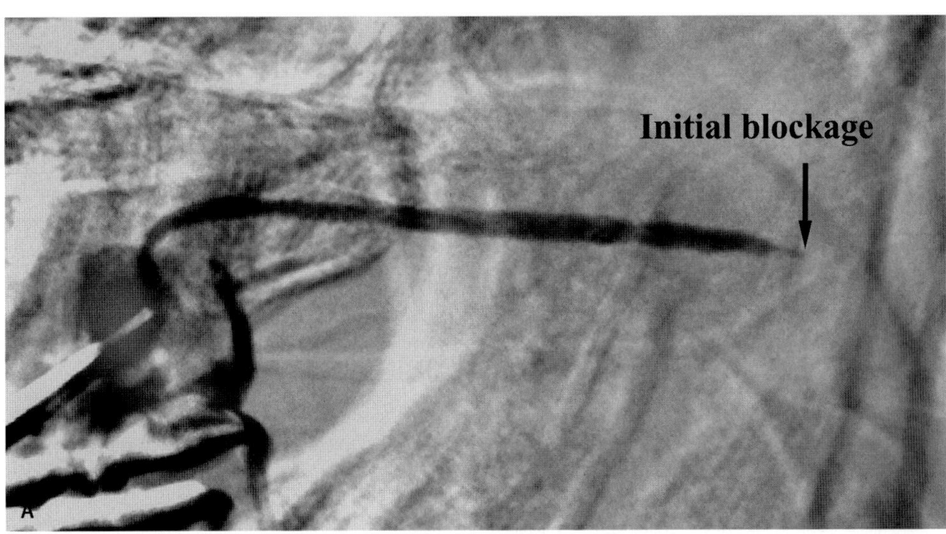

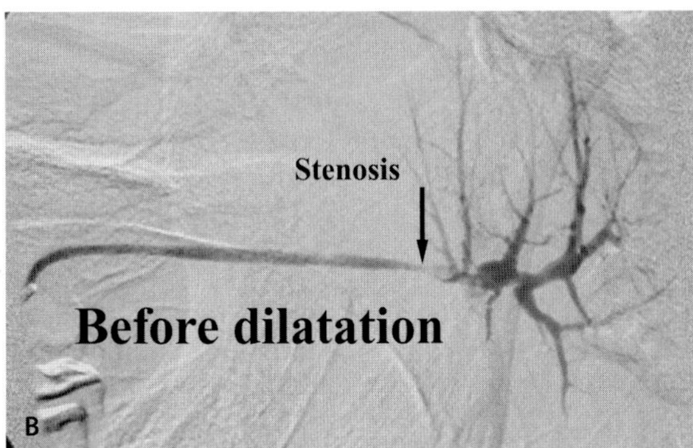

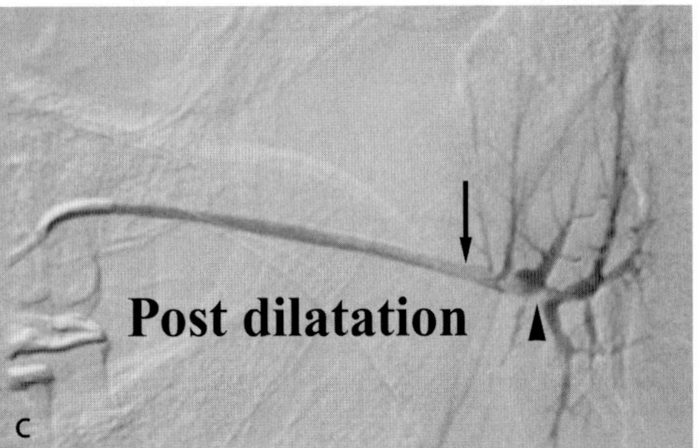

Figure 14.8

Parotid sialography; occlusion of Stensen's duct and no filling of parenchyma before successful duct ballooning. A Digital subtraction parotid sialography; stricture occluding Stensen's duct (*arrow*). B Subtraction sialography after probing through duct with guide wire shows stenosis (*arrow*) but filling of parenchyma. C Subtraction sialography after dilatation shows widening of stricture (*arrow*). A small filling defect in gland (*arrowhead*) may be mucus or residual stone. Patient did well after procedure and no further intervention was needed

Biopsy

Definition

Either tissue or cellular material for pathologic diagnosis.

Clinical Features

- With an image-guided procedure deep lesions in the maxillofacial area can often be reached with minimal morbidity.

Imaging Features

- Fine needle aspiration provides cytologic information.
- Core biopsy gives a solid tissue core which is fixed in formalin and embedded for traditional pathologic studies with light microscopy.
- Typically 22-gauge needles are used for fine needle aspiration and 16-, 18-, or 20-gauge core biopsy needles are used for core biopsies.
- Negative fine needle aspiration findings are difficult to interpret since they may be due sampling error.
- Core biopsy gives higher percentage of positive answers and easier to trust when negative. Core biopsy is however more invasive since the needle size is larger.
- For bone biopsies 13-gauge bone biopsy needles are used.
- CT fluoroscopy reduces radiation and improves efficiency over regular CT imaging as guidance.

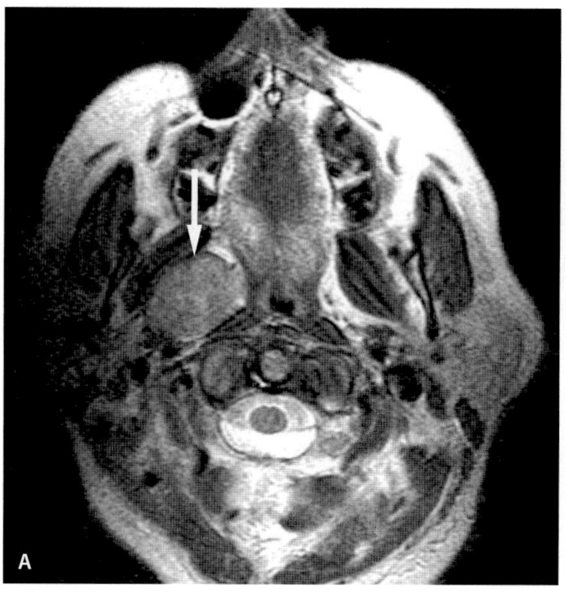

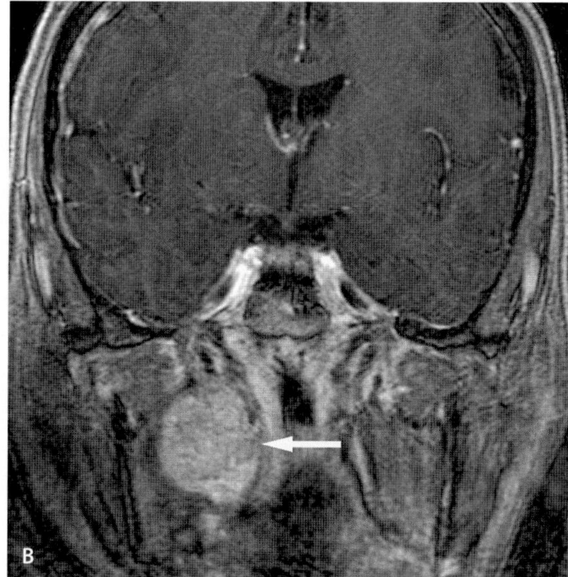

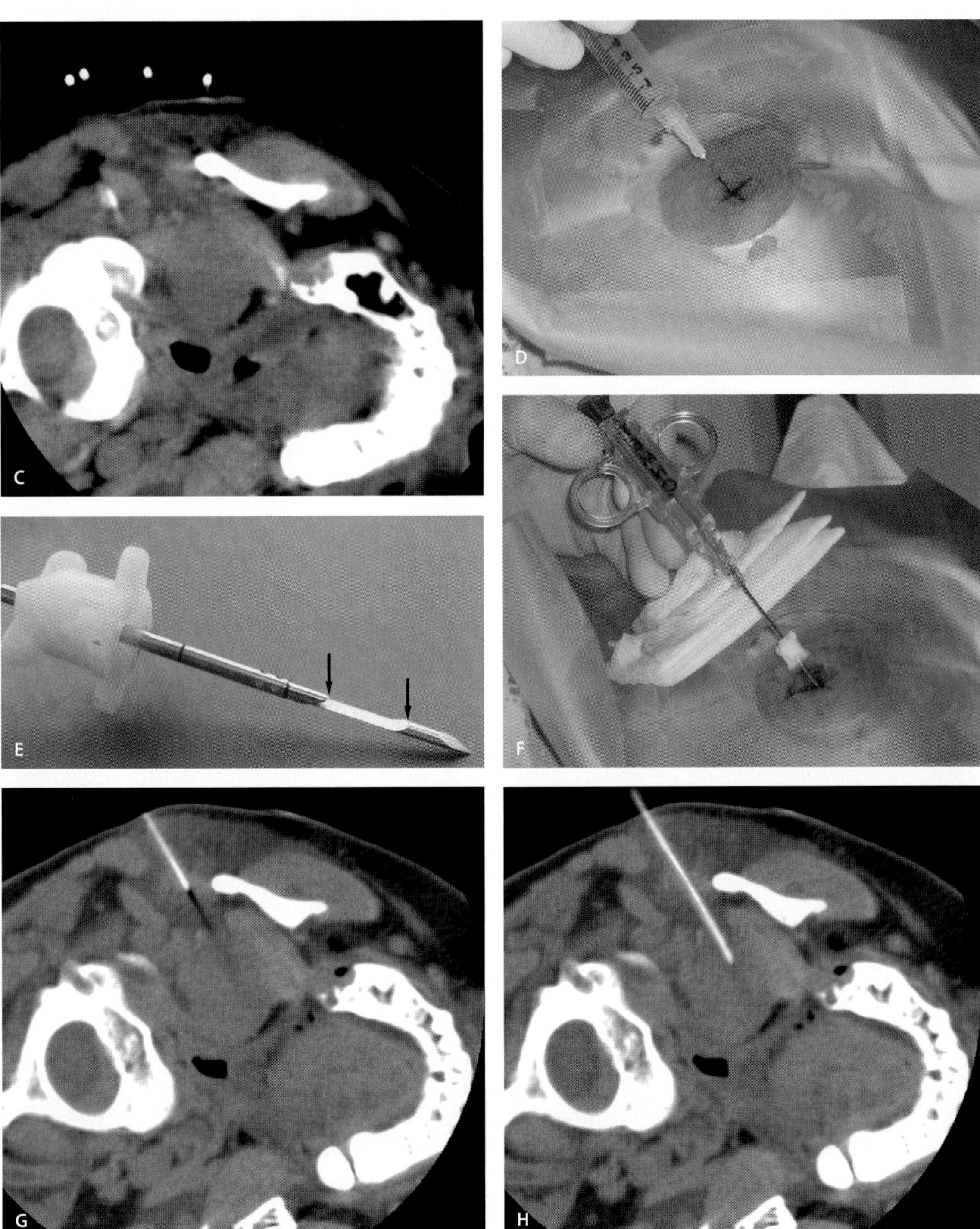

Figure 14.9

CT fluoroscopy guided biopsy of parapharyngeal mass. **A** Axial T2-weighted MRI shows deep parapharyngeal mass (*arrow*). **B** Coronal T1-weighted post-Gd MRI shows mass (*arrow*) medial to ramus of mandible. **C** Patient placed in lateral decubitus. Markers, white dots, are placed on skin to guide an oblique posterior approach. **D** Local anesthesia is induced. **E** 16-gauge Temno core biopsy needle; tissue core is obtained in cut-out on needle (between arrows). **F** Temno biopsy needle inserted through a small skin incision. **G** CT fluoroscopy shows biopsy needle at correct angle. **H** CT fluoroscopy confirms correct position of needle within mass

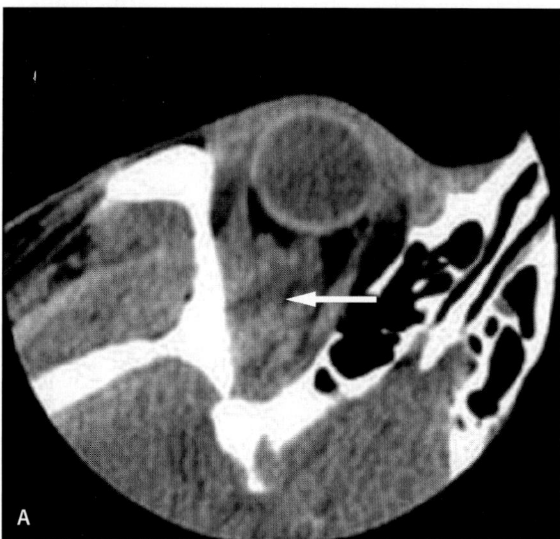
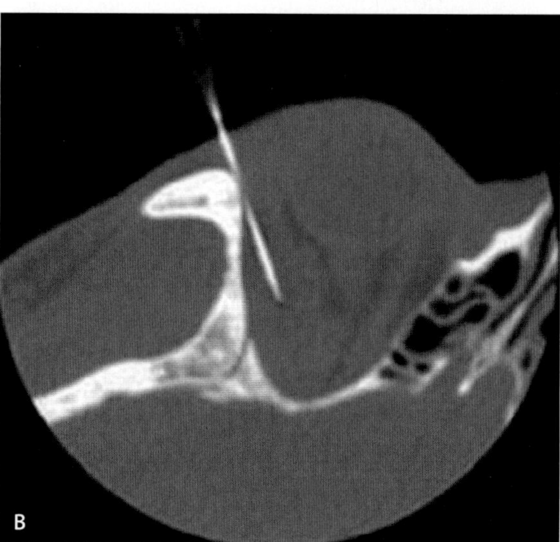

Figure 14.10

CT fluoroscopy guided biopsy of orbital mass. A Axial CT image shows intraorbital mass (*arrow*) in posterior lateral aspect of right orbit. B Axial CT image, bone window, shows fine needle, 25-gauge, in correct position; aspiration revealed signs of hemangioma

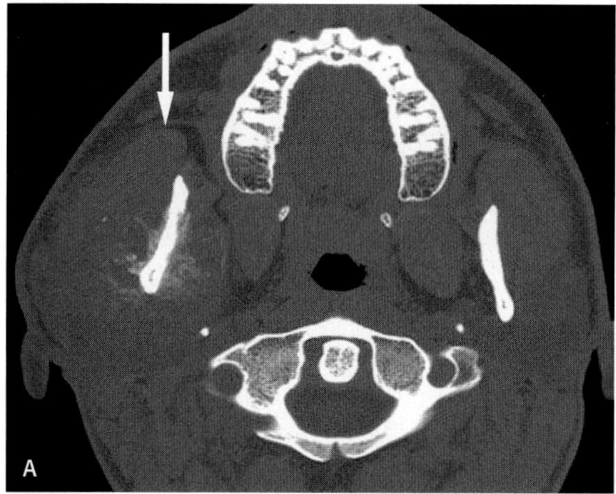
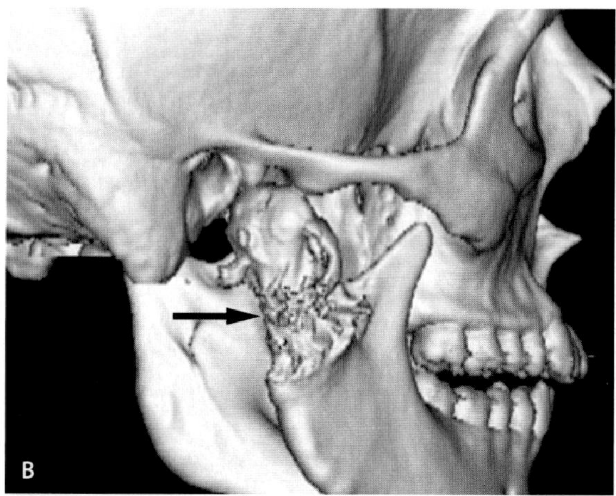
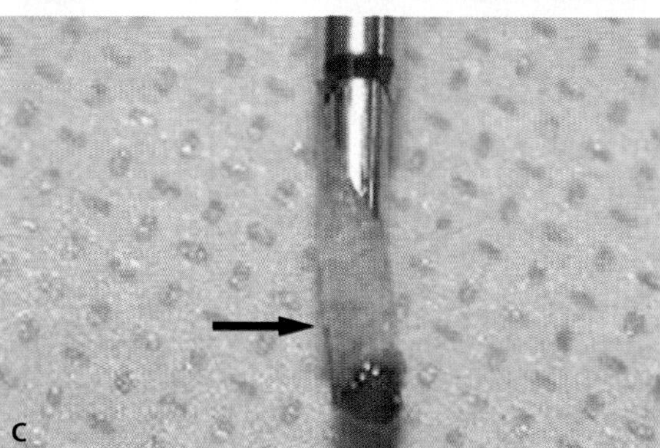

Figure 14.11

Bone biopsy of mass around mandibular ramus. A Axial CT image shows soft-tissue mass with extensive sunburst periosteal bone reaction (*arrow*). B 3D CT image depicts relationship between tumor and ramus of mandible (*arrow*). C Bone core (*arrow*) obtained using a 13-gauge bone biopsy needle demonstrated chondrosarcoma

Facial Hemangioma Embolization

Definition

Percutaneous treatment of facial hemangioma by injection of absolute alcohol.

Clinical Features

- Hemangiomas of face often regress with time.
- Image-guided alcohol embolization is often less invasive than surgery which is difficult because of intricate nature of hemangiomas.

Imaging Features

- Using general anesthetics percutaneous injection of alcohol can be used to reverse hemangiomas. Other substances can also be used.

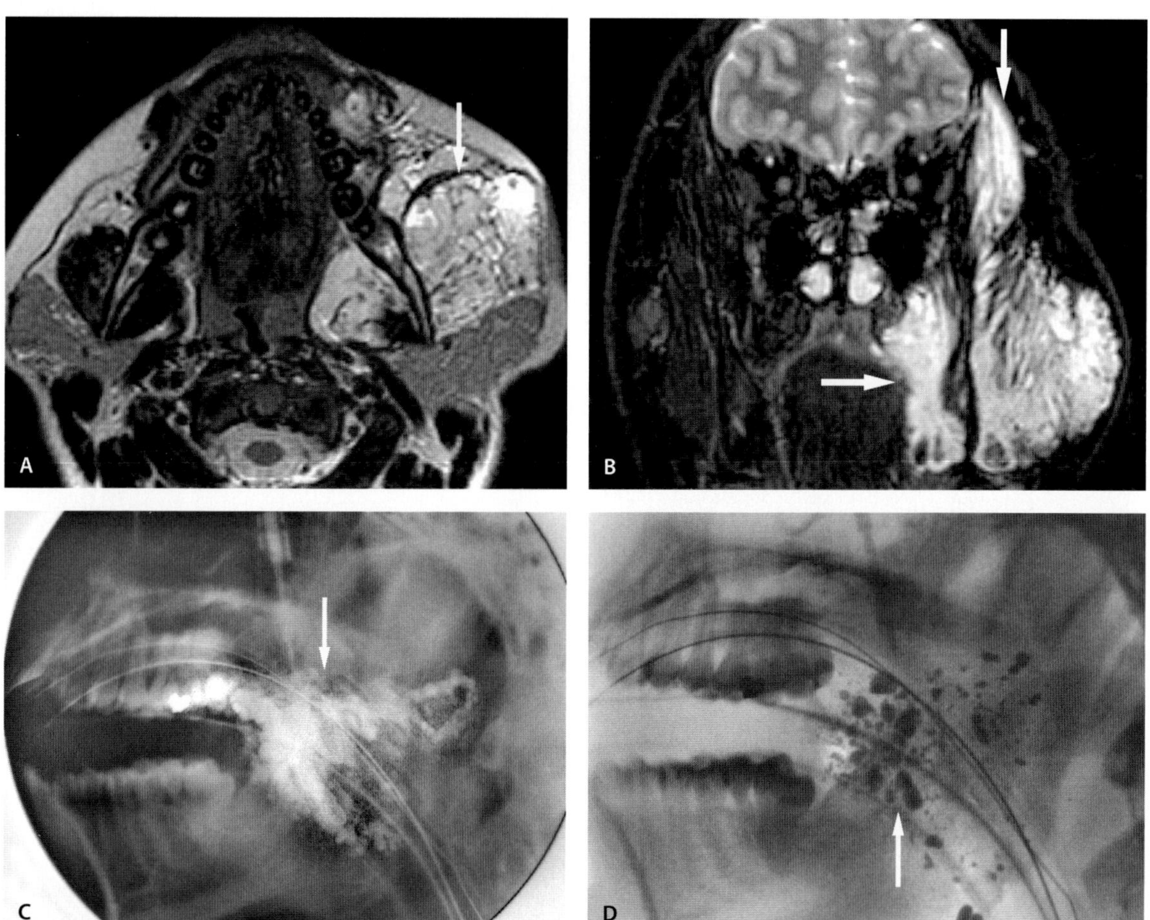

Figure 14.12

Facial hemangioma embolization. A Axial T1-weighted fat-suppressed post-Gd MRI shows hemangioma located in left masticator space (*arrow*). B Coronal T2-weighted fat-suppressed MRI shows large mass of infiltrating nature (*arrows*). C Lateral view (fluoroscopy) shows percutaneous injection of hemangioma (*arrow*) using a mixture of Ethiodol and absolute alcohol. D Post-injection lateral view (fluoroscopy) shows residual contrast material (*arrow*) as an indicator of the injection site (treatment courtesy of Dr. H. Wang, University of Rochester Medical Center, NY)

Nose Bleed Embolization

Definition

Using interventional angiographic technique to embolize small vessels leading to nose bleed using particles or spheres.

Clinical Features

- Most nose bleeds can be stopped by packing and conservative measures.
- Nose bleed may be life-threatening if it is not stopped by conservative measures. Either surgery or interventional techniques may be used to block bleeding vessels.
- Interventional techniques are less invasive than open surgery.

Imaging Features

- High-quality digital subtraction angiography in two planes often necessary.
- Microcatheter technique needed to embolize specific vessels.
- Risk of blindness if retinal arteries are embolized.
- Often performed by interventional neuroradiologists.

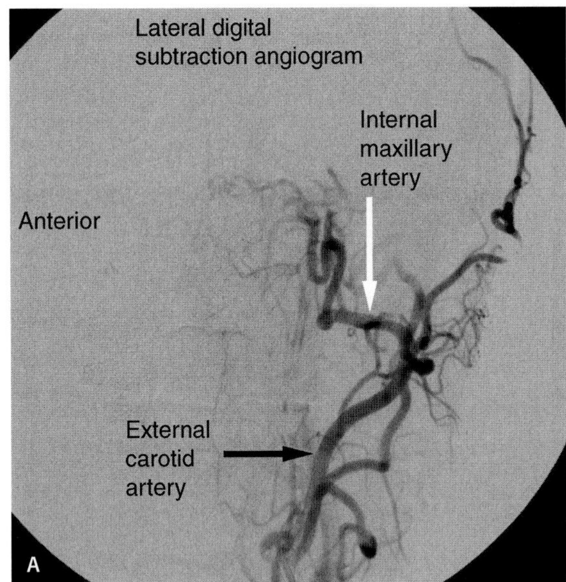

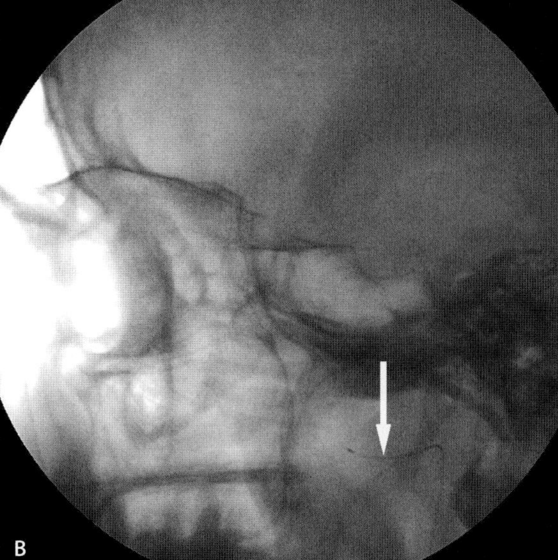

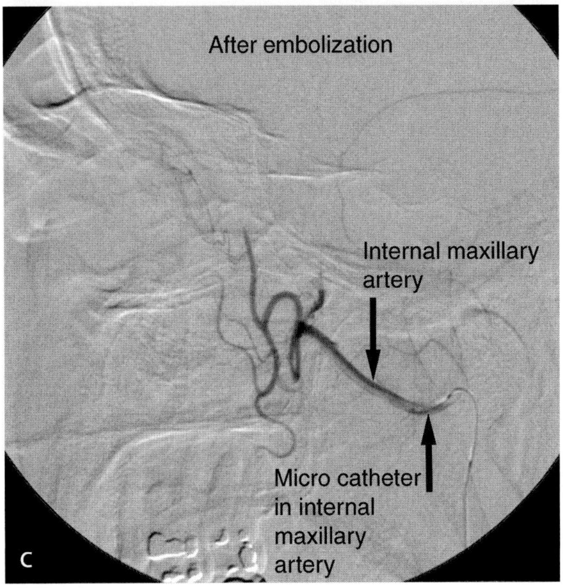

Figure 14.13

Nose bleed embolization. **A** Digital subtraction angiography (fluoroscopy) shows external carotid artery and internal maxillary artery (*arrows*). Internal maxillary artery is main feeder for nose bleeds. **B** Lateral view (fluoroscopy) shows microcatheter (*arrow*) placed in internal maxillary artery. **C** Lateral digital subtraction angiography (fluoroscopy) after embolization shows microcatheter in internal maxillary artery (*arrows*) and marked reduction of small vessels in nasal region (treatment courtesy of Dr. H. Wang, University of Rochester Medical Center, Rochester, NY)

Juvenile Angiofibroma Embolization

Definition

Juvenile angiofibroma is a benign locally aggressive vascular tumor which is often supplied from branches of the internal maxillary artery and foramen rotundum, arteries in the Vidian canal, the sphenomaxillary artery and occasionally also from the ophthalmic artery. Standard treatment is surgery after preoperative embolization which effectively reduces intraoperative bleeding.

Using minimally invasive interventional radiographic techniques, small vessels are embolized by means of a microcatheter in the angiofibroma.

Clinical Features

- Primarily a disease of adolescent males; only a few cases reported in females.
- Usually progressive growth but occasional regression has been reported.
- Located in the nose, nasopharynx and parapharyngeal space.
- Often presents with nasal obstruction and epistaxis.

Imaging Features

- Very vascular.
- Locally aggressive.
- Will often arise in sphenopalatine foramen.
- T1-weighted MRI: intermediate signal.
- T2-weighted MRI: high signal.
- T1-weighted post-Gd MRI: intense enhancement.
- MRI often shows flow voids.

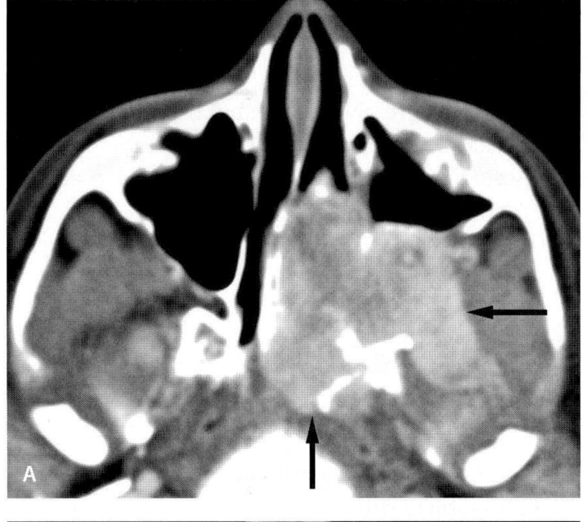

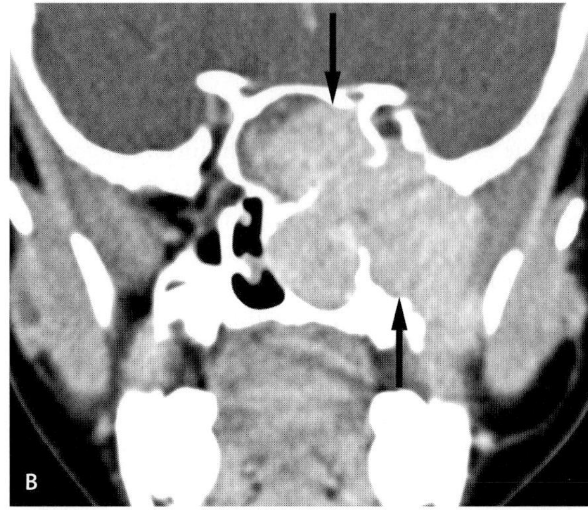

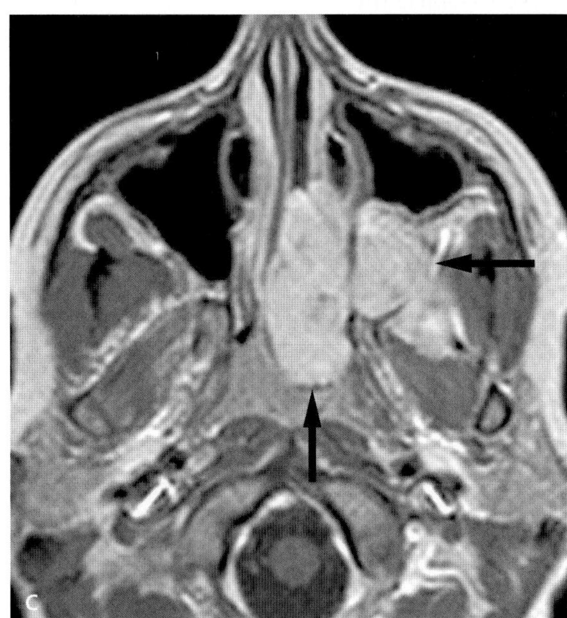

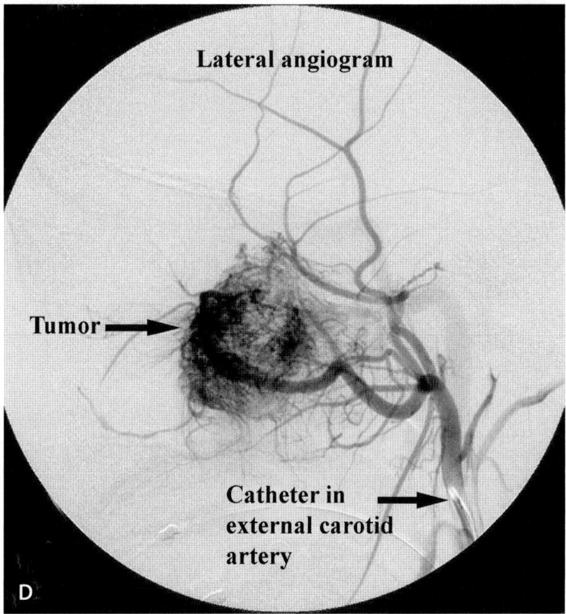

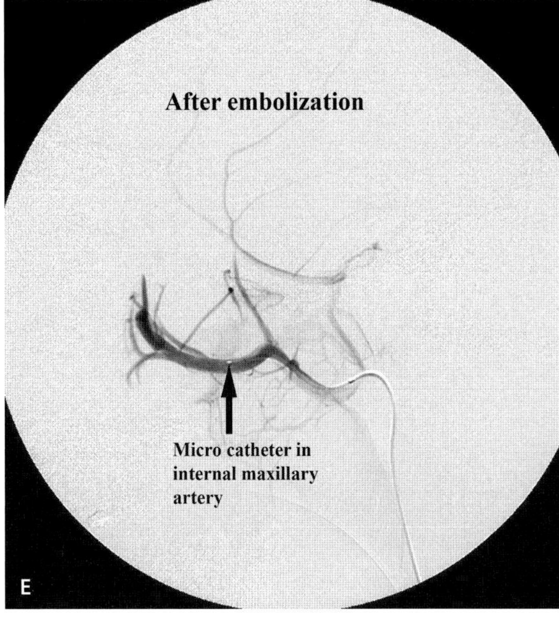

Figure 14.14

Juvenile angiofibroma embolization. **A** Axial post-contrast CT image shows enhancing mass (*arrows*) in left nasal cavity, nasopharynx, maxillary sinus, and infratemporal fossa with bone destruction. **B** Coronal post-contrast CT image shows enhancing mass (*arrows*) in left sphenoid sinus, left nasal cavity, left maxillary sinus, and left infratemporal fossa. **C** Axial T1-weighted post-Gd MRI shows intensely enhancing mass (*arrows*). **D** Digital subtraction angiography in lateral projection with catheter in left external carotid artery (*arrow*) showing dramatic tumor vascularity of juvenile angiofibroma (*arrow*). **E** Digital subtraction angiography in lateral projection after embolization, with microcatheter in left internal maxillary artery (*arrow*). Using particles, tumor vascularity has been almost completely eliminated (treatment courtesy of Dr. H. Wang, University of Rochester Medical Center, NY, USA)

Suggested Reading

Barsotti JB, Westesson P-L, Ketonen LM (1992) Diagnostic and interventional angiographic procedures in the maxillofacial region. In: Westesson P-L (ed) Oral and maxillofacial surgery clinics of North America: contemporary maxillofacial imaging. WB Saunders, Philadelphia, pp 35–49

Brown JE (2002) Minimally invasive techniques for treatment of benign salivary gland obstruction. Cardiovasc Intervent Radiol 25:345–351

Brown JE, Drage NA, Escudier MP, et al (2002) Minimally invasive radiologically guided intervention for the treatment of salivary calculi. Cardiovasc Intervent Radiol 25:352–355

Drage NA, Brown JE, Escudier MP, et al (2002) Balloon dilatation of salivary duct strictures: report on 36 treated glands. Cardiovasc Intervent Radiol 25:356–359

Garcia-Cervigon E, Bien S, Rüfenacht D, et al (1988) Pre-operative embolization of naso-pharyngeal angiofibromas. Report of 58 cases. Neuroradiology 30:556–560

Jacobsson M, Petruson B, Svendsen P, et al (1988) Juvenile nasopharyngeal angiofibroma. A report of eighteen cases. Acta Otolaryngol 105:132-139

Kandarpa K, Aruny JE (eds) (2001) Handbook of interventional radiologic procedures, 3rd edn. Williams & Wilkins, Philadelphia

McGurk M, Makdissi J, Brown JE (2004) Intra-oral removal of stones from the hilum of the submandibular gland: report of technique and morbidity. J Oral Maxillofac Surg 33: 683–686

McGurk M, Escudier MP, Brown JE (2005) Modern management of salivary calculi. Br J Surg 92:107–112

Natvig K, Skalpe IO (1984) Pre-operative embolization of juvenile nasopharyngeal angiofibromas with gelfoam. J Laryngol Otol 98:829–833

Stansbie JM, Phelps PD (1986) Involution of residual juvenile nasopharyngeal angiofibroma (a case report). J Laryngol Otol 100:599–603

Zenk J, Constantinidis J, Al-Kadah B, et al (2001) Transoral removal of submandibular stones. Arch Otolaryngol Head Neck Surg 127:432–436

Subject Index

C

D

E

F

N

O

P

R

S

T

U

V

W

X

Z